1995
YEAR BOOK OF
MEDICINE®

The 1995 Year Book Series

Year Book of Allergy and Clinical Immunology: Drs. Rosenwasser, Borish, Gelfand, Leung, Nelson, and Szefler

Year Book of Anesthesiology and Pain Management: Drs. Tinker, Abram, Chestnut, Rothenberg, Roizen, and Wood

Year Book of Cardiology®: Drs. Schlant, Collins, Engle, Gersh, Kaplan, and Waldo

Year Book of Chiropractic: Dr. Lawrence

Year Book of Critical Care Medicine: Drs. Parrillo, Balk, Calvin, Franklin, and Shapiro

Year Book of Dentistry®: Drs. Meskin, Berry, Currier, Kennedy, Leinfelder, Roser, and Zakariasen

Year Book of Dermatologic Surgery®: Drs. Swanson, Glogau, and Salasche

Year Book of Dermatology®: Drs. Sober and Fitzpatrick

Year Book of Diagnostic Radiology®: Drs. Federle, Clark, Gross, Madewell, Maynard, Latchaw, and Young

Year Book of Digestive Diseases®: Drs. Greenberger and Moody

Year Book of Drug Therapy®: Drs. Lasagna and Weintraub

Year Book of Emergency Medicine®: Drs. Wagner, Dronen, Davidson, King, Niemann, and Roberts

Year Book of Endocrinology®: Drs. Bagdade, Braverman, Horton, Kannan, Landsberg, Molitch, Morley, Nathan, Odell, Poehlman, Rogol, and Ryan

Year Book of Family Practice®: Drs. Berg, Bowman, Davidson, Dexter, Dietrich, and Scherger

Year Book of Geriatrics and Gerontology®: Drs. Beck, Reuben, Burton, Small, Whitehouse, and Goldstein

Year Book of Hand Surgery®: Drs. Amadio and Hentz

Year Book of Hematology®: Drs. Spivak, Bell, Ness, Quesenberry, Wiernik, and Blume

Year Book of Infectious Diseases®: Drs. Keusch, Barza, Bennish, Gelfand, Klempner, Skolnik, and Snydman

Year Book of Infertility and Reproductive Endocrinology®: Drs. Mishell, Lobo, and Sokol

Year Book of Medicine®: Drs. Bone, Cline, Epstein, Greenberger, Malawista, Mandell, O'Rourke, Utiger

Year Book of Neonatal and Perinatal Medicine®: Drs. Fanaroff and Klaus

Year Book of Nephrology®: Drs. Coe, Favus, Henderson, Kashgarian, Luke, and Curtis

Year Book of Neurology and Neurosurgery®: Drs. Bradley and Wilkins

Year Book of Neuroradiology: Drs. Osborn, Eskridge, Grossman, Hudgens, and Ross

Year Book of Nuclear Medicine®: Drs. Gottschalk, Blaufox, McAfee, Wacker, and Zubal

Year Book of Obstetrics and Gynecology®: Drs. Mishell, Kirschbaum, and Morrow

Year Book of Occupational and Environmental Medicine®: Drs. Emmett, Frank, Gochfeld, and Hessl

Year Book of Oncology®: Drs. Simone, Bosl, Glatstein, Ozols, and Steele

Year Book of Ophthalmology®: Drs. Cohen, Adams, Augsburger, Benson, Eagle, Flanagan, Grossman, Laibson, Nelson, Rapuano, Reinecke, Sergott, Tasman, Tipperman, and Wilson

Year Book of Orthopedics®: Drs. Sledge, Cofield, Dobyns, Griffin, Poss, Springfield, Swiontkowski, and Wilson

Year Book of Otolaryngology–Head and Neck Surgery®: Drs. Paparella and Holt

Year Book of Pain: Drs. Gebhart, Haddox, Jacox, Marcus, Rudy, Shapiro, and Janjan

Year Book of Pathology and Laboratory Medicine®: Drs. Mills, Bruns, Gaffey, and Stoler

Year Book of Pediatrics®: Dr. Stockman

Year Book of Plastic, Reconstructive, and Aesthetic Surgery: Drs. Miller, Cohen, McKinney, Robson, Ruberg, and Whitaker

Year Book of Podiatric Medicine and Surgery®: Dr. Kominsky

Year Book of Psychiatry and Applied Mental Health®: Drs. Talbott, Breier, Frances, Meltzer, Schowalter, Tasman, and Yudofsky

Year Book of Pulmonary Disease®: Drs. Bone and Petty

Year Book of Rheumatology®: Drs. Sergent, LeRoy, Meenan, Panush, and Reichlin

Year Book of Sports Medicine®: Drs. Shephard, Drinkwater, Eichner, Torg, Col. Anderson, and Mr. George

Year Book of Surgery®: Drs. Copeland, Bland, Deitch, Eberlein, Howard, Luce, Seeger, Souba, and Sugarbaker

Year Book of Thoracic and Cardiovascular Surgery®: Drs. Ginsberg, Lofland, and Wechsler

Year Book of Transplantation®: Drs. Sollinger, Eckhoff, Hullett, Knechtle, Longo, Mentzer, and Pirsch

Year Book of Ultrasound®: Drs. Merritt, Babcock, Carroll, Fagin, Finberg, and Fleischer

Year Book of Urology®: Drs. DeKernion and Howards

Year Book of Vascular Surgery®: Dr. Porter

Statement of Purpose

The YEAR BOOK Service

The YEAR BOOK series was devised in 1901 by practicing health professionals who observed that the literature of medicine and related disciplines had become so voluminous that no one individual could read and place in perspective every potential advance in a major specialty. In the final decade of the 20th century, this recognition is more acutely true than it was in 1901.

More than merely a series of books, YEAR BOOK volumes are the tangible results of a unique service designed to accomplish the following:

- to *survey* a wide range of journals of proven value
- to *select* from those journals papers representing significant advances and statements of important clinical principles
- to provide *abstracts* of those articles that are readable, convenient summaries of their key points
- to provide *commentary* about those articles to place them in perspective

These publications grow out of a unique process that calls on the talents of outstanding authorities in clinical and fundamental disciplines, trained literature specialists, and professional writers, all supported by the resources of Mosby, the world's preeminent publisher for the health professions.

The Literature Base

Mosby subscribes to nearly 1,000 journals published worldwide, covering the full range of the health professions. On an annual basis, the publisher examines usage patterns and polls its expert authorities to add new journals to the literature base and to delete journals that are no longer useful as potential YEAR BOOK sources.

The Literature Survey

The publisher's team of literature specialists, all of whom are trained and experienced health professionals, examines every original, peer-reviewed article in each journal issue. More than 250,000 articles per year are scanned systematically, including title, text, illustrations, tables, and references. Each scan is compared, article by article, to the search strategies that the publisher has developed in consultation with the 270 outside experts who form the pool of YEAR BOOK editors. A given article may be reviewed by any number of editors, from one to a dozen or more, regardless of the discipline for which the paper was originally published. In turn, each editor who receives the article reviews it to determine whether or not the article should be included in the YEAR BOOK. This decision is based on the article's inherent quality, its probable usefulness to readers of that YEAR BOOK, and the editor's goal to represent a balanced picture of a given field in each volume of the YEAR BOOK. In addition, the editor indicates when to include figures and tables from the article to help the YEAR BOOK reader better understand the information.

Of the quarter million articles scanned each year, only 5% are selected for detailed analysis within the YEAR BOOK series, thereby assuring readers of the high value of every selection.

The Abstract

The publisher's abstracting staff is headed by a physician-writer and includes individuals with training in the life sciences, medicine, and other areas, plus extensive experience in writing for the health professions and related industries. Each selected article is assigned to a specific writer on this abstracting staff. The abstracter, guided in many cases by notations supplied by the expert editor, writes a structured, condensed summary designed so that the reader can rapidly acquire the essential information contained in the article.

The Commentary

The YEAR BOOK editorial boards, sometimes assisted by guest commentators, write comments that place each article in perspective for the reader. This provides the reader with the equivalent of a personal consultation with a leading international authority—an opportunity to better understand the value of the article and to benefit from the authority's thought processes in assessing the article.

Additional Editorial Features

The editorial boards of each YEAR BOOK organize the abstracts and comments to provide a logical and satisfying sequence of information. To enhance the organization, editors also provide introductions to sections or individual chapters, comments linking a number of abstracts, citations to additional literature, and other features.

The published YEAR BOOK contains enhanced bibliographic citations for each selected article, including extended listings of multiple authors and identification of author affiliations. Each YEAR BOOK contains a Table of Contents specific to that year's volume. From year to year, the Table of Contents for a given YEAR BOOK will vary depending on developments within the field.

Every YEAR BOOK contains a list of the journals from which papers have been selected. This list represents a subset of the nearly 1,000 journals surveyed by the publisher and occasionally reflects a particularly pertinent article from a journal that is not surveyed on a routine basis.

Finally, each volume contains a comprehensive subject index and an index to authors of each selected paper.

1995

The Year Book of MEDICINE®

Editors

Roger C. Bone, M.D.
Martin J. Cline, M.D.
Franklin H. Epstein, M.D.
Norton J. Greenberger, M.D.
Stephen E. Malawista, M.D.
Gerald L. Mandell, M.D.
Robert A. O'Rourke, M.D.
Robert D. Utiger, M.D.

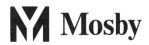 Mosby

St. Louis Baltimore Boston Carlsbad Chicago Naples New York Philadelphia Portland
London Madrid Mexico City Singapore Sydney Tokyo Toronto Wiesbaden

Vice President and Publisher, Continuity Publishing: Kenneth H. Killion
Director, Editorial Development: Gretchen C. Murphy
Manager, Continuity–EDP: Maria Nevinger
Developmental Editor: Kelly Poirier
Acquisitions Editor: Linda Steiner
Illustrations and Permissions Coordinator: Lois Ruebensam
Project Manager, Editing: Tamara L. Smith
Project Supervisor, Editing: Rebecca Nordbrock
Senior Production Editor: Wendi Schnaufer
Senior Project Manager, Production: Max F. Perez
Proofreading Supervisor: Barbara M. Kelly
Manager, Literature Services: Edith M. Podrazik, R.N.
Senior Information Specialist: Terri Santo, R.N.
Information Specialist: Nancy R. Dunne, R.N.
Senior Medical Writer: David A. Cramer, M.D.
Vice President, Professional Sales and Marketing: George M. Parker
Marketing and Circulation Manager: Barry J. Bowlus
Marketing Coordinator: Lynn Stevenson

1995 EDITION
Copyright © July 1995 by Mosby-Year Book, Inc.

Printed in the United States of America
Composition by International Computaprint Corporation
Printing/binding by Maple-Vail

Mosby-Year Book, Inc.
11830 Westline Industrial Drive
St. Louis, MO 63146

Editorial Office:
Mosby-Year Book, Inc.
200 North LaSalle Street
Chicago, IL 60601
International Standard Serial Number: 0084-3873
International Standard Book Number: 0-8151-7268-0

Contributing Editors

Robert S. Brown, M.D.
Associate Professor of Medicine, Harvard Medical School; Clinical Chief, Renal Unit, Beth Israel Hospital, Boston

Terry Strom, M.D.
Professor of Medicine, Harvard Medical School; Director, Division of Clinical Immunology, Beth Israel Hospital, Boston

Special Article By:
David Y. Graham, M.D.
Department of Medicine, Division of Molecular Virology, Veterans Affairs Medical Center; Baylor College of Medicine, Houston

Table of Contents

Mosby Document Express

Copies of the full text of the original source documents of articles abstracted or referenced in this publication are available by calling Mosby Document Express, toll-free, at **1 (800) 55-MOSBY.**

With Mosby Document Express, you have convenient, 24-hour-a-day access to literally every article on which this publication is based. In fact, through Mosby Document Express, virtually any medical or scientific article can be located and delivered by FAX, overnight delivery service, international airmail, electronic transmission of bitmapped images (via Internet), or regular mail. The average cost of a complete, delivered copy of an article, including up to $4 in copyright clearance charges and first-class mail delivery, is $12.

For inquiries and pricing information, please call the toll-free number shown above. To expedite your order for material appearing in this publication, please be prepared with the code shown next to the bibliographic citation for each abstract.

Journals Represented

Mosby subscribes to and surveys nearly 1,000 U.S. and foreign medical and allied health journals. From these journals, the Editors select the articles to be abstracted. Journals represented in this YEAR BOOK are listed below.

ASAIO Journal
Acta Cytologica
Alimentary Pharmacology and Therapeutics
American Heart Journal
American Journal of Cardiology
American Journal of Clinical Pathology
American Journal of Gastroenterology
American Journal of Hematology
American Journal of Kidney Diseases
American Journal of Medicine
American Journal of Pediatric Hematology/Oncology
American Journal of Physiology
American Journal of Public Health
American Journal of Respiratory and Critical Care Medicine
American Journal of Roentgenology
American Review of Respiratory Disease
Annals of Internal Medicine
Annals of Rheumatic Diseases
Annals of Surgery
Archives of Disease in Childhood
Archives of Internal Medicine
Archives of Pathology and Laboratory Medicine
Arthritis and Rheumatism
Blood
Bone and Mineral
British Journal of Clinical Pharmacology
British Medical Journal
Canadian Journal of Public Health
Cancer
Chest
Circulation
Clinical Biochemistry
Clinical Endocrinology
Clinical Infectious Diseases
Clinical Nephrology
Critical Care Medicine
Diabetes
Diabetes Care
Diabetologia
Dialysis and Transplantation
European Heart Journal
European Journal of Endocrinology
European Journal of Haematology
European Respiratory Journal
Experimental Hematology
Gastroenterology
Gut
Hepatology
Infection Control and Hospital Epidemiology
Intensive Care Medicine

International Journal of Artificial Organs
International Journal of Cancer
International Journal of Fertility
Journal of Applied Physiology: Respiratory, Environmental and Exercise Physiology
Journal of Clinical Endocrinology and Metabolism
Journal of Clinical Investigation
Journal of Clinical Oncology
Journal of Experimental Medicine
Journal of Human Hypertension
Journal of Hypertension
Journal of Immunology
Journal of Infectious Diseases
Journal of Internal Medicine
Journal of Nuclear Medicine
Journal of Occupational Medicine
Journal of Rheumatology
Journal of Thoracic and Cardiovascular Surgery
Journal of the American College of Cardiology
Journal of the American Geriatrics Society
Journal of the American Medical Association
Journal of the American Society of Nephrology
Journal of the National Cancer Institute
Kidney International
Lancet
Medicine
Modern Pathology
Nature
Nephron
New England Journal of Medicine
Obstetrics and Gynecology
Pain
Pediatric Infectious Disease Journal
Science
Southern Medical Journal
Stroke
Surgery
Thorax
Thrombosis and Haemostatis
Transfusion
Transplantation

STANDARD ABBREVIATIONS

The following terms are abbreviated in this edition: acquired immunodeficiency syndrome (AIDS), cardiopulmonary resuscitation (CPR), central nervous system (CNS), cerebrospinal fluid (CSF), computed tomography (CT), deoxyribonucleic acid (DNA), electrocardiography (ECG), health maintenance organization (HMO), human immunodeficiency virus (HIV), intensive care unit (ICU), intramuscular (IM), intravenous (IV), magnetic resonance (MR) imaging (MRI), and ribonucleic acid (RNA).

Helicobacter pylori: Current Status in Diagnosis, Therapy, Pathophysiology, and Thinking*

DAVID Y. GRAHAM, M.D.

Department of Medicine, and the Division of Molecular Virology, Veterans Affairs Medical Center, and Baylor College of Medicine, Houston, Texas

Introduction

The lay literature has been brimming with articles about *Helicobacter pylori* and its relationship to peptic ulcer disease and gastric carcinoma; patients are often better informed than their physicians. Physicians as a group are only now beginning to accept that peptic ulcer is one manifestation of a treatable, curable, and possibly preventable infectious disease. Acceptance has been rapid now that sufficient data are available to show that what appeared at the outset to be an outrageous idea was fact. We are now in the midst of a true revolution in the practice of gastroenterology (1). What is going to happen is relatively clear; how it is going to happen is much less so. Physicians have begun to look to soothsayers to interpret the omens and predict the future.

H. pylori as a Pathogen

Helicobacter pylori is a pathogen. *Helicobacter pylori* infection causes acute and chronic inflammation with progressive destruction of the gastric mucosa. Approximately 1 in 6 individuals infected with *H. pylori* have peptic ulcer disease develop, and probably between 1 and 2 per 1,000 individuals will have gastric carcinoma or gastric lymphoma. As there is no recognizable benefit from having the infection, we can predict that one of the goals will be to eliminate *H. pylori* infection from mankind. That will probably be difficult to achieve and may require treatment of active cases, identification of weak links in the transmission chain, and possibly vaccination to prevent or reduce the rate of acquisition of the infection in the population.

H. pylori Disease Associations

The field of *H. pylori* is beginning to mature. In February 1994, an NIH Consensus Development Conference concluded that *H. pylori* was the cause of most cases of peptic ulcer disease and that all patients with *H. pylori* infection should receive antimicrobial therapy (2). Cure of *H. pylori* infection cures peptic ulcer. In June, the International Agency for Research on Cancer Working Group of the World Health Organization defined *H. pylori* as a group I, or definite, human carcinogen. The role of *H. pylori* in cancer has broadened as it has also become increasingly recognized that cure of *H. pylori* infection results in remission of many, if not most, cases of primary B-cell gastric lymphoma (3). Thus, *H. pylori* has moved from being an obscure cause of gastritis to playing a pivotal role in the pathogenesis of peptic ulcer disease, gastric carcinoma, and primary B-cell gastric lymphoma. The relationship of *H. pylori* infec-

* This work was supported by the Department of Veterans Affairs and by the generous support of Hilda Schwartz.

tion to dyspepsia not associated with peptic ulcer disease remains unclear.

Epidemiology and Transmission

Human beings are the only known hosts for H. pylori, although there have been examples of animals, such as monkeys and cats, who have been in contact with humans, from whom H. pylori has been recovered. Such examples probably represent a humanosis (animal infection required from a human, the opposite of a zoonosis).

Helicobacter pylori infection has a higher prevalence among inhabitants of developing rather than developed countries (4). Even within developed countries, there are marked differences in prevalence among different groups. For example, in the United States, H. pylori infection is approximately twice as frequent in blacks and Hispanics than in age-matched whites (5, 6). Initially, the high prevalence of H. pylori in blacks appeared to be independent of socioeconomic status. Recently, the increase in prevalence was resolved as being only apparent by adjusting for the socioeconomic class of the individual's family during his or her childhood (4), because H. pylori infection is typically acquired in childhood. The H. pylori infection typically clusters in families with small children (7, 8), suggesting that infants or young children amplify the infection and may be important in H. pylori transmission (10). It appears to be infrequently transmitted between couples without children (9). The ability to reliably type H. pylori strains as well as to isolate H. pylori from stools will be required before the question of the direction of transmission as well as the source of the infection within a family or group can be completely understood.

One method to examine the genetic influences on a disease is to study the prevalence in twins. The frequency of H. pylori infection in monozygotic and dizygotic twins and in the subgroups of twins that were separated at birth and reared in entirely different environments can be compared. That study design allows estimation of the relative importance of environmental and genetic factors.

Studies of the prevalence of H. pylori in monozygotic and dizygotic twins have revealed good evidence for genetic susceptibility to H. pylori infection (11). The genetic factors that contribute to the differences in susceptibility remain unknown. A recent paper suggested that blood group antigens may serve as an important adhesin for H. pylori to the human gastric mucosa (12). This conclusion is probably in error, as previous studies had shown no relationship between the prevalence of H. pylori infection and the blood group or the secretor status of an individual (13–16). In addition, the putative adhesin could only be identified in late growth cultures and on formalin-fixed tissues, suggesting that the observation may not have an in vivo counterpart.

Pathogenesis of *H. pylori*–Related Diseases

Although there is little new hard evidence to address the question of how *H. pylori* infection leads to such markedly different diseases (e.g., duodenal ulcer compared with gastric cancer), 2 different but not necessarily exclusive hypotheses have emerged (17). One hypothesis is that host or environmental factors are the key; the other is that the different diseases result from infection with different clones of *H. pylori*. There are data to support both.

H. pylori and Acid Secretion

It has long been known that duodenal ulcer was associated with excessive secretion of gastric acid. Since the early 1970s, it has been recognized that duodenal ulcer disease was associated with perturbations in the regulation of gastrin release (18). Because gastrin is trophic for gastric mucosa, 1 hypothesis was that the exaggerated gastrin response to meals present in patients with duodenal ulcer might be responsible for the observed increase in parietal cell mass.

When it was discovered that *H. pylori* infection was responsible for the abnormal regulation of gastrin secretion seen in patients with peptic ulcer, the question became whether *H. pylori* infection was the cause of the increased parietal cell mass in patients with duodenal ulcer. It now appears that it is not. Cure of *H. pylori* infection results in reversal of the abnormalities in gastrin secretion but rarely with a reduction in maximum acid output (19, 20). Maximum acid output is directly related to parietal cell mass, so the failure of maximum acid output to return to normal after cure of the infection suggests that the increased acid secretion was not the result of *H. pylori*–induced hypergastrinemia but rather it preexisted the infection and the duodenal ulcer disease. Thus, individuals with high intrinsic rates of gastric acid secretion may be the ones who are at risk for duodenal ulcer if they become infected with *H. pylori*.

Current data support the hypothesis that the abnormalities in gastrin release result from the interaction between the chronic inflammatory response to the infection and somatostatin-containing D cells (21). Somatostatin release is a pivotal feature of the inhibitory limb of the pathway gastrin secretion with chronic inflammation inhibiting somatostatin release. Further confirmation that *H. pylori* itself is not directly involved is suggested by experiments showing that the reversal of exaggerated meal-stimulated gastrin release occurs in all groups of individuals with *H. pylori* infection (e.g., asymptomatic gastritis, nonulcer dyspepsia) and that the reversal occurs much later than the disappearance of both the bacteria and the acute inflammatory cell response (22).

One confusing aspect of the issue is the report that treatment of *H. pylori* infection was associated with a decline in gastric acid secretion (23). Further experiments and a better understanding of the experiments have resolved the confusion. *Helicobacter pylori* infection causes a leftward shift of the dose-response curve for acid secretion to infusion of gastrin-releasing peptide (GRP) but not with an increase in the maximum acid output. The study suggesting a decline in acid secretion after cure of the infection used a submaximal dose of GRP. It is now thought that because cure of the infection restores the dose response to normal without reducing the parietal cell mass, the changes in regulation of gastrin secretion associated with *H. pylori* infection are not pivotal events in the pathogenesis of duodenal ulcer disease. *

Virulence Factors

A search for virulence factors that may promote duodenal ulcer or gastric cancer is under way. A number of putative virulence factors have been identified. Urease and the ammonium produced topically in the stomach were early candidates, but their role appears unlikely. A gene, *cagA*, has been found to be absent in some strains of *H. pylori* but has been found in all or most isolates from patients with peptic ulcer, duodenal ulcer, most isolates from patients with asymptomatic gastritis (90%), and many if not most isolates from patients with gastric cancer (24-30). These findings cast doubt on a significant pathologic role for *cagA*. The fact that it is found in only some isolates is possible evidence for disease-specific genes or gene products. It has long been thought that duodenal ulcer disease protects against gastric carcinoma. Recent data confirm this (31). As both duodenal ulcer and gastric cancer are related to *H. pylori* infection, any critical factor in one should be absent in the other. One approach emphasized that researchers might be able to focus on features that are unique to either duodenal ulcer or gastric carcinoma to identify disease-specific factors. For example, it has long been known that the gastric histology in patients with duodenal ulcer is markedly different from that in patients with gastric ulcer. The question is, "Why?" Figure 1 shows a comparison of factors in patients with gastric cancer and with duodenal ulcer disease. The high acid secretion is a feature only of duodenal ulcer disease, and advanced intestinal metaplasia

FACTOR	DU	CA
H. pylori infection	√	√
H. pylori urease	√	√
◆ Gastric ammonium	√	√
*cag*A, *vac*A genes	√	√
Low gastric ascorbate	√	√
High acid output	√	--
Corpus atrophy	--	√
Type III intestinal metaplasia	--	√

Fig 1.—Relation between factors suggested to be important in the pathogenesis of the *H. pylori*-related diseases, duodenal ulcer *(DU)* and gastric carcinoma *(CA).* (Courtesy of Dr. Graham.)

in pangastritis is a unique feature of gastric carcinoma. Therefore, many factors that are currently being evaluated as putative virulence factors for ulcer or cancer are common to both diseases and clearly cannot be the unique factor(s) being sought. As there is currently little evidence to support the hypothesis that excess gastric acid secretion is related to *H. pylori,* one might focus on identifying the factor that restricts gastritis (but not the infection) to the antrum of patients with duodenal ulcer. It seems most likely that this will be a host factor. In contract, low gastric juice ascorbic acid concentrations are found in all forms of gastritis (32, 33).

Although pangastritis with atrophy and advanced intestinal metaplasia is related to gastric carcinoma, the prevalence and age of onset vary remarkably in different regions of the world. This wide variability and rapid change suggest that there are either major differences in the prevalence of disease-specific clones of *H. pylori,* or that other environmental factors, such as intake of dietary salt or nitrates, or fresh fruits and vegetables, are the important factors. We predict that study of the current popular putative virulence factors will lead to a better understanding of the biology of *H. pylori* but not of the *H. pylori*–associated diseases.

Identification of the Presence of *H. pylori* Infection

Confirming the diagnosis of *H. pylori* infection has been greatly simplified by the introduction of a number of serologic tests. Available tests include those that can be ordered from central laboratories and rapid tests designed for use in the office.

One caveat regarding serologic testing is that at least one of the national reference laboratories uses its own "in-house" enzyme-linked immunosorbent assay, which is of unknown specificity and sensitivity and has not been approved by the Food and Drug Administration (FDA). Therefore, one should demand that if serum samples are sent out for *H. pylori* serology, the test used should be one that is approved for use.

Current tests that examine for the presence of anti–*H. pylori* IgG as well as IgA and IgM titers have not been found to correlate as well with the presence or absence of *H. pylori* infection. Follow-up after therapy to confirm cure is still problematic. Although IgG titers decline after successful therapy of the *H. pylori* infection, they do so slowly. It often takes 12–18 months before the titer of an individual patient falls enough that one can be confident that the therapy has been successful.

The noninvasive, nonradioactive ^{13}C urea breath test can detect the presence of active infection and therefore is potentially useful for diagnosis of *H. pylori* infection both before and after therapy. The test is based on the extremely high levels of urease present in *H. pylori.* A simple office-based version of the test has been submitted to the FDA and should be available soon.

The gold standard for the presence of *H. pylori* infection has been endoscopy with multiple biopsies of the gastric mucosa. Introduction of

Here? ———▶

H₂-antagonist

Acid Pump Inhibitor

Here? ——▶

Antacids

Topical agents

Prostaglandin

Here? ———▶

Fig 2.—There was considerable debate concerning where to place antimicrobial within the pantheon of therapies for peptic ulcer disease. (Courtesy of Dr. Graham.)

the Genta stain (a combination of the hematoxylin and eosin, Alcian blue, and Steiner silver stains), which allows identification of the bacteria, detailed histology of the inflammation, as well as detection of the presence of intestinal metaplasia, has greatly simplified the histopathologist's task of identifying whether an infection is present (34). Nevertheless, the average pathologist does rather poorly in identifying whether *H. pylori* infection is present or absent. Hopefully, new atlases will rapidly correct these deficiencies.

Treatment of *H. pylori* Infection

There was some initial confusion about where antimicrobial therapy belonged in the armamentarium of the treatment of peptic ulcer disease. A wide variety of successful therapies proved to accelerate ulcer healing and, if given as maintenance therapy after healing, reduced the rate of ulcer recurrence. It was not clear whether antimicrobial therapy should be recommended as the initial therapy, only after more traditional therapies had failed, or only for a specific subgroup of patients (Fig 2). Two events clarified the issue. First, effective antimicrobial therapies for *H. pylori* infection were devised and, more important, peptic ulcer disease was recognized to be an infectious disease. Thus, the question about

Acid Disease	Infectious Disease
H₂-blocker	Antibiotics
Acid pump inhibitor	
Antacids	
Topical agent	
Prostaglandin	

Fig 3.—Recognition that *H. pylori* infection was an infectious disease and a cause of peptic ulcer changed the issue from where to place therapy to an understanding that the goals of the 2 types of therapy were different. For example, antisecretory is aimed at healing the wound, whereas antimicrobial therapy focuses on the underlying cause of the disease. (Courtesy of Dr. Graham.)

where to place antimicrobial therapy among the therapies for peptic ulcer disease became moot. Antimicrobial therapy should be used to treat the infection, and antisecretory therapy might also be used to accelerate ulcer healing and to achieve rapid pain relief (Fig 3).

The expectations regarding antimicrobial therapy have also changed. We have now come to demand that the antimicrobial therapies be as effective as they are in other infectious diseases. We will no longer consider therapies that yield cure rates of 40% to 50% and should be hesitant to use one that yields a cure rate of less than 80%.

Successful treatment of the *H. pylori* infection currently requires combinations of antimicrobials. A number of antimicrobial combinations will achieve cure rates between 80% and 100% (Table 1). Unfortunately, they can still be considered as "recipes." We use the word recipe instead of regimen because changes in dosing interval or dose often result in significantly poorer results. Also, the stomach is a very hostile place for antibiotics to function. *Helicobacter pylori* organisms are outside the body, encased in thick mucus, and in an environment where the low pH can adversely affect antimicrobial effectiveness. Tetracycline, bismuth, and metronidazole appear to be largely pH-independent antimicrobials, whereas the effectiveness of amoxicillin and the macrolides (clarithromycin and possibly azithromycin) is enhanced by increasing the pH.

Table 1 shows current recommendations and the results that can be anticipated. Several caveats are in order. Tetracycline hydrochloride is the effective tetracycline; doxycycline is not (35). Combinations of an acid pump inhibitor (omeprazole or lansoprazole) and 2 antimicrobials are more effective than using 1 antimicrobial. The combination of omeprazole and amoxicillin appears to be very sensitive to external factors. For example, with this therapy, smokers have markedly lower cure rates than nonsmokers (36). More reliable results with this combination have been attained when very high doses of omeprazole (120 mg) have been administered with 2 to 3 g of amoxicillin, suggesting that for maximum effectiveness with this therapy, the intragastric pH must be close to 7 (37). In contrast, the combination of clarithromycin and amoxicillin yields cure rates in the range of 90% without omeprazole (38).

The reader must be cognizant that the data regarding individual therapies for *H. pylori* have generally been reported from small trials, and direct comparisons between different regimens are still unavailable. Standard triple therapy (500 mg of tetracycline-HCl q.i.d., 250 mg of metronidazole t.i.d., and 2 bismuth-containing tablets, such as Pepto-Bismol, q.i.d., with meals and at bedtime for 14 days with or without an antisecretory drug) has been used in a number of studies with 90 or more patients and has consistently yielded cure rates in the range of 85% to 95% (39–43). Metronidazole-resistant *H. pylori* will respond less well, with cure rates between 60% and 70%, but will not greatly affect the outcome unless they are very prevalent in the population (43–46). In addition, the pharmacist may need to be alerted, and patients educated, that the regimen includes tetracycline both with meals and with bismuth.

TABLE 1.—Antimicrobial Combinations and Results

Therapy	Hp Drug 1	Hp Drug 2	Hp Drug 3	Notes*	Success
Triple	tetracycline HCl 500 mg q.i.d.	metronidazole 250 mg t.i.d.	bismuth subsalicylate† 2 tablets q.i.d.	with meals for 14 days plus an antisecretory drug	>90%
Triple	tetracycline HCl 500 mg q.i.d.	clarithromycin 500 mg t.i.d.	bismuth subsalicylate 2 tablets q.i.d	with meals for 14 days plus an antisecretory drug	>90%
Triple	amoxicillin 500 mg q.i.d.	clarithromycin 500 mg t.i.d.	bismuth subsalicylate 2 tablets q.i.d	with meals for 14 days plus an antisecretory drug	>90%
Triple	amoxicillin 500 mg q.i.d.	metronidazole 250 t.i.d.	bismuth subsalicylate 2 tablets q.i.d.	with meals for 14 days plus an antisecretory drug	>80%
Dual	clarithromycin 250 mg b.i.d.	metronidazole 500 mg b.i.d.	omeprazole 20 mg b.i.d.	for 7 to 14 days	>90%
Dual	amoxicillin 750 mg t.i.d.	clarithromycin 500 mg t.i.d.		with meals for 14 days plus an antisecretory drug	>90%
Dual	amoxicillin 750 mg t.i.d.	metronidazole 500 mg t.i.d.		with meals for 14 days plus an antisecretory drug	>85%
Dual	clarithromycin 500 mg t.i.d	omeprazole 40 mg q.a.m.		with meals for 14 days	75% to 85%
Dual	amoxicillin 750 mg t.i.d.	omeprazole 40 mg t.i.d.		with meals for 14 days	>90%
Dual‡	amoxicillin 1 gm t.i.d.	omeprazole 20 mg b.i.d.		with meals for 14 days	35% to 60%

* Generally, one should continue an antisecretory drug for 6 weeks to ensure ulcer healing.
† Bismuth subcitrate can be substituted.
‡ This outcome is based on Dr. Graham's impressions and estimates based on review of the available data as well as on the results of clinical trials. This particular combination at these or lower dosages is not recommended.
(Courtesy of Dr. Graham.)

Although, both meals and bismuth will theoretically reduce the effectiveness of tetracycline, the prescription is correct and should be followed as such. It is also important to educate patients about the importance of taking all of the medication rather than stopping when they feel better. They should also be informed that bismuth may turn their stool black. Physicians must be educated that sequential addition of agents may lead to an increase in the frequency of metronidazole-resistant *H. pylori* (i.e.,

TABLE 2.—Recommendations for Therapy of *H. pylori* Disease

1. Confirm the presence of the infection by one or more tests: serology, urea breath test, or histology.
2. Treat the patient for 2 weeks with one of the therapies shown to yield a cure rate of 90% or greater.
3. Four to 6 weeks after the end of antimicrobial therapy confirm cure with a urea breath test or histology.

(Courtesy of Dr. Graham.)

to follow the recipe). Table 2 shows the overall approach from diagnosis to confirmation of cure. To avoid false results, it is important to wait 4–6 weeks after ending the antimicrobial therapy before confirming a cure.

The 95% confidence limits of the reported cure rate of a trial, rather than the percentage reported cured, may give a better estimation of the results that may be achieved. For example, if a therapy resulted in a 90% cure rate, what range of values might one encounter if the study were repeated? The 95% confidence limits for a cure rate of 90% are shown in Table 3 when the sample size is increased from 10 to 200. Meta-analyses have been done using results reported largely in abstracts of studies with very small sample sizes, and these meta-analyses are also commonly used as examples in speeches by opinion leaders (47). It should be evident that the range of results to be expected depends on sample size. For example, a sample size of about 30 is required to be at all hopeful that a therapy reporting a 90% cure will consistently achieve a cure rate of 70% or more. This is a different calculation from that required to compare 2 therapies. To prove that a therapy that yielded a 95% cure rate was statistically better than one with an 80% cure rate would require

TABLE 3.—Expected Range of Results if a Study
That Reports a Cure Rate of 90% or 100%
Is Repeated

	Cure Rate Reported	
Sample size	90%	100%
10	55% to 99%	69% to 100%
20	68% to 99%	83% to 100%
30	73% to 98%	88% to 100%
50	78% to 96%	93% to 100%
100	82% to 95%	96% to 100%
150	84% to 94%	97% to 100%
200	85% to 94%	98% to 100%

(Courtesy of Dr. Graham.)

88 patients per group (80% power, $P = .05$); a comparison of cures of 95% and 85% would require 160 patients per group. One can therefore not rely on intuition or small studies to choose between therapies.

Poor compliance has been shown to be the major factor predicting poor results with triple therapy (40, 48). One must remember that in patients with ulcers, side effects have rarely necessitated stopping therapy, and none of the "simpler" therapies have shown a better rate of compliance. Even with the "difficult" therapies, compliance is generally excellent as patients with ulcer disease are used to taking medications as prescribed because they are very desirous of getting rid of the disease.

The Future

The medical research and funding establishments have not yet made the adjustments necessary to focus research on methods to prevent the transmission of, reduce the rate of acquisition of, and cure the *H. pylori* infection. Requests for research proposals stress pathogenesis and are seemingly oblivious to the fact that, if the infection is prevented or cured, *H. pylori*–associated diseases will disappear. At the same time, gastric infection with *Helicobacter* species may ultimately provide excellent models for the study of topics such as mucosal inflammation, bacteria–mucosal interactions, and mucosal-associated lymphoma. How *H. pylori* infection causes peptic ulcer is of intellectual interest but may have little practical application, because elimination of *H. pylori* from humankind will make the problem moot. One might ask whether the current emphasis on "basic" questions will actually prolong the association of *H. pylori* with humankind.

References

1. Graham DY: Evolution of concepts regarding *Helicobacter pylori*: From a cause of gastritis to a public health problem. *Am J Gastroenterol* 89:469–472, 1994.
2. NIH Consensus Conference: *Helicobacter pylori* in peptic ulcer disease. NIH Consensus Development Panel on *Helicobacter pylori* in Peptic Ulcer Disease. *JAMA* 272:65–69, 1994.
3. Isaacson PG: Gastric lymphoma and *Helicobacter pylori*. *N Engl J Med* 330:1310–1311, 1994.
4. Malaty HM, Graham DY: Importance of childhood socioeconomic status on the current prevalence of *Helicobacter pylori* infection. *Gut* 35:742–745, 1994.
5. Malaty HM, Evans DG, Evans DJ, Jr., Graham DY: *Helicobacter pylori* in Hispanics: Comparison with blacks and whites of similar age and socioeconomic class. *Gastroenterology* 103:813–816, 1992.
6. Graham DY, Malaty HM, Evans DG, Evans DJ, Jr, Klein PD, Adam E: Epidemiology of *Helicobacter pylori* in an asymptomatic population in the United States. Effect of age, race, and socioeconomic status. *Gastroenterology* 100:1495–1501, 1991.
7. Drumm B, Perez Perez GI, Blaser MJ, Sherman PM: Intrafamilial clustering of *Helicobacter pylori* infection. *N Engl J Med* 322:359–363, 1990.
8. Malaty HM, Graham DY, Klein PD, Evans DG, Adam E, Evans DJ: Transmission of *Helicobacter pylori* infection. Studies in families of healthy individuals. *Scand J Gastroenterol* 26:927–932, 1991.

9. Perez-Perez GI, Witkin SS, Decker MD, Blaser MJ: Seroprevalence of *Helicobacter pylori* infection in couples. *J Clin Microbiol* 29:642–644, 1991.

10. Graham DY, Klein PD, Evans DG, et al: *Helicobacter pylori*: Epidemiology, relationship to gastric cancer and the role of infants in transmission. *Eur J Gastroenterol Hepatol* 4:S1–S6, 1992.

11. Malaty HM, Engstrand L, Pedersen NL, Graham DY: *Helicobacter pylori* infection: Genetic and environmental influences. A study of twins. *Ann Intern Med* 120:982–986, 1994.

12. Boren T, Falk P, Roth KA, Larson G, Normark S: Attachment of *Helicobacter pylori* to human gastric epithelium mediated by blood group antigens. *Science* 262:1892–1895, 1993.

13. Mentis A, Blackwell CC, Weir DM, Spiliadis C, Dailianas A, Skandalis N: ABO blood group, secretor status and detection of *Helicobacter pylori* among patients with gastric or duodenal ulcers. *Epidemiol Infect* 106:221–229, 1991.

14. Hook Nikanne J, Sistonen P, Kosunen TU: Effect of ABO blood group and secretor status on the frequency of *Helicobacter pylori* antibodies. *Scand J Gastroenterol* 25:815–818, 1990.

15. Loffeld RJ, Stobberingh E: *Helicobacter pylori* and ABO blood groups. *J Clin Pathol* 44:516–517, 1991.

16. Dickey W, Collins JS, Watson RG, Sloan JM, Porter KG: Secretor status and *Helicobacter pylori* infection are independent risk factors for gastroduodenal disease. *Gut* 34:351–353, 1993.

17. Go MF, Graham DY: Determinants of clinical outcome of *H. pylori* infection: Duodenal ulcer, in Hunt RH, Tytgat GNJ (eds): *Helicobacter pylori* Basic Mechanisms to Clinical Cure. Dordrecht: Kluwer Academic Publishers, 421–428, 1994.

18. McGuigan JE, Trudeau WL: Differences in rates of gastrin release in normal persons and patients with duodenal-ulcer disease. *N Engl J Med* 288:64–66, 1973.

19. Graham DY: *Helicobacter pylori*: Its epidemiology and its role in duodenal ulcer disease. *J Gastroenterol Hepatol* 6:105–113, 1991.

20. McColl KE, Fullarton GM, Chittajalu R, et al: Plasma gastrin, daytime intragastric pH, and nocturnal acid output before and at 1 and 7 months after eradication of *Helicobacter pylori* in duodenal ulcer subjects. *Scand J Gastroenterol* 26:339–346, 1991.

21. Moss SF, Legon S, Bishop AE, Polak JM, Calam J: Effect of *Helicobacter pylori* on gastric somatostatin in duodenal ulcer disease. *Lancet* 340:930–932, 1992.

22. Graham DY, Go MF, Lew GM, Genta RM, Rehfeld JF: *Helicobacter pylori* infection and exaggerated gastrin release: Effects of inflammation and progastrin processing. *Scand J Gastroenterol* 28:690–694, 1993.

23. el-Omar E, Penman I, Dorrian CA, Ardill JES, McColl KEL: Eradicating *Helicobacter pylori* infection lowers gastrin mediated acid secretion by two thirds in patients with duodenal ulcer. *Gut* 34:1060–1065, 1993.

24. Figura N, Guglielmetti P, Rossolini A, et al: Cytotoxin production by *Campylobacter pylori* strains isolated from patients with peptic ulcers and from patients with chronic gastritis only. *J Clin Microbiol* 27:225–226, 1989.

25. Tummuru MK, Cover TL, Blaser MJ: Cloning and expression of a high-molecular-mass major antigen of *Helicobacter pylori*: Evidence of linkage to cytotoxin production. *Infect Immun* 61:1799–1809, 1993.

26. Crabtree JE, Taylor JD, Wyatt JI, et al: Mucosal IgA recognition of *Helicobacter pylori* 120 kDa protein, peptic ulceration, and gastric pathology. *Lancet* 338:332–335, 1991.

27. Pretolani S, Figura N, Gatto MRA, et al: The San Marino *H. pylori* study II: A population-based study on the prevalence of endoscopic lesions and its association with *H. pylori* and anticytotoxin-protein (CagA) antibodies. (Abstract) *Am J Gastroenterol* 89:1307, 1994.

28. Go MF, Versalovic J, Graham DY: Is PCR a reliable technique to detect the presence of putative *H. pylori* virulence genes? (Abstract) *Am J Gastroenterol* 89:78, 1994.

29. Crabtree, JE, el-Omar E, Bugnoli M, et al: Serum CagA antibodies in *Helicobacter pylori* positive healthy volunteers and patients with dyspeptic disease. (Abstract) *Am J Gastroenterol* 89:206, 1994.

30. Labigne A, Lamouliatte H, Birac C, Sedallian A, Megraud F: Distribution of the cagA gene among *Helicobacter pylori* strains with peptic ulcer. (Abstract) *Am J Gastroenterol* 89:166, 1994.

31. Parsonnet J, Friedman GD, Vandersteen DP, et al: *Helicobacter pylori* infection and the risk of gastric carcinoma. *N Engl J Med* 325:1127-1131, 1991.

32. Axon ATR: The ascorbic acid story, in Hunt RH, Tytgat GNJ, (eds): *Helicobacter pylori* Basic Mechanisms to Clinical Cure. Dordrecht: Kluwer Academic Publishers, 469-474, 1994.

33. Freeman JT: Hafkesbring R: Comparative studies of ascorbic acid levels in gastric secretion and blood. III. Gastrointestinal diseases. *Gastroenterology* 32:878-886, 1957.

34. Genta RM, Robason GO, Graham DY: Simultaneous visualization of *Helicobacter pylori* and gastric morphology: A new stain. *Hum Pathol* 25:221-226, 1994.

35. Borody TJ, George LL, Brandl S, et al: *Helicobacter pylori* eradication with doxycycline-metronidazole-bismuth subcitrate triple therapy. *Scand J Gastroenterol* 27:281-284, 1992.

36. Zala G, Wirth HP, Giezendanner S, et al: Omeprazole/amoxicillin: Impaired eradication of *H. pylori* by smoking but not by omeprazole pretreatment. (Abstract) *Gastroenterology* 106:A215, 1994.

37. Bayerdörffer E, Miehlke S, Mannes GA, et al: Double-blind trial of omeprazole (120 mg) + amoxicillin for *Helicobacter pylori* eradication in duodenal ulcer patients. (Abstract) *Am J Gastroenterol* 89:1364, 1994.

38. Al-Assi MT, Genta RM, Karttunen TJ, Graham DY: Clarithromycin-amoxycillin therapy for *Helicobacter pylori* infection. *Ailment Pharmacol Therap* 8:453-456, 1994.

39. Cutler AF, Schubert TT: Patient factors affecting *Helicobacter pylori* eradication with triple therapy. *Am J Gastroenterol* 88:505-509, 1993.

40. Graham DY, Lew GM, Malaty HM, et al: Factors influencing the eradication of *Helicobacter pylori* with triple therapy. *Gastroenterology* 102:493-496, 1992.

41. Hosking SW, Ling TK, Yung MY, et al: Randomised controlled trial of short term treatment to eradicate *Helicobacter pylori* in patients with duodenal ulcer. *BMJ* 305:502-504, 1992.

42. Borody TJ, Andrews P, Shortis NP, Bae H, Brandl S: Optimal *H. pylori* (HP) therapy—A combination of omeprazole and triple therapy (TT). (Abstract) *Gastroenterology* 106:A55, 1994.

43. de Boer WA, Driessen WMM, Potters VPJ, Tytgat GNJ: Randomized study comparing 1 and 2 weeks of quadruple therapy for eradicating *Helicobacter pylori*. *Am J Gastroenterol* 89:1993-1997, 1994.

44. Bell GD, Powell K, Burridge SM, et al: Experience with 'triple' anti-*Helicobacter pylori* eradication therapy: Side effects and the importance of testing the pretreatment bacterial isolate for metronidazole resistance. *Aliment Pharmacol Ther* 6:427-435, 1992.

45. Rautelin H, Seppala K, Renkonen OV, Vainio U, Kosunen TU: Role of metronidazole resistance in therapy of *Helicobacter pylori* infections. *Antimicrob Agents Chemother* 36:163-166, 1992.

46. Seppala K, Farkkila M, Nuutinen H, et al: Triple therapy of *Helicobacter pylori* infection in peptic ulcer. A 12-month follow-up study of 93 patients. *Scand J Gastroenterol* 27:973-976, 1992.

47. Mohamed AH, Chiba A, Wilkerson J, Hunt RH: Eradication of *Helicobacter pylori* (Hp): A meta-analysis. (Abstract) *Gastroenterology* 106:142A, 1994.

48. Graham DY: Determinants of antimicrobial effectiveness in *H. pylori* gastritis, in Hunt RH, Tytgat GNJ, (eds): *Helicobacter pylori* Basic Mechanisms to Clinical Cure. Dordrecht: Kluwer Academic Publishers, 531-537, 1994.

PART ONE

INFECTIOUS DISEASES

GERALD L. MANDELL, M.D.

Introduction

There is both good news and bad news to report. New therapies are being developed and evaluated. Agents discussed include itraconazole for fungal disease, famcyclovir for viral disease, and interferon-γ as an immune modulator. New aspects of the common cold have been described, which raises interesting therapeutic possibilities. We now have a good understanding of the clinical picture of both ehrlichiosis and Hantavirus pulmonary syndrome, with effective treatment for the former.

On the downside are the increasing incidence of resistant pneumococcal and enterococcal infection and the lack of clinical success in several trials of antiviral therapy for patients with HIV infection.

Gerald L. Mandell, M.D.

1   Common Cold

Introduction

Things used to be relatively simple in cold management. Up-to-date physicians knew that antibiotics were not effective for viral colds, but such complications as sinusitis were considered clear-cut indications for antibacterial therapy. Read on and, perhaps, get more confused.

Gerald L. Mandell, M.D.

Computed Tomographic Study of the Common Cold
Gwaltney JM Jr, Phillips CD, Miller RD, Riker DK (Univ of Virginia Health Science Ctr, Charlottesville; Procter & Gamble Co, Cincinnati, Ohio)
N Engl J Med 330:25–30, 1994   119-95-1–1

Objective.—Despite the prevalence of colds, the changes they produce in the nasal passages and sinuses remain incompletely understood. A CT study was therefore done in 31 generally healthy adults (mean age, 24 years) who had had a self-diagnosed cold for 2–4 days. Seventy-nine other patients were evaluated but did not undergo CT scanning.

Methods.—Computed tomographic scans were made of the nasal passages, ostiomeatal complex, and paranasal sinuses. As many as 20 images were acquired in a direct coronal plane. In addition, the nasal secretions were cultured for viruses, and nasal airway resistance was measured by anterior rhinomanometry. Nasal mucociliary clearance was quantified by using indigo carmine dye, saccharin, and sorbitol.

Findings.—Rhinovirus was isolated from the nasal secretions in 27% of patients. Abnormal nasal airway resistance was nearly invariable; it correlated with CT findings of swollen turbinates and thickened nasal walls. Mucosal transport was delayed in most patients, and transport times correlated with the severity of illness. Congestion of the nose or head correlated with occlusion of the ethmoid infundibulum. Some patients without ethmoid abnormalities did have changes in the maxillary sinuses. Radiopaque material in the sinus cavities had the density of soft tissue or fluid. Several anatomical variations were visualized, including marked septal deviation, infraorbital air cells, and enlarged ethmoid bullae.

Follow-Up.—Both mucosal transport times and sinus abnormalities resolved in patients who were followed and reported feeling well (Fig

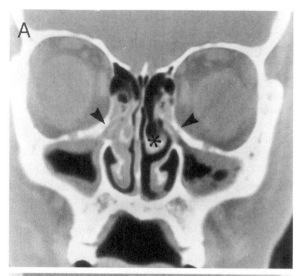

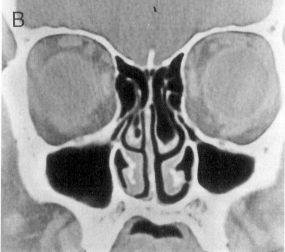

Fig 1–1.—Initial and follow-up sinus CT scans in an untreated adult (subject 1) with the common cold. **A,** the initial scan, obtained on day 4 of illness, shows bilateral occlusion of the ethmoid infundibulum (*arrows*), the passage draining the maxillary sinus; abnormalities of the ethmoid sinuses (**right,** 4 mm; **left,** 4 mm) and maxillary sinuses (**right,** 4 mm; **left,** 7 mm); and bilateral pneumatization of the middle turbinate (concha bullosa [*asterisk*]). **B,** the scan obtained on day 13 shows minimal residual infundibular occlusion and a residual abnormality of the right maxillary sinus (2 mm). (Courtesy of Gwaltney JM Jr, Phillips CD, Miller RD, et al: N Engl J Med 330:25–30, 1994.)

1–1). Nasal airway resistance remained abnormal in patients with persistent symptoms.

Discussion.—The upper airways are more broadly involved in the common cold than has been thought. Ostiomeatal and sinus abnormalities are frequently seen on CT studies in adults with colds. Reversible changes appear to be more significant than anatomical variations.

▶ The conclusion is definite and simple. From 70% to 80% of patients with acute uncomplicated colds had CT evidence of sinus involvement. In some ways, this is not surprising, because patients frequently state that they have congested sinuses and changes in voice character, which may reflect sinus involvement. This study provides definitive documentation of that phenomenon. Patients improved systematically and by CT scan without antibiotic treatment. The problem, of course, is to differentiate viral sinusitis from bacterial sinusitis. In a patient with cold and sinus symptoms, fever is probably the most useful finding that indicates the likelihood of bacterial sinusitis. I would be hard-pressed to document that hypothesis in a definitive study, but Jack Gwaltney has repeatedly told me that the common cold in adults rarely results in significant fever (more than 100.5°F).—G.L. Mandell, M.D.

Effect of Inhalation of Hot Humidified Air on Experimental Rhinovirus Infection
Hendley JO, Abbott RD, Beasley PP, Gwaltney JM Jr (Univ of Virginia Health Sciences Ctr, Charlottesville)
JAMA 271:1112–1113, 1994   119-95-1–2

Background.—Nasal inhalation of steam decreases nasal obstruction in many patients and may provide sustained benefit up to 7 days in patients with coryza. Steam inhalation raises the temperature of the nasal mucosa and thereby may reduce viral replication. The effect of steam inhalation on rhinovirus shedding was investigated.

Methods.—After intranasal inoculation with an untyped rhinovirus, 20 volunteers subsequently underwent 30-minute intranasal steam treatments at 24 and 48 hours. Active vapor temperature was 42–44°C, and placebo vapor was 22°C. Viral titers in nasal washings were assessed on each of 5 days after inoculation.

Results.—All volunteers shed the challenge rhinovirus 1 or more days after inoculation. Antibody titer increased in 9 patients treated with active vapor and in 8 treated with placebo. Area under the curve, average viral titers for all 5 follow-up days, and viral shedding velocity were similar for the 2 groups. Mean titers did not differ significantly between groups on any day. The daily proportion of participants shedding virus was also similar between groups.

Conclusion.—Two 30-minute treatments with steam did not affect rhinovirus replication assessed by viral titer in nasal washings. Any sustained effect of nasal inhalation of steam on rhinovirus symptoms is not mediated by reduction in viral replication.

Effect of Inhaling Heated Vapor on Symptoms of the Common Cold

Forstall GJ, Macknin ML, Yen-Lieberman BR, VanderBrug Medondorp S
(Cleveland Clinic Found, Ohio)

JAMA 271:1109–1111, 1994   119-95-1–3

Background.—Heated humidified air raises nasal mucosal temperature and may relieve symptoms of the common cold. However, studies of the benefit of nasal steam inhalation in patients with the common cold have produced conflicting results. Whether thermal and temporal conditions that inactivate rhinovirus in vitro improve common cold symptoms was investigated.

Methods.—Thirty-two volunteers with symptoms of the common cold underwent a 60-minute treatment of steam that raised intranasal temperature to 43°C. A placebo group of 36 volunteers received ambient air at 20–24°C. During a 7-day follow-up, patients and investigators rated subjective symptoms, and objective nasal resistance was evaluated.

Results.—Patients' and investigators' symptom index scores were virtually identical for both treatments. Symptoms decreased significantly from baseline in both groups, but changes over time were comparable. By day 7, improvement in nasal resistance was significantly greater after placebo treatment than after steam treatment, possibly reflecting higher baseline nasal resistance rather than effect of treatment.

Conclusion.—Steam inhalation had no beneficial effect on common cold symptoms in this group of volunteers.

▶ These 2 selections provide a double whammy to steam treatment of the common cold. The Cleveland Clinic group found no benefit for symptoms, and the University of Virginia group found no reduction in viral shedding. I will omit the obligatory discourse on chicken soup.—G.L. Mandell, M.D.

2 Urinary Tract Infection

Introduction

Urinary tract infections are extremely common, especially in women. Despite this, many questions remain unanswered. Rigid adherence to the requirement for 10^5 organisms per milliliter of urine to make a diagnosis has been shown to be incorrect. Young women frequently have true infection, with 10^2 or 10^3 organisms per milliliter. There seems to be very little relationship between urinary tract infections and subsequent development of chronic renal disease; therefore, the primary goal in therapy is to relieve symptoms and prevent acute problems, such as urosepsis. Two groups of patients are somewhat special: pregnant women and elderly individuals.

Gerald L. Mandell, M.D.

Urinary Tract Infection During Pregnancy: Its Association With Maternal Morbidity and Perinatal Outcome
Schieve LA, Handler A, Hershow R, Persky V, Davis F (Univ of Illinois, Chicago)
Am J Public Health 84:405–410, 1994   119-95-2–1

Introduction.—Although an association has been established between antepartum urinary tract infection and perinatal mortality or pyelonephritis, other associations with maternal and infant morbidity are unclear. The relationship between untreated urinary tract infection and adverse pregnancy outcomes was examined in a retrospective cohort analysis.

Methods.—The data for 25,746 mother–infant pairs from a university perinatal registry were examined. Of these women, 1,988 had antepartum urinary tract infection. Associations with perinatal and maternal outcomes were studied with univariate and multivariate logistic analysis.

Results.—Women with antepartum urinary tract infection were significantly more likely than those who were uninfected to have adverse maternal outcomes (premature labor, hypertension–preeclampsia, anemia, and amnionitis) and adverse perinatal outcomes (low-birth-weight infants, premature infants, preterm infants with low birth weight, and infants small for gestational age). The risks for perinatal mortality and endometritis were also elevated, but not significantly, in the women with infection. Multivariate analysis revealed a significant association between urinary tract infection and perinatal death for women aged 20–29 years, and the association of infection with infants who were small for gestational age was no longer significant.

Discussion.—Associations between antepartum urinary tract infection and several adverse maternal and perinatal outcomes were established, underscoring the need for prenatal screening. The mechanisms by which urinary tract infection affects these outcomes require further study.

▶ There is a clear-cut association between urinary tract infection during pregnancy and problems in both the mother and infant. The logical leap is to suggest that elimination of the infection during pregnancy will reduce the incidence of the associated adverse outcomes. The data are not clear here, although they strongly support the finding that elimination of bacteriuria markedly reduces the incidence of acute pyelonephritis during that pregnancy. This is a compelling reason to search for and eradicate bacteria of pregnancy.—G.L. Mandell, M.D.

A Study of Various Tests to Detect Asymptomatic Urinary Tract Infections in an Obstetric Population

Bachman JW, Heise RH, Naessens JM, Timmerman MG (Mayo Clinic and Found, Rochester, Minn)
JAMA 270:1971–1974, 1993   119-95-2–2

Introduction.—Undetected asymptomatic urinary tract infection (AUTI) during pregnancy is associated with significant maternal and infant morbidity. Three rapid screening techniques used to detect AUTI in obstetric patients were compared.

Methods.—A total of 1,047 consecutive obstetric patients were assessed for the presence of AUTI on their initial visits. Urine culture, urinalysis sediment microscopy, urine Gram's staining, and urine dipstick testing were used. Only urinalysis and dipstick testing were used to test urine samples on subsequent visits; positive test results were verified with urine culture.

Results.—Twenty-four patients had positive urine cultures at the initial visit. Of the rapid screening techniques, Gram's staining was clearly superior, with a sensitivity of 91.7% and a specificity of 89.2%. The dipstick test had a sensitivity of 50% and a specificity of 96.9% and detected either leukocyte activity or nitrites. Using urinalysis to detect leukocytes produced a 25% sensitivity and a 99% specificity; using urinalysis to detect bacteria produced a 75% sensitivity and a 59.7% specificity. On subsequent visits, a positive predictive value of 3% for urinalysis and 5% for dipstick testing was noted. In patients with nitrites, the predictive value of dipstick testing rose to 36.8%, whereas the presence of leukocytes lowered the predictive value of dipstick testing to 1.9%.

Conclusion.—Urinalysis was clearly inferior to urine dipstick testing and Gram's stain in detecting AUTI. Gram's stain is more expensive than dipstick testing but provides the most sensitive same-day screening results. Dipstick testing for nitrites, however, is a cost-effective screening method for follow-up visits.

▶ How should pregnant women be screened for AUTIs? Cost rears its ugly head again. Urine culture is still considered the gold standard. However, that test is relatively expensive. The major points that I gleaned from this study are that urinalysis is expensive and insensitive in detecting bacteriuria. Urine dipstick, which detects leukocyte esterase and nitrites, was the best of the nonmicroscopic tests but was only 50% sensitive. Gram's stain was sensitive and specific. Bacteriuria incidence in this study was only 2.3%. This rate would be expected to be much greater in an area in which patients were from a lower socioeconomic strata.—G.L. Mandell, M.D.

Does Asymptomatic Bacteriuria Predict Mortality and Does Antimicrobial Treatment Reduce Mortality in Elderly Ambulatory Women?
Abrutyn E, Mossey J, Berlin JA, Boscia J, Levison M, Pitsakis P, Kaye D (Med College of Pennsylvania, Philadelphia; Veterans Affairs Med Ctr, Philadelphia; Univ of Pennsylvania, Philadelphia)
Ann Intern Med 120:827–833, 1994   119-95-2-3

Introduction.—Some studies have found an association between asymptomatic bacteriuria and increased mortality in elderly individuals. The findings of a 9-year study designed to evaluate this association in elderly ambulatory women and to determine whether antimicrobial therapy can improve longevity in those patients with asymptomatic bacteriuria were evaluated.

Methods.—The study was carried out in a geriatric center and 21 continuing care retirement communities. All female residents without urinary tract catheters were eligible to participate in an observational study of mortality. In a double-blind, controlled clinical trial, antimicrobial therapy or placebo was administered to patients with bacteriuria to assess whether treatment of asymptomatic bacteriuria decreases mortality. Midstream urine specimens were obtained on enrollment and every 6 months thereafter.

Results.—Of the participants, 1,173 were found to be uninfected, and 318 had bacteriuria. Women who were infected were older, sicker, and had higher mortality (18.7 vs. 10.1 per 100,000 resident-days) than those who were uninfected. Multivariate Cox analysis, however, revealed that infection was not related to mortality, whereas age at entry and self-rated health were strong predictors of subsequent death. In the clinical trial, patients with bacteriuria who received antimicrobial therapy had a mortality rate comparable to that of untreated patients with bacteriuria (13.8

and 15.1 per 100,000 resident-days, respectively). Overall cure rates were 82.9% for treated patients and 15.6% for untreated patients.

Conclusion.—Neither the observational study nor the clinical trial confirmed an association between asymptomatic bacteriuria in elderly women and increased mortality. The 192 treated patients and the 166 control patients did not differ in baseline characteristics. Although antimicrobial therapy was effective in curing infection, treatment did not reduce mortality. Increased mortality in elderly women can be predicted by means of a simple, subjective measure, self-rated health.

▶ In 1981, Dontas et al. reported that "bacteriuria in old age is associated with a reduction in survival of 30–50%" (1). This dramatic report, along with several others, motivated the Medical College of Pennsylvania group to examine the question. These investigators confirmed the observation that there was an association between bacteriuria and poor prognosis. They went a step further and treated patients and found that resolution of asymptomatic bacteriuria did not alter prognosis. This finding is important because it strongly suggests that screening for asymptomatic bacteriuria in elderly patients is not justified. If presented with an elderly patient who has bacteriuria without symptoms, there is no justification for therapy.—G.L. Mandell, M.D.

Reference

1. Dontas AS, et al: N Engl J Med 304:939–943, 1981.

Bladder Irrigation With Amphotericin B for Treatment of Fungal Urinary Tract Infections
Jacobs LG, Skidmore EA, Cardoso LA, Ziv F (Albert Einstein College of Medicine, Bronx, NY)
Clin Infect Dis 18:313–318, 1994   119-95-2–4

Background.—There is uncertainty regarding the differentiation of fungal infection vs. colonization of the urinary tract, as well as the indications for and timing of treatment. Bladder irrigation with amphotericin B is a widely used treatment, despite the lack of controlled trials. Because of the availability of new oral antifungal agents, this therapy was reexamined.

Patients and Methods.—The outcome of amphotericin B bladder irrigation in 71 women and 24 men (mean age, 75 years) who had been hospitalized for treatment of funguria in 1989 and 1990 was studied retrospectively. Half the patients had been admitted from a nursing home. More than 90% had been receiving broad-spectrum antibiotics; three fourths had indwelling bladder catheters. All patients had urine yielding more than 10,000 colony-forming units of fungi/mL and/or had funguria on microscopic examination of the urine.

The hospital in this study had not been using oral antifungal agents at the time the patients were admitted. All patients were treated with a standard protocol of amphotericin B administration: 25 mg of amphotericin B in 500 mL of 5% dextrose in water in a continuous infusion of 42 mL/hr. Outcome was assessed by culturing of urine samples after treatment.

Results.—Treatment was based on the findings of 2 consecutive culture samples in 43 patients and 1 sample in 37. Three fourths of patients had *Candida albicans,* two thirds had pyuria, and one third had bacteriuria. Half the patients had fever at the start of treatment. The median duration of treatment was 5 days, and there were no apparent adverse effects.

Funguria was eradicated in 80% of patients. No significant differences were noted between patients with diabetes and those without or between patients with catheters and those without. The findings of fever and pyuria were unrelated to treatment response. The hospital mortality rate was 39% in the study group.

Conclusion.—Amphotericin B bladder irrigation successfully eradicates funguria in 80% of frail, elderly patients in an acute care setting. Risk factors for fungal urinary tract infection include old age, female sex, diabetes mellitus, indwelling bladder catheterization, and broad-spectrum antibiotic treatment. A controlled, prospective study of oral fluconazole vs. amphotericin B bladder irrigation for such infections is under way.

▶ One weakness of this study is the method of patient selection. Potential subjects were identified only from pharmacy records of drug orders for amphotericin B bladder irrigation. Thus, patients who were not treated and those treated by other means were not evaluated. Nonetheless, there is some useful information in this paper. Funguria was eradicated in 80% of patients, but we don't know what receiving no treatment would have done. Note the very high mortality rate of 39%. These were very sick patients. There is no indication about whether the funguria was a marker of severe illness or actually led to mortality. A reasonable approach for management of funguria without evidence of bloodstream or disseminated infection is as follows: remove the indwelling catheter, which is nearly always present, and treat with bladder irrigation and/or a course of systemic therapy with amphotericin B or fluconazole. We eagerly await controlled studies to answer these questions better. Transplant patients and patients with neutropenia probably should receive systemic therapy. Another consideration for therapy is oral 5-fluorocytosine, which results in high urine levels.—G.L. Mandell, M.D.

3 Tuberculosis

Introduction

Who would have imagined that, in 1995, the Editor of the Infectious Diseases section would select 9 articles on tuberculosis? All physicians are by now aware of the resurgence of tuberculosis in the United States and the convergence of tuberculosis and HIV infection. The flurry of activity has resulted in some good, solid laboratory and clinical research that will be useful to us in dealing with this disease.

Gerald L. Mandell, M.D.

The Epidemiology of Tuberculosis in San Francisco: A Population-Based Study Using Conventional and Molecular Methods
Small PM, Hopewell PC, Singh SP, Paz A, Parsonnet J, Ruston DC, Schecter GF, Daley CL, Schoolnik GK (Stanford Univ, Calif; Univ of California, San Francisco; San Francisco Dept of Public Health)
N Engl J Med 330:1703–1709, 1994   119-95-3–1

Introduction.—The recent resurgence of tuberculosis in urban areas of the United States is attributed to a combination of biological and social factors. In a population-based epidemiologic study conducted in San Francisco, conventional techniques were combined with molecular fingerprinting by restriction-fragment–length polymorphism (RFLP) analysis. The incidence of cases resulting from recently transmitted infection was investigated, and some of the risk factors for transmission of *Myobacterium tuberculosis* were identified.

Methods.—All patients reported to the tuberculosis registry in San Francisco during 1991 and 1992 were included. Routine demographic data and specific information concerning tuberculosis were collected. The registries for tuberculosis and AIDS were crossmatched to identify all patients reported to have both diseases as of September 1993. The isolates of *M. tuberculosis* were studied by using RFLP, and patients infected with the same strains were identified according to their RFLP patterns. Patients with identical patterns were grouped in clusters for risk factor analysis.

Results.—There were 585 confirmed cases of tuberculosis during the study period. Viable isolates of *M. tuberculosis* were not available from 89 patients, and other patients were excluded for technical reasons; 473

patients were therefore included for analysis. Active tuberculosis appeared to have resulted from a recent infection in 191 patients. Although conventional methods of tracing patient contacts identified links among only 10% of these patients, molecular fingerprinting identified 44 clusters. Twenty clusters comprised only 2 persons; the largest cluster consisted of 30 persons. Patients in clusters were compared with those not in clusters to identify risk factors for recent infection. For patients younger than age 60 years, Hispanic ethnicity, black race, birth in the United States, and a diagnosis of AIDS were independently associated with being in a cluster. Twelve patients in the largest cluster were living in or were employed by a residential facility for patients with AIDS. Noncompliance with therapy by a single patient was implicated as a factor for disease transmission in the 3 largest clusters.

Conclusions.—Nearly one third of the new cases of tuberculosis in San Francisco were the result of recent infection. Because noncompliance with therapy is an important factor in the spread of the disease, prompt and effective treatment is needed to reduce the incidence of tuberculosis. Molecular fingerprinting techniques are more useful than conventional epidemiologic methods in tracing of contacts.

▶ In the past, we always had to guess whether active tuberculosis was caused by activation of an older, latent infection or was the result of a newly acquired microbe. Now; using the tools of molecular fingerprinting, the California team could show that one third of the patients studied who had new tuberculosis infection in San Francisco had recently acquired the organisms from other infected patients. The points to emphasize are that strategically located patients can infect a large number of contacts and that standard epidemiologic contact tracing may not detect this connection.—G.L. Mandell, M.D.

Transmission of Tuberculosis in New York City: An Analysis by DNA Fingerprinting and Conventional Epidemiologic Methods
Alland D, Kalkut GE, Moss AR, McAdam RA, Hahn JA, Bosworth W, Drucker E, Bloom BR (Albert Einstein College of Medicine; Bronx, NY; Univ of California, San Francisco; City Univ of New York, Bronx)
N Engl J Med 330:1710–1716, 1994   119-95-3–2

Introduction.—The incidence of tuberculosis in the United States is rising, and drug resistance is increasing. Whether the rise in the number of cases is attributable to reactivation of latent infection or to an increase in transmission was investigated.

Methods.—Demographic, social, and household information was collected for 104 adult patients from the Bronx who had a positive culture for *Mycobacterium tuberculosis*. Susceptibility testing was performed, and restriction-fragment–length polymorphism (RFLP) analysis was conducted and confirmed.

Results.—Unique RFLP strains were found in 65 patients (group 1), and strains comparable to other isolates were found in 39 patients (group 2). Isolates were categorized into 12 clusters. Patients in group 2 were significantly more likely than those in group 1 to be young and Hispanic, to have HIV infection, to have lower median income, and to have multiple drug resistance. Group 2 patients were less likely to be foreign-born and were more likely to have recently transmitted disease.

Discussion.—Although the recent increase in incidence of tuberculosis infection is thought to be caused by reactivation of infection, DNA fingerprinting demonstrates that recent transmission is the mode of infection in inner-city patients, such as those in group 2, but reactivation is the mode of infection for those in group 1. Recent transmission accounts for approximately 40% of inner-city cases of tuberculosis and approximately two thirds of the drug resistance found.

▶ Amazingly, the results of the New York study were very similar to those of the San Francisco study (see Abstract 119-95-3-1). Newly acquired infection made up approximately 40% of the incidence cases. Of special interest was the fact that approximately two thirds of patients with drug-resistant disease appeared to have acquired recently transmitted tuberculosis. The reason that DNA fingerprinting with RFLP analysis is effective is that there is a very large diversity of patterns in *M. tuberculosis* found to cause disease. Thus, cases of tuberculosis caused by strains with identical RFLP patterns are very likely to be recently transmitted disease.—G.L. Mandell, M.D.

Transmission of Multidrug-Resistant *Mycobacterium tuberculosis* Among Persons With Human Immunodeficiency Virus Infection in an Urban Hospital: Epidemiologic and Restriction Fragment Length Polymorphism Analysis

Coronado VG, Beck-Sague CM, Hutton MD, Davis BJ, Nicholas P, Villareal C, Woodley CL, Kilburn JO, Crawford JT, Frieden TR, Sinkowitz RL, Jarvis WR (Ctrs for Disease Control and Prevention, Atlanta, Ga; New York City Dept of Health; Elmhurst Hosp, New York)
J Infect Dis 168:1052–1055, 1993   119-95-3-3

Background.—Reports of hospital outbreaks of multidrug-resistant (MDR) tuberculosis in immunocompromised patients have recently increased. Using restriction-fragment–length polymorphism (RFLP) analysis, the relatedness of epidemiologically linked isolates was examined for 1 outbreak of MDR tuberculosis in a New York hospital.

Methods.—Hospital medical records and health department records for a 2-year period were reviewed to identify cases of tuberculosis that were resistant to isoniazid, rifampin, and streptomycin. The comparison group was composed of cases of tuberculosis that were not resistant to these drugs from the same hospital during the same 2 years. A cohort study of patients with HIV infection who were hospitalized on implicated medical wards and who had no history of tuberculosis was done.

Results.—From 1989 to 1991, the percentage of patients who had tuberculosis with MDR isolates rose from .6% to 10%. Of the 16 patients with MDR tuberculosis, 2 had received previous antituberculosis therapy. Fourteen of these patients died between 14 and 381 days of onset of symptoms. Patients with MDR tuberculosis were significantly more likely to have HIV infection and to have been admitted to that same hospital previously. In 8 patients with MDR tuberculosis, previous hospitalization coincided with hospitalization on the same ward of a patient with infectious MDR tuberculosis. Seven of these 8 patients appear to have been in 1 chain of transmission from a single patient. Four spent at least 1 day across the hall from the ambulatory patient with MDR tuberculosis. Three of these 4 were smear-positive inpatients on a ward where 2 more of the 8 (both with HIV) were admitted. The remaining patient was exposed to a patient with MDR tuberculosis who had been transferred from the facility from which patient 8 had come.

One hundred seventeen patients who were infected with HIV and survived 4 months or longer after admission were housed on wards with patients who had MDR tuberculosis. In 7% of this group, MDR tuberculosis subsequently developed. The incidence of MDR tuberculosis was significantly higher among white than nonwhite patients. Proximity (within 3 rooms) and duration (> 10 days) of exposure to patients with MDR tuberculosis were significant factors for increased risk of the disease.

Restriction-fragment–length polymorphism banding patterns from 6 of the theoretical chain of 8-patient transmission (including the source patient) and from 4 other patients (including 1 hospital employee) were identical. Isolates from 1 other patient in the chain and 2 other patients with MDR tuberculosis had unique RFLP patterns. None of the isolates from patients with nonresistant tuberculosis had RFLP patterns matching those of patients with MDR tuberculosis. The predominant strain linked to MDR tuberculosis from this outbreak was also implicated at 3 other New York institutions. Patients with tuberculosis were isolated in single rooms without special ventilation. Most did not have private bathroom facilities. Compliance with isolation precautions was inconsistent.

Discussion.—These data highlight the risk of nosocomial tuberculosis in patients who are infected with HIV. The interval from exposure to disease was 2.5–4 months. An inadequate medical regimen and incomplete adherence to isolation protocols contributed to risk. Patients with tuberculosis should be isolated in rooms with negative air pressure. Outbreaks of MDR tuberculosis illustrate the importance of surveillance for drug-resistant *Mycobacterium tuberculosis* so that clusters can be recognized. Careful adherence to isolation guidelines is essential.

▶ This study focused on tuberculosis transmission in a large city hospital. There was significant transmission of MDR tuberculosis to patients who were infected with HIV. The factors that can predict this were obvious and included proximity of the rooms and longer duration of hospitalization for the patient with HIV infection. There has been much written and said about the need for special masks and isolation procedures for patients with tuberculosis. This study indicates that the ultimate in precautions should be applied when the infected patients harbor MDR tuberculosis and susceptible patients are infected with HIV. Negative-pressure isolation rooms and the use of effective masks are essential. Ultraviolet light air treatment should be considered.—G.L. Mandell, M.D.

Risk for Developing Tuberculosis Among Anergic Patients Infected With HIV

Moreno S, Baraia-Etxaburu J, Bouza E, Parras F, Pérez-Tascón M, Miralles P, Vicente T, Alberdi JC, Cosín J, López-Gay D (Hosp Gen Gregorio Maranón and Consejería de Salud de la Comunidad Autónoma, Madrid)
Ann Intern Med 119:194–198, 1993   119-95-3–4

Background.—Past studies have revealed a significant incidence of tuberculosis in patients infected with HIV and in those with AIDS. Most patients with AIDS are found to have anergy on multiple antigen skin testing, and latent tuberculosis infection may pass undetected. In Madrid, disseminating tuberculosis has been the AIDS defining disease in 18% of patients with HIV infection. The risk of contracting tuberculosis was evaluated among anergic and nonanergic individuals infected with HIV. The advantages of extending the indications of chemoprophylaxis to patients with anergy in the area were considered.

Method.—Over 3 years, patients admitted with HIV infection underwent delayed-type hypersensitivity skin testing, including positive protein purified derivative test (PPD), and CD4+ cell count. Development of tuberculosis was monitored. Diagnosis was considered certain on isolation of *Mycobacterium tuberculosis* from any clinical specimen.

Results.—Of 374 patients, 29% showed positive results to the PPD test. Forty-one percent had negative PPD tests but no skin anergy, and 30% had anergy. Fifteen percent of patients with previously negative PPD tests and no anergy converted to a positive test result in the 26-month follow-up. Patients who had not received isoniazid chemoprophylaxis were at similar risk of contracting tuberculosis as those who had positive PPD test results and those with anergy. The risk was greater in the latter 2 groups than in patients without anergy who had a negative PPD test result. Drug users who had not received isoniazid treatment were more commonly found to have tuberculosis than homosexual men or patients infected with HIV in other categories.

Conclusion.—The risk of contracting tuberculosis is high in anergic patients with HIV infection. These patients, along with those who have positive results of PPD tests, should be offered preventive therapy if they live in areas of high incidence of tuberculosis or if their CD4 count drops to fewer than 500 CD4 cells/mm^3.

▶ This study addresses a common clinical dilemma. A patient with HIV infection undergoes a skin test and is found to be PPD negative. If the patient is PPD positive, it is agreed that preventive therapy should be started. However, the negative PPD is negated by the fact that the patient has anergy. What to do? These investigators found that the risk of active tuberculosis was similar in anergic patients who were PPD negative compared with those who were PPD positive. Thus, they suggest that anergic patients with AIDS be treated with isoniazid. Here is where clinical judgment comes into play. If the patient has resided in an area of low prevalence of tuberculosis and will not come into contact with patients with tuberculosis, then it seems reasonable not to institute therapy. However, patients who come from high-prevalence areas, patients with contact with inner-city populations, prison populations, and IV drug abusers should all probably receive preventive therapy, even in the face of a negative PPD and anergy.—G.L. Mandell, M.D.

Bacille Calmette-Guérin Immunization in Normal Healthy Adults
Brewer MA, Edwards KM, Palmer PS, Hinson HP (Vanderbilt Univ, Nashville, Tenn)
J Infect Dis 170:476–479, 1994   119-95-3-5

Background.—The incidence of tuberculosis is increasing in the United States. The disease is spread by the aerosol route and can disseminate rapidly. In addition, the proportion of *Mycobacterium tuberculosis* isolates that are multiply resistant to available antituberculosis medications is increasing. Both these factors put health care workers at particular risk for contracting the disease. Accordingly, the role of Bacille Calmette-Guérin (BCG) immunization, a live, attenuated vaccine that has been used against *M. tuberculosis* for many years, is being reassessed in health care personnel. The reactogenicity and immunogenicity of the Glaxo strain of BCG was investigated in a vaccine trial.

Participants and Methods.—The BCG vaccine was given to 20 healthy employees or relatives of employees at the Vanderbilt University Medical Center. Participants were aged 18–65 years. All results of the purified protein derivative (PPD) skin test were negative, and all participants were HIV serology-negative. Local adverse reactions were monitored, and intermediate-strength PPD skin test responses were assessed at 2 and 12 months after the vaccination.

Results.—Erythema, induration, and tenderness at the vaccination site were reported by all participants. Fifteen participants complained of muscular soreness. Local ulceration with drainage occurred in 14, and tender regional adenopathy was reported by 2. Bacille Calmette-Guérin organisms were isolated from the ulcer of the only participant who underwent culture. In all participants, the PPD skin tests demonstrated induration.

Conclusion.—Normal, healthy adults at risk of occupational exposure to tuberculosis should be advised about the local reactions that can occur after administration of BCG and the high rate of persistent PPD skin test responses, if such vaccinations are being considered. In those receiving vaccination, the vaccination site should be covered to reduce nosocomial transmission of the vaccine strain.

▶ There is a resurgence in interest in BCG vaccine for prevention of tuberculosis. This study documents the experience of BCG administration to 20 healthy adults. I was surprised to see that 14 of the participants had local ulceration and drainage, and most had positive PPDs at 12 months. I was taught that a very strongly positive PPD after BCG probably meant reinfection with tuberculosis, but there was no evidence for that in these patients, and some had PPDs with 33 mm of induration. The authors do indicate that chest radiographs were not taken in those participants with increased skin response, but I assume that they were not sick. I've never used BCG myself, nor have I seen patients who have recently received BCG. This particular strain appears to be fairly "hot" and probably will result in effective immunization, but at a price of local reaction.—G.L. Mandell, M.D.

Post-BCG Tuberculin Testing: Interpreting Results and Establishing Essential Baseline Data
Skotniski EM (Health and Welfare Canada, Hamilton, Ont, Canada)
Can J Public Health 84:307–308, 1993   119-95-3–6

Purpose.—Bacille Calmette-Guérin (BCG) vaccination is generally thought to render the tuberculin skin test useless. Conversion to positive skin test after vaccination has been considered a sign of effective vaccination. To establish the rate of tuberculin reactivity among children vaccinated with BCG and to assess the value of the tuberculin skin test as a diagnostic tool in such a population, data collected as a portion of a case-finding program in Northern Saskatchewan were analyzed.

Methods.—In a small native community, all children aged 2 months to 2 years who had received BCG vaccine at birth were reviewed. Excluding those who may have exhibited false results (because of other vaccines, for example), the children were tested with 5tu purified protein derivative (PPD), and induration was measured in millimeters 48–72 hours later. Any child with an induration greater than 5 mm was referred to the TB Control Centre.

Results.—Of the 65 children tested, approximately 55% were nonreactive. Six children had induration of 5–9 mm, and 23 had induration of 10 mm or more. On follow-up at the TB Control Centre, 25 of 29 children had confirmed cases of primary tuberculosis. The other 4 had no sign of infection.

Discussion.—In this immunized population, a positive skin test correlated significantly with primary tuberculosis but not with vaccination. Many factors can affect tuberculin reactivity after BCG vaccine, including dose and route, manufacturer and vaccine technique, age of the patient, time elapsed since vaccine, and presence of a BCG scar. One large study found that 97% of children had positive skin test results 6–9 weeks after vaccination and continued to have positive test results 4 years later. Others have found as few as 12.6% converted to positive skin test. Although this study was small and not the primary focus of the data collection process, it is noteworthy because of the high percentage of the population found to have primary infection. A previous study of Inuit children yielded similar results. In interpreting skin test results, it is important to remember that cross-reactions to BCG vaccine tend to be small and wane rapidly with age. A positive mantoux skin test in a rural aboriginal child is highly predictive, whether or not the child has received BCG.

▶ This study population is very different from that in Abstract 119-95-3–5, which included Vanderbilt hospital employees. Here, native communities in northern Canada were assessed, and, in this group, all 23 children with a post-BCG skin test reaction of greater than 10 mm had primary tuberculosis. This is the clinical rule of thumb by which I operate: a positive PPD test result in a patient who previously received BCG should be treated as any other positive. It would be very interesting to follow the Vanderbilt group to see whether, at 2 and 5 years, the BCG-induced PPD positivity wanes.—G.L. Mandell, M.D.

Bacillus Calmette-Guérin Infection After Vaccination of Human Immunodeficiency Virus-Infected Children

Besnard M, Sauvion S, Offredo C, Gaudelus J, Gaillard J-L, Veber F, Blanche S (Hôpital Necker Enfants Malades, Paris; Hôpital Jean Verdier, Bondy, France)
Pediatr Infect Dis J 12:993–997, 1993   119-95-3–7

Background.—Tuberculosis is one of the most serious complications of HIV type I infection. The efficacy of the *Mycobacterium bovis/Bacillus Calmette-Guérin* (BCG) vaccination is still controversial, and its risk-benefit ratio in patients infected with HIV has not been fully assessed. However, this live vaccine, which persists in the body for several months or years, theoretically exposes patients with progressive immunologic deficiencies to disseminated BCG infection. The long-term complications of the vaccine in children infected with HIV were reported.

Method.—Clinical BCG infections developed after vaccination in 352 children with HIV infection. Sixty-eight of the children were vaccinated with BCG before HIV infection was diagnosed. All 68 children were infected by HIV during the perinatal period or at birth and were vaccinated with BCG within 2 months of birth.

Results.—In 9 children, a complicated BCG infection developed 3–35 months after vaccination. Seven children had large satellite adenopathy from which BCG was isolated. Two children had disseminated BCG infection beyond the satellite ganglion; infection involved the spleen and mesenteric and mediastinal lymph nodes in 1 patient and the liver and lungs in the other. All the children were asymptomatic at the time of vaccination. Development of antimycobacterial cellular immunity was retrospectively confirmed by at least 1 positive patch test result in 4 of 7 children 1–6 months after vaccination. All patch test results were consistently negative for the remaining children. At the time of vaccination, results of intradermal tests and lymphocyte transformation tests to tuberculin were also constantly negative for all children. All but 1 patient had a severe cellular immunodeficiency when BCG infection was diagnosed.

Conclusion.—The increasing incidence of tuberculosis in the United States has brought a renewed interest in vaccinating children who have HIV infection with BCG. However, the risks clearly call for caution and should be weighed against the possible benefits of vaccination. The local risk for tuberculosis and the resistance phenotypes of the strains likely to be encountered also need to be considered. The prognosis of HIV infection must also be considered, and children at risk for the development of early and severe forms of HIV disease, particularly those with a high viral replication at birth, should not be vaccinated with BCG.

▶ This is a problem in institutions in which BCG vaccination is routinely given to children. The vaccine was inadvertently given to 68 children infected with HIV. Several of these children had significant, vaccine-related complications. Also remember that BCG vaccination in normal, healthy individuals frequently resulted in ulcerative lesions that shed the organism (see Abstract 119-95-3–5). Thus, health care workers and family members who come in contact with the immunosuppressed patients may be a source of transmission of live mycobacteria. Bacillus Calmette-Guérin is an *M. bovis* strain that has been attenuated by multiple in vitro passages.—G.L. Mandell, M.D.

The Effect of Directly Observed Therapy on the Rates of Drug Resistance and Relapse in Tuberculosis
Weis SE, Slocum PC, Blais FX, King B, Nunn M, Matney GB, Gomez E, Foresman BH (Univ of North Texas Health Science Ctr, Fort Worth; Fort Worth–Tarrant County Health Dept, Tex; John Peter Smith Hosp, Fort Worth, Tex)
N Engl J Med 330:1179–1184, 1994   119-95-3–8

Background.—Tuberculosis is once again an important public health problem. Poor compliance with medical regimens is a major reason for

Rates of Relapse and Resistance Among Cases of
M. *tuberculosis*, According to Treatment

VARIABLE	TRADITIONAL THERAPY (N = 407)	DIRECTLY OBSERVED THERAPY (N = 581)	P VALUE
	number (percent)		
Relapse			
Total	85 (20.9)	32 (5.5)	<0.001
Multidrug resistant	25 (6.1)	5 (0.9)	<0.001
During therapy	18 (4.4)	7 (1.2)	0.003
Primary resistance			
No. of drugs	114 (28.0)	51 (8.8)	<0.001
No. of cases	53 (13.0)	39 (6.7)	0.001
Acquired resistance			
No. of episodes	57 (14.0)	12 (2.1)	<0.001
No. of patients	39 (10.3)	8 (1.4)	<0.001

Note: The 407 cases treated by traditional therapy occurred in 379 patients from January 1980 through October 1986, and the 581 cases treated under direct observation occurred in 578 patients from November 1986 through December 1992.
(Courtesy of Weis SE, Slocum PC, Blais FX, et al: N Engl J Med 330:1179–1184, 1994.)

the development of resistant infections and relapse. The outcomes of a program of universal, directly observed treatment for tuberculosis in Tarrant County, Texas, were studied.

Methods.—Data were obtained on all patients with positive cultures for *Mycobacterium tuberculosis* in Tarrant County between 1980 and 1992. Through October 1986, a traditional, unsupervised drug regimen was used. Thereafter, almost all patients were given treatment under direct observation by health care personnel.

Findings.—Four hundred seven episodes in which patients were given traditional treatment were compared with 581 episodes in which therapy was under direct observation. In this 13-year period, the frequency of primary drug resistance declined from 13% to 6.7% after the direct observation program was begun. The frequency of acquired resistance decreased from 14% to 2.1%. The relapse rate dropped from 20.9% to 5.5%. The number of relapses with multidrug-resistance organisms declined from 25 to 5 (table).

Conclusion.—Universal, direct observation of treatment for tuberculosis was associated with reduced relapse, multidrug-resistant relapse, and acquired resistance rates. The program was also cost-effective.

▶ This is such a simple and obvious concept that one wonders why it is not adopted more universally. There is a very high concordance of drug-resistant tuberculosis and patients who are noncompliant. This can easily be fixed with directly observed therapy (DOT). This study nicely documented a very significant decline in development of resistance and lower relapse rates when DOT was used.—G.L. Mandell, M.D.

Evaluation of Rooms With Negative Pressure Ventilation Used for Respiratory Isolation in Seven Midwestern Hospitals

Fraser VJ, Johnson K, Primack J, Jones M, Medoff G, Dunagan WC (Washington Univ, St Louis, Mo; Barnes Hosp, St Louis, Mo)
Infect Control Hosp Epidemiol 14:623–628, 1993   119-95-3–9

Background.—The incidence of tuberculosis (TB) is increasing, and numerous nosocomial outbreaks have been described. Many of these outbreaks appear to be related to inadequate infection control measures and the improper functioning of isolation rooms. The adequacy of respiratory isolation rooms was evaluated in 7 major hospitals in a major metropolitan area not currently in the midst of a TB epidemic.

Method.—Infection control personnel from all 7 hospitals provided information relating to respiratory isolation policies and frequency of ventilation tests. Actual direction of airflow was evaluated in the isolation rooms using smokesticks, and direction of airflow was measured from the hallway and from the anteroom (if present) with all possible combinations of open and closed doors.

Results.—Four of the 7 hospitals were teaching hospitals, 2 were private community nonteaching hospitals, and 1 was a pediatric teaching hospital. The percentage of isolation rooms in each hospital ranged from .4% to 93%. Only 3 hospitals had intensive care respiratory isolation rooms, and none had isolation rooms in the emergency department. None of the hospitals had a program of systematic evaluation of airflow in the negative pressure rooms, and the frequency of air exchanges in these rooms was not measured. Of 3,574 rooms examined, 121 were designed to have negative pressure suitable for respiratory isolation. Of these, 96% were tested and 55% were considered truly negative pressure with all doors closed and airflow measured from the hallway. A significant difference was found among hospitals in the percentage of designated isolation rooms that had truly negative pressure from 3 of 18 to 11 of 12. Hospital age, size, and type correlated with correct direction of airflow ($P < 0.0001$). Presence or absence of an anteroom, however, did not significantly affect results.

Conclusion.—Only a small number of rooms evaluated in 7 major hospitals were designated for respiratory isolation, and the performance of these was not routinely monitored. High-risk areas, such as ICUs and emergency departments, were not provided with respiratory isolation facilities. The direction of airflow in respiratory isolation rooms was revealed to not always be correct. To prevent the growing risk of TB transmission, the correction and maintenance of baseline engineering controls for respiratory isolation should be standard in all health care facilities.

▶ Do you remember the hospital in New York in which patient-to-patient transmission was documented (see Abstract 119-95-3–3)? This study examined airflow patterns to see whether negative pressure rooms truly were negative relative to hallways. It is frightening to note that half the negative pressure rooms actually demonstrated positive airflow from the room with the infected patient to the hallways and corridors. This can be fixed relatively simply, but the step before fixing it is knowing that you have the problem. Thus, a strong plea for evaluating the direction of airflow, especially in areas of high prevalence of TB.—G.L. Mandell, M.D.

4 Nontuberculous Mycobacterial Infection

Introduction

"Nontuberculous mycobacterial infection" is a better term than atypical mycobacteria and encompasses a wide range of organisms. A strong association between *Mycobacterium avium* complex disease and AIDS has focused much attention on this organism. These selections highlight an increasingly recognized pathogen and a new form of treatment.

Gerald L. Mandell, M.D.

Clinical and Epidemiologic Characteristics of *Mycobacterium haemophilum* , an Emerging Pathogen in Immunocompromised Patients

Straus WL, Ostroff SM, Jernigan DB, Kiehn TE, Sordillo EM, Armstrong D, Boone N, Schneider N, Kilburn JO, Silcox VA, LaBombardi V, Good RC (Ctrs for Disease Control and Prevention, Atlanta, Ga; Mem Sloan-Kettering Cancer Ctr; St. Luke's –Roosevelt Hosp Ctr, NY; et al)
Ann Intern Med 120:118–125, 1994   1 1 9-95-4–1

Background.—*Mycobacterium haemophilum* is a rare pathogen that was first reported in 1978 in an Israeli woman with Hodgkin's disease. More recently, infections with M. *haemophilum* have been reported in patients with AIDS. Thirteen cases of M. *haemophilum* infection were described.

Methods.—Cases were obtained from 7 New York City hospitals and represented all patients who were found to have M. *haemophilum* infections between January 1989 and September 1991 and were followed through September 1992.

Findings.—*Mycobacterium haemophilum* infection caused disseminated cutaneous lesions, bacteremia, and diseases of the bones, joints, lymphatic system, and lungs. Time from initiation of laboratory assessment to definitive identification of M. *haemophilum* infection ranged from 14 to 495 days (mean, 124 days). Once the diagnosis was established, various treatments were used. The drug susceptibilities for 9 M. *haemophilum* isolates were determined. All isolates were susceptible to ciprofloxacin, cycloserine, and rifabutin and were completely resistant to ethambutol and pyrazinamide.

Conclusion.—*Mycobacterium haemophilum* infection can cause a severe, sometimes fatal, multisystem infection in severely immunocompromised hosts. *Mycobacterium haemophilum* infections will probably be recognized more often as the number of susceptible immunocompromised hosts increases and appropriate laboratory procedures are used. Because infections often respond to treatment, accurate diagnosis is important.

▶ Cutaneous lesions in immunocompromised hosts are the hallmark of this microbe. Optimal therapy has not been established in comparative studies; however, in vitro sensitivity patterns and clinical experience suggest that rifampin, amikacin, and ciprofloxacin are effective (see reference below).—G.L. Mandell, M.D.

Reference

1. Kiehn TE, et al: *Eur J Clin Microbiol Infect Dis* 12:114–118, 1993.

Treatment of Refractory Disseminated Nontuberculous Mycobacterial Infection With Interferon Gamma: A Preliminary Report

Holland SM, Eisenstein EM, Kuhns DB, Turner ML, Fleisher TA, Strober W, Gallin JI (Natl Inst of Allergy and Infectious Diseases, Bethesda, Md; Natl Cancer Inst, Bethesda, Md; Warren Grant Magnuson Clinical Ctr, Bethesda, Md)
N Engl J Med 330:1348–1355, 1994   119-95-4–2

Introduction.—The host defenses involved in protection against mycobacteria appear to include T cell and monocyte or macrophage functions. Experimental studies suggest an important role for the cytokine signals that pass between these cells, particularly those produced by interferon-γ. Seven patients with nontuberculous disseminated mycobacterial infection resistant to chemotherapy were treated with interferon-γ.

Patients and Methods.—Four patients had idiopathic CD4+ T-lymphocytopenia, and 3 patients were from a family predisposed to the development of *Mycobacterium avium* complex infection. None were positive for HIV. All mycobacterial infections involved at least 2 organ systems. Peripheral blood cells were assessed for cellular proliferation, cytokine production, and phagocyte function. In addition to antimycobacterial agents, the patients received interferon-γ administered subcutaneously 2 or 3 times weekly in a dose of 25–50 $\mu g/m^2$ of body surface area. This therapy was planned for 1 year and was continued if patients continued to improve.

Results.—Cells from patients produced significantly less interferon-γ and interleukin-2 than did cells from normal individuals after phytohemagglutinin stimulation. Stimulation with ionomycin and phorbol myristate acetate led to normal production of interferon-γ in both groups of patients. All 7 patients had marked clinical improvement within 8 weeks of the start of interferon therapy. Blood cultures cleared, fever and night sweats abated, and the number of skin lesions was reduced. There was also radiographic improvement and a reduction in the need for paracentesis. Interferon-γ treatment did not result in a dramatic change in CD4+ T-cell counts or cell-activation markers during the treatment period.

Conclusion.—Interferon-γ may prove to be a powerful adjunct to standard regimens in the treatment of mycobacterial infections. There were no serious side effects in these patients.

▶ Interferon-γ was previously known as a macrophage activating factor. It is approved in the United States for prevention of infection in patients with chronic granulomatous disease of childhood, as it apparently increases the ability of phagocytes to kill ingested organisms. A series of in vitro and animal studies has demonstrated that interferon-γ can potentiate destruction of a variety of pathogens by macrophages. Investigators examined 6 patients with *M. avium* complex infections and one with *Mycobacterium kansasii* infection and found that interferon-γ, along with appropriate antimicrobial therapy, appeared to be very effective. In only 1 patient was anergy reversed by interferon-γ therapy. There was no specific measurement of microbicidal capacity of the patient's monocytes or macrophages for mycobacteria, but one would guess that this is the basis for the effectiveness of the therapy. Because these patients were chronically ill and had not previously responded to antimicrobial therapy alone, the authors were impressed with the efficacy of interferon-γ. Despite this, it would be more convincing to see a placebo-controlled trial to demonstrate efficacy.—G.L. Mandell, M.D.

5 Viral Infection

Introduction

Hantavirus pulmonary syndrome burst onto the medical scene in 1993. My home state of Virginia just reported its first indigenous case. This syndrome is nicely reviewed in the selection. Also discussed are a new vaccine and new therapy for varicella disease.

Gerald L. Mandell, M.D.

Hantavirus Pulmonary Syndrome: A Clinical Description of 17 Patients With a Newly Recognized Disease

Duchin JS, Koster FT, Peters CJ, Simpson GL, Tempest B, Zaki SR, Ksiazek TG, Rollin PE, Nichol S, Umland ET, Moolenaar RL, Reef SE, Nolte KB, Gallaher MM, Butler JC, Breiman RF, and the Hantavirus Study Group (Ctrs for Disease Control and Prevention, Atlanta, Ga; Univ of New Mexico Hosp, Albuquerque; New Mexico Dept of Health, Santa Fe; et al)
N Engl J Med 330:949–955, 1994   119-95-5–1

Background.—A previously undescribed hantavirus recently was proven responsible for an outbreak of severe respiratory illness in the Four Corners area of New Mexico, Arizona, Colorado, and Utah. Although hantaviruses are a recognized cause of hemorrhagic fever and renal disease in Asia, there have been no previous reports of acute illness resulting from hantavirus infection acquired in North America. The clinical, laboratory, and autopsy findings of the first 17 patients with confirmed hantavirus infection were examined.

Findings.—Prodromal symptoms included fever and myalgia in all patients. Seventy-six percent also had cough or dyspnea, 76% also had gastrointestinal symptoms, and 71% also had headache. All patients had tachypnea, 94% had tachycardia, and 50% had hypotension. Leukocytosis, with a median peak cell count of 26,000/mm^3, was often accompanied by myeloid precursor cells, thrombocytopenia, prolonged prothrombin and partial thromboplastin times, elevated serum levels of lactate dehydrogenase, decreased serum levels of protein, and proteinuria. Pathologic examination revealed large, serous pleural effusions with severe edema of the lungs. Microscopic findings included intra-alveolar edema with scant to moderate numbers of hyaline membranes and interstitial lymphoid infiltrates. Eighty-eight percent of patients had a rapidly progressive acute pulmonary edema. Thirteen patients, all of whom had profound hypotension, died.

Discussion.—The recently reported outbreak of hantavirus pulmonary syndrome features a brief prodromal illness followed by a rapidly progressive, noncardiogenic pulmonary edema. A total of 53 cases in 14 states had been identified by the end of 1993. Pending further study of this particular epidemic, prevention strategies will include modification of behavior or lifestyle and control of rodents.

▶ Think of hantavirus in patients with potential contact with mouse feces; a brief, influenza-like illness; and pulmonary edema syndrome associated with leukocytosis and thrombocytopenia. Ribavirin therapy (obtainable from the Centers for Disease Control and Prevention) is offered to patients, but the drug does not appear to be dramatically effective. The most important feature of management is adequate oxygenation and support of hemodynamic function in the face of tremendous pulmonary fluid loss.—G.L. Mandell, M.D.

Cost-Effectiveness of a Routine Varicella Vaccination Program for US Children

Lieu TA, Cochi SL, Black SB, Halloran ME, Shinefield HR, Holmes SJ, Wharton M, Washington AE (Univ of California, San Francisco; Ctrs for Disease Control and Prevention, Atlanta, Ga; Kaiser Permanente Pediatric Vaccine Study Ctr, Oakland, Calif; et al)
JAMA 271:375–381, 1994   119-95-5-2

Purpose.—Routine varicella vaccination of healthy children could prevent most of the 3.7 million cases of chickenpox that occur in the United States every year. Whether such a policy would be cost-effective, especially in light of the most recent information on the efficacy of varicella vaccine, was addressed, and the economic consequences of routine varicella vaccination of healthy children were evaluated.

Methods.—A decision analysis model was used to compare the costs, outcomes, and cost-effectiveness of routine vaccination vs. no intervention. A mathematical model of vaccine efficacy that used published and unpublished data, as well as expert opinion, was also used. Some sources of empirical data on the costs of medical utilization and work loss from varicella were used, and the effects of expected changes in the age distribution of disease were assessed.

Results.—Assuming 97% vaccination coverage at the age of school entry, the model indicated that a program of routine varicella vaccination would avoid 94% of potential cases of chickenpox. The estimated cost of the vaccine, with each child receiving a single dose at a cost of $35, was $162 million per year. From a societal perspective, including considerations of work-loss and medical costs, the program would save $5 for every $1 invested. From a health care payer's perspective, however, the cost of the program would be approximately $2 per case of chickenpox prevented, or $2,500 per life-year saved. Variations in rate of coverage and price of vaccine affected the medical cost of disease prevention, but efficacy of vaccine did not, at least within the plausible range of assumptions. A catch-up vaccination program for 12-year-old children would result in net savings only if the coverage rate of preschool children decreased to 50%.

Conclusion.—From a societal perspective, a routine varicella vaccination program for healthy children would save money, including work-loss and medical costs. Although it would not save money from the health payer's perspective, it would still be cost-effective compared with other prevention programs. Policy decisions regarding this issue should consider not only cost-effectiveness but also qualitative judgments, including the relative value of preventing morbidity and mortality from varicella vs. other diseases.

▶ The authors make a strong point that routine varicella vaccination for healthy children would be extremely beneficial and cost-effective. The debate about acyclovir therapy for patients seen in the first 24 hours continues. It appears that this therapy will get the child back to school and the parents back to work 1 day earlier. As of this writing, varicella vaccine still is not approved for general use in the United States but is currently licensed in Japan.—G.L. Mandell, M.D.

A Randomized Trial of Acyclovir for 7 Days or 21 Days With and Without Prednisolone for Treatment of Acute Herpes Zoster
Wood MJ, Johnson RW, McKendrick MW, Taylor J, Mandal BK, Crooks J (Birmingham Heartlands Hosp, England; Bristol Royal Infirmary, England; Royal Hallamshire Hosp, Sheffield, England; et al)
N Engl J Med 330:896–900, 1994   119-95-5–3

Purpose.—Among immunocompetent patients, herpes zoster—caused by reactivation of the latent varicella-zoster virus—is predominantly a disease of elderly individuals. The incidence of postherpetic neuralgia is difficult to determine, but up to 57% of patients may have persistent pain for at least 1 month. Controlled studies have shown that 7–10 days of acyclovir can hasten healing and reduce pain in patients with herpes zoster; however, its effectiveness in the prevention of postherpetic neuralgia is controversial. Studies of oral corticosteroids for the same indications have given conflicting results. The effects of a longer course of antiviral therapy and concurrent steroid administration were evaluated.

Methods.—The analysis included 349 of 400 enrolled adult patients without immune dysfunction who had a clinical diagnosis of herpes zoster. The patients were randomized to receive either acyclovir therapy alone for 7 or 21 days, 800 mg orally, 5 times/day; acyclovir plus prednisolone for 21 days; or acyclovir for 7 days plus prednisolone for 21 days. The dose of prednisolone was started at 40 mg/day and was tapered over 3 weeks. The patients were assessed over 28 days for progression of rash and intensity of pain, then over 6 months for postherpetic neuralgia.

Results.—There were no significant differences in terms of progression of rash, either between groups or on subgroup analyses. Although there were no significant differences in percentage of rash healed on days 7, 14, and 21, pooled group analysis showed that patients receiving steroids were more likely to show greater healing by days 7and 14. In the acute phase, patients receiving 21 days of acyclovir were 6% to 8% more likely to have relief of pain than those receiving 7 days of acyclovir. Intensity of pain was also lower in patients receiving the longer course of acyclovir and in those receiving steroid. There were no significant differences in prolonged zoster-associated pain, although pain tended to cease earlier in patients receiving the longer course of acyclovir. Sixteen percent of patients reported at least 1 adverse event, and a higher incidence was reported in the steroid groups. There were 3 serious adverse events, although only 1—hematemesis in a patient taking the long course of acyclovir plus steroid—was considered to result from the study medication.

Conclusion.—In immunocompetent patients with acute herpes zoster, adding prednisolone to acyclovir may help in healing the rash and in reducing the incidence and severity of pain during the first few weeks. There is no apparent reduction in the incidence or severity of postherpetic neuralgia. Given the adverse effects of prednisolone, its use is not recommended. Neither is extending acyclovir therapy recommended, as it is expensive and has only a modest clinical benefit.

▶ The goals of treatment of patients with acute herpes zoster are to shorten the acute illness and prevent postherpetic neuralgia. Acyclovir will shorten the acute illness, but its effect on postherpetic neuralgia is unclear. This study was instructive because there was a comparison of 7 and 21 days of therapy with acyclovir with or without prednisolone. Of course, it would have been nice to have had a placebo group, but antiviral therapy has become a standard for herpes zoster because of the definite shortening of the course of the acute illness. A new agent, famciclovir, has been shown to be as effective as acyclovir in the treatment of acute herpes zoster and to shorten the duration of postherpetic neuralgia significantly as compared with placebo.—G.L. Mandell, M.D.

6 Therapy

Introduction

One of the exciting elements of dealing with patients who have infectious diseases is that effective therapy is usually (but sadly not always) available. The choice of optimal therapy can be problematic because of newly recognized pathogens, changes in susceptibility patterns of old pathogens, and development of new agents. In addition, adjunctive agents that modulate the immune system are becoming more frequently used (see the article on interferon-γ in the Nontuberculous Mycobacterial Infection chapter).

Gerald L. Mandell, M.D.

Elimination of *Staphylococcus aureus* Nasal Carriage in Health Care Workers: Analysis of Six Clinical Trials With Calcium Mupirocin Ointment

Doebbeling BN, Breneman DL, Neu HC, Aly R, Yangco BG, Holley HP Jr, Marsh RJ, Pfaller MA, McGowan JE Jr, Scully BE, Reagan DR, Wenzel RP, and the Mupirocin Collaborative Study Group (Univ of Iowa, Iowa City; Univ of Cincinnati, Ohio; Columbia Univ, New York; et al)
Clin Infect Dis 17:466–474, 1993   119-95-6-1

Objective.—Colonization of the anterior nares with *Staphylococcus aureus* may be present in approximately one third of healthy adults, with up to half being intermittent carriers. Efforts to eliminate nasal carriage, even when successful, are typically followed by recolonization shortly after the end of treatment. The unique antibiotic mupirocin, produced by subfermentation of *Pseudomonas fluorescens*, has excellent in vitro activity against a broad range of gram-positive bacteria, including methicillin-susceptible and methicillin-resistant *S. aureus*. Six double-blind, randomized studies that assessed the efficacy and safety of calcium mupirocin ointment to eliminate nasal *S. aureus* carriage among health care workers were reported.

Methods.—An identical protocol was used in the 6 studies, which included 339 healthy personnel with stable nasal carriage of *S. aureus*. The patients were independently randomized to receive either calcium mupirocin ointment or placebo ointment, with instructions to apply a 1-cm length of ointment to each nostril twice a day for 5 days. Bacteriologic status was assessed by culture samples taken 48–96 hours after the completion of therapy, with additional samples taken at 1, 2, and 4 weeks.

Results.—Carriage of *S. aureus* was eliminated at the initial post-treatment culture in 91% of the mupirocin group vs. 6% of the placebo group. By the 4-week follow-up culture, 82% and 12%, respectively, remained culture negative. Seventy-four percent of the mupirocin group remained culture negative throughout follow-up, compared with 13% of the placebo group. Results were similar regardless of methicillin resistance. Mupirocin-resistant *S. aureus* developed in a few patients although all isolates were judged susceptible with broth microdilution. All adverse effects were minor, with no difference between groups in their incidence.

Conclusions.—Intranasal calcium mupirocin ointment appears to be a safe and effective treatment for the elimination of nasal carriage of *S. aureus* among health care workers. Mupirocin resistance appears to develop slowly. Its use should be limited, however, to settings in which it has been shown to be beneficial and when other treatment options are not as effective.

▶ There are certain situations in which elimination of staphylococcal nasal carriage appears to be beneficial. One is in patients with recurrent furunculosis, in whom the source of the infection is frequently the anterior nares. Another is in health care workers who have been epidemiologically associated with staphylococcal infections in their patients. A third situation is in patients who are found to be staphylococcal carriers and are candidates for nasal or transsphenoidal intracranial surgery. Various creams and ointments have been tried over the years, but none have been very effective. Perhaps the most effective regimen has been the combination of an antistaphylococcal β-lactam agent, such as cloxacillin plus rifampin, both taken orally for about 1 week. However, this regimen has drawbacks in that adverse reactions from the systemic administration of the agents may occur. Mupirocin is effective and very well tolerated; however, resistance may develop, and resistant organisms may spread to susceptibles (see Abstract 119-95-7-2).—G.L. Mandell, M.D.

Treatment of Sporotrichosis With Itraconazole
Sharkey-Mathis PK, Kauffman CA, Graybill JR, Stevens DA, Hostetler JS, Cloud G, Dismukes WE, and Other Members of the NIAID Mycoses Study Group (Univ of Texas Health Science Ctr, San Antonio; Univ of Michigan, Ann Arbor; Stanford Univ, San Jose, Calif; et al)
Am J Med 95:279–285, 1993   119-95-6-2

Background.—Sporotrichosis, a mycotic infection caused by the dimorphic fungus *Sporothrix schenckii*, can be classified as either systemic or cutaneous inoculation sporotrichosis, with the latter being most common. Current treatment regimens for this condition, including amphotericin B, ketoconazole, or a saturated solution of potassium iodide, are of limited value in more recalcitrant instances and may present difficulties with tolerance, toxicity, and administration. Other therapeutic alternatives of equal or greater efficacy are therefore needed. Studies using itraconazole, a new oral triazole antifungal agent, have reported clinical efficacy in treatment of sporotrichosis. The use of itraconazole for treatment of this condition was described.

Patients and Methods.—Twenty-seven patients, aged 22–86 years, were included. Study criteria mandated that all patients have positive cultures for *S. schenckii* or histopathology compatible with this infection. Patients with either systemic or cutaneous sporotrichosis were treated. Over 3–18 months, patients received a daily dose of itraconazole ranging from 100 to 600 mg. After treatment, patients were grouped as responders or nonresponders, with responders further classified as remaining on treatment, relapsed, or free from disease.

Results.—Thirty courses of itraconazole were given. Alcoholism and diabetes mellitus were frequent underlying diseases, noted in 7 and 8 patients, respectively. Involved sites included lymphocutaneous only in 9 patients, articular/osseous in 15 (multifocal in 3), and lung in 3. Eleven patients had undergone previous therapy without success. There were 25 responders and 5 nonresponders. All nonresponders had received at least 200 mg of itraconazole daily over 6–18 months. Seven of the 25 responders relapsed 1–7 months after treatment periods of 6–18 months. Of these, 2 are responding to a second course. After 10 months of treatment, 1 responder was lost to follow-up. Of the remaining 17, 3 are currently on treatment, and 14 are disease-free at follow-up of 6–42 months. Overall, patients tolerated treatment with itraconazole, and few side effects were noted.

Conclusion.—Itraconazole represents an effective treatment for patients with either cutaneous or systemic sporotrichosis.

▶ Sporotrichosis is usually limited to the skin, but systemic and disseminated disease is seen, especially in patients with such risk factors as alcoholism, diabetes, and chronic obstructive pulmonary disease. Itraconazole is the newest of the antifungal azole drugs. These agents inhibit ergosterol biosynthesis. This study indicates that itraconazole is effective therapy for sporotrichosis. It probably is better tolerated than standard therapy with either saturated solutions of potassium iodide or amphotericin. Like ketoconazole, itraconazole blood levels are reduced in patients who are taking drugs that decrease gastric acidity.—G.L. Mandell, M.D.

Dexamethasone Therapy for Bacterial Meningitis in Children: 2-Versus 4-Day Regimen

Syrogiannopoulos GA, Lourida AN, Theodoridou MC, Pappas IG, Babilis GC, Economidis JJ, Zoumboulakis DJ, Beratis NG, Matsaniotis NS (Univ of Patras, Greece; Karamandanion Children's Hosp, Patras, Greece; Univ of Athens, Greece; et al)
J Infect Dis 169:853–858, 1994   119-95-6-3

Background.—A 4-day regimen of dexamethasone is beneficial in meningitis resulting from *Streptococcus pneumoniae, Haemophilus influenzae* type b, and *Neisseria meningitidis*. Nevertheless, acceptance of this treatment is limited because of concerns about steroid-related complications. Two- and 4-day regimens of dexamethasone in patients with bacterial meningitis were compared.

Methods.—Of 118 children, aged 2.5 months to 15 years, who had bacterial infections treated with conventional IV antimicrobial therapy, 62 received IV dexamethasone, .15 mg/kg, every 6 hours for 2 days, and 54 received dexamethasone therapy for 4 days.

Results.—The dexamethasone regimens provided comparable clinical responses, with similar numbers of days to resolution of fever, neck stiffness, and irritability; return to normal consciousness; and completion of antibiotic therapy. The mean time to defervescence was 1.8 days for the 2-day group and 1.6 days for the 4-day group. Overall, the incidences of complications with the 2 regimens were similar during hospitalization and relative to the 3 principal etiologic agents, N. *meningitidis*, H. *influenzae*, and *S. pneumoniae*. One patient in the 2-day group and 3 in the 4-day group had gross gastrointestinal bleeding. In all 4 patients, the bleeding subsided within 24 hours without the need for blood transfusion. At the 6-week follow-up, 3.3% of assessed patients in the 2-day group and 5.7% of those in the 4-day group had neurologic sequelae. These sequelae persisted in only 2 patients in the 4-day group after 6 and 19 months.

Conclusion.—Two- and 4-day regimens of dexamethasone therapy adjunctive to standard antibiotic therapy for bacterial meningitis provide similar outcomes, but gastrointestinal bleeding occurs less frequently with the shorter regimen. The 2-day regimen is therefore appropriate for treating *H. influenzae* and meningococcal meningitis.

▶ Many pediatricians have accepted dexamethasone as a standard adjunct for therapy of *H. influenzae* meningitis in children. Fewer data exist and there is less acceptance of the role of corticosteroids in meningitis caused by the pneumococcus and the meningococcus. *Haemophilus influenzae* meningitis is becoming much less common because of the effectiveness of childhood immunization for *H. influenzae* type b disease. In addition, the increase in incidence of penicillin-resistant pneumococci has changed the equation somewhat. The reason for this statement is that animal data indicate that corticosteroid therapy reduces CNS inflammation (the good news) but decreases penetration of antibiotics into the spinal fluid (the bad news). Before the problem of penicillin resistance in pneumococci, there were such high levels in the spinal fluid that partial reduction had no real effect. Now, however, there is the fear that reduction of CSF antibiotic levels may affect the outcome of certain infections. This appears to be the greatest potential problem with children treated with vancomycin in whom CSF levels are barely adequate (see Abstract 119-95-7-1).—G.L. Mandell, M.D.

Ciprofloxacin and Trimethoprim-Sulfamethoxazole Versus Placebo in Acute Uncomplicated *Salmonella* Enteritis: A Double-Blind Trial
Sánchez C, García-Restoy E, Garau J, Bella F, Freixas N, Simó M, Lite J, Sánchez P, Espejo E, Cobo E, Rodriguez M (Hospital de Mútua de Terrassa, Barcelona; Universitat Politécnica de Catalunya, Barcelona)
J Infect Dis 168:1304–1307, 1993   119-95-6–4

Introduction.—Various antibacterial agents have failed to alter the course of acute *Salmonella* enteritis. The new fluorinated quinolones, however, have exhibited excellent activity in vitro against salmonellae and possess favorable pharmacokinetic properties.

Study Plan.—Sixty-five patients with acute, culture-confirmed *Salmonella* enteritis but no complications were randomized to receive ciprofloxacin at a dose of 500 mg, trimethoprim–sulfamethoxazole (TMP-SMZ) at 160 and 800 mg, or placebo. All medications were given orally twice a day for 5 days in a double-blind design.

Results.—There were no treatment-related differences in the duration of diarrhea, abdominal pain, vomiting, or fever. Neither active treatment led to a complete resolution of symptoms more rapidly than did placebo. Also, the rate of clearance of salmonellae from the stools did not differ significantly among the groups.

Interpretation.—Why neither ciprofloxacin nor TMP-SMZ has proven effective in the treatment of *Salmonella* enteritis is unclear. Resistance and a lack of compliance are not valid explanations, and it is not likely that diarrhea prevented adequate drug absorption.

▶ There continues to be debate about the wisdom of treating uncomplicated *Salmonella* enteritis. Data with such agents as ampicillin have suggested that treatment has little or no clinical effect and actually prolongs the carrier state. However, there is no question that a few patients experience devastating complications of this usually self-limited disease. Therefore, significant host impairment or especially severe or prolonged disease is considered to be a valid indication for treatment in the hope of avoiding metastatic infections. The quinolones, such as ciprofloxacin, have been reported to be efficacious, and many infectious disease consultants have recommended the quinolones as the therapy of choice for uncomplicated *Salmonella* enteritis.

This study suggests caution in that neither ciprofloxacin nor TMP-SMZ affected the clinical course of the disease or rate of clearance of the organism from the stools. I would still favor therapy for patients who are severely ill and those who have impairments of host defense. Ciprofloxacin (or ofloxacin) is an attractive agent because of its activity against other diarrheal pathogens, including *Shigella* and *Campylobacter* species.—G.L. Mandell, M.D.

Empiric Parenteral Antibiotic Treatment of Patients With Fibromyalgia and Fatigue and a Positive Serologic Result for Lyme Disease: A Cost–Effectiveness Analysis

Lightfoot RW Jr, Luft BJ, Rahn DW, Steere AC, Sigal LH, Zoschke DC, Gardner P, Britton MC, Kaufman RL (Univ of Kentucky, Lexington; State Univ of New York, Stony Brook; Med College of Georgia, Augusta; et al)
Ann Intern Med 119:503–509, 1993   119-95-6-5

Background.—Testing for antibodies to *Borrelia burgdorferi*, the causative agent in Lyme disease, is being done increasingly in patients with nonspecific somatic complaints or fatigue. There have been no reports of the efficacy of empirical, IV antibiotic treatment in patients with nonspecific complaints and a positive antibody titer for Lyme disease. Several reports have suggested that such treatment is ineffective. The cost-effectiveness of empirical, parenteral antibiotic therapy in patients who have chronic fatigue, myalgia, and a positive serologic result for Lyme disease but do not have its classic manifestations was investigated.

Methods.—Data were derived from peer-reviewed journals, expert opinion, and published epidemiologic research. The costs and benefits of empirical parenteral treatment for patients with positive serologic results were compared with those of treatment for only patients with classic symptoms of Lyme disease.

Findings.—In endemic areas, the incidence of false positive serologic results in patients with nonspecific myalgia or fatigue is 4 times greater than the incidence of true positive results in patients with nonclassical infections. Treatment of the former group costs $86,221 for each patient with a true positive result who is treated. In the empirical treatment strategy, there are 29 cases of drug toxicity for every case in the more conservative strategy.

Conclusions.—The costs and risks of empirical parenteral antibiotic treatment exceeded the benefits for most patients with a positive Lyme antibody titer whose only symptoms are nonspecific myalgia or fatigue. The empirical strategy is cost-effective only when patient anxiety about nontreatment exceeds the cost of treatment.

▶ Lyme disease has captured the public's attention. Patients with a variety of complaints, including aches and pains and fatigue, will often undergo serologic studies for Lyme disease as part of their evaluation. The tests for

Lyme disease are clearly not perfect, and their sensitivity and specificity are evolving. In their analysis, the authors assumed that the test was 100% sensitive (no cases were missed) and had a specificity of 98%, that is, 2% of the normal population would have a positive test result for Lyme disease. With that as a starting point, the authors found a false positive–to–true positive ratio in the most endemic region of the country of about 3 to 1 and in the least endemic region of about 1,000 to 1. In evaluating patients with nonspecific complaints compatible with fibromyalgia, heavy emphasis has to be placed on the prevalence of Lyme disease in that geographic area, history of tick exposure, and, perhaps the most important, the presence of the characteristic erythema migrans rash. Oral therapy, such as 100 mg of doxycycline twice per day for 10–30 days is usually adequate. Usually, IV therapy should initially be used only in those patients with objective neurologic abnormalities or those with atrioventricular heart block.—G.L. Mandell, M.D.

7 Resistance

Introduction

Microbial resistance to antimicrobial agents has been a fact of life ever since the introduction of antibiotics into clinical practice. Two new developments have especially concerned infectious disease physicians. First, the pneumococcus, which like *Streptococcus pyogenes* was considered to be so universally susceptible to penicillin that most laboratories did not do susceptibility tests, has now developed significant penicillin resistance. Second, we are, for the first time in recent memory, encountering organisms for which we have no (and I emphasize *no*) effective therapy available.

Gerald L. Mandell, M.D.

Emergence of Drug-Resistant Pneumococcal Infections in the United States
Breiman RF, Butler JC, Tenover FC, Elliott JA, Facklam RR (Ctrs for Disease Control and Prevention, Atlanta, Ga)
JAMA 271:1831–1835, 1994   119-95-7–1

Background.—Empiric drug treatment of *Streptococcus pneumoniae* infection may be complicated by drug resistance. Reports of drug-resistant pneumococcal infections from a wide geographic area suggest that resistance is spreading rapidly. In recent years, serious drug-resistant pneumococcal infections have been reported in the United States. Drug susceptibility patterns of *S. pneumoniae* in selected hospitals in the United States were estimated.

Methods.—Pneumococcal isolates from normally sterile sites from 544 patients were submitted to the Centers for Disease Control and Prevention. Minimum inhibitory concentrations for a variety of commonly used antimicrobial drugs were determined for these isolates.

Results.—More than 5% of the isolates were resistant to penicillin, erythromycin, and/or trimethoprim–sulfamethoxazole. The prevalence of resistance to these agents was substantially higher for 1991 and 1992 compared with 1979 through 1987 (Fig 7–1). In all, 16.4% of all strains were resistant to at least 1 of the following agents: penicillin, erythromycin, trimethoprim–sulfamethoxazole, and chloramphenicol. Six serotypes

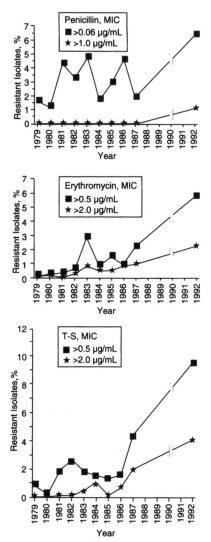

Fig 7–1.—Percentages of pneumococcal isolates resistant to penicillin, erythromycin, and combination trimethoprim–sulfamethoxazole (T-S) from 1979 through 1992. Minimum inhibitory concentration (MIC) testing was not performed from 1988 to 1991. (Courtesy of Breiman RF, Butler JC, Tenover FC, et al: *JAMA* 271:1831–1835, 1994.)

comprised 85% of the resistant strains: serotypes 6B, 23F, 14, 9V, 19A, and 19F.

Conclusion.—The emergence of drug-resistant pneumococcal infections will challenge clinicians who treat patients with pneumococcal disease. Widened, intensified surveillance for drug resistance is needed to provide useful data to clinicians making empirical therapeutic choices for treatment of infections commonly caused by pneumococci. Routine screening for drug resistance should be done in microbiology laboratories that culture pneumococci. Use of 23-valent pneumococcal capsular polysaccharide vaccines should be used aggressively in patient groups that have an increased risk of disease.

▶ This paper documents and emphasizes the increase in prevalence of *S. pneumoniae* that are resistant to multiple antibiotics. Of note is the fact that these isolates were from normally sterile sites and, thus, should be considered true pathogens. Also note that many of these strains are resistant to commonly used agents, such as erythromycin and trimethropim–sulfamethoxazole, as well as penicillin. There are 2 practical points to be emphasized. First, microbiology laboratories should test and report the susceptibility profiles of pneumococci so that physicians are aware of the local patterns. Second, serious pneumococcal infections should nearly always be treated as if the organisms are resistant until proven otherwise. This usually means that infections outside the CNS can be treated with high doses (approximately 20 million units per day for adults) of penicillin or the third-generation cephalosporins, cefotaxime or ceftriaxone. Infections of the CNS should be treated initially with cefotaxime or ceftriaxone plus rifampin. If it is highly suspected or known that the organism is resistant to the third-generation cephalosporins, vancomycin may be used (usually with a third-generation cephalosporin), although vancomycin appears to be less effective than the β-lactam agents.—G.L. Mandell, M.D.

An Outbreak of Mupirocin-Resistant *Staphylococcus aureus* on a Dermatology Ward Associated With an Environmental Reservoir
Layton MC, Perez M, Heald P, Patterson JE (Yale Univ, New Haven, Conn)
Infect Control Hosp Epidemiol 14:369–375, 1993   1 19-95-7-2

Background.—The epidemiology of *Staphylococcus aureus* in hospitals, including methicillin-resistant (MRSA) and borderline methicillin-susceptible (BMSSA) strains, continues to change with time. During a prospective epidemiologic survey of MRSA at 1 center, an outbreak of mupirocin-resistant BMSSA occurred on the dermatology ward.

Methods and Findings.—The outbreak occurred in the 12-bed inpatient dermatology ward in a university hospital. Most of these inpatients had severe, exfoliating disorders. Over 12 months, MRSA or BMSSA strains were isolated from 13 patients on the ward. Eighty-five percent of the isolates were mupirocin-resistant. In 9 patients (81.8%), isolates were present on admission; 8 of these patients had been hospitalized on the same ward in the preceding 2 months. The results of nasal and hand cultures performed on 36 hospital personnel were negative. Extensive environmental cultures were done, and a blood pressure cuff and the patients' communal shower were found to be positive for mupirocin-resistant BMSSA. Pulsed-field gel electrophoresis of all mupirocin-resistant isolates showed that the 9 patients with isolates present on admission and both environmental sources had identical DNA typing patterns. After policies of changing blood pressure cuffs between patients and requiring more stringent cleaning of communal areas were initiated, repeat environmental cultures proved negative.

Conclusion.—Outbreaks of *S. aureus* are usually not associated with an environmental reservoir. On this ward, however, all patients had severe desquamation, which might have prolonged environmental contamination.

▶ *Staphylococcus aureus* is usually considered a person-to-person bug, but this study indicates that the microbe can be found in the environment. It is probable that severe desquamation from patients on this dermatology ward promoted this somewhat unusual pattern of microbial distribution. Mupirocin has been very effective in eradicating the staphylococcal nasal carriage state (see Abstract 119-95-6-1), but topical agents can and do promote resistance, and this study is a good example of that.—G.L. Mandell, M.D.

Urinary Tract Infection With an *Enterococcus faecalis* Isolate That Requires Vancomycin for Growth
Fraimow HS, Jungkind DL, Lander DW, Delso DR, Dean JL (Thomas Jefferson Univ, Philadelphia)
Ann Intern Med 121:22–26, 1994   119-95-7-3

Introduction.—Highly resistant microorganisms, including the multiple-drug–resistant *Enterococcus*, often find ideal growing conditions in the hospital ICU. In 1 case, an *Enterococcus faecalis* isolate required an antimicrobial agent to grow.

Case Report.—Woman, 46, was hospitalized for acute cholecystitis, cholangitis, and fulminant pancreatitis complicated by sepsis and adult respiratory distress syndrome. She was transferred to the surgical ICU on day 30 of hospitalization. Nosocomial pneumonias subsequently developed, and prolonged mechanical ventilation was required. She received broad-spectrum antimicrobial therapy, which included vancomycin from days 14 through 61 and 74 through 150. Cultures from several sites yielded vancomycin-resistant *E. faecalis.* The nutritional requirement of the organism was specifically for the glycopeptide antimicrobial agent vancomycin. Vancomycin therapy was discontinued when bacteremia and sepsis with vancomycin-resistant *E. faecalis* developed in the patient. Imipenem therapy cleared the enterococci from the urine and other sites, and the woman's fever and pyuria resolved.

Discussion.—The *E. faecalis* isolate, strain TJ310, was isolated repeatedly from the patient's urine. This strain grew in primary culture but not on subculture and appeared to be closely related to other vancomycin-resistant *E. faecalis* isolates with the *vanB* genotype previously isolated from the same patient. Unlike other isolates, however, strain TJ310 was dependent on vancomycin for growth. Production of the *vanB* ligase may be the critical factor required for growth of the vancomycin-dependent strain. This unusual clinical phenomenon shows the remarkable adaptive ability of bacterial organisms to the intense antimicrobial pressure of the ICU setting.

▶ If you thought that microbes were diabolical in developing resistance to potent antimicrobial agents, consider this report. The organism went mere resistance one step further and actually became dependent on vancomycin for growth. The exact mechanism of the vancomycin dependence is unknown. Vancomycin resistance is mediated by a change in enzymes that construct the bacterial cell wall. In this vancomycin-dependent strain, the change that conveyed resistance was lethal but could be compensated for by the induction of another enzyme by vancomycin. The authors noted that colonies would not grow on subculture, and this finding suggested a fastidious or nutritionally deficient organism. They note, "ultimately we found that the nutritional requirement was specifically for the glycopeptide antimicrobial agent vancomycin." The key clue was the fact that the isolate grew only around a vancomycin-impregnated disk.—G.L. Mandell, M.D.

8 HIV

Introduction

A pall of pessimism has descended on some physicians who care for patients with HIV. Some of this pessimism is an appropriate reaction to studies that have indicated that, at best, antiretroviral agents are effective for only a limited time, and this positive effect is often counterbalanced by adverse reactions. In contrast, we are doing better in preventing opportunistic infections and, thus, are providing a longer and better quality of life for many patients with HIV infection.

Gerald L. Mandell, M.D.

The Association Between Circumcision Status and Human Immunodeficiency Virus Infection Among Homosexual Men
Kreiss JK, Hopkins SG (Univ of Washington, Seattle; Seattle–King County Dept of Public Health)
J Infect Dis 168:1404–1408, 1993   119-95-8–1

Background.—Studies in Africa have shown that the presence of a foreskin enhances the efficiency of female-to-male transmission of HIV. Further, uncircumcised men have an increased risk of genital ulcerative diseases, which facilitate transmission of HIV. To evaluate the relationship between circumcision status and HIV infection, HIV-seropositive and HIV-seronegative homosexual men were examined.

Methods.—Men from an HIV screening center and 2 HIV treatment clinics were included. A standard questionnaire was administered, and charts were reviewed to determine status of HIV serology.

Results.—Three hundred sixteen participants were seropositive, and 186 were seronegative. Infection with HIV was significantly associated with nonwhite race, IV drug use (IVDU), sexual partners with histories of IVDU, higher than average number of male partners per year, higher frequency of unprotected receptive anal intercourse, genital herpes, syphilis, and uncircumcised status. Uncircumcised men tended to be older and nonwhite. A history of syphilis was more prevalent among uncircumcised men. After adjusting for age, number of male partners, and frequency of receptive anal intercourse, uncircumcised status was independently associated with HIV infection, race, IVDU, and syphilis.

There was a 2 times increased risk of HIV infection associated with uncircumcised status.

Discussion.—Several potential sources of bias were inherent. Circumcision status and history of syphilis and herpes were taken as reported and not verified. All participants who were seronegative came from a single clinic, and most of those who were seropositive came from 1 other clinic. Analysis of the data by site confirmed the association of uncircumcised status with HIV infection. A study of men seen at a sexually transmitted disease (STD) clinic in Kenya found a 2.7-fold increase in HIV-seropositivity among uncircumcised men. In another study of men with STDs after contact with prostitutes, circumcision status was the strongest predictor of subsequent conversion to seropositivity. Initial results of 2 studies in the United States link uncircumcised status with HIV infection in heterosexual men.

The association between uncircumcised status and HIV infection of the insertive partner during rectal intercourse was confirmed. White men were 4 times as likely to be circumcised as nonwhite men. Minority populations in the United States are disproportionately infected with HIV, and lower circumcision rates may be a contributing factor. The circumcision rate of newborns has declined in recent years. Several health benefits result from circumcision, including prevention of phimosis, paraphimosis, and balanoposthitis and reduced risk of penile cancer. Decreased rate of urinary tract infections, STDs, and cervical cancers in female partners have also been noted. Circumcision also offers protection with respect to risk of HIV infection.

▶ Because circumcision is tied to socioeconomic and religious factors, it is hard to obtain data without confounding variables. This Seattle group did an excellent job in trying to sort out risks and came to a conclusion that is supported by several other studies. After exposure, infection with HIV is less likely to develop in circumcised men than in noncircumcised men. The logical connection appears to be that the foreskin itself may serve as a site of initial viral entry; the moist glans in the uncircumcised patient may be more hospitable to the virus; other STDs are more common in uncircumcised men, and these may be cofactors; and finally, trauma to the glans may be more common in uncircumcised men as compared with circumcised men who have a glans that is covered with a stratum corneum layer. Cast my vote for circumcision.—G.L. Mandell, M.D.

The Duration of Zidovudine Benefit in Persons With Asymptomatic HIV Infection: Prolonged Evaluation of Protocol 019 of the AIDS Clinical Trials Group
Volberding PA, for the AIDS Clinical Trials Group of the National Institute of

Allergy and Infectious Diseases (Univ of California, San Francisco)
JAMA 272:437–442, 1994   1 19-95-8–2

Background.—Zidovudine therapy is known to delay the clinical progression of HIV in both symptomatic and asymptomatic patients, although the durability of this benefit has not yet been established. Given the large number of patients with HIV infection who might be considered for zidovudine treatment, such information is important. The zidovudine-induced delay in clinical progression of asymptomatic HIV was therefore evaluated for its durability. In addition, the relationship between this effect and the entry CD4+ cell count was determined.

Patients and Methods.—A total of 1,565 asymptomatic patients with HIV infection who participated in the protocol 019 AIDS Clinical Trials were evaluated. All patients had entry CD4+ counts of less than .50 × 10⁹/L (500 µL). Patients were offered a total daily dose of 500 mg of open-label zidovudine after the original randomized 1989 trial was unblinded. The initial treatment groups had included placebo and 500 mg or 1,500 mg of zidovudine daily in divided doses. The duration of the effect of zidovudine was determined by conducting 3 separate analyses: an analysis of all extended follow-up data from all patients; an analysis of all patients, using follow-up of the initial placebo-assigned participants censored at the time open-labeled zidovudine was begun; and an analysis of the effect of beginning zidovudine in patients originally assigned to placebo.

Results.—During a mean follow-up of 2.6 years, 232 patients progressed to AIDS or died. In all 3 conducted analyses, zidovudine was correlated with a significant decrease in the risk of disease progression. A decreasing placebo:zidovudine relative risk with duration of use was noted, however, indicating a nonpermanent effect. A relationship between duration of benefit and entry CD4+ cell count was observed, with greater benefit seen in patients with higher counts at entry. No significant differences in survival were noted between patients initially assigned to zidovudine or placebo.

Conclusions.—A significant delay in progression of disease was noted with use of zidovudine. Earlier use of zidovudine, however, was not correlated with an additional prolongation of survival compared with delayed initiation. The delay in progression diminished over time, particularly in patients with lower CD4+ cell counts. Treatment strategies that alter drug regimens before the loss of zidovudine benefit need to be investigated.

▶ This major study from the AIDS Clinical Trials Group of the National Institute of Allergy and Infectious Diseases indicates that there is no advantage in using zidovudine (ZDV or AZT) therapy early in symptomatic disease. It is now clear that there is a high viral load in patients with HIV infection, even during the asymptomatic period. A key therapy question then is, "Would early therapy be beneficial in the long run?" It is logical to assume that reduction in viral counts during the asymptomatic period would delay the onset of symptoms and death; on the other hand, prolonged exposure to a drug such as ZDV may result in viral resistance to the agent and escape from therapy. This study followed a large number of patients with CD4 counts less than 500/μL. There was a 2-year window of benefit for most patients, and no benefit to early therapy.

Expert groups have analyzed these results and have concluded that it is reasonable to institute ZDV therapy in asymptomatic patients who have counts of 500 CD4 cells or less. It is also reasonable to wait for symptoms to develop before instituting therapy or to wait for counts to fall to lower levels (i.e., 200 CD4 cells/μL). For patients receiving ZDV, they suggest switching to ddl (didanosine) or adding ddl or ddC (zalcitabine) when the patient either worsens clinically or demonstrates a significant drop below 200 CD4 cells/μL. If the patient is clinically stable, the advice is to make no change (1).
—G.L. Mandell, M.D.

Reference

1. Sande MA, et al: *JAMA* 270:2583–2589, 1993.

The Effect of the Interaction of Acyclovir With Zidovudine on Progression to AIDS and Survival: Analysis of Data in the Multicenter AIDS Cohort Study
Stein DS, for the Multicenter AIDS Cohort Study (Albany Med Ctr, NY)
Ann Intern Med 121:100–108, 1994   119-95-8-3

Introduction.—Zidovudine is the chief antiviral agent used to treat patients who have HIV infection. It significantly delays the progression of disease but does not prevent it. Consequently, other agents, such as acyclovir, are frequently used with zidovudine to enhance or prolong its effect.

Method.—The effects of acyclovir were examined in 515 individuals seropositive for HIV who participated in the Multicenter AIDS Cohort Study. Zidovudine had been prescribed for these patients before AIDS was clinically diagnosed. The trial was a prospective multicenter study of homosexual and bisexual men who were followed semiannually. The findings at study visits 7 to 17, which occurred from 1987 to 1992, were analyzed.

Findings.—Acyclovir therapy did not significantly alter the time to progression to AIDS and did not influence the development of clinical cytomegalovirus infection. Compared with zidovudine alone, the use of acyclovir along with zidovudine was associated with a 26% reduction in rate of mortality. When acyclovir was used explicitly for HIV infection, the rate of mortality declined 36%. Survival appeared to be prolonged after AIDS developed. Initiation of acyclovir treatment before AIDS was diagnosed did not enhance survival.

Conclusion.—Acyclovir, added to zidovudine therapy, can significantly prolong the survival of patients with HIV infection who have been exposed to herpesvirus infections.

▶ Opportunistic infections are thought to make the patient sicker directly and possibly enhance the growth of HIV in part by inducing HIV growth promoters, such as tumor necrosis factor. The benefit of acyclovir was to increase survival time significantly. There is no good evidence that acyclovir plus zidovudine has enhanced anti-HIV activity, and the best guess is that the positive result was caused by the effect of acyclovir on herpes viruses, including herpes simplex virus and cytomegalovirus. It is important to emphasize that this was not a placebo-controlled, randomized study, and, although the results are interesting, they need to be confirmed in a randomized, controlled trial before specific therapeutic recommendations can be made.—G.L. Mandell, M.D.

A Randomized Pilot Study of Alternating or Simultaneous Zidovudine and Didanosine Therapy in Patients With Symptomatic Human Immunodeficiency Virus Infection
Yarchoan R, Lietzau JA, Nguyen B-Y, Brawley OW, Pluda JM, Saville MW, Wyvill KM, Steinberg SM, Agbaria R, Mitsuya H, Broder S (Natl Cancer Inst, Bethesda, Md)
J Infect Dis 169:9–17, 1994   119-995-8–4

Background.—Zidovudine or didanosine can individually benefit patients with HIV infection, but the long-term use of these drugs is often precluded by toxicity and/or resistance. Theoretically, combination therapy may result in drug synergy, reduced toxicity, less likelihood of resistance, and an ability to affect a variety of cell populations simultaneously. Didanosine and zidovudine have exhibited synergistic anti-HIV effect in vitro and have not been found to confer cross-resistance. The simultaneous receipt of these 2 agents and a regimen of alternating therapy with the 2 were compared.

Methods.—All randomized patients had AIDS or symptomatic HIV infection and less than 3 months of previous therapy with anti-HIV agents. All abstained from antiretroviral and immunomodulatory therapy for 4 weeks before the study. The simultaneous treatment group received zidovudine at 100 mg every 8 hours and didanosine at 250 mg every 24 hours. In the alternating therapy arm, patients started with zidovudine at 100 mg every 4 hours for 3 weeks, then didanosine at 250 mg every 12 hours for 3 weeks and continued to alternate in that pattern. Results were reviewed for significant differences between the 2 groups every 6 months.

Results.—Enrollment over 1 year yielded 21 evaluable patients in the simultaneous arm and 18 in the alternating arm. One year after completing enrollment, a significant difference between the groups prompted an offering of simultaneous therapy to all patients who had been randomized to alternating therapy. At baseline, 10 patients in the simultaneous group and 4 in the alternating group had detectable serum p24 antigen. Patients were followed from 33 to 104 weeks. Two patients in the alternating arm died of advanced HIV infection. One patient in the simultaneous arm died of pancreatitis, which probably resulted from medications. Patients in the simultaneous arm had more sustained and significantly greater increases in CD4 cells, with the maximum increase (at 9 weeks) being 108 ± 16 cells/mm^3. The maximun increase for patients in the alternating group was 44 ± 17 above baseline. Both arms showed comparable improvement in delayed-type hypersensitivity. All patients in the simultaneous arm with detectable serum p24 antigen were negative for it by week 6, and 3 of these patients remained negative throughout the study. Two patients in the alternating arm transiently reverted to negative, and 2 more who were negative at entry became positive. Both groups had peak weight gain at 27 weeks, but it was significantly greater in the simultaneous arm (5.8 kg) than in the alternating arm (1.9 kg) and lasted longer (63 vs. 45 weeks). There was a trend toward fewer infections in the simultaneous arm, which was consistent with the trend in increased CD4s. The incidence of hiatus from therapy caused by toxicity was similar for both arms.

Conclusion.—Evidence indicates that simultaneous therapy results in delayed resistance, but the early (by week 6) difference in CD4 cell counts between the 2 groups suggests some other mechanism for the superiority of simultaneous therapy. These agents may each act preferentially on different cell populations. Simultaneous therapy was not demonstrated to be better than either agent used alone. However, the dosing schedule of combined anti-HIV therapies is an important variable. Simultaneous therapy with zidovudine and didanosine may warrant larger controlled trials.

▶ We know that zidovudine (ZDV) therapy has a time-limited beneficial effect, in part because of development of resistance. Would alternating ZDV and didanosine therapy therefore be more effective than combination therapy? This was a small study (only 17 patients in the alternating group), and it used a surrogate end point of CD4 cell levels. The good news is that after little more than 1 year of therapy, patients on the alternating regimen had slightly higher CD4 counts. However, it is difficult to evaluate the study because no patients were untreated and no patients were treated with either drug alone. While awaiting definitive data, physicians treating patients with HIV infection have several alternatives when the patients are failing: first, switch to another agent; second, use combination therapy; and finally, use alternating therapy. The next abstract addresses 1 potential problem with combination therapy.—G.L. Mandell, M.D.

Convergent Combination Therapy Can Select Viable Multidrug-Resistant HIV-1 *In Vitro*

Larder BA, Kellam P, Kemp SD (Wellcome Research Labs, Kent, England)
Nature 365:451–453, 1993   119-95-8–5

Introduction.—Previous studies have found that HIV-1 resistance to 3'-azido-3'-deoxythymidine, zidovudine (AZT) did not predict resistance to 2 reverse transcriptase inhibitors, 2', 3'-dideoxyinosine (ddI) and non-nucleoside reverse transcriptase inhibitors (NNRTIs). The possible development of cross-resistant viral strains was explored with in vitro experiments.

Methods.—By site-specific mutagenesis, the ddI resistance mutation (74V), and then the NNRTI-resistant mutation (181C) were introduced into an AZI-resistant viral strain. Next, cultured virus, resistant to AZT and ddI, were exposed to nevirapine alone, then nevirapine plus AZT, and finally AZT, ddI, and nevirapine together.

Results.—On introduction of 74V, the AZT-resistant strain developed a new strain resistant to both AZT and ddI, but subsequent introduction of 181C produced a strain that was resistant to both ddI and NNRTI but was sensitive to AZT. The viral cultures, initially resistant to AZT and ddI, when passaged with nevirapine alone, developed nevirapine resistance and reduced AZT resistance because of a Y181-C mutation. When passaged with nevirapine and AZT, the AZT resistance returned, as a result of a V106-A mutation. The final passage with all 3 agents produced increasing nevirapine and AZT resistance, caused by the V106-A mutation appearing in the reverse transcriptase and a wild-type codon 181. Resistance to ddI was persistent in all passages.

Conclusion.—Highly triply resistant strains of HIV-1 can be developed quickly in vitro. The triple resistance to AZT, ddI, and nevirapine is caused by a single mutation at codon 184 in the reverse transcriptase. Therefore, combination therapy will likely produce multiple-drug resistance, particularly in patients who already have dual-resistant viral strains. However, synergistic drug combinations that reestablish AZT sensitivity should be further studied.

▶ With certain infections, combination antimicrobial therapy decreases the development of resistance. This has been well documented for therapy of patients with tuberculosis, in whom a single drug, such as isoniazid, frequently fails because resistance develops. When isoniazid is combined with rifampin, however, the development of resistance to either agent during therapy is rare. In contrast, *Pseudomonas aeruginosa* can develop resistance to imipenem when used as monotherapy or when combined with gentamicin. The question for therapy of HIV infection is: Will combination therapy prevent development of resistance? Based on this in vitro study, the answer is no. The in vivo implications are that combination therapy could result in highly resistant strains of HIV, and this could occur with both simultaneous and alternating therapies.—G.L. Mandell, M.D.

9 Opportunistic Infections

Introduction

The prevention and management of opportunistic infections in patients with HIV infection is one of the few medical success stories of the pandemic. Experts on AIDS agree that the single most important and effective medication for patients with HIV infection is trimethropim-sulfamethoxazole. Not only is this the most effective preventive treatment for *Pneumocystis carinii* pneumonia, but it appears to decrease the incidence of toxoplasmic encephalitis. These selections consider toxoplasmic encephalitis and infections caused by *Mycobacterium avium* complex and *Candida albicans*.

Gerald L. Mandell, M.D.

Toxoplasmic Encephalitis in Patients With the Acquired Immunodeficiency Syndrome
Luft BJ, Hafner R, Korzun AH, Leport C, Antoniskis D, Bosler EM, Bourland DD III, Uttamchandani R, Fuhrer J, Jacobson J, Morlat P, Vilde J-L, Remington JS, and Members of the ACTG 077p/ANRS 009 Study Team (State Univ of New York, Stony Brook; Natl Inst of Allergy and Infectious Diseases, Bethesda, Md; Harvard School of Public Health, Boston; et al)
N Engl J Med 329:995–1000, 1993   119-95-9–1

Background.—Toxoplasmic encephalitis in patients with AIDS is generally a presumptive diagnosis based on clinical manifestation, a positive antitoxoplasma antibody titer, and characteristic neuroradiologic abnormalities. The diagnosis is confirmed by clinical and radiologic response to therapy, but the time frame for treatment response has not been established. The course of patients treated for acute toxoplasmic encephalitis was analyzed and the objective clinical criteria for making an empirical diagnosis were evaluated.

Methods.—Forty-nine patients with AIDS and toxoplasmic encephalitis underwent neurologic assessment. The degree of severity of 23 signs or symptoms was scored from 0 (normal) to 6. Language fluency, language comprehension, and repetition were assessed as either normal or abnormal.

Results.—Based on neurologic assessment, 35 patients responded to treatment, and 12 did not. Eighteen patients who responded improved by day 3; 30, by day 7; and 32, by day 14. By day 7 of treatment, 26 patients demonstrated improvement in half their baseline abnormalities; by day 14, 32 demonstrated such improvement. Two patients who did not respond had persistent new abnormalities during the first week of treatment but had good or complete radiologic response at the end of treatment. Patients who responded to treatment improved in all neuroanatomical categories, whereas those who did not either did not improve or deteriorated in all categories except nonlocal abnormalities.

Conclusion.—Brain biopsy for definitive diagnosis should be considered if a patient with apparent toxoplasmic encephalitis continues to show neurologic deterioration despite appropriate antitoxoplasma therapy or does not improve after 10–14 days of treatment.

▶ Central nervous system toxoplasmosis in patients with AIDS is usually diagnosed clinically because of characteristic CNS findings on CT or MRI and a positive serologic test result for toxoplasmosis. The standard therapy for CNS toxoplasmosis in patients infected with HIV is pyrimethamine given as a loading dose of 200 mg followed by 50–100 mg by mouth daily. In addition, sulfadiazine, 1–1.5 g by mouth every 6 hours, and folinic acid, 10 mg by mouth daily for 6 weeks, are given. High fluid intake should be encouraged to prevent crystalluria and renal damage. Forty percent of patients will have adverse reactions to this therapy; thus, alternative therapies are being studied. The study group used oral clindamycin, 600 mg 4 times daily, and pyrimethamine, 75 mg daily for 6 weeks. Although this was not a comparative study, the group concluded that the efficacy was comparable to that reported with the standard regimen. Analysis of the patients in this study indicated that if signs and symptoms do not improve within 10–14 days, this is an atypical course for toxoplasmosis, and brain biopsy should be considered. Note that toxoplasmosis was less likely to develop in patients who had received trimethropim–sulfamethoxazole for pneumocystis prophylaxis (see reference below).—G.L. Mandell, M.D.

Reference

1. Carr A, et al: *Ann Intern Med* 117:106–111, 1992.

Primary Prophylaxis With Pyrimethamine for Toxoplasmic Encephalitis in Patients With Advanced Human Immunodeficiency Virus Disease: Results of a Randomized Trial

Jacobson MA, Besch CL, Child C, Hafner R, Matts JP, Muth K, Wentworth DN, Neaton JD, Abrams D, Rimland D, Perez G, Grant IH, Saravolatz LD, Brown LS, Deyton L, and the Terry Beirn Community Programs for Clinical Research on AIDS (Univ of California, San Francisco; San Francisco Gen

Hosp; Tulane Univ, New Orleans, La; et al)
J Infect Dis 169:384–394, 1994   119-95-9–2

Background.—Toxoplasmic encephalitis (TE), probably caused by reactivation of latent *Toxoplasma gondii,* causes considerable morbidity and mortality among patients with AIDS and is reportedly the most common cause of intracerebral mass lesions in such patients. To evaluate pyrimethamine and clindamycin as prophylaxis against TE, a multicenter, placebo-controlled, double-blind trial was initiated.

Methods.—Eligible patients from 16 centers were initially randomized into 4 groups: pyrimethamine, placebo for pyrimethamine, clindamycin, and placebo for clindamycin. After an interim analysis revealed an increased incidence of dose-limiting toxicity in the clindamycin group, randomization to clindamycin or placebo for it was halted. Some of those patients were rerandomized. Patients received either 25 mg of pyrimethamine or matching placebo 3 times per week. Prophylaxis for *Pneumocystis carinii* pneumonia (PCP) was limited to 1 of 3 agents. Patients were seen at 2 and 4 weeks and then at 2-month intervals.

Results.—At entry, there were significantly more patients in the pyrimethamine group than in the placebo group with a history of AIDS-defining opportunistic infection. Median follow-up was 254 days. The incidence of TE was low and comparable in both the pyrimethamine and placebo groups. The mortality rate was significantly higher in the pyrimethamine group (28.9/100 person-years) than in the placebo group (15.7/100 person-years), a difference that grew progressively from 6 months of follow-up to the end of the study. The mortality rate in the placebo group was similar to that of similar large groups of nonstudy patients. Analyses by center, PCP prophylactic agent, and several other variables did not reveal other potential explanations for the increased mortality rate with pyrimethamine. The incidence of TE was significantly higher among patients with baseline CD4 counts less than $50/\mu L$ and those receiving aerosolized pentamidine PCP prophylaxis (rather than trimethoprim–sulfamethoxazole).

Discussion.—The efficacy of pyrimethamine as TE prophylaxis could not be judged because of the unexpectedly low rate of TE. Pyrimethamine at this dose appears to have a negative effect on survival, especially in light of the increased cumulative mortality rate with increased duration of pyrimethamine exposure. However, a direct etiologic relationship could not be established. This effect may be caused by antifolate activity. Concomitant leucovorin therapy could have attenuated the risk. The group with the lowest baseline value of hemoglobin had excess pyrimethamine-associated death; within this subgroup, patients receiving zidovudine and pyrimethamine accounted for most deaths. A decreased risk of TE, death, or both was associated with trimethoprim-sulfamethoxazole. This agent reportedly has activity against *T. gondii.* For patients with HIV infection who receive trimethoprim-sulfamethoxazole prophylaxis for PCP, additional prophylaxis for TE may be unnecessary.

▶ Because pyrimethamine is the mainstay of treatment of toxoplasmosis, it was thought that low doses (25 mg twice weekly) would be effective prophylaxis. The authors could not reach a conclusion about the efficacy of the pyrimethamine, but there was an unexplained higher death rate in that group. Of interest was the fact that trimetropim–sulfamethoxazole was shown to be effective in reducing the development of TE. Toxoplasmic encephalitis developed in only 1 of 218 patients who received trimethroprim–sulfamethoxazole, as compared with 7 of 117 of those who used aerosolized pentamidine for prophylaxis against PCP.—G.L. Mandell, M.D.

Two Controlled Trials of Rifabutin Prophylaxis Against *Mycobacterium avium* Complex Infection in AIDS
Nightingale SD, Cameron DW, Gordin FM, Sullam PM, Cohn DL, Chaisson RE, Eron LJ, Sparti PD, Bihari B, Kaufman DL, Stern JJ, Pearce DD, Weinberg WG, LaMarca A, Siegal FP (Univ of Texas, Dallas; Ottawa Gen Hosp, Ont, Canada; Veterans Affairs Med Ctr, Washington, DC; et al)
N Engl J Med 329:828–833, 1993   119-95-9–3

Background.—In most patients with AIDS, disseminated *Mycobacterium avium* complex infection eventually develops. This infection is associated with substantial morbidity and decreases survival by approximately 6 months. Two controlled trials of rifabutin prophylaxis against this infection were reported.

Methods.—The 2 randomized, double-blind, multicenter trials were identical in design. Patients received rifabutin, 300 mg, or placebo. All had AIDS, with CD4 cells counts of 200/mm³ or less.

Findings.—In the first trial, *M. avium* complex bacteremia developed in 17% of the 298 patients given placebo and in 8% of the 292 given rifabutin. In the second study, bacteremia developed in 18% of the 282 patients given placebo and in 9% of the 274 given rifabutin. The active treatment significantly delayed the onset of fatigue, fever, decline in Karnofsky performance score, decline in level of hemoglobin, increased alkaline phosphatase, and hospitalization. Rifabutin did not produce more adverse effects than placebo did. Although there were fewer deaths in the groups given rifabutin than in the groups given placebo during the double-blind phase of the trials, overall survival among groups did not differ. Groups also did not differ significantly in the distribution of minimal inhibitory concentrations of rifabutin among the isolates of *M. avium* complex (Fig 9-1).

Conclusion.—Although there was no overall survival benefit associated with rifabutin prophylaxis, there was a trend toward improved survival with rifabutin in the analysis limited to the double-blind phase.

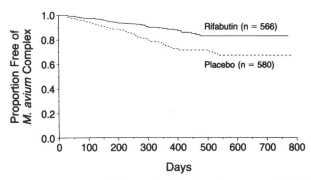

Fig 9–1.—Time to M. *avium* complex bacteremia in the intention-to-treat analysis of the combined study populations. The relative risk of bacteremia in the rifabutin group as compared with the placebo group was .45 (95% confidence interval, .32 to .63; P < .001). (Courtesy of Nightingale SD, Cameron DW, Gordin FM, et al: *N Engl J Med* 329:828–833, 1993.)

Rifabutin prophylaxis reduced the frequency of disseminated M. *avium* complex infection in this patient population. Because rifabutin in patients with active tuberculosis may promote the development of rifampin-resistant strains, active tuberculosis must be excluded in patients with HIV infection before rifabutin monotherapy is initiated.

▶ Although rifabutin is effective in preventing disseminated M. *avium* complex infections in patients with AIDS, it is not universally used. There are several reasons for this. First, there was no overall survival benefit: Second, although bacteremia was reduced by half, it was still a somewhat uncommon complication (17% in the placebo group). Finally, there is the fear that rifabutin given inadvertently to patients infected with *Mycobacterium tuberculosis* may result in development of resistance to both rifabutin and rifampin. If rifabutin prophylactic therapy is used, it is suggested that it be used only for those patients with CD4 counts less than 100/mm^3, in whom the incidence of M. *avium* complex bacteremia is higher. In addition, it should be used only in patients who are blood-culture negative for the organism. Therapy of M. *avium* complex bacteremia with rifabutin alone has a high rate of failure. If the patient is found to have bacteremia, treatment should be instituted with combination therapy, including clarithromycin plus ethambutol plus or minus another agent, such as ciprofloxacin.—G.L. Mandell, M.D.

Resistance of *Candida albicans* to Fluconazole During Treatment of Oropharyngeal Candidiasis in a Patient With AIDS: Documentation by In Vitro Susceptibility Testing and DNA Subtype Analysis
Redding S, Smith J, Farinacci G, Rinaldi M, Fothergill A, Rhine-Chalberg J, Pfaller M (Univ of Texas Health Science Ctr, San Antonio; Oregon Health Sciences Univ, Portland)
Clin Infect Dis 18:240–242, 1994   119-95-9–4

Background.—Fluconazole has been shown to treat oral thrush effectively in patients with AIDS. Infection persists, however, in a significant number of patients at the end of therapy, causing relapse and recurrent infections. Development of resistance to fluconazole among isolates of *Candida* species is cause for concern. Although actual resistance is rare, treatment of some patients with oropharyngeal and esophageal candidiasis has failed in spite of initial favorable responses to fluconazole. A patient who was treated for recurrent infections of oropharyngeal candidiasis and required increasingly higher doses of fluconazole to control the infections was described.

Case Report.—Man, aged 30 years, who had AIDS was treated for 2 years for 14 infections of oropharyngeal candidiasis. Each infection was treated for 14 days with doses of fluconazole that ranged from 100 to 800 mg/day. After the 14th infection, the patient did not respond to 800 mg of fluconazole and received parenteral therapy with amphotericin B at 30 mg/day. In vitro susceptibility testing revealed development of resistance to fluconazole. Molecular epidemiologic techniques confirmed the persistence of the same strain of *Candida albicans* throughout 12 of the episodes.

Discussion.—The persistence of a single DNA subtype of C. *albicans* for 2 years is remarkable and shows that resistance to fluconazole can arise within a single strain of *Candida*. Because this resistance may develop, fluconazole should only be used with a clear therapeutic goal. Diagnosis of infections should be made clinically and by examination of smears.

▶ Fluconazole is widely used for treatment of oropharyngeal candidiasis in patients with AIDS and has been used with some efficacy to prevent cryptococcal meningitis. It is important to realize that resistance to *Candida* can and does develop.—G.L. Mandell, M.D.

10 Nosocomial Infection

Introduction

The hospital is still a dangerous place when it comes to acquiring infection. The 2 abstracts in this chapter consider the most common nosocomial infection for many hospitals, *Clostridium difficile* diarrhea, and that potentially lethal nosocomial infection, nosocomial pneumonia.

Gerald L. Mandell, M.D.

***Clostridium difficile* Colonization and Diarrhea at a Tertiary Care Hospital**
Samore MH, DeGirolami PC, Tlucko A, Lichtenberg DA, Melvin ZA, Karchmer AW (Harvard Med School, Boston)
Clin Infect Dis 18:181–187, 1994   119-95-10–1

Background.—*Clostridium difficile* is the major infectious cause of nosocomial diarrhea. The incidence of C. *difficile* diarrhea at New England Deaconess Hospital increased from 10.2 cases per 1,000 patients discharged in 1989 to 14.7 cases per 1,000 patients discharged in 1990, despite infection control interventions. Risk factors for C. *difficile* and incidence of infection in different wards were investigated prospectively.

Methods.—Specimens were obtained from patients from 2 wards and 3 ICUs. Rectal swab cultures were obtained weekly until patients were discharged. Risk factors were evaluated for culture positivity at admission and for C. *difficile* acquisition.

Results.—At least 1 culture for C. *difficile* was positive for 18% of 496 patient admissions. The prevalence of culture positivity for initial cultures performed within 72 hours of admission was 11%. Risk factors for culture positivity at admission were previous instances of C. *difficile* diarrhea, renal insufficiency, and recent hospitalization. Significant risk factors for C. *difficile* acquisition were admission to the vascular surgery service and liver transplantation. Fifteen percent of patients who had initial negative cultures acquired C. *difficile*. Patients found to have asymptomatic colonization at admission had a low risk of later development of C. *difficile* diarrhea, but C. *difficile* diarrhea developed later in 47% of 19 patients who acquired toxigenic strains.

Discussion.—Progression to diarrhea could occur early after acquisition or not at all. Because of increasing prevalence of infection in referring hospitals and the community, a high percentage of patients who are admitted to tertiary care hospitals may already be infected with C. *difficile.*

▶ Much of what we call antibiotic-associated diarrhea is now known to be caused by *C. difficile* and its toxins. It is interesting that diarrhea rarely developed in the patients who were found to have colonization on admission, whereas diarrhea did develop in nearly half of those who were documented to acquire the organism during hospitalization. The conclusion is that disease occurs immediately after acquisition or not at all. This is somewhat similar to that which is seen with the carrier state of organisms, such as the meningococcus. We should make every effort to decrease the spread of this pathogen from patient to patient. That is more easily said than done.—G.L. Mandell, M.D.

Nosocomial Pneumonia in Mechanically Ventilated Patients Receiving Antacid, Ranitidine, or Sucralfate as Prophylaxis for Stress Ulcer: A Randomized Controlled Trial
Prod'hom G, Leuenberger P, Koerfer J, Blum A, Chiolero R, Schaller M-D, Perret C, Spinnler O, Blondel J, Siegrist H, Saghafi L, Blanc D, Francioli P (Centre Hospitalier Universitaire Vaudois, Lausanne, Switzerland)
Ann Intern Med 120:653–662, 1994   119-95-10–2

Background.—There is concern that the benefits of prophylaxis for stress ulcers that use agents that raise the gastric pH in patients in the ICU may be outweighed by the risk of nosocomial pneumonia. Sucralfate can prevent stress ulcers effectively without raising gastric pH, but it remains to be seen whether it can decrease the risk of nosocomial pneumonia. Three regimens of prophylaxis for stress ulcer—antacid, ranitidine, and sucralfate—were compared in terms of bacterial colonization, nosocomial pneumonia, and gastric bleeding.

Methods.—The analysis included 244 consecutive patients in the medical or surgical ICU who had mechanical ventilation and a nasogastric tube in place. All patients were intubated for longer than 24 hours. They were randomized to receive stress-ulcer prophylaxis with an aluminum hydroxide–magnesium hydroxide antacid suspension, 20 mL every 2 hours; ranitidine, 150 mg in a continuous IV infusion; and sucralfate, 1 g every 4 hours. Predefined criteria were used to measure the incidence of gastric bleeding and colonization and of early- and late-onset nosocomial pneumonia. Two hundred thirteen patients were observed for more than 4 days.

Results.—Macroscopic evidence of gastric bleeding was observed in 10% of the sucralfate group, 4% of the antacid group, and 6% of the ranitidine group. There were no differences among the groups in the incidence of early-onset pneumonia. However, late-onset pneumonia developed in only 5% of patients in the sucralfate group who were observed for more than 4 days, compared with 16% of patients in the antacid group and 21% of those in the ranitidine group. Gastric pH was lower, and gastric and oropharyngeal colonization were less frequent in patients receiving sucralfate. There were no differences among the groups in mortality rates. Molecular typing studies found that 84% of patients with late-onset, gram-negative bacillary pneumonia had gastric colonization with these organisms before pneumonia developed.

Conclusion.—Prophylaxis for stress ulcers with sucralfate appears to be more effective than antacid or ranitidine in reducing the risk of late-onset nosocomial pneumonia in patients who are mechanically ventilated. It is also just as effective in preventing gastric bleeding. Many of these patients have median gastric pH values greater than 4; they will not benefit from the "protective" effects of sucralfate.

▶ A few years ago, several articles presented data supporting an attractive hypothesis. Treatments that decreased gastric acidity allowed greater bacterial growth in the stomach and were associated with higher levels of nosocomial pneumonia caused by aspiration. Sucralfate, which does not change gastric pH, was shown to be associated with fewer instances of pneumonia. Other studies refuted this hypothesis. Perhaps this is the final word, as 244 patients were evaluated. Sucralfate was effective in reducing the incidence of gastric bleeding and did result in fewer episodes of pneumonia. It makes sense and it is logical. Sucralfate probably should be adopted if stress-ulcer prevention is used in patients who are mechanically ventilated.—G.L. Mandell, M.D.

11 Ehrlichiosis

Introduction

The first case of human ehrlichiosis in the United States was recognized in 1986. We are learning much about this illness and find that it has a broader spectrum of possible presentations than originally recognized. Here, at the University of Virginia, we have seen patients thought to have Rocky Mountain "spotless" fever, toxic shock syndrome, and fever of unknown origin.

Gerald L. Mandell, M.D.

Human Ehrlichiosis in the United States, 1985 to 1990
Fishbein DB, Dawson JE, Robinson LE (Natl Ctr for Infectious Diseases, Atlanta, Ga; Ctrs for Disease Control and Prevention, Atlanta, Ga)
Ann Intern Med 120:736–743, 1994   119-95-11-1

Background.—Ehrlichiosis is an uncommon new disease that was first recognized in the United States in 1986. Because only 40 cases have been reported, characterization of the illness has been prevented. The clinical features in 237 serologically confirmed cases of human ehrlichiosis from 1985 through 1990 were described.

Methods.—Patients whose serum had a fourfold increase or decrease in antibodies to *Ehrlichia canis* or *Ehrlichia chaffeensis* were interviewed. Presumptive diagnoses and clinical findings were derived from medical records.

Results.—Patients sought medical attention a median of 4 days after onset of symptoms. Among 185 patients for whom information about clinical diagnosis at the first medical visit was available, rickettsial infection was the most common initial diagnosis. Only 22.2% of patients, however, were suspected of having a rickettsial illness. The most common symptoms were fever, malaise, and headache; no symptom was present in more than 75% of patients on the first day (table). Rash was noted in 36.2% of patients a median of 5 days after onset of symptoms. The rash was most often macular or papular or both, but petechial and erythematous rashes were also reported. More than 60% of patients were hospitalized a median 7 days after onset of symptoms for a mean of 5 days. The mean duration of illness was 23 days. Three patients died, and 28 had 1 or more serious manifestations or clinical complications.

Percentage of Patients with Specific Symptoms or Signs, and Day Symptoms Were First Noted

Symptom or Sign	Total Number with Information,* n	Median Day of Onset	Percentage with Symptom or Sign during Illness†		
			First Day	First Week	At Any Time
Fever	211	1	73.7	96.6	97.2
Malaise	188	1	65.0	79.0	84.0
Headache	193	1	59.9	75.5	81.3
Myalgia	191	1	44.1	57.9	68.1
Rigor	180	1	41.6	53.0	61.1
Arthralgia	181	1	21.1	34.2	41.4
Nausea	174	1	19.9	42.3	48.3
Diaphoresis	156	2	24.1	45.1	53.2
Anorexia	183	2	21.9	51.6	66.1
Pharyngitis	172	2	7.9	15.2	25.6
Vomiting	188	3	9.3	26.7	37.2
Cough	172	3	5.2	17.5	26.2
Abdominal pain	166	3	4.0	13.3	21.7
Diarrhea	167	4	3.9	17.1	24.6
Rash	212	5	6.0	25.1	36.2
Lymphadenopathy	171	5	3.3	15.1	24.6
Confusion	167	6	1.3	13.5	19.8

* Case patients for whom information was not available were excluded for these calculations.
† Symptoms or signs reported by fewer than 10% of the case patients were ataxia, arthritis, decreased hearing, epistaxis, hepatomegaly, jaundice, meningismus, seizures, and stupor.
(Courtesy of Fishbein DB, Dawson JE, Robinson LE: Ann Intern Med 120:736–743, 1994.)

Renal dysfunction or failure occurred in 16 patients; laboratory evidence indicated disseminated intravascular coagulation in 15.

Conclusion.—Prompt diagnosis of human ehrlichiosis is hindered by its nonspecific clinical presentation and varied clinical manifestation. Future studies of this disease should focus on identifying methods to prevent infection.

▶ This is an excellent overview of a large group of patients with serologically confirmed ehrlichiosis. A point to be emphasized is that the triad that should trigger high suspicion includes exposure to ticks, febrile illness, and pancytopenia. To these 3, I would add the commonly seen increase in liver alanine aminotransferase and aspartate aminotransferase and the surprisingly frequent occurrence of rash (approximately one third of patients). Both tetracycline and chloramphenicol appear to be effective therapy.—G.L. Mandell, M.D.

Ehrlichiosis Presenting as a Life-Threatening Illness With Features of the Toxic Shock Syndrome
Fichtenbaum CJ, Peterson LR, Weil GJ (Washington Univ, St Louis, Mo)
Am J Med 95:351–357, 1993   119-95-11–2

Objective.—More than 250 cases of human ehrlichiosis have been reported in the United States since 1986. Most have been seen as acute self-limited febrile illnesses. Nine patients treated at Washington University Medical Center during a 3-year period were reviewed.

Methods.—Cases were identified through records of the infectious disease services and serology laboratories. Clinical and laboratory data were obtained from hospital records. Sera were also tested at the Centers for Disease Control and Prevention, and standard criteria were applied to define toxic shock syndrome (TSS).

Results.—Eight definite cases and 1 probable case were identified. All patients had exposure to ticks. The mean time from exposure to onset of symptoms was 11 days. The mean duration of symptoms before hospitalization was 5.9 days. All had fevers (38.4°–40.9° C) at admission. Eight had rashes, including 6 patients with diffuse erythema, 1 with purpura, 1 with a transient macular rash, and 3 with petechiae. Most had conjunctival hemorrhage or erythema, pulmonary edema or diffuse infiltrates, and hypotension. Other manifestations occurring in at least 5 patients were anorexia, malaise, myalgias, meningeal irritation, headache, hyponatremia, and anemia. Changes in mental status, abdominal pain, diarrhea, and nausea with vomiting each occurred in 3 patients. Two patients had hyperbilirubinemia, and 2 patients with hypotension had pronounced thrombocytopenia and disseminated intravascular coagulation. The average time from first physician contact to initiation of appropriate antibiotic therapy was 6.9 days. On average, defervescence transpired 3 days later. The mean hospital stay was 12 days. Survivors had no sequelae at discharge. Five patients met the criteria for TSS. All 5 had diffuse sunburn-like rash, conjunctival involvement, hypotension, and dysfunction of at least 3 organ systems. Four were treated in ICUs. Two patients with TSS required mechanical ventilation, and 1 child died.

Comments.—Previous reports have indicated that ehrlichiosis is a mild to moderately severe illness that is less serious than Rocky Mountain spotted fever. More recently, reports of renal failure, adult respiratory distress syndrome, hepatitis, neurologic impairment, and requirements of mechanical ventilation have appeared. Three adult deaths have been attributed to ehrlichiosis. Ehrlichiosis has not yet been listed in the differential diagnosis of TSS. In the present review, all patients with TSS and 2 others had conjunctival erythema or hemorrhage. This feature is not commonly associated with ehrlichiosis. The severity of these cases may be a reflection of the tertiary care setting, which serves more critically ill patients, or it may be attributable to delays in diagnosis and therapy. Animal studies have shown that early treatment with tetracycline can decrease the severity of disease. Additional underlying host factors, such as age or immunosuppression, may affect severity. This series of patients was too small to assess such effects accurately. One case is thought to be the first report of fatal ehrlichiosis in a child. Clinicians in endemic areas should be aware of the potential severity of ehrlichiosis and act promptly to begin tetracycline or chloramphenicol when indicated. Patients with fever and headache should be asked about exposure to ticks, and ehrlichiosis should be added to the list of diseases that can cause TSS.

▶ We have to expand our list of differential diagnoses for the patient with the TSS pattern. This would include staphylococcal and streptococcal toxic shock, Rocky Mountain spotted fever, bacterial sepsis syndrome, and now ehrlichiosis. It is said that one of the distinguishing features between Rocky Mountain spotted fever and ehrlichiosis is the lack of vasculitis in the latter. Because severe ehrlichiosis may be complicated by disseminated intravascular coagulation pancytopenia and hemorrhage, this distinction may be impossible to make during life.—G.L. Mandell, M.D.

Human Ehrlichiosis in Adults After Tick Exposure: Diagnosis Using Polymerase Chain Reaction
Everett ED, Evans KA, Henry RB, McDonald G (Univ of Missouri Health Sciences Ctr, Columbia; Harry S Truman Mem Veterans Hosp, Columbia, Mo)
Ann Intern Med 120:730–735, 1994   119-95-11–3

Background.—Human ehrlichiosis was first documented in the United States in 1986. A new pathogen, *Ehrlichia chaffeensis,* was characterized by polymerase chain reaction and 16S rRNA gene-sequencing techniques from a cultured blood sample from a patient with ehrlichiosis. A rapid, accurate diagnostic test for ehrlichiosis, polymerase chain reaction, was then developed. Laboratory findings associated with human ehrlichiosis were characterized.

Methods.—Thirty adult patients with acute febrile illness or with unexplained fevers and cytopenias, abnormal profiles, or both underwent se-

Abnormal Laboratory Findings

Variables *	Patients n/N(%)	Median Value	Range
Lymphopenia (<1000×10⁶/L)	22/29 (76)	66×10^6	Normal to 192×10^6
Platelets (<150×10⁹/L)	21/30 (70)	119×10^9	48 to $3i1 \times 10^9$
Leukopenia (<4.3×10⁹/L)	17/30 (57)	4.2×10^9	1.6 to 12.2×10^9
Fibrin degradation products, *mg/L*	6/8 (75)	...	Normal to >40
Activated partial thromboplastin time, *s*	8/15 (53)	...	Normal to 50
Prothrombin time	1/14 (7)	...	...
Fibrinogen	0/4 (0)	...	...
Lactic dehydrogenase (>4.2 μkat/L)	17/18 (94)	6.2	Normal to 35.4
Aspartate aminotransferase (>0.8 μkat/L)	23/27 (85)	1.43	Normal to 22.2
Alanine aminotransferase (>1.1 μkat/L)	17/23 (74)	1.65	Normal to 16.0
Alkaline phosphatase (>2.3 μkat/L)	11/25 (44)	2.0	Normal to 18.8
Total bilirubin (>20.4 mmol/L)	6/25 (24)	15.4	Normal to 92.3
Hyponatremia (>136 mmol/L)	15/29 (52)	134	Normal to 126
Blood urea nitrogen, creatinine	1/26 (4)	...	...

Note: Laboratory values were obtained within 24–48 hours of patient encounter. Three patients who had normal values or were not initially evaluated went on to have thrombocytopenia, leukopenia, and abnormal liver profiles develop during hospitalization and before the diagnosis was considered.
* Normal values are in parentheses, which also contain units for the median and range.
(Courtesy of Everett ED, Evans KA, Henry RB, et al: *Ann Intern Med* 120:730–735, 1994.)

rial clinical examinations, hematologic profiles, liver profiles, electrolyte determinations, and chest radiographs.

Results.—The pattern of abnormal laboratory findings indicated that human ehrlichiosis commonly involved the hematologic, hepatic, and central nervous systems (table). Minimal hypocalcemia, trace to 1+proteinuria, and mild anemia were also common. Five of 8 patients whose CSF was examined because of neurologic symptoms had results compatible with meningeal inflammation. Only 2 of 25 patients who underwent chest radiographs had abnormal findings. One, who had asthma, had an atelectasis that cleared the next day; the other had an exudative pleural fusion possibly related to the *Ehrlichia* infection. Three patients underwent bone marrow examinations to evaluate leukopenia and thrombocytopenia; the results were normal. Twenty of 23 patients tested by the polymerase chain reaction using E. *chaffeensis* sequences and whole blood samples were positive for the organism.

Conclusion.—Ehrlichiosis should be considered in the differential diagnosis of patients with febrile illness after known or possible exposure to ticks, particularly if accompanying cytopenias, abnormal liver profiles, or both are present. The polymerase chain reaction applied to whole blood samples may provide confirmation of the diagnosis within 24–48 hours.

▶ The polymerase chain reaction was used to confirm the diagnosis of human ehrlichiosis. The causative organism is now called *E. chaffeensis*. It is interesting that 2 patients had leukocyte inclusions seen on smear that were compatible with the *Ehrlichia* morulae. Inclusions were not described in the Centers for Disease Control and Prevention series (see Abstract 119-95-11-1). Eight of the 30 patients underwent CSF examination because of mental status change, photophobia, or intense headaches. Of 5 patients who had inflammatory cells in the CSF, 4 showed a mild lymphocytic pleocytosis.—G.L. Mandell, M.D.

PART TWO

THE CHEST

———————

ROGER C. BONE, M.D.

Introduction

In my Introduction to the 1994 YEAR BOOK OF MEDICINE, I described my ordeal with a hypernephroma, which resulted in a nephrectomy performed at the Medical College of Ohio Hospital just after Christmas in 1993. I thought the YEAR BOOK'S Introduction was an appropriate forum for a physician to analyze his own illness and his adjustments to that illness. It was a harrowing experience; however, fortunately, a year later the results of a CT scan are negative for metastasis. I realize that an individual in my situation is always at risk, but I am thankful for each passing day, month, and year.

My wife, Rosemary, and I recently received the Courage Award from the American Cancer Society. The award dinner was attended by other cancer survivors. Because I told you my story in the 1994 YEAR BOOK, this year I would like to tell you Rosemary's story.

At the awards ceremony, Rosemary gave a talk, and then I was to follow with a presentation. Rosemary, however, left me speechless. She survived breast cancer and, after surgery and postoperative radiation, had a recurrence locally. Her lumpectomy then became a radical mastectomy. Her courage has been an inspiration to me. We are both savoring every sunset together.

Rosemary's recollections reminded me of a play I read as a teenager. It is only now that I understand one of the play's most important messages. The play was *Our Town*, written by Thornton Wilder in 1935. It was a contemporary play about ordinary people in an American small town. The characters, like all of us, are letting life pass them by. In the first act, the audience is introduced by the Stage Manager to the people of Grover's Corners, New Hampshire, a mythical New England town that represents American small-town values. The theme of the first act is birth; the second, marriage; and the third, death. Emily, a character who is married in the second act, dies during childbirth in the third act. She returns as a spirit and becomes the focus of the play's conclusion. After her death, Emily observes the living and discovers how little time people take to enjoy their lives. She asks to return to her grave, saying, "They really don't understand, do they?" The Stage Manager then closes the play.

A similar theme is expressed in an American classic, *Walden*, by Henry David Thoreau. From his retreat on Walden Pond, Thoreau observes that men "become like machines whose sole purpose is to make a living. These men lead lives of quiet desperation."

The point I am making is how precious life is, especially life that can be lived in good health. Physicians are the select few in our society who have the knowledge and skill to return good health to those who are ill. A physician with the ability to assist others to recover from disease and cope with illness has a privilege that all physicians should appreciate. To be sure, it is a privilege that has monetary and social rewards. However, the greatest reward of all is to see sick and injured individuals cured and returned to active and productive lives.

It is with renewed vigor that I present this edition of Mosby's YEAR BOOK OF MEDICINE. To achieve that goal of good health for our patients, we as physicians must be as informed and as knowledgeable as possible. This YEAR BOOK features the best of this year's research results, including studies of clinical and basic research. I have selected articles that I believe are particularly applicable to the clinical practice of pulmonary medicine. The Chest section is separated into 20 chapters, which encompass the major clinical entities of pulmonary and critical care medicine. Significant events in pulmonary and critical care medicine presented in this year's YEAR BOOK include:

- the increasing incidence of multidrug-resistant *Mycobacterium tuberculosis*
- the introduction of a new, long-acting bronchodilator, salmeterol
- the incidence of silent pulmonary embolism in patients with deep venous thrombosis
- the introduction of low-molecular-weight heparin for prophylaxis against deep venous thrombosis
- the recognition that it is important to use the international normalized ratio for monitoring anticoagulant therapy and other issues regarding the use of coumarin
- the increasing survival of patients who undergo lung transplantion
- the lack of benefit of methotrexate in patients with steroid-dependent asthma
- the effect of inhaled corticosteroids on short-term bone growth
- the potential role of a leukotriene blocker in antigen-induced bronchospasm
- the prediction of who will and who will not be able to quit cigarette smoking with the use of the nicotine patch
- the diagnosis of idiopathic giant bullous emphysema
- the predictability of bronchodilator reversibility with inhaled β-agonist and ipratropium bromide
- survival after sleeve resection for lung cancer
- the prospective evaluation of unilateral adrenal masses in patients with operative non–small-cell carcinoma
- the role of preoperative chemotherapy plus surgery compared with surgery alone in patients with non–small-cell cancer
- the predictability of compliance with nasal continuous positive airway pressure in patients with sleep apnea
- the role of uvulopharyngoplasty or nasal continuous positive airway pressure (CPAP) in the long-term survival of patients with obstructive sleep apnea
- the compliance of patients with nasal CPAP

- the use of percutaneous, intracavitary installation of amphotericin-B in the treatment of hemoptysis from cavitary aspergilloma of the lung
- liver–lung interactions in endotoxemia
- the poor utility of extracorporeal removal of carbon dioxide in the treatment of adult respiratory distress syndrome (ARDS)
- the use of corticosteroids for treating the chronic fibroproliferative process in patients with late ARDS
- a new consensus on ARDS and the criteria for diagnosis
- the use of low-dose nitric oxide to improve oxygenation in patients with ARDS
- the use of surfactant in patients with ARDS
- the high incidence of pulmonary aspiration in patients with tracheostomies who are mechanically ventilated
- the use of nebulized ipratropium bromide in patients who are mechanically ventilated
- the role of the left ventricle during weaning in patients with chronic obstructive pulmonary disease
- risk factors for the development of pneumonia in trauma patients
- the effect of an increase in oxygen delivery on mortality in surgical patients who are critically ill
- the stability of choices regarding life-sustaining therapy
- the withdrawal of care in the medical ICU.

As one of the editors of this YEAR BOOK, I review the best literature in the field. This is an honor. In addition, I also have the privilege of being able to converse with colleagues who have similar interests, concerns, and aspirations. Finally, I enjoy tracing the yearly progress that is being made in our medical specialties.

Roger C. Bone, M.D.

12 Asthma

Introduction

The virtual epidemic of asthma that has occurred over the past 10–20 years has yet to be explained fully; however, it has gotten research going to the extent that we know much more about the disease. Probably the most important revelation has been the importance of the underlying inflammatory response. This fact alone has given us a wealth of avenues to follow in our research efforts. Yet, this may not be all we need. Although many have been loudly advocating the increased use of inhaled corticosteroids in the treatment of moderate-to-severe asthma, this advice is not yet universally adopted. Another, little-recognized problem that thwarts our treatments is the frequency with which health care personnel fail to teach patients how to treat themselves. This critically important aspect is addressed in 1 of this year's abstracts.

This edition of the YEAR BOOK OF MEDICINE also contains hopeful new information about the use of inhaled corticosteroids by young patients, a group that has been particularly hard hit in the asthma epidemic: Not only are inhaled corticosteroids effective, but their effects on growth are apparently minimal or insignificant. The role of inflammation in asthma provides diverse directions. For instance, a new leukotriene receptor blocker, ICI 204,219, can block bronchoconstriction. However, the stories are not all good. The nonsteroidal anti-inflammatory agent methotrexate is shown not to be effective as an adjuvant to steroid treatment for asthma.

Recent information from the Centers for Disease Control and Prevention shows that the age-adjusted rate of mortality caused by asthma has increased 46% from 1980 through 1989. The greatest increase in rate of mortality was among women (54%), compared with 23% among men; the age-adjusted frequency increased by 38%. Interestingly, the prognosis of childhood asthma in female patients is less favorable than it is in male patients. All these data are disturbing. Importantly, the increasing frequency and severity of asthma symptoms in women also warrants further study.

Roger C. Bone, M.D.

Chronic Sinusitis: Relationship of Computed Tomographic Findings to Allergy, Asthma, and Eosinophilia

Newman LJ, Platts-Mills TAE, Phillips CD, Hazen KC, Gross CW (Univ of Virginia Health Sciences Ctr, Charlottesville)

JAMA 271:363–367, 1994
119-95-12-1

Objective.—A system for quantifying the severity of chronic sinusitis was developed. The severity was correlated with the presence of allergy, asthma, and eosinophilia.

Study Population.—One hundred four patients with symptoms of chronic sinusitis that had failed to respond adequately to medical measures were seen at a university hospital otolaryngology clinic. They had received an average of 5 courses of antibiotics in the past 2 years. Asthma had been identified in 38% of the group.

Methods.—Computed tomographic scans were available for review from 21 patients who had a history of wheezing and from 47 who lacked this symptom. A score of 0 to 3 was assigned for the degree of obstruction to the nasal passages and each osteomeatal complex. The maximum degree of mucosal thickening was measured at 7 sinus sites: the frontal, maxillary, and ethmoid areas and the sphenoid region. A total of 30 points was possible. Sera were assayed for total IgE and specific IgE antibodies to common inhalant allergens. Surgical biopsy specimens were examined for eosinophils and cultured.

History of Wheezing, Markers of Allergy, or Eosinophilia as Predictive Factors for Extensive Sinus Disease

	No.	Prevalence of CT Score ≥12, %*	Sensitivity, %	Specificity, %	OR (95% CI)†
History of wheezing					
Yes	21	71§	55	85	6.25 (1.8-22)
No	47	26	...	...	...
IgE antibodies to inhalants‡					
RAST ≥40 U/mL	14	78§	43	93	9.2 (2.0-49)
RAST <40 U/mL	53	28	...	...	...
Total IgE					
≥240 µg/L	14	57‖	44	85	2.5 (0.67-10)
<240 µg/L	53	34	...	...	...
Peripheral eosinophilia					
≥0.3×10⁶/L	15	87¶	65	93	24 (3.7-204)
<0.3×10⁶/L	33	21	...	...	...
Tissue eosinophilia					
Positive	34	65§	81	68	9.5 (2.5-38)
Negative	31	16	...	...	...

* Significance judged by Mantel-Haenszel χ^2 test.
† OR indicates odds ratio; CI, confidence interval.
‡ RAST indicates radioallergosorbent test.
§ $P < .005$.
‖ Prevalence was not significant.
¶ $P < .001$.
(Courtesy of Newman LJ, Platts-Mills TAE, Phillips CD, et al: *JAMA* 271:363–367, 1994.)

Findings.—Patients who had a history of wheezing had significantly higher CT scores than those who did not; the respective mean scores were 15.4 and 7.3. The serum IgE titer and eosinophilia also correlated closely with the presence of extensive sinus disease, but neither these parameters nor wheezing precluded the need for CT examination (table). Sixty-five percent of patients with extensive sinus disease and only 7% of those with a CT score less than 12 had eosinophilia. Tissue eosinophilia also correlated with extensive sinus disease. All sinus cultures yielded at least 1 aerobic organism.

Implications.—This method of quantifying chronic sinusitis shows that associations between sinusitis and both asthma and allergic disorder are limited to patients who have extensive involvement. Peripheral blood eosinophilia signifies that extensive sinusitis probably is present.

▶ Sinusitis is remarkably common, affecting nearly 30 million Americans (1). Sinusitis becomes chronic when it lasts more than 3 months. Although the association between asthma and sinus disease is well accepted—we often see it in our patients—the mechanisms of the association are not understood entirely. However, the view that sinusitis contributes directly to asthma is strengthened by studies that found that performing sphenoethmoidectomy on these patients can aid in the management of asthma (2). The pathophysiology of chronic asthma is typified by eosinophil-rich inflammation of the bronchial tree. Because paranasal infiltration of eosinophilia and extracellular deposition of major basic protein have been shown to relate to mucosal damage in patients with chronic sinusitis, as well as in patients with asthma, it is thought that eosinophils may also act as effector cells in chronic sinusitis (3).

In the current study, however, the results suggest that the association of asthma, allergy, and eosinophilia is present only in patients with extensive sinus disease. Further, these authors found that the association between asthma and chronic sinusitis was strong only in those patients with extensive disease and that patients with positive radioallergosorbent test (RAST) results are at greater risk of having extensive sinus disease and are more likely to have coexisting asthma than patients who are nonallergic. Previous studies have also shown an increased incidence of sinusitis in individuals with allergies and have demonstrated that challenge with nasal allergens can result in both symptoms and radiographic findings of sinusitis (4, 5).

The most remarkable association found by these authors was that of peripheral eosinophilia and extent of chronic sinusitis. Importantly, this correlation was highly significant among patients with no history of wheezing and among those whose RAST results were negative, as well as among those patients with histories of allergy and asthma. This finding suggests that sinus inflammation, rather than coexisting asthma or allergy, is the stimulus for eosinophilia and that chronic sinusitis is more important in causing eosinophilia than has been thought. This study also makes it clear that the search for the causes of sinusitis or the associated wheezing should include an investigation of T-cell–mediated mechanisms of eosinophil recruitment as well as IgE-mediated mechanisms.—R.C. Bone, M.D.

References

1. *NIH Data Book 1990.* Bethesda, Md, US Department of Health and Human Services, publication 90-1261, 1990.
2. Slavin RG: Relationship of nasal disease to sinusitis to bronchial asthma. *Ann Allergy* 49:76-80, 1982.
3. Harlin SL, Ansel DG, Lane SR, et al: A clinical and pathologic study of chronic sinusitis: The role of the eosinophil. *J Allergy Clin Immunol* 81:867-875, 1988.
4. Van Dishoeck HAE, Franssen MGC: The incidence and correlation of allergy and chronic maxillary sinusitis. *Adv Otorhinolaryngol* 10:1-29, 1961.
5. Pelikan Z, Pelikan-Filipek M: Role of nasal allergy in chronic maxillary sinisitis: Diagnostic value of nasal challenge with allergen. *J Allergy Clin Immunol* 86:484-491, 1990.

Medical Personnel's Knowledge of and Ability to Use Inhaling Devices: Metered-Dose Inhalers, Spacing Chambers, and Breath-Actuated Dry Powder Inhalers

Hanania NA, Wittman R, Kesten S, Chapman KR (Univ of Toronto)
Chest 105:111–116, 1994   119-95-12–2

Introduction.—Self-administered inhalation therapy is commonly prescribed for patients with asthma and chronic obstructive pulmonary disease (COPD). There is evidence, however, that many, if not most, patients misuse their metered-dose inhalers (MDIs). Proposed solutions to this problem have included evaluation by medical personnel and a variety of alternative inhaler devices. The ability of medical personnel to use the newer devices was evaluated.

Methods.—Three groups of 30 medical personnel—respiratory therapists, registered nurses, and medical house staff physicians—were surveyed to determine their knowledge of and ability to use various common inhaling devices. The devices examined were the MDI, the Aerochamber MDI with a spacing chamber, and the Turbuhaler breath-actuated multidose dry powder inhaler. The medical professionals were asked to demonstrate each device using a placebo inhalant and to answer questions relevant to their use and maintenance.

Results.—The mean knowledge scores of the respiratory therapists were significantly higher than those of the physicians or nurses. The percent mean demonstration scores ranged from 60% to 98% for the respiratory therapists, 21% to 69% for the physicians, and 60% to 82% for the nurses; the lowest scores were all achieved for the Turbuhaler (Fig 12-1). Knowledge of and practical skills with the Turbuhaler were also lowest, proportional to the times the devices had been in use. Seventy-seven percent of respiratory therapists had received formal instruction in these devices at school, compared with only 43% of the physicians and 30% of the nurses.

▶ In the 1994 YEAR BOOK OF MEDICINE, the issue of physician knowledge of MDI use was addressed in a study by Interiano (1). The surprising finding of

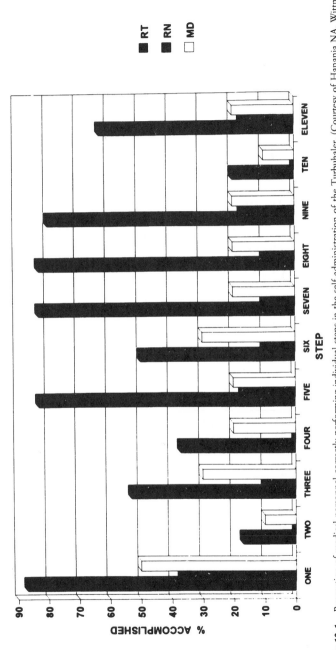

Fig 12-1.—Proportion of medical personnel correctly performing individual steps in the self-administration of the Turbuhaler. (Courtesy of Hanania NA, Wittman R, Kesten S, et al: *Chest* 105:111-116, 1994.)

that study was that house staff physicians often do not know how to use MDIs correctly; rather, respiratory care practitioners knew best how to use them. Unfortunately, it does not appear that this failing is changing very fast. The results of this study indicate that many health care providers still lack a fundamental knowledge of the use of these devices. Although considerable study has gone into patterns of drug deposition in the lung that result from MDI use, this knowledge is for naught as long as treating physicians do not use or teach their patients correct technique with the MDI. Research indicates that only 10% to 15% of a properly administered MDI dose reaches the lung, a figure that may drop significantly with improper usage.

This study of medical personnel's knowledge of MDI use is no more encouraging. It indicates that the situation may be getting worse, with the newly introduced drug-administration devices, such as the Aerochamber and the Turbuhaler (a dry powder inhaler), being used with even less proficiency. As in last year's study, house staff physicians and nurses fared worst, whereas respiratory therapists were most likely to perform well in using and training patients to use the MDI.

This is bad news given our emphasis on in-home maintenance therapy with inhaled corticosteroids. It is embarrassing for physicians not to know this critical aspect of treatment; the training of all physicians should include full instruction on MDIs and their use. Before patients are going to use MDIs appropriately, they must be correctly trained by their treating physician or respiratory therapist.—R.C. Bone, M.D.

Reference

1. 1994 YEAR BOOK OF MEDICINE, pp 9–12.

Effect of Beclomethasone Dipropionate on Bone Mineral Content Assessed by X-Ray Densitometry in Asthmatic Children: A Longitudinal Evaluation

Baraldi E, Bollini MC, De Marchi A, Zacchello F (Univ of Padova, Italy)
Eur Respir J 7:710–714, 1994   119-95-12–3

Introduction.—Although studies suggest that children with asthma who are treated with inhaled corticosteroids (ICS) may have impaired bone density, little information is available on the effect of long-term ICS therapy. The effect of 6 months of beclomethasone dipropionate (BDP) therapy on bone metabolism in children with asthma was examined.

Methods.—Fourteen children, aged 5–14 years, with moderate asthma were treated with 300–400 μg of inhaled BDP daily for at least 6 months. The control group consisted of 16 age-matched children with mild asthma who were not treated with ICS. Measurements of the recti-

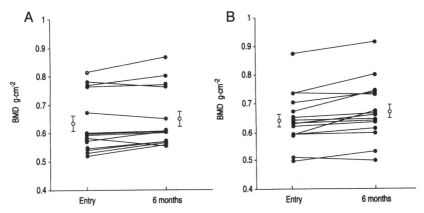

Fig 12–2.—Individual results of bone mineral density in children treated with BDP (group 1) (**A**) and in controls (group 2) (**B**) at the initiation and at termination of the study. During the observation period, mean BMD increased significantly both in the BDP group ($P < .05$) and in the control group ($P < .01$). *Open circles* indicate mean values and *vertical bars* represent ± SEM. *Abbreviation: BMD,* bone mineral density. (Courtesy of Baraldi E, Bollini MC, De Marchi A, et al: *Eur Respir J* 7:710–714, 1994.)

linear lumbar spine were made with a dual energy x-ray absorptiometry densitometer. Lung function, including forced expiratory volume in 1 second (FEV$_1$), was evaluated using a dry bell spirometer.

Results.—There was no significant difference in bone mineral density between the 2 groups after 6 months of treatment (Fig 12-2). After 6 months, the FEV$_1$ for group 1 had increased significantly from baseline values.

Discussion.—The use of BDP for 6 months in children with asthma did not result in bone density loss, but a slowdown in skeletal maturation cannot be ruled out. Additional studies should be done to evaluate longer term safe use of inhaled BDP in children.

▶ The effects of long-term ICS treatment on children have become an issue of increasing interest. These anti-inflammatory agents may be literal lifesavers for children with severe asthma; unfortunately, the side effects of this treatment have not been thoroughly investigated and may be more important than we thought. Much of the safety research has centered around the not-unexpected effects of this treatment on the hypothalamic–pituitary–adrenocortical axis. The authors of this study, however, chose to examine bone mineralization, because a recent study of individuals without asthma indicated that BDP, 400μg/day, significantly reduced serum osteocalcin (1). This result is confounded by another study, however, which showed that asthma itself may have the same effect on children (2). The effects of bone mass accumulation in childhood have been shown to carry through a lifetime, later affecting the risk of osteoporosis. Thus, the authors of this study examined the mineral content of bone with x-ray absorptiometry to determine the effects of a 6-month treatment with BDP. Bone in the lumbar spine was used, because this metabolically active trabecular bone appears to be most affected by higher-dose corticosteroid treatments.

The results of this study are good news, as far as they went. No significant loss of bone density was seen during the 6-month treatment. The authors point out, however, that this result does not rule out an effect on skeletal maturation. Such an effect is hinted at in the average percent gain in bone density: it was 2.3% for children with asthma who received BDP and 4% for the control group. The statistical significance of this measure was questionable, however, and the clinical relevance was even less clear. It is clear, however, that the question of decreased bone growth must be approached more thoroughly. With the increasing incidence of serious asthma among children, long-term ICS treatment may become more common, and it is important to know what effects this may have on growth (see Abstract 119-95-12-4 for more on this subject).—R.C. Bone, M.D.

References

1. Teelucksingh S, Padfield PL, Tibi L, Gough KJ, Holt PR: Inhaled corticosteroids, bone formations, and osteocalcin. *Lancet* 338:60–61, 1991.
2. Konig P, Hillman L, Cervantes C, et al: Bone metabolism in children with asthma treated with inhaled beclomethasone dipropionate. *J Pediatr* 122:219–226, 1993.

Short Term Growth During Treatment With Inhaled Fluticasone Propionate and Beclomethasone Diproprionate
Wolthers OD, Pedersen S (Kolding Hosp, Højbjerg, Denmark)
Arch Dis Child 68:673–676, 1993   119-95-12-4

Introduction.—Inhaled glucocorticosteroids that are used prophylactically in children with asthma can cause suppression of growth. In a randomized, double-blind, crossover trial, linear growth was compared in children treated with 2 inhaled glucocorticosteroids.

Methods.—After a run-in period (period 1), 19 children were treated for three 15-day periods (periods 2, 4, and 6) separated by two 15-day washout periods (periods 3 and 5) with 200 μg of fluticasone propionate and 400 and 800 μg of beclomethasone dipropionate per day. Knemometry measurements of the lower right leg were made twice per week.

Results.—There were no significant differences between the 2 treatments for the 17 patients who completed the study. Growth velocities slowed significantly during period 6, and the use of beclomethasone dipropionate significantly slowed growth velocity compared with fluticasone propionate (Fig 12–3).

Discussion.—The 2 medications were chosen because they are therapeutically equivalent. Growth results indicate that fluticasone propionate exerts a significantly lower systemic effect than does beclomethasone

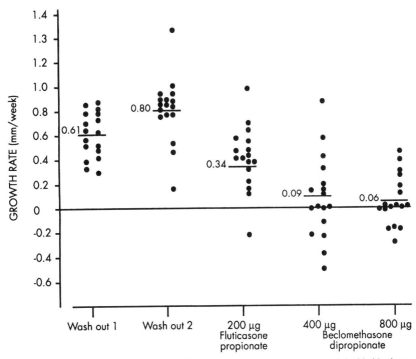

Fig 12–3.—Rates of lower leg growth in 17 children during washout periods and double-blind treatment with fluticasone propionate, 200 μg/day; beclomethasone dipropionate, 400 μg/day; and beclomethasone dipropionate, 800 μg/day. (Courtesy of Wolthers OD, Pedersen S: *Arch Dis Child* 68:673–676, 1993.)

dipropionate. Although studies of dose response are needed, fluticasone propionate may be a desirable alternative to beclomethasone dipropionate in children with asthma.

▶ In this study, the use of inhaled fluticasone propionate, a synthetic glucocorticosteroid currently under development, was compared with the use of beclomethasone dipropionate, which has been used to control asthma for many years. These authors have shown previously that knemometry is a useful tool to measure the effect of glucocorticosteroids on linear growth in children (1, 2). Knemometry, which comes from the Greek word meaning lower leg, makes it possible to measure changes in the length of the lower leg with great accuracy.

Efficacy studies by the drug manufacturer suggest that a dose of 200 μg/day of fluticasone propionate is clinically equivalent to a dose of 400 μg/day of beclomethasone dipropionate with regard to control of pulmonary symptoms (Glaxo, personal communication). The authors, therefore, compared these doses and added a dose of 800 μg/day of beclomethasone, which they expected would have a significant effect on growth rate (1). Although there were no significant differences in pulmonary function or severity of symptoms among the treatments, children receiving 400 μg and 800 μg of beclomethasone dipropionate had statistically significantly lowered growth velocity. The systemic effects of another inhaled glucocorticosteroid, budesonide, are known to be dose related and become significant at doses of 800 μg/day, when administered in a conventional metered dose inhaler with a spacer (1, 2). The finding that 400 μg/day of beclomethasone produced growth rates similar to the 800-μg/day dose of both beclomethasone and budesonide was surprising, and these authors liken the effect to that seen in children receiving 2.5 mg/day of prednisone.

The effect of fluticasone propionate on long-term growth has not been fully investigated. There have been reports, however, that beclomethasone dipropionate in doses from 100 to 800 μg/day does not effect statural growth (3–5). Most of these studies were both retrospective and not controlled, and the children received the drug by means of a conventional metered-dose inhaler.

To what extent short-term lower leg growth relates to overall statural growth is unclear. What is clear is that the incidence of asthma in children is growing at an alarming rate, and safe methods for long-term control are needed. Despite the existence of some effect on growth in children, inhaled corticosteroids are an essential treatment modality in many, if not most, patients with asthma. The alternative is oral corticosteroids with their profound effects on growth, as well as other well-known and debilitating side effects.—R.C. Bone, M.D.

References

1. Wolthers OD, Pedersen S: Growth of asthmatic children during treatment with budesonide: A double-blind trial. *BMJ* 303:163–165, 1991.
2. Wolthers OD, Pedersen S: Controlled study of linear growth in asthmatic children during treatment with inhaled glucocorticosteroids. *Pediatrics* 89:839–842, 1992.
3. Godfrey S, Balfour-Lynn L, Tooley M: A three- to five-year follow-up of the use of the aerosol steroid, beclomethasone dipropionate, in childhood asthma. *J Allergy Clin Immunol* 62:335–339, 1978.
4. Graff-Lonnevig V, Kraepelien S: Long term treatment with beclomethasone dipropionate aerosol in asthmatic children with special reference to growth. *Allergy* 34:57–61, 1979.
5. Nassif E, Weinberger M, Sherman B, et al: Extra-pulmonary effects of maintenance corticosteroid therapy with alternate-day prednisone and inhaled beclomethasone in children with chronic asthma. *J Allergy Clin Immunol* 80:518–529, 1987.

The Role of Methotrexate in the Management of Steroid-Dependent Asthma

Coffey MJ, Sanders G, Eschenbacher WL, Tsien A, Ramesh S, Weber RW, Toews GB, McCune WJ (Univ of Michigan, Ann Arbor)

Chest 105:117–121, 1994   119-95-12–5

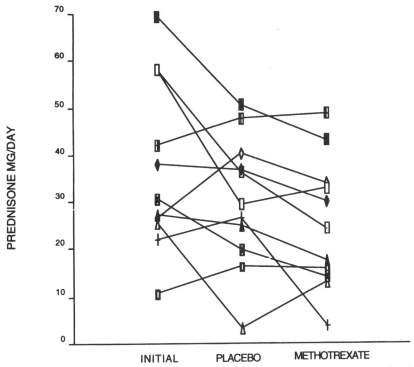

Fig 12–4.—Average daily prednisone dose in 11 corticosteroid-dependent asthmatics treated with low-dose methotrexate during the initial placebo and methotrexate phases. A different notation is used for each patient. Prednisone dose was calculated from the last 2 weeks of the initialization phase and the last 4 weeks of the placebo and methotrexate phase, respectively. (Courtesy of Coffey MJ, Sanders G, Eschenbacher WL, et al: *Chest* 105:117–121, 1994.)

Introduction.—Because patients with severe asthma who require high-dose, long-term steroid therapy commonly experience debilitating side effects, other anti-inflammatory agents have been used to reduce dependence on corticosteroids. There have been mixed reports on the efficacy of methotrexate as a steroid-sparing agent in patients with asthma. Methotrexate was compared with placebo in the management of steroid-dependent asthma.

Methods.—Eleven patients participated in the double-blind crossover trial. Entry criteria required participants to be nonsmokers between 18 and 50 years of age with severe asthma and no history of kidney or liver disease. None of the patients had a seasonal variation in their asthma. During an initial phase, pulmonary function was maximized while patients received the lowest steroid dose. They were then randomized into either the methotrexate phase or the placebo phase for 12 weeks, followed by crossover to a second 12-week period. The minimum cumulative dose of methotrexate was 150 mg.

Results.—All patients were severely steroid-dependent, requiring a mean prednisone dose of greater than 30 mg/day. In addition, they were receiving maintenance asthma medications, including theophylline, an inhaled β-agonist, and high-dose inhaled steroids. The patients' required mean dose of prednisone decreased compared with the initial period during both methotrexate and placebo periods (Fig 12–4). Methotrexate was not superior to placebo, and only 3 of 11 patients responded to the drug. Eight patients who kept accurate diary cards during the study showed no significant difference in peak flow rates during the 2 treatment phases.

Conclusion.—Low-dose methotrexate did not have a significant steroid-sparing effect in these patients with severe asthma. Because patients were carefully monitored, greater compliance with medications may explain the observed reductions in steroid dosage during the study. Three patients did respond, suggesting that a subgroup of patients with steroid-dependent asthma may benefit from methotrexate.

▶ The side effects of prolonged steroid therapy are well documented and include many debilitating problems, such as infection, hypertension, and peptic ulceration (1). To avoid these complications, other anti-inflammatory agents have been studied in the control of steroid-dependent asthma. The use of methotrexate, which acts as an anti-inflammatory agent when given in low doses, seems reasonable in these patients, whose asthma would presumably be associated with the greatest inflammatory involvement (2).

Although the initial report found that the concurrent steroid dose could be reduced significantly in 4 of 6 patients treated with adjuvant methotrexate and increased in only 1 of 6 patients (3), this study, as well as a subsequent study, found no overall benefit in the use of methotrexate for steroid-dependent asthma (4). What Coffey and colleagues did find was that the dose of steroid could be decreased in patients taking both methotrexate and placebo, and there was no significant difference in the amount of reduction between the 2 treatment phases. There was a 20% mean decrease in dose in patients receiving placebo alone. Eight patients who kept accurate diary cards showed no significant difference between patients taking methotrexate and those taking placebo. Ten cases of asthma exacerbation occurred that required a boost and then a tapering of prednisone therapy; these cases were equally divided between the methotrexate and placebo groups. Side effects of methotrexate therapy included nausea, abdominal cramps, and diarrhea; the incidence of side effects was the same for both groups. Only 1 patient was withdrawn from the study when alopecia developed during the first phase of treatment. This patient was later found to be receiving placebo. Three patients did respond to methotrexate therapy and could reduce their steroid dose by 33% or greater during the active phase of treatment. However, no common factors could be found to predict responders and nonresponders.

A very interesting and important point is made by the authors, who cite a previous study in which patient compliance was found to improve by study enrollment alone because it increased the patient's awareness of the disease and gave the patient more confidence that therapy was beneficial (5). Although a small number of patients whose asthma was more drug responsive were helped by methotrexate, the authors of this study suggested that intensified conventional therapy and more frequent visits to the physician were more important than the addition of methotrexate.

Clearly, the issue of anti-inflammatory therapy for steroid-dependent asthma needs a great deal more study with greater numbers of patients. In the interim, I would call your attention to an article reviewed in the 1993 YEAR BOOK OF MEDICINE (6). The study was a randomized, placebo-controlled trial of cyclosporine in patients with corticosteroid-dependent chronic severe asthma. In that study, cyclosporine therapy resulted in a significant mean increase of 12% above that of placebo in peak expiratory flow rate, with a nearly 50% decrease in disease exacerbations requiring prednisolone. Based on the available data, I plan to use cyclosporine rather than methotrexate for such patients. In the cyclosporine study, side effects were mostly minor in both groups, but included hypertrichosis, hypertension, tremor, headache, nausea, and paresthesia.—R.C. Bone, M.D.

References

1. Adinoff A, Hollister J: Steroid-induced fractures and bone loss in patients with asthma. N Engl J Med 309:265–268, 1983.
2. Snapper JR: Inflammation and airway function: The asthma syndrome (editorial). Am Rev Respir Dis 141:531–533, 1990.
3. Mullarkey MF, Webb R, Pardee NE: Methotrexate in the treatment of steroid-dependent asthma. Ann Allergy 56:347–350, 1986.
4. Erzurum SC, Leff JA, Cochran JE, Ackerson LM, Szefler SJ, Martin RJ, Cott GR: Lack of benefit of methotrexate in severe, steroid-dependent asthma: A double-blind, placebo-controlled study. Ann Intern Med 114:353–360, 1991.
5. Woods J, Williams J, Travel M: The two-period crossover design in medical research. Ann Intern Med 110:560–566, 1989.
6. 1993 YEAR BOOK OF MEDICINE, pp 91–92.

Inhaled ICI 204,219 Blocks Antigen-Induced Bronchoconstriction in Subjects With Bronchial Asthma

Nathan RA, Glass M, Minkwitz MC (Allergy Assoc, Colorado Springs, Colo; ZENECA Pharmaceuticals Groups, Wilmington, Del)
Chest 105:483–488, 1994   119-95-12–6

Background.—ICI 204,219 is a selective, orally active leukotriene antagonist that is being assessed in clinical trials. Oral formulations of ICI 204,219 have demonstrated inhibition of antigen-induced bronchoconstriction during allergen-challenge studies in patients with asthma. The antagonism of antigen-induced bronchoconstriction by 3 inhalation formulations of ICI 204,219 was evaluated.

Patients and Methods.—Sixteen patients, aged 20–43 years, were evaluated. All patients showed reproducible hypersensitivity to allergen dur-

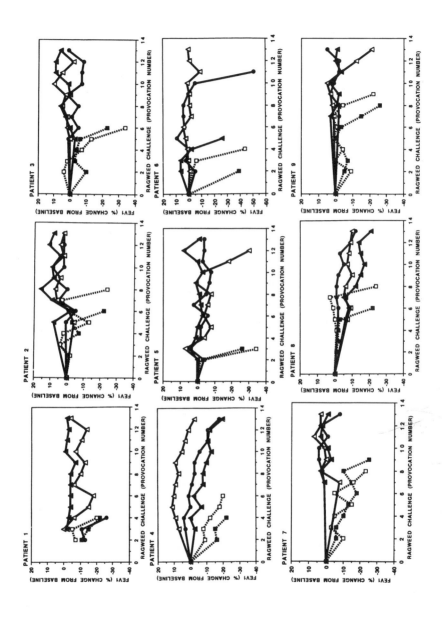

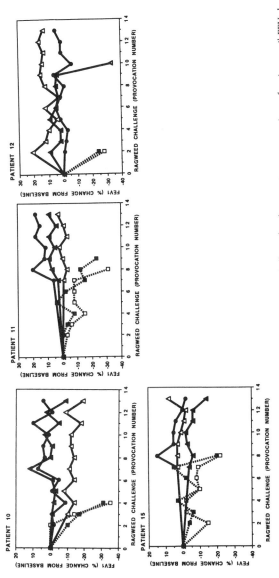

Fig 12-5.—Forced expiratory volume in 1 second of patients with asthma who were challenged with increasing concentrations of antigen until FEV₁ decreased 20% or the maximum allergen concentration was reached. *Shaded box with dotted line* indicates first screening period; *open box with dotted line,* second screening period; *open triangle with solid line,* challenge 30 minutes after receiving 4 actuations of formulation 1 (.05 mg per actuation); *shaded triangle with solid line,* challenge 30 minutes after receiving 4 actuations of formulation 2 (.05 mg per actuation); *shaded circle with solid line,* challenge 30 minutes after receiving one actuation of formulation 3 (.2 mg per actuation). (Courtesy of Nathan RA, Glass M, Minkwitz MC: *Chest* 105:483–488, 1994.)

ing screening challenges. A single, .2-mg dose of each of the 3 ICI 204,219 formulations was administered to each patient. After 30 minutes, a ragweed challenge was performed until forced expiratory volume in 1 second (FEV_1) decreased by 20% or the maximum allergen concentration (100 $\mu g/mL$) was achieved.

Results.—Most patients tolerated 10 $\mu g/mL$ of allergen without a 20% decrease in FEV_1 (Fig 12-5). Twenty-seven mild-to-moderate adverse events were noted. The most common events were headache in 6 patients, rhinitis in 4, and cough in 3. No serious or unexpected adverse reactions were associated with use of ICI 204,219.

Conclusion.—The inhalation formulations of ICI 204,219 inhibited bronchoconstriction in patients with reproducible sensitivity to ragweed challenges.

▶ It appears that endogenous mediators may play many roles in the pathogenesis of asthma. For instance, interleukin-8 has been found to act as an attractant to neutrophils in a number of disease states, including asthma. These authors examined the role of arachidonic acid metabolites, the sulfidopeptide leukotrienes (LTC_4, LTD_4, and LTE_4), in asthma. This study was made possible by the availability of a leukotriene receptor blocker, ICI 204,219, which has already been found to reduce bronchoconstriction in allergen challenge tests (1–3). The agent has also been found to reduce bronchoconstriction in patients with asthma (4). This study examined the ability of this antagonist to block bronchoconstriction in patients with reproducible responses to challenges with ragweed.

When administered 30 minutes before a ragweed challenge, a single, .2-mg dose of ICI 204,219 administered as an inhalant totally inhibited bronchoconstriction in 31 of 39 attempts in 13 patients with mild asthma. This result is in contrast with those of some other studies of leukotriene antagonists, although those authors admitted that dosing may have been a problem (4). The use of an inhaled form of antagonist in this study may have optimized the dose within the lung to provide these favorable results. This is an interesting class of drugs that, with further study, may provide pulmonologists with a method of blocking the acute effects of allergens on airway function.—R.C. Bone, M.D.

References

1. Findlay SR, Barden JM, Easley CB, Glass M: Effect of the oral leukotriene antagonist, ICI 204,219, on antigen-induced bronchoconstriction in subjects with asthma. *J Allergy Clin Immunol* 89:1040–1045, 1992.
2. Taylor IK, O'Shaughnessy KM, Fuller RW, Dollery CT: Effect of cysteinyl-leukotriene receptor antagonist ICI 204,219 on allergin-induced bronchoconstriction and airway hyperreactivity in atopic subjects. *Lancet* 337:690–694, 1991.
3. Nathan RA, Storms WW, Bodman SF, Minkwitz MC, Glass M: Inhibition by aerosolized ICI 204,219, LTD4 receptor antagonist, of allergen-induced bronchoconstriction. *J Allergy Clin Immunol* 87:256, 1991.
4. Rasmussen JB, Eriksson L-O, Andersson K-E: Reversal and prevention of airway response to antigen challenge by the inhaled leukotriene D4 antagonist (L-648,051) in patients with atopic asthma. *Allergy* 46:266–273, 1991.

13 Smoking Cessation

Introduction

Recent reports about smoking in the United States are very encouraging. In certain groups, such as black women, significant decreases in the number of smokers have been noted. Further legislation has been contemplated to reduce the number of available smoking areas. One article selected for this year's YEAR BOOK OF MEDICINE notes significant decreases in the number of health care workers who smoke cigarettes—with physicians leading the way. For those who are addicted to smoking and want to quit, the 1995 YEAR BOOK contains some new advice. It seems that the form of counseling that accompanies the use of the nicotine patch may be more important than the patch itself, with patients who receive 8 weeks of 60-minute group counseling sessions achieving the greatest reduction in smoking. Even in the best group, however, the 6-month abstinence rate was only 20%, pointing to the true difficulty of kicking the habit.

Another study this year started with the concept that not all patients are able to quit. However, by finding indicators of the ultimate potential success of cessation efforts for individual patients, the authors of this study have made it possible for physicians to identify patients likely to achieve smoking cessation. With this information available, it will be possible to target difficult cases for special treatment, such as the above-described counseling. Smoking remains one of the most popular yet dangerous habits of people worldwide, and there remains no cure for the most common effect of smoking, chronic obstructive pulmonary disease. Smoking will continue to take a heavy toll through the end of this century. One can only hope that people will someday realize that this destructive habit has no real merits.

Roger C. Bone, M.D.

Predicting Smoking Cessation: Who Will Quit With and Without the Nicotine Patch

Kenford SL, Fiore MC, Jorenby DE, Smith SS, Wetter D, Baker TB (Univ of Wisconsin, Madison)

JAMA 271:589–594, 1994   119-95-13–1

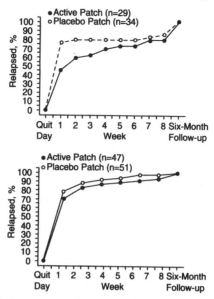

Fig 13–1.—The cumulative proportion of patients smoking at 6-month follow-up for study 1 (**top**) and study 2 (**bottom**), presented as a function of the week at which they smoked their first cigarette (i.e., when relapsers started to smoke). (Courtesy of Kenford SL, Fiore MC, Jorenby DE, et al: JAMA 271:589–594, 1994.)

Introduction.—Although the transdermal nicotine patch has proven effective in helping individuals quit smoking, there is considerable variation in rates of cessation. These differences may be caused by the heterogeneity in the general population of smokers. Studies have sought to identify factors that might predict the success or failure of attempts to quit smoking with and without the nicotine patch.

Methods.—Two independent, randomized, double-blind, placebo-controlled studies of the nicotine patch were reported. Both studies assessed outcome at the end of treatment and at 6 months' follow-up. The first study, which included 87 patients, provided 8 weeks of 22-mg nicotine patch therapy plus intensive group counseling. The second study, which included 112 patients, provided 4 weeks of 22-mg nicotine patch therapy, 2 weeks of 11-mg nicotine patch therapy, and brief individual therapy. Factors that could predict smoking cessation, based on measures assessed before and during treatment, in both the nicotine and placebo patch groups were sought.

Results.—None of the pretreatment markers examined could predict success in smoking cessation consistently. These markers included the Fagerstrom Tolerance Questionnaire score, number of cigarettes smoked per day, years smoked, expired air carbon monoxide level, and baseline blood levels of nicotine and cotinine. The intratreatment markers of severity of withdrawal and levels of nicotine replacement were also nonpredictive. However, 83% of patients in study 1 and 97% of those in study 2 who used nicotine patches and who smoked at all during the second week of treatment were still smoking at 6 months, whereas 46% and 41%, respectively, of those who abstained from smoking through the second week were still abstinent at follow-up. Three fourths of patients using the nicotine patch who were smoking at follow-up had started during the first or second week of treatment. The same was true for 86% of patients using the placebo who were smoking at follow-up (Fig 13–1).

Conclusion.—Whether the patient smokes during the first 2 weeks of nicotine or placebo patch therapy appears to be an important predictor of the success of smoking cessation. The traditional markers of dependence on tobacco are not good predictors of success in quitting. For patients who are trying to quit, the clinician should stress total abstinence and follow-up within the first 2 weeks of the attempt. If the patient has smoked during this time, more aggressive therapy might be considered.

▶ The essential point of this study is that, without an indication of the likelihood of success in getting a patient to quit smoking, there is no way to determine the intensity of the programs needed to achieve withdrawal from cigarette smoking. There are, in fact, a variety of programs that can be used as adjuvants to the nicotine patch to increase the odds of successful smoking cessation. To date, several studies have addressed this question of the likelihood of quitting—but without clear and confirmable results (1–4). By limiting the number of variables and increasing the sample to include 2 groups of smokers, this study has appropriately addressed the question of whether intensive group counseling or brief individual counseling is an appropriate adjuvant to use of the nicotine patch.

The most powerful predictor of success observed in this trial was the occurrence of smoking during the first 2 weeks of treatment. If a smoker regresses during that period, the likelihood of both long- and short-term success is greatly diminished. Thus, an assessment of smoking during the second week of a program could become a yardstick for treating physicians. A number of potential predictors, including the number of cigarettes smoked per day, the Fagerstrom Tolerance Questionnaire, and the number of years of smoking, were shown to have low reliability in this study. Nonpredictive biochemical parameters included the level of carbon monoxide in the expired air, pretreatment blood levels of nicotine and cotinine, and the levels of nicotine and cotinine achieved by the nicotine patch. Unfortunately, none of the pretreatment measures identified in this study had the ability to predict treatment success.

Although this study may not have used completely typical groups of smokers and may have suffered from inaccurate assessment or the use of inappropriate measures of dependence, the authors felt justified in concluding the following: It should be stressed at the outset of smoking cessation treatment that total abstinence is of critical importance for most smokers. Additionally, it should be propitious to time the heaviest interdictive efforts, such as adjuvant counseling, during the first 2 weeks of treatment. Assessments during the second week should be predictive of later success. In the event that smoking recurs during the 2-week period, it is still possible to change the treatment method or to add other adjuvant treatments.—R.C. Bone, M.D.

References

1. Tiffany ST, Baker TB: The role of aversion and counseling strategies in treatments for cigarette smoking. In: Baker TB, Cannon DE (eds): *Assessment and Treatment of Addictive Disorders.* New York, NY: Praeger; 238–289, 1988.
2. West DW, Graham S, Swanson M, Wilkinson G: Five-year follow-up of a smoking withdrawal clinic population. *Am J Public Health* 67:536–544, 1977.
3. Horwitz MB, Hindi-Alexander MI, Wagner TJ: Psychosocial mediators of abstinence, relapse, and continued smoking: A one-year follow-up of a minimal intervention. *Addict Behav* 10:29–39, 1985.
4. Garvey AJ, Bliss RE, Hitchcock JL, Heinhold JW, Rosner B: Predictors of smoking relapse among self-quitters: A report from the normative aging study. *Addict Behav* 17:367–371, 1992.

Trends in Cigarette Smoking Among US Physicians and Nurses
Nelson DE, Giovino GA, Emont SL, Brackbill R, Cameron LL, Peddicord J, Mowery PD (Natl Ctr for Chronic Disease Prevention and Health Promotion, Atlanta, Ga; Natl Inst for Occupational Safety and Health, Atlanta, Ga; Batelle, Inc, Arlington, Va)
JAMA 271:1273–1275, 1994   119-95-13–2

Introduction.—Recent trends in smoking among physicians and nurses have not been reported. Because health care workers can serve as models and educators for appropriate health behavior, it is expected that they would have a lower smoking prevalence than the general population.

Methods.—Data from the National Health Interview Survey (NHIS) were analyzed to determine trends in smoking for 1974 through 1991. Questions on smoking prevalence were asked on 12 NHISs during this period: 1974, 1976 through 1980, 1983, 1985, 1987, 1988, 1990, and 1991. Physicians, nurses, and licensed practical nurses were classified as "ever smokers," "current smokers," or "former smokers." Quit ratios were calculated by dividing the number of former smokers by the number of ever smokers.

Results.—When data from 1974, 1976, and 1977 were compared with those from 1990 and 1991, the prevalence of cigarette smoking was found to have declined from 18.8% to 3.3% among physicians, from 31.7% to 18.3% among registered nurses, and from 37.1% to 27.2% among licensed practical nurses. Quit ratios increased substantially during the study. The average annual declines were 1.15% for physicians, .88% for registered nurses, and .62% for licensed practical nurses.

Discussion.—Most physicians in the United States who have ever smoked have quit. Although both registered and licensed practical nurses had a lower smoking prevalence in 1990 and 1991 than in the 1970s, they have quit at a lower rate than physicians. Until recently, smoking prevalence among licensed practical nurses has been higher than among all adults. However, older health care workers, many of whom smoked, are being replaced by younger individuals who are less likely to smoke. The decline in smoking is encouraging and shows that physicians and nurses are following the advice that they give to patients.

▶ It is fairly surprising that any physician—or for that matter, anyone involved in health care—would continue to smoke, but of course some do. Studies have shown that both physicians and nurses are significant role models with regard to appropriate health behavior, and smoking clearly undermines these important roles (1–3). Using data from 1990 and 1991, these authors estimate that 18,000 physicians, 322,000 registered nurses, and 128,000 licensed practical nurses in the United States smoke. Compared with previous data, however, the 1990–1991 data showed that cigarette smoking had declined from 18.8% to 3.3% among physicians, from 31.7% to 18.3% among registered nurses, and from 37.1% to 27.2% among licensed practical nurses.

The decline in the number of physicians and nurses who smoke is the result of a number of factors. Increased media attention to the dangers of smoking has persuaded many individuals, both health care workers and the general population, to quit, with more rapid decline occurring among more educated individuals (4). In addition, more nonsmokers are entering the health care professions. Part of the reason for this may be self-selection and part may be the pressure on students in medical and nursing schools to discourage smoking. There has also been a general decline in smoking among younger persons, and as older persons (many of whom smoked) leave the workforce and are replaced by younger (nonsmoking) workers, smoking prevalence declines (5).

The findings of this study are in agreement with those of previous studies, showing that physicians are less likely to smoke than the rest of the population (2, 6). Among registered nurses, smoking prevalence was higher than that of the general population during the late 1960s; since the mid-1970s, however, smoking has been less common in this group than in the general population (7). In marked contrast to the trends seen among physicians and registered nurses, the prevalence of smoking among licensed practical nurses has been higher than that of the general population until recently (7). This difference may reflect the association between lower level of education and higher prevalence of smoking, because the educational level of these workers is usually lower than that of physicians and registered nurses (8). Special efforts should be directed toward this group to further lower their incidence of smoking.

Studies have shown that physicians and nurses stop smoking for the same reasons mentioned by the general population, including adverse health effects, pressure from family and friends, and cost. Health care professionals also often cite the desire to set a better example for both their adult and younger patients as another reason for stopping, and of course, seeing patients who have adverse health problems related to smoking may be an additional motivator to quit.

Physicians and nurses have an important role as health care educators and exemplars of good health-related behavior. Smoking subverts that role and sends the wrong message to patients who smoke. It has also been shown that physicians and nurses who smoke are much less likely than others to perceive their importance as health care educators and are less likely to encourage their patients to quit smoking (9, 10). The decline in smoking prevalence among physicians and nurses is encouraging because it shows that most of them are taking their own advice not to smoke.—R.C. Bone, M.D.

References

1. US Department of Health, Education, and Welfare: *Smoking and Health: A Report of the Surgeon General.* Rockville, Md, US Public Health Service, 1979.
2. National Clearinghouse for Smoking and Health: *Survey of Health Professionals: Smoking and Health, 1975.* Rockville, Md, US Public Health Service, 1976.
3. Kottke TE, Hill C, Heitzig C, et al: Smoke-free hospitals. *Minn Med* 68:53–55, 1985.
4. Pierce JP, Fiore MC, Novotny TE, et al: Trends in cigarette smoking in the United States: Educational differences are increasing. *JAMA* 261:56–60, 1989.
5. National Cancer Institute: *Strategies to Control Tobacco Use in the United States: A Blueprint for Public Health Action in the 1990s.* Bethesda, Md, National Cancer Institute, 1991.
6. Harvey L: *Physician Opinion on Health Care Issues 1987.* Chicago, American Medical Association, 1987.
7. Cigarette smoking among adults—United States, 1990. *Morb Mortal Wkly Rep* 42:230–233, 1993.
8. Fiore MC, Novotny TE, Pierce JP, et al: Trends in cigarette smoking in the United States. *JAMA* 261:49–55, 1989.
9. Levitt EE, DeWitt KN: A survey of smoking behavior and attitudes of Indiana physicians. *J Indiana Med Assoc* 63:336–339, 1970.
10. Dalton JA, Swenson I: Nurses and smoking: Role modeling and counseling behaviors. *Oncol Nurse Forum* 13:45–48, 1986.

14 Chronic Obstructive Pulmonary Disease

Introduction

The most important news in the field of chronic obstructive pulmonary disease (COPD) over the past year has been the availability of a new, long-acting β-adrenergic agonist, salmeterol, which can be used for the treatment of asthma or COPD. Additionally, ipratropium bromide, which has been available for the treatment of obstructive lung disease with a metered-dose inhaler, is now also available in a nebulized form. Both of these agents are important adjuncts to therapy in selected patients. A discussion of both agents is presented in the commentaries to articles selected for this chapter. Other selections for this chapter include the diagnosis and treatment of idiopathic giant bullous emphysema, the inability of a bronchodilator response to distinguish between asthma and COPD, theophylline withdrawal and its effects on patients with COPD, and, lastly, the current status of replacement therapy for hereditary α_1-antitrypsin deficiency.

Roger C. Bone, M.D.

Idiopathic Giant Bullous Emphysema (Vanishing Lung Syndrome): Imaging Findings in Nine Patients
Stern EJ, Webb WR, Weinacker A, Müller NL (Univ of Washington, Seattle; Univ of California, San Francisco; Vancouver Gen Hosp, BC, Canada)
AJR 162:279–282, 1994   119-95-14–1

Introduction.—Since Burke first described a patient with "vanishing lungs" caused by giant bullae in 1937, scattered reports have appeared of what has been referred to as "vanishing lung syndrome." This progressive disorder may be associated with various forms of emphysema and is found mainly in young men who smoke.

Patients.—The findings on high-resolution CT scanning were reviewed in 9 men in whom 1 or more bullae occupied at least one third of a hemithorax. The patients had a mean age of 41 years; all but 1 smoked.

Findings.—The bullae usually were 2–8 cm in diameter and involved the lungs asymmetrically. The upper lobes were consistently involved, and 6 patients also had bullae at the lung bases. The largest bullae could

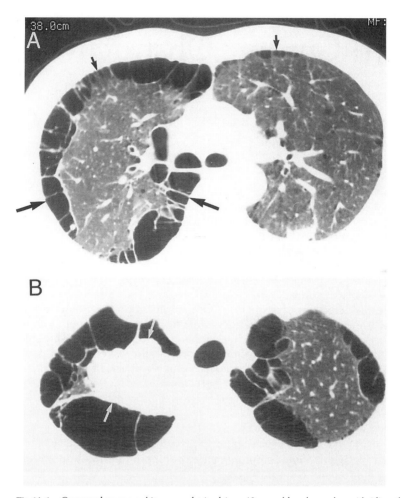

Fig 14–1.—Computed tomographic scans obtained in a 40-year-old male smoker with idiopathic giant bullous emphysema. **A,** asymmetric paraseptal emphysema (*small arrows*) and subpleural bullae (*large arrows*) are evident, and minimal centrilobular emphysema also is apparent. **B,** further cephalad, large right-sided apical adenocarcinoma (*arrows*) is evident. (Courtesy of Stern EJ, Webb WR, Weinacker A, et al: *AJR* 162:279–282, 1994.)

be confused with pneumothorax. All patients had subpleural bullae. All but 2 also had intraparenchymal bullae, which were not larger than 2–3 cm in diameter. In the apical region, the bullae occupied most of the thorax. All patients had evidence of paraseptal emphysema that was contiguous with the larger subpleural bullae (Fig 14–1). Eight patients also had some degree of centrilobular emphysema. One patient had a pneumothorax that had not been noted on chest radiographs.

Conclusion.—The predominant finding in these patients with vanishing lung syndrome was the presence of extensive paraseptal emphysema that coalesced into giant bullae.

▶ First described in 1937, this baffling, emphysema-like condition is rare, although it is progressive and may be fatal. In more recent studies, vanishing lung has been termed type I bullous disease or primary bullous disease of the lung. Patients are initially seen with dyspnea and radiographic findings of large bullae that may occupy the upper two thirds of both hemithoraces; the condition occurs most often in young men who smoke. In this study of 9 patients with giant bullae, a closer look at the vanishing lung was obtained by using CT.

The criteria for vanishing lung in this study included bullae that occupy at least one third of a hemithorax. In these patients, multiple giant bullae with diameters usually ranging from 2 to 8 cm, but up to 20 cm, were seen; the distribution of the bullae was often asymmetrical, and no single bulla was seen to dominate in terms of volume. The bullae compress adjacent tissues, further compromising pulmonary function. The development of vanishing lung appears to begin with paraseptal emphysema that merges into giant bullae. Although this event may take place in both smokers and nonsmokers, smokers who have complications of centrilobar emphysema become symptomatic.

In treating this malady, surgical bullectomy can provide clinical improvement, and other, less invasive, operative techniques are now being evaluated that, if validated, may result in fewer complications than more invasive techniques. However, underlying and associated disorders may have serious implications in treatment. The additional data provided by CT can assist in elucidating these factors; for instance, Gaensler and associates concluded that the best surgical results can be obtained when the bullae are associated with paraseptal emphysema (1), which can be seen in CT scans and may be considered a positive indication for surgery. On the other hand, the presence of centrilobular emphysema has been associated with poor outcome after bullectomy. Other conditions that may accompany vanishing lung and can be better assessed with CT are bronchiectasis, infected cysts, pleural disease, pulmonary artery enlargement, and pneumothorax.—R.C. Bone, M.D.

Reference

1. Gaensler E, Jederlinic P, FitzGerald M: Patient work-up for bullectomy. *J Thorac Imaging* 1:75–93, 1986.

Is the Short-Term Response to Inhaled β-Adrenergic Agonist Sensitive or Specific for Distinguishing Between Asthma and COPD?
Kesten S, Rebuck AS (Toronto Hosp)
Chest 105:1042–1045, 1994   119-95-14-2

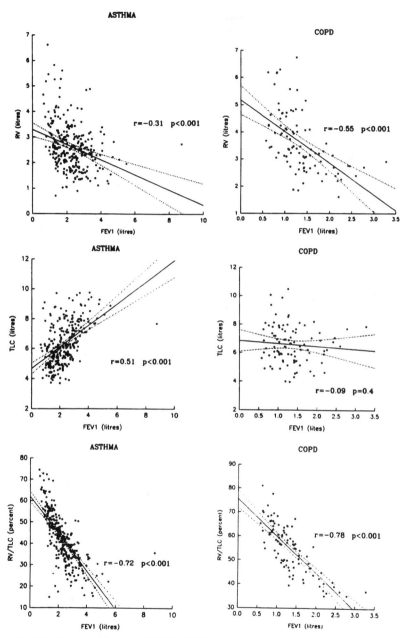

Fig 14–2.—Correlation between RV, TLC, RV:TLC ratio, and FEV₁. (Courtesy of Kesten S, Rebuck AS: *Chest* 105:1042–1045, 1994.)

Introduction.—There is no agreement regarding clinical standards for distinguishing chronic obstructive pulmonary disease (COPD) from asthma, although bronchodilator responsiveness is frequently used. Other laboratory indices that might be useful in diagnosing and evaluating COPD were examined retrospectively. In addition, the usefulness of forced vital capacity (FVC), forced expiratory volume in 1 second (FEV_1), residual volume (RV), and total lung capacity (TLC) in distinguishing between COPD and asthma was assessed.

Methods.—Pulmonary function studies were conducted in 287 patients, aged 48–50 years, with a diagnosis of asthma, and 108 patients, aged 63–67 years, with a diagnosis of COPD. Forced expiratory volume in 1 second and FVC were measured.

Results.—Although FEV_1 was significantly larger in patients with asthma than in those with COPD, FVC was similar for the 2 groups. Sensitivities and specificities of FEV_1 were generally low for the diagnosis of asthma; FEV_1 correlated with RV in patients with COPD, and with TLC in those with asthma (Fig 14–2). There was a correlation between FEV_1 and the RV–TLC ratio, which was similar for both groups.

Summary.—Stable COPD responds better to anticholinergic agents and infrequently to steroids, whereas asthma is better managed with β-agonists and steroids. Bronchodilator responses failed to distinguish between COPD and asthma. Changes in FEV_1 and FVC after inhalation of bronchodilators were neither sensitive nor specific enough to distinguish between COPD and asthma. Lung volume correlated better with the RV–TLC ratio than with either RV or TLC alone.

▶ The reversibility of airflow obstruction has always been a key criterion for resolving asthma from COPD. Studies of asthma often require the presence of approximately 15% reversibility of airway obstruction as proof of the presence of asthma, whereas studies of COPD may make the absence of reversibility an entrance condition. However, a recent study by Meslier and colleagues found that the reversibility criterion could not be used to discriminate between a small group of patients with asthma and one with chronic bronchitis, showing a lack of both specificity and sensitivity (1). The authors of this study enrolled 395 patients with either asthma or COPD into an evaluation of airway response to bronchodilator treatment. In addition to the standard measure of FEV_1, the authors also chose to assess the additional pulmonary function values of FVC, RV, and TLC in the differentiation of asthma from COPD.

If an increase in the FEV_1 of 20% or more, in the face of a 200-mL minimum increase, is used as a criterion, the sensitivity in diagnosing asthma is 29% and the specificity is 87%; when the percentage increase is lowered to 10% or more, the sensitivity is 58% and the specificity is 77%. When the percent predicted FEV_1 was used as a criterion, the results were much the same, with very low sensitivities and somewhat better specificities. In looking at other measures of pulmonary function, the authors found that the FEV_1

correlated with the RV, TLC, and RV–TLC in patients with asthma but only with the RV and RV–TLC in those with COPD.

The results of this study indicate that the response of the airway to bronchodilator is of little use in differentiating asthma from COPD. This fact should be carefully considered by those designing studies of these disease conditions and by the physicians who use the results of those studies to guide their treatment of patients who have asthma or COPD.

I guess it comes down to "what's in a name?" Names give physicians and patients a label that they can associate with symptoms—I imagine that makes both feel better about the state of their knowledge. Unfortunately, in many patients, it is essentially a false security and may actually be misleading. I would rather call the entities obstructive lung disease that are responsive to treatment with bronchodilators (β-agonists, ipratropium bromide, or both) and/or steroids. That way, patients would not be denied therapeutic trials with specific agents just because they were mislabeled. Remember, 15% to 20% of all patients who are described as having COPD by experienced physicians respond to corticosteroids. Thus, many patients who are labeled with COPD and might respond are denied a therapeutic trial of corticosteroids.—R.C. Bone, M.D.

Reference

1. Meslier N, Racineux JL, Six P, Lockhart A: Diagnostic value of reversibility of chronic airway obstruction to separate asthma from chronic bronchitis. *Eur Respir J* 2:497–505, 1989.

In Chronic Obstructive Pulmonary Disease, a Combination of Ipratropium and Albuterol Is More Effective Than Either Agent Alone: An 85-Day Multicenter Trial
Bone R, for the COMBIVENT Inhalation Aerosol Study Group (Med College of Ohio, Toledo)
Chest 150:1411–1419, 1994   119-95-14-3

Objective.—Studies have shown that patients with chronic obstructive pulmonary disease (COPD) respond better to a combination of β-agonists and anticholinergic bronchodilators than to either agent used alone. This combination is used everywhere but in North America. In a double-blind, randomized, parallel-group, 12-week prospective study, the long-term effects of concurrent administration of albuterol-ipratropium inhalation therapy vs. administration of either drug alone were evaluated.

Methods.—Five hundred thirty-four patients with COPD, aged 40–88 years, with a minimum 10-year history of smoking were included. In addition to corticosteroids and theophylline, the patients received either 100 μg of albuterol, 21 μg of ipratropium, or a combination of the 2 drugs an average of 4 times a day for 85 days. Tests of pulmonary function tests were conducted on days 1, 29, 57, and 85 at 15, 30, and 60 minutes after inhalation and hourly for a total of 8 hours.

Results.—Fewer patients who received combination therapy than those who received either drug alone withdrew because of adverse effects, the most common of which were lower respiratory tract symptoms. Total and 4-hour dosing forced expiratory volume in 1 second (FEV_1) values and mean peak responses showed that the combination was better than either drug alone. The mean peak increases over baseline for FEV_1 on the 4 test days were 31% to 33% for the combination, 24% to 27% for albuterol, and 24% to 25% for ipratropium. Area under the curve and forced vital capacity values were significantly higher for the combination than for either of the drugs alone.

Conclusion.—The combination is as safe as, and significantly more effective than, either drug alone and provides 20% to 40% more bronchodilation, possibly by decreasing the rate of decline of FEV_1.

▶ Although the relative irreversibility of airway obstruction has long been considered a hallmark of COPD, it has also been known that the airways in this disease do respond to both β-adrenergic agonist and anticholinergic bronchodilators, the latter being the most effective. Because these 2 drugs work by different mechanisms, it is reasonable to assume that their effects might be additive and, indeed, 5 of 7 studies comparing albuterol plus ipratropium have indicated that the combination is better than either agent alone (1–7). These were generally poorly controlled studies, however, with few patients and too low a power to find significant improvements. Nonetheless, combination therapy has been approved and made available in most countries for some time. This study is a double-blind, randomized, parallel-group design, multicenter study that enrolled 534 patients in an effort to understand the effects of combination therapy better. Therapy consisted of 2 puffs from a dual-drug, metered-dose inhaler containing 21 μg of ipratropium bromide and 120 μg of albuterol sulfate.

The results of this study confirm the benefits of combination therapy. An additional bronchodilation of 20% to 40% over that of single agents characterized the combination. In addressing the important question of whether long-term bronchodilator therapy slows the rate of pulmonary function decline in patients with COPD, no change was seen in baseline patient characteristics during the 3-month course of this study. Much longer studies would be needed to confirm any such effect. The safety of this dual-drug treatment appeared to be better than that which would be expected from the additive effects of the 2 agents—more patients dropped out of the single-drug arms of the study than the combination arm. The dual-drug metered-dose inhaler is easy to use and should improve patient compliance. A determination of the long-term effects of this therapy is awaited.—R.C. Bone, M.D.

References

1. Casali L, Grassi C, Rampulla C, Rossi A: Clinical pharmacology of a combination of bronchodilators. *Int J Clin Pharmacol Biopharm* 7:277–280, 1979.
2. Lees AW, Allan GW, Smith J: Nebulised ipratropium bromide and salbutamol in chronic bronchitis. *Br J Clin Pract* 3:340–342, 1980.
3. Leitch AG, Hopkin JM, Ellis DA, Merchant S, McHardy GJR: The effect of aerosol ipratropium bromide and salbutamol on exercise tolerance in chronic bronchitis. *Thorax* 33:711–713, 1978.
4. Petrie GR, Palmer KNV: Comparison of aerosol ipratropium bromide and salbutamol in chronic bronchitis and asthma. *BMJ* 1:430–432, 1975.
5. Lightbody IM, Ingram CG, Legge JS, Johnston RN: Ipratropium bromide, salbutamol and prednisolone in bronchial asthma and chronic bronchitis. *Br J Dis Chest* 72:181–186, 1978.
6. Easton PA, Jadue C, Dhingra S, Anthonisen NR: A comparison of the bronchodilating effects of a beta-2 adrenergic agent (albuterol) and an anticholinergic agent (ipratropium bromide) given by aerosol alone or in sequence. *N Engl J Med* 315:735–739, 1985.
7. Lloberes P, Ramis L, Montserrat JM, Serra J, Campistol J, Picdo C, et al: Effect of three different bronchodilators during an exacerbation of chronic obstructive pulmonary disease. *Eur Respir J* 1:536–539, 1988.

Bronchodilator Reversibility to Low and High Doses of Terbutaline and Ipratropium Bromide in Patients With Chronic Obstructive Pulmonary Disease

Newnham DM, Dhillon DP, Winter JH, Jackson CM, Clark RA, Lipworth BJ
(Univ of Dundee, Scotland; King's Cross Hosp, Dundee, Scotland)
Thorax 48:1151–1155, 1993   119-95-14-4

Introduction.—There is no general agreement on whether combining anticholinergic drugs with β-agonists is beneficial to patients with chronic obstructive pulmonary disease (COPD) or on the use of forced expiratory in volume in 1 second (FEV_1), forced vital capacity (FVC), or relaxed vital capacity (RVC) as measures of bronchodilator response in these patients. The responses of patients with COPD to low and high doses of terbutaline and ipratropium were examined, and different measures of bronchodilator response were evaluated.

Methods.—Twenty-seven patients with COPD (average age, 69 years) who were smokers or former smokers and had chronic bronchitis and an FEV_1 of less than 60% of normal received inhalation therapy. In sequence 1, all patients received 500 μg of terbutaline, 5,000 μg of terbutaline, 40 μg of ipratropium bromide, and 200 μg of ipratropium bromide on consecutive days. In sequence 2, low and high doses of ipratropium bromide were administered and followed by low and high doses of terbutaline. Measurements of FEV_1, FVC, and RVC were recorded at baseline and at 30 minutes after each dose.

Results.—Measurements of FEV_1, RVC, and FVC did not differ significantly from baseline. Improvement in bronchodilator responses was seen in approximately 75% of patients in sequence 1 and 81% of those

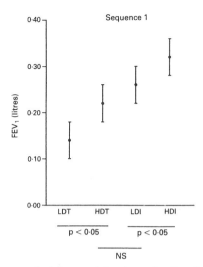

Fig 14–3.—Effects of sequential inhalation with low-dose terbutaline, 500 μg (*LDT*), high-dose terbutaline, 5,000 μg (*HDT*), low-dose ipratropium, 40 μg (*LDI*), and high-dose ipratropium, 200 μg (*HDI*) as sequence 1 and the reverse order (LDI, HDI, LDT, HDT) as sequence 2 on FEV_1 responses. Responses are shown as means and 95% confidence intervals of change from baseline for all 27 patients. (Courtesy of Newnham DM, Dhillon DP, Winter JH, et al: *Thorax* 48:1151–1155, 1993.)

in sequence 2 (Fig 14–3). When ipratropium was given first, high-dose terbutaline did not yield an improvement over low-dose terbutaline. When low-dose terbutaline was given first, however, high-dose terbutaline gave rise to a significant improvement, particularly as assessed by RVC.

Discussion.—Relaxed vital capacity, FEV_1, and PVC were all good indicators of response to combined therapy. Other studies have shown that patients with COPD respond better to low doses of inhaled ipratropium bromide than to inhaled β_2-agonist.

Conclusion.—There was no significant benefit from high-dose terbutaline administered after ipratropium bromide. Although all bronchodilator response measures detect responders, RVC appears to be particularly useful for detecting responses in patients with COPD who do not have a significant FEV_1 response.

▶ Although many studies have indicated that combination therapy consisting of β-adrenergic agonists and cholinergic antagonists is the best that one can do for the patients with COPD, the matter is not without controversy. Even when just 2 forms of drugs are examined, questions of dosing, order, and specific drug have confounded the results. For instance, many studies have examined either high or low doses of both drugs rather than some of the other likely permutations, including order of treatment.

The authors of this study also address an additional controversy regarding the question of assessment of obstructive disease: should forced or relaxed lung volumes be used? In assessing obstruction, the FVC and FEV_1 have generally been considered as the standard. However, the RVC, which is an indicator of relaxed lung volume, may also be useful in this assessment. The results of this study support both the forced and relaxed lung methods, finding that all 3 measurements were equally useful in assessing the effects of drugs examined.

Patients in this study had just recovered from an acute exacerbation of COPD, requiring hospitalization and treatment with nebulized salbutamol, but were considered to have stable COPD. Each patient received 2 different sequences of the drugs on 2 different days after the acquisition of stable baseline measurements of pulmonary function. Sequence 1 consisted of 500 μg of terbutaline administered in 2 puffs, followed by 500 μg of terbutaline administered in 5 puffs, 40 μg of ipratropium administered in 2 puffs, and 200 μg of ipratropium administered in 5 puffs. The second sequence was the reverse of the first, starting with low-dose ipratropium, followed by high-dose ipratropium, low-dose terbutaline, and high-dose terbutaline. Thirty minutes after each drug was administered, each of the 3 assessment methods was applied. Improvements were seen after each sequential dose, except when high-dose terbutaline was administered as the last drug in the series. In other words, the higher doses and the combination drug effect were beneficial in these patients except when high-dose terbutaline followed administration of ipratropium. The authors speculate that this may occur as the dose-response curve for terbutaline is flattened by the inhibition of vagal tone caused by ipratropium. The failure of high-dose terbutaline to improve ventilatory function further can only be seen clearly in the measurements of RVC, validating that method as an adjunctive method to the determination of FEV_1 in the assessment of bronchodilator dosing.

Although experience in COPD is limited, the recent release of salmeterol may be a very important addition to our treatment regimen for COPD. I believe this longer-acting β-adrenergic agonist may be very suitable for patients with COPD, as well as for patients with asthma (1, 2). Why? Its prolonged activity. In vitro and in vivo evidence indicates that activity continues for 12 hours—a major advantage. Also, whereas salmeterol and albuterol produce similar maximal bronchodilation in patients with asthma (3), salmeterol does so at lower doses (2). In fact, salmeterol (42 μg twice daily) produced results superior to 180 μg of albuterol given 4 times a day in patients with asthma. Additionally, salmeterol may be a more effective and less toxic alternative to theophylline in patients with recurrent nocturnal airway obstruction (see the commentary for Abstract 119-95-14–3 about mislabeling patients with asthma and those with COPD).

Another recent addition to our therapeutic armamentarium is the recent approval of a nebulizer solution of ipratropium bromide (IB). In fact, nebulized IB (500 μg) was recently compared with nebulized albuterol (5 mg) (4). One third of the patients responded to neither, one third responded to both, and one third responded to only 1 agent or the other. In another study, when patients were given both albuterol and IB by nebulizer, the majority requested the combination therapy (6). I believe we should be treating obstructive lung disease with both agents. Today we can't, except by nebulizer. Hopefully, the Food and Drug Administration will someday approve a combination inhaler.—R.C. Bone, M.D.

References

1. Frew AJ, Kennedy SM, Chan-Yeung M: Methacholine responsiveness, smoking and atopy as risk factors for accelerated FEV_1 decline in male working populations. *Am Rev Respir Dis* 146:878–883, 1992.
2. Pearlman DS, Cherirnsky P, LaForce C, et al: A comparison of salmeterol with albuterol in the treatment of mild-to-moderate asthma. *N Engl J Med* 327:1420–1425, 1992.
3. Midgren B, Melander B, Persson G: Formoterol, a new long-acting β_2 agonist inhaled twice daily in stable asthma subjects. *Chest* 101:1019–1022, 1992.
4. Palmer JBD, Stuart AM, Shephard GL, Viskum K: Inhaled salmeterol in the treatment of patients with moderate to severe reversible obstructive airways disease—A 3-month comparison of the efficacy and safety of twice-daily salmeterol (100 µg) with salmeterol (50 µg). *Respir Med* 86:409–417, 1992.
5. Nisar M, Earis JE, Pearson MG, Calverley PMA: Acute bronchodilator trials in chronic obstructive pulmonary disease. *Am Rev Respir Dis* 146:555–559, 1992.
6. O'Driscoll BR, Kay EA, Taylor RJ, et al: A long-term prospective assessment of home nebulizer treatment. *Respir Med* 86:317–325, 1992.

Effects of Theophylline Withdrawal in Severe Chronic Obstructive Pulmonary Disease
Kirsten DK, Wegner RE, Jörres RA, Magnussen H (Hosp Grosshansdorf, Germany)
Chest 104:1101–1107, 1993   119-95-14-5

Introduction.—Although theophylline, cholinergic receptor antagonists, and β_2-agonists are used to treat patients with chronic obstructive pulmonary disease (COPD), no controlled study has examined the efficacy of theophylline in combined therapy. In a randomized, double-blind, placebo-controlled trial, the effect of theophylline withdrawal was studied in patients with COPD.

Methods.—Thirty-eight patients with COPD, aged 40–80 years, received either theophylline or placebo by inhalation over a 6-day period. In 18 patients, theophylline was withdrawn and replaced by placebo from day 3 on. Serum levels of theophylline, blood gases, and pulmonary function were measured. Exercise performance was tested, and clinical rating, quality of life, and dyspnea were assessed.

Results.—When exercise performance was tested and clinical symptoms, dyspnea, and quality of life were rated, there was no significant difference between groups (table). Lung function, partial pressure of CO_2 in arterial blood ($PaCO_2$), symptom scores, and breathing scores in 72% of placebo recipients decreased significantly after theophylline therapy was withheld. Thirteen patients in the placebo group were considered theophylline responders.

Six-Minute Walking Distance, Results of CRQ, Clinical Ratings
of Overall Dyspnea, and Clinical Scoring of Symptoms and
Auscultation Findings Before and 2 Days After Withdrawal
of Theophylline

	Placebo Group Withdrawn		Theophylline Group Continued	
	Days 1 & 2	Days 5 & 6	Days 1 & 2	Days 5 & 6
6 min walking distance (m)	357 ± 124	337 ± 116	419 ± 145	446 ± 139 †
CRQ *	97.9 ± 11.4	95.4 ± 16.6	101.7 ± 18.1	103.1 ± 20.8
BDI *	4.4 ± 2.2	—	4.5 ± 2.7	—
TDI *		−0.9 ± 1.9	—	0.4 ± 2.6 †
OCD *	53.0 ± 15.6	52.9 ± 15.4	49.2 ± 16.3	51.2 ± 18.1
MRC scale *	1.9 ± 1.0	2.1 ± 1.1	2.1 ± 1.0	1.9 ± 1.1
Symptom score	3.4 ± 1.7	4.2 ± 1.7 †	2.8 ± 1.6	2.8 ± 1.9
Auscultation score	5.8 ± 2.8	6.7 ± 3.5 †	5.9 ± 2.0	5.6 ± 1.8

Abbreviations: CRQ, chronic respiratory disease questionnaire; BDI, baseline
dyspnea index; TDI, transition dyspnea index; OCD, oxygen cost diagram; MRC,
Medical Research Council.
Note: Values are means ± 1 SD. Significance levels are given for comparisons of
assessments on days 5 and 6 vs. days 1 and 2 within groups, and the comparison of
TDI in the theophylline group vs. the placebo group.
* $n = 35$ patients (19 in theophylline group).
† $P < .05$.
(Courtesy of Kirsten DK, Wegner RE, Jörres RA, et al: *Chest* 104:1101–1107,
1993.)

Discussion.—Although the improvement seen with theophylline was
small, it was significant. Patients with more serious COPD are more
likely to benefit from theophylline therapy. Approximately half of the
patients were categorized as theophylline responders. Because theophylline withdrawal was not directly correlated with lung function, effects in
addition to bronchodilation may be at work. Because the response of
patients with COPD to theophylline therapy is speculative at best, patients must be evaluated individually.

▶ And it's another big rematch: theophylline, β_2-adrenergic agonists, cholinergic receptor antagonists, and combinations of the 3 in the treatment of
patients with COPD. Despite the fact that the strengths of these agents have
been tested many times before, often with discrepant results, these high-
powered combination therapies are, once again, head to head in a trial that
examines the effects of optimal doses of the specific receptor effectors. The
question to be asked is as follows: When dosages of the 2 receptor effectors
are truly optimized, will withdrawal from ongoing theophylline treatments
have deleterious effects on the patient's condition? This is a unique approach to the question of the effectiveness of theophylline that provides a

direct answer to a question being voiced by physicians, as theophylline is currently included in the therapeutic regimen of many patients with COPD.

And, in this matchup, the theophylline combination regimen is, once again, a winner. Two days after the substitution of placebo, study participants underwent small but significant detrimental changes in lung function, Paco$_2$, exercise performance, dyspnea, and other symptoms. In at least half the patients in this group, these changes manifested in a clinically relevant fashion, including changes in the 6-minute test of walking distance. Theophylline responders and nonresponders could not be distinguished by their forced expiratory volume in 1 second response to inhaled β-agonist. This ties in with our lack of knowledge about the ultimate therapeutic effect of theophylline in obstructive lung disease. It may not only produce bronchodilation but it may also work through some effect on the CNS by changing breathing patterns or, among several theories, by altering the hypoxic drive.

The toxic nature of theophylline and its side effects, however, which were noted and not uncommon in this study, should always be remembered when determining dosing of this drug. Because theophylline is often used in patients with advanced disease, this may be a delicate balance. The results of this study indicate that about half the patients with COPD will respond favorably to theophylline. Thus, trial withdrawals from theophylline treatment for individual patients may be a recommended method of determining whether treatment with a potentially toxic drug should be continued or curtailed.—R.C. Bone, M.D.

Replacement Therapy for Hereditary Alpha$_1$-Antitrypsin Deficiency: A Program for Long-Term Administration
Barker AF, Siemsen F, Pasley D, D'Silva R, Buist AS (Oregon Health Sciences Univ, Portland)
Chest 105:1406–1410, 1994   119-95-14–6

Background.—Short-term studies have demonstrated the biological efficacy of weekly and monthly IV infusion of human α_1-antitrypsin (AAT) in individuals with hereditary AAT deficiency, PiZ phenotype, and emphysema. The long-term effects of AAT infusion on functional capacity and pulmonary function were evaluated.

Methods.—Fourteen patients with AAT deficiency, PiZ phenotype, and chronic obstructive pulmonary disease (COPD) began weekly infusion of AAT, 60 mg/kg, and were subsequently maintained at 120–180 mg/kg every 2-3 weeks. Patient charts were reviewed.

Results.—Duration of treatment was 12–48 months. Functional status stabilized in 12 patients, and hospitalizations were reduced in 4. Pulmonary function stabilized in 13 patients, even though 11 patients had demonstrated a steady decrease in forced expiratory volume in 1 second (FEV$_1$) during the 12–20 months before treatment (Fig 14-4). Bronchodilator response exceeded 12% in 7 of 12 patients tested, a small but important change in those patients with severe obstruction. Three patients

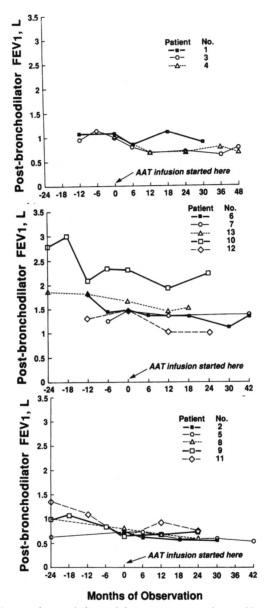

Fig 14-4.—Pulmonary function before and during augmentation therapy. (Courtesy of Barker AF, Siemsen F, Pasley D, et al: *Chest* 105:1406-1410, 1994.)

experienced self-limited adverse reactions to AAT; 1 required brief hospitalization.

Conclusion.—Augmentation therapy with AAT may stabilize lung function in patients with AAT deficiency and COPD. Whether these effects are derived directly from augmentation therapy or are the result of the close follow-up associated with therapy will be determined with more experience.

▶ In 1988, replacement therapy for individuals deficient in AAT became available in the United States. However, only short-term studies of this therapy have been performed to date. The authors of this study saw the need for confirmation that the long-term benefits of this therapy match those that are seen in the shorter term. They examined pulmonary function and side effects in patients with moderate-to-severe COPD who were treated with AAT for 1–4 years. This treatment is not recommended for patients who smoke, and none of the patients in this study had smoked for at least 1 year. This study was done with the caveat that a full clinical trial of this question would require more patients and funds than were available at the time. This study involved 14 patients with COPD who were treated with infusions of AAT, 120–180 mg/kg, every 2–3 weeks, such that trough levels of AAT were maintained above 60 mg/dL. Each patient was examined by the same physicians and pulmonary function laboratories during the study.

Patients treated with AAT remained stable through the course of the study. The FEV_1 remained relatively unchanged, although no statistical significance could be shown because of the short time period and small number of patients. The number of hospitalizations required for these patients decreased from the period previous to the infusion, although, again, no statistical significance was ascribed to this effect. Only 4 adverse reactions were seen. These effects were associated with 2 lots of the drug that apparently contained adulterants. Ecchymosis, reported in some previous studies, was not seen in these patients.

As has been previously reported (1), a response of greater than 12% to bronchodilator treatment was seen in most of these patients, making such treatment a recommended mode when conditions are appropriate. This is a curious finding, however, in a disease that is theoretically irreversible. Further study of this phenomenon may be warranted to determine how this can occur.—R.C. Bone, M.D.

Reference

1. Tobin MJ, Cook PJL, Hutchison DCS: Alpha₁-antitrypsin deficiency: The clinical and physiological features of pulmonary and emphysema in subjects homozygous for features Pi type Z: A survey by the British Thoracic Association. *Br J Dis Chest* 77:14–27, 1983.

15 Cystic Fibrosis

Introduction

Remarkable advances have been made in our treatment of cystic fibrosis. These strides have added to longevity of patients with this disease. In fact, the median survival in 1992 was 32 years for men and 27.9 years for women (1). This increase in longevity probably has resulted from such treatments as aggressive antibiotic therapy and improved nutritional management. Hopefully, further increases in longevity will result from our increased understanding of the genetics of cystic fibrosis. The recent advances in our understanding of cystic fibrosis that have resulted from such research are astonishing. Many of these advances have been reviewed in the 1993 and 1994 volumes of the YEAR BOOK OF MEDICINE. At present, we know that the gene responsible for the disease has been identified and mapped to chromosome 7. Researchers also have been able to produce the abnormal protein that causes cystic fibrosis. Such studies have determined that this protein is an intramembranous chloride channel that regulates the conductance of chloride through the cell membrane. In patients with cystic fibrosis, the respiratory epithelium absorbs excess sodium and secretes chloride in a defective manner. The hope is that gene therapy soon may be possible. The gene has been inserted into rat tracheal cells in vivo using a retrovirus, and expression of the functional channel has continued for 6 months. In the 1993 YEAR BOOK OF MEDICINE, we reviewed the next step in this process, the development of an appropriate animal model of cystic fibrosis.

In the 1994 YEAR BOOK OF MEDICINE, we discussed the possibility of human gene therapy for patients with cystic fibrosis because of the availability of safe and effective aerosol delivery systems. In fact, researchers at the University of Iowa have recently inserted a healthy copy of the cystic fibrosis gene into an adenovirus and inserted the genetically altered virus into the nasal passages of volunteers with cystic fibrosis, thereby correcting the chloride flow defect in the nasal passages of these patients. What is left is the repair of malfunctioning cells in the intrapulmonary airways. This year's Cystic Fibrosis chapter takes the next step and analyzes the expression of the cystic fibrosis gene in the adult human lung. The results of that article show that cystic fibrosis has important implications for lung function through effects on the small airways and alveoli. These advances are pivotal, because they should soon lead us to therapies that are more than just supportive for this lethal disease.

Roger C. Bone, M.D.

Reference

1. Cystic Fibrosis National Registry. Bethesda, Md, Cystic Fibrosis Foundation, 1992.

Expression of the Cystic Fibrosis Gene in Adult Human Lung

Engelhardt JF, Zepeda M, Cohn JA, Yankaskas JR, Wilson JM (Univ of Pennsylvania, Philadelphia; Duke Univ, Durham, NC; Univ of North Carolina, Chapel Hill)
J Clin Invest 93:737–749, 1994   119-95-15–1

Introduction.—Cystic fibrosis (CF) causes life-threatening pathology in the lung. To understand the pathophysiology of CF lung disease better, the pattern of CF transmembrane conductance regulator (CFTR) expression and the localization of CFTR messenger RNA and protein in the lung were studied.

Methods.—Lung tissue specimens were obtained from the lungs of 8 adults with CF. At least 6 random fields each from the proximal bronchiole, terminal bronchiole, respiratory bronchiole, and alveoli were examined. In situ hybridization and immunocytochemical analysis were used to identify the cells expressing exceptional amounts of CFTR messenger RNA and CFTR protein. Three tissue samples with high levels of CFTR expression were also analyzed for CC10 expression, a gene that identifies the presence of a subtype of Clara cells.

Results.—A higher number of epithelial cells expressing CFTR messenger RNA were found in the respiratory and terminal bronchioles than in the proximal bronchioles and alveoli. Higher expression occurred in alveolar cells with a cuboidal shape, suggesting that expression occurred in type II pneumocytes rather than squamous type I pneumocytes or intra-alviolar macrophages. Cystic fibrosis transmembrane conductance regulator protein was localized to the apical surface of primarily nonciliated airway epithelial cells, but no cell type could be identified. The 3 samples expressing high levels of CFTR also demonstrated high expression of CC10 in more than half the cells of the proximal bronchioles and much lower or no expression of CC10 in the terminal and respiratory bronchioles and the alveolar regions. Expression of CFTR occurred in a subset of the regions expressing CC10 in the proximal bronchioles and occurred without expression of CC10 in the terminal and respiratory bronchioles and the alveoli.

Discussion.—These findings indicate that CFTR RNA and protein are expressed in certain of the epithelial cells in all of the distal airway structures. The strongest expression occurred equally in the terminal and respiratory bronchioles, suggesting that these structures may have a shared mechanism for facilitating transport of CFTR-mediated chloride. The partial concordance between CFTR and CC10 expression suggests that expression of CFTR occurs in either a subpopulation of Clara cells or in some other nonciliated cell type. Further study of the specific cell type expressing CFTR will have important implications for gene therapy strategies.

▶ The most deadly effects of the CF gene mutation occur within the lung. Impaired pulmonary function can result in malnutrition, clubbing, and inhibited growth. Although much has been learned about the exact underlying genetic and molecular causes of CF, the accepted treatment modes to date have not changed dramatically. The essential effect of the CF gene is a dysfunctional chloride channel—the CFTR—which results in abnormal secretions. In the lung, these secretions cause obstruction and promote the development of infection. A number of molecular biological techniques are now being used with high expectations in an effort to correct the deficiency, although no panacea is available.

To understand better how CF affects pulmonary function, the authors of this study have examined the distribution of CFTR messenger RNA transcripts within the lung to determine the distribution of expression of the abnormal gene. Previous studies have shown little CFTR expression on the surface epithelium of the bronchus, whereas high levels of expression have been seen in the submucosal glands within the cartilage-supported proximal airways (1). Little is known, however, about CFTR expression in the bronchioles and alveoli. Nonciliated secretory cells, or Clara cells, which produce a marker known as CC10, are found largely in the smaller bronchioles and were used in this study to aid in the localization of CFTR expression.

The findings indicate that considerable expression of CFTR occurs in the distal regions of the respiratory tree, particularly in the respiratory bronchioles and the alveoli. Much variability was seen between individual study participants and between individual cells within a locality. For instance, the ciliated cells within the smaller bronchioles do not appear to express the protein. Such a finding suggests a greater degree of heterogeneity of the cells at this level of the bronchial tree than had previously been shown. It was also seen that the distribution of CFTR expression does not match that of CC10 expression, indicating possible heterogeneity among the nonciliated cells. These results indicate that CF may have important implications for lung function, even down to the level of the smaller bronchioles and the alveoli.—R.C. Bone, M.D.

Reference

1. Engelhardt JF, Yankaskas JR, Ernst SA, Yang Y, Marino CR, Boucher JA, Cohn JA, Wilson JM: Submucosal glands are the predominant site of CFTR expression within the human bronchus. *Nat Genet* 2:240–248, 1992.

16 Lung Cancer

Introduction

Lung cancer is one frustrating disease: its cause is known in 90% of cases (cigarette smoking); operative techniques have markedly improved; and genetic markers of disease susceptibility and metastatic potential are now being appreciated. Paradoxically, while researchers are continuing to make inroads into our understanding of lung cancer, we are finding that the incidence and overall mortality attributed to lung cancer continue to increase worldwide. Currently in the United States, lung cancer produces more deaths than any other type of cancer.

Hopefully, our science will translate into improved survival someday. Because lung cancer is so often disseminated at discovery, this will probably only result from improvements in prevention and earlier diagnoses and, possibly, through the use of our new understanding of the genetics associated with lung cancer to assist in prevention, diagnosis, and treatment. The first study in this chapter examines the potential relationship of pulmonary hamartomas and malignancy. The frequency of such a relationship is more than 6 times greater than that which is expected in the general population. Because adrenal metastases are frequently found in non–small-cell lung cancer, the accuracy of CT scanning and MRI in detecting both enlargement and potential metastasis is evaluated in the second abstract. Survival after either sleeve lobectomy or pneumonectomy is evaluated in the third abstracted article. The fourth abstract describes a randomized trial comparing preoperative chemotherapy plus surgery with surgery alone in patients who have IIIA non–small-cell lung cancer, as staged by the tumor-node-metastasis system. The study found that patients with non–small-cell lung cancer who undergo preoperative chemotherapy have an increased median survival rate compared with those who undergo surgery only.

Roger C. Bone, M.D.

Pulmonary Hamartoma and Malignancy
Ribet M, Jaillard-Thery S, Nuttens MC (Hôpital Calmette, Lille, France; Centre Hospitalier Universitaire, Lille, France)
J Thorac Cardiovasc Surg 107:611–614, 1994   119-95-16–1

Introduction.—Pulmonary hamartomas are considered benign. They have been associated with malignancy, however, especially with bronchial carcinoma. The nature of the association between pulmonary hamartomas and lung cancer was explored retrospectively.

Methods.—The records of 61 patients undergoing surgery for a pulmonary or endobronchial hamartoma were studied. Medical histories, chest radiographs, operative findings, and pathologic reports were reviewed. The incidence of bronchial carcinoma during a mean follow-up of 9 years (range, 1–22 years) was compared with the incidence in the general population in the same area at the same time.

Results.—Ten patients with a hamartoma also had a malignancy. In 2 of these patients, the pulmonary hamartomas were associated with an incomplete Carney's triad. Eight patients had various forms of carcinoma affecting the skin, esophagus, stomach, thyroid, and tongue, and 3 had bronchial squamous carcinomas, which appeared synchronously or preceded or followed the hamartoma. All the patients with bronchial carcinomas were smokers. The incidence of bronchial carcinoma was 6.66 times higher than that in the general population.

Discussion.—Hamartomas are clearly associated with bronchial carcinomas, and the association can be either synchronous or metachronous. These findings, however, do not establish a causal association. A multicenter prospective study using multivariate analysis of risk factors is needed to establish the significance of the association. Nevertheless, patients with pulmonary hamartomas should be closely followed.

▶ The presence of pulmonary hamartoma has been associated with certain forms of pulmonary and extrapulmonary malignancy. Although hamartomas are nearly always harmless, this association with more serious disease needs to be confirmed and, if confirmed, its significance should be closely examined. Answers to these questions may come more easily when the origin of hamartoma is understood. Hamartoma is commonly considered a developmental dysfunction. There is some controversy, however, with that idea—some think that the nodules may arise as a result of external factors or inflammatory activity. Although they have the appearance of neoplasms, hamartomas generally consist of elements of the tissue in which they are situated and do not usually compress the surrounding tissues. Because of this and the fact that they have not previously been associated with malignancy, they are often managed with simple observation. However, resection may be necessary if the airway is restricted; such surgery rarely results in recurrence.

In this study, patients with surgically treated hamartoma were examined. Their cases were reviewed, and they received extensive follow-up. Approximately half of these cases were identified after the patient complained; others were discovered by chance on chest radiographs. As determined from patients with previous radiographs, the hamartomas, which ranged in size from .5–30 cm in diameter, were slowly enlarging, with a doubling rate of 2–26 years. Just more than half the hamartomas were treated with enucleation; the rest were resected through a variety of techniques. The mean follow-up was 9 years. Of 61 patients with hamartoma, 10 had an associated malignancy.

The frequency of squamous cell bronchial carcinomas in this study was 6.66 times greater than would be expected in the general population, a number that closely matched those obtained in a previous study (1). In assessing some demographic features of lung cancer and hamartoma (frequency and age), the authors found that they did not match as well as might be expected, given the above finding. This may decrease the significance of any association between hamartoma and lung cancer. As is so often the case in such a study, the issue of cause and effect is critical here. Although the authors advocate a multicenter trial to resolve this complicated issue, they also recommend that patients with hamartoma receive a complete evaluation with follow-up, based on the frequency of simultaneous occurrences of hamartoma and malignancy. This is sound advice: although this may not be a cause-and-effect association, nothing has been proven. Additionally, it is possible that certain external factors may predispose individuals to both conditions.—R.C. Bone, M.D.

Reference

1. Karasik A, Modan M, Jacob C, et al: Increased risk of lung cancer in patients with chondromatous hamartoma. *J Thorac Cardiovasc Surg* 80:216–220, 1980.

Prospective Evaluation of Unilateral Adrenal Masses in Patients With Operable Non-Small-Cell Lung Cancer: Impact of Magnetic Resonance Imaging

Burt M, Heelan RT, Coit D, McCormack PM, Bains MS, Martini N, Rusch V, Ginsberg RJ (Mem Sloan-Kettering Cancer Ctr, New York)

J Thorac Cardiovasc Surg 107:584–589, 1994   119-95-16–2

Background.—In a previous study, most unilateral adrenal masses in patients with otherwise operable non–small-cell lung cancer (NSCLC) were found to be benign. The ability of MRI to predict malignant or benign adrenal masses in such patients was investigated.

Methods.—Sixteen women and 11 men, aged 42–75 years, with a unilateral adrenal mass were enrolled. Twenty-three patients had adenocarcinoma, and 4 had epidermoid cancer of the lung. When a unilateral adrenal mass was found on CT, respiratory-compensated and cardiac-gated thin-section MRI of the adrenal glands was performed. The adrenal mass was judged malignant or benign by a radiologist. Percutaneous needle biopsy of the adrenal mass was then done if technically possible. If the biopsy specimen was nondiagnostic or a biopsy was not feasible, an adrenalectomy was done through a posterior approach.

Findings.—The clinical locoregional stage was I in 9 patients, II in 1, IIIA in 16, and IIIB in 1. Twenty-five patients completed MRI. Nineteen percent of adrenal masses were metastatic NSCLC; 81% were benign

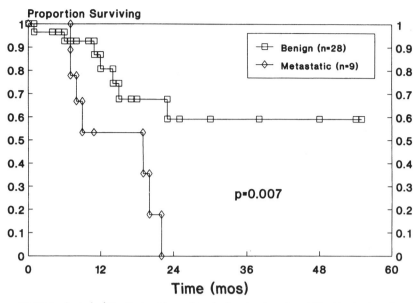

Proportion Surviving

Fig 16–1.—Survival of 9 patients with a unilateral adrenal metastasis and 28 with a benign adrenal mass. Patients were in operable condition except for the adrenal mass. The survival of patients with benign disease was significantly longer than that of patients with metastatic disease. (Courtesy of Burt M, Heelan RT, Coit D, et al: *J Thorac Cardiovasc Surg* 107:584–589, 1994.)

(Fig 16-1). Patients with benign and malignant lesions did not differ in age, sex, histologic type, or locoregional stage. The malignant lesions, however, were significantly larger than the benign ones. Magnetic resonance imaging correctly predicted mass malignancy in the 4 patients with a histologically confirmed metastasis from NSCLC. In the 21 patients with histologically benign masses, however, MRI was interpreted as benign in 5, malignant in 14, and indeterminate in 2. Thus, the false negative rate was 0% and the false positive rate was 67%.

Conclusion.—The best available MRI scanning techniques could not consistently predict whether a unilateral mass was malignant or benign. Magnetic resonance imaging, therefore, cannot replace biopsy in the assessment of unilateral adrenal masses in patients with operable NSCLC.

▶ One of the more common complications of NSCLC is metastasis to the adrenal gland; reports variously indicate that this occurs with a frequency of 18% to 42%. In the case of operable lung cancer, however, these figures may be different; 1 study found that 8% of all patients with operable cancers had enlarged adrenal glands, as determined by CT (1). Of those patients, 26% had metastatic deposits on examination by needle biopsy or additional CT scanning. Among 10 patients examined in this study who had operable NSCLC and adrenal swelling, as determined by CT scanning, 4 had biopsy-proven metastases to the adrenal gland. These studies indicate that 60% to 74% of the adrenal masses associated with NSCLC will ultimately prove to be benign. Thus, the ability to distinguish benign from malignant adrenal masses is critically important. The central purpose of this study was the use of new advances in MRI in prospectively evaluating adrenal swelling to determine whether it represents malignant or benign disease. It was believed that the development of new, higher-power magnets (1.5 T) might permit such a discrimination.

Unfortunately, these authors found that even state-of-the-art MRI techniques cannot be used to determine accurately whether swollen lymph glands associated with NSCLC are malignant. In 21 cases of histologically confirmed benign masses, only 5 were correctly diagnosed; 14 were considered malignant by MRI analysis. The technique was, however, highly sensitive (100%) in finding metastases.

Researchers continue to develop new modes of MRI, and one day it may be used to confirm benign adrenal disease accurately. Until then, however, the use of percutaneous needle aspiration biopsy in cases of adrenal masses associated with NSCLC is recommended. Although the authors noted that no mass of less than 2 cm was malignant, such an observation needs to be confirmed before clinicians can make treatment decisions based on that assumption.—R.C. Bone, M.D.

Reference

1. Oliver TW Jr, Bernardino ME, Miller JI, Mansour K, Greene D, David WA: Isolated adrenal masses in non–small-cell bronchogenic carcinoma. *Radiology* 153:217–218, 1991.

Survival Related to Nodal Status After Sleeve Resection for Lung Cancer
Mehran RJ, Deslauriers J, Piraux M, Beaulieu M, Guimont C, Brisson J (Laval Univ, Ste-Foy, Quebec, Canada)
J Thorac Cardiovasc Surg 107:576–583, 1994   119-95-16–3

Background.—Sleeve lobectomy, a lung-saving procedure indicated for central tumors, can be done instead of pneumonectomy. The relationship between survival and nodal status, however, is controversial. In most series, the presence of N1 disease adversely affects the prognosis, with few or no long-term survivors. A comparative analysis was based on nodal status.

Methods.—From 1972 to 1992, 142 patients, aged 11–78 years, underwent sleeve resection at 1 center (Fig 16–2). Surgery was indicated by a central tumor in 79% of patients, a peripheral tumor in 13%, and compromised pulmonary function in 8%. Histologic type was squamous in 72.5%, nonsquamous in 24.6%, and carcinoid in 2.8%.

Findings.—Resection was complete in 87% of patients. The operative mortality rate was 2.1%. Survival rates at 5 and 10 years were 46% and 33%, respectively. The 73 patients with N0 status had 5- and 10-year sur-

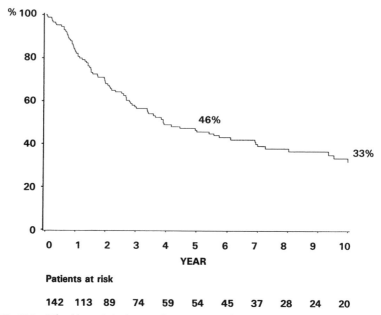

Fig 16–2.—Life-table analysis showing the percentage of all patients remaining alive after sleeve resection of bronchogenic carcinoma. (Courtesy of Mehran RJ, Deslauriers J, Piraux, et al: *J Thorac Cardiovasc Surg* 107:576–583, 1994.)

vival rates of 57% and 46%, respectively. Corresponding rates in the 55 patients with N1 status were 46% and 27%, respectively. None of the 14 patients with N2 status survived 5 years. Twenty-three percent of patients had local recurrences, but the prevalence did not differ significantly between those with N0 and N1 disease.

Conclusion.—Sleeve resection is an adequate treatment for patients with resectable lung cancer and N0 or N1 status. An N2 status makes the prognosis significantly worse and may be a contraindication for this procedure.

▶ The removal of diseased lung tissue via sleeve resection reduces the damage to the remaining lung tissue; hence, it was originally considered a technique to be used in patients for whom a normal pneumonectomy might result in inadequate pulmonary function. Recent reports have indicated, however, that sleeve lobectomy may be just as effective for removing cancerous tissues as other methods of resection. This technique may have the additional benefits of lower rates of operative mortality and improved quality of life.

The primary indication for sleeve resection is a lesion in the right upper lobe. An anatomical justification for this technique is derived from the fact that upper lobe lymphatic drainage tends to cause metastases to the nodes below the right upper lobe bronchus rather than lobes associated with the bronchus of the middle or lower lobes.

Previous studies have compared the effects of pneumonectomy, lobectomy, and sleeve lobectomy in patients with cancer. Patients with stages I and II non–small-cell lung cancers that had been resected had an overall 5-year survival rate of 45%, although the stage II disease 5-year survival rate was only 14%. Studies indicate that local recurrences may occur in 18% to 23% of these patients, whereas distant recurrences occur in 19% to 26%. Studies of sleeve resection indicate that its overall 5-year survival rate is 40%, whereas sleeve resection in stages I, II, and III disease are associated with 5-year survival rates of 63%, 37%, and 21%, respectively. Additionally, it has been noted that the absence of nodal involvement may improve survival to 60%. These figures for the 5-year survival rates of patients who undergo either lobectomy or sleeve lobectomy are better than those for patients who undergo pneumonectomy.

Controversy also remains over whether sleeve resection is appropriate when lymph nodes are involved. In 1 study, 5- and 10-year survival rates changed from 71% and 48.5% to 17% and 10%, respectively, when the nodes were involved. In another study, the same numbers were 59% and 47% (N0) and 21% and 0% (N1). The results of this study agreed most closely with a study by Naruke, who found a 5-year survival rate after sleeve resection of 50% for patients without nodal involvement and 45.9% for those with N1 disease (1). Naruke stated that sleeve resection is appropriate in N1 disease if it can be *completely* resected. Therein lies the rub. The best way to assure complete resection is the intraoperative evaluation of frozen lobar, hilar, and mediastinal lymph node sections, although there are no foolproof methods. The results of this study (46% 5-year survival rate for N0 disease, 57% for N1) indicate that lymph node involvement may not be significant in N1 disease. However, N2 disease carries a poorer prognosis, and, in this study, there were no 5-year survivors. The use of sleeve resection appears to provide similar results as conventional lobectomy in terms of survival. In addition, more functional lung tissue remains available to the patient or, should recurrent disease strike the region, for resection.—R.C. Bone, M.D.

Reference

1. Naruke T: Bronchoplastic and bronchovascular procedures of the tracheobronchial tree in the management of primary lung cancer. *Chest* 96:S53–S56, 1989.

A Randomized Trial Comparing Preoperative Chemotherapy Plus Surgery With Surgery Alone in Patients With Non–Small-Cell Lung Cancer

Rosell R, Gómez-Codina J, Camps C, Maestre J, Padille J, Cantó A, Mate JL, Li S, Roig J, Olazábal A, Canela M, Ariza A, Skácel Z, Morera-Prat J, Abad A (Univ of Barcelona; Hosp La Fe, Valencia, Spain; Hosp Gen, Valencia, Spain)
N Engl J Med 330:153–158, 1994   119-95-16-4

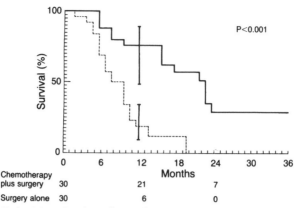

Fig 16–3.—Kaplan–Meier plot of overall survival in patients with stage IIIA lung cancer treated with surgery (*dashed line*) or chemotherapy and surgery (*solid line*). Ninety-five percent confidence intervals at 12 months are indicated (*bars*). The number of patients at risk is shown below the graph. (Courtesy of Rosell R, Gómez-Codina J, Camps C, et al: N Engl J Med 330:153–158, 1994.)

Objective.—Whether preoperative chemotherapy is a worthwhile addition to resection for patients with non–small-cell lung cancer (NSCLC) was determined.

Patients.—Fifty-nine men and 1 woman with histologically confirmed stage IIIA NSCLC were included. Patients were randomly assigned to surgery only or to 3 courses of preoperative chemotherapy. All patients received mediastinal irradiation after surgery in a cumulative dose of 50 Gy. Chemotherapy consisted of mitomycin (6 mg/m²), ifosfamide (3 g/m²), and cisplatin (50 mg/m²), all given intravenously at 3-week intervals. The patient groups were comparable in most respects.

Results.—Sixteen patients given chemotherapy had a partial radiographic response to treatment, and 2 had a complete response. The median disease-free survival time was 5 months for the surgical group and 20 months for patients given chemotherapy. The respective median overall survival times were 8 and 26 months. Among the surviving patients, the median follow-up was 19 months for those treated only surgically and 2 years for those given combined treatment. Relapses developed during follow-up in 56% of patients given combined treatment and in 74% of those who had only surgery. Overall survival is shown in Figure 16–3.

Tumor Characteristics.—The prevalence of mutated K-*ras* oncogenes was more than twice as great in the surgical group. These patients tended to have aneuploid tumor cells, whereas most of those given chemotherapy had tumors consisting of diploid cells.

Conclusion.—Preoperative chemotherapy prolongs the survival of patients undergoing resection of NSCLC.

▶ This study approaches an important question in the treatment of NSCLC: Should surgical resection be preceded by a chemotherapeutic regimen? The question of treatment for stage IIIA (N2) cancers has previously been studied with equivocal results, some of which may have resulted from nonstandardized techniques and definitions. It has also been reported that tumor size and location and the number of N2 levels involved may be predictive of outcome. A summary of the numbers obtained by several recent studies, in which a total of 1,180 patients were treated with surgery, yielded an overall 5-year survival rate of only 14% to 30% (1–4).

On the other hand, studies that included preoperative treatment with chemotherapy have found a 17% to 40% survival rate (5–11). Although it appears that benefits may accrue from pretreatment, their significance is unclear. The authors of this study have chosen to examine this issue carefully in a phase-3 trial of patients with stage IIIA cancers. The pretreatment regimen consisted of mitomycin, ifosfamide, and cisplatin sufficient to obtain a 60% response rate. This level was also associated with low toxicity.

The results of the trial indicate that preoperative chemotherapy is beneficial in this type of cancer. The mean period of disease-free survival was 5 months in the non–chemotherapy-treated group and 20 months in the treated group; the median overall survival of the former was 8 months, whereas mean survival in the treated group was 26 months. The results also indicated that the location or size of the tumor and the number of N2 levels involved were predictive of outcome. In a side analysis, the authors searched for the K-*ras* oncogene with oligonucleotide probes specific for known point mutations in tumor specimens from each of these patients. Twenty percent of the patients had such mutations; previous studies have shown that these patients form a subgroup that does not respond well to treatment and has poor survival. In this study, however, that correlation did not hold up: survival among the treated patients who underwent complete tumor resection was not influenced by K-*ras* status.

The results of this prospective, randomized study appear to support the use of presurgical chemotherapy in patients with stage IIIA NSCLC. However, a caveat should be noted in that differences between the groups could have had an effect on these results: The frequencies of aneuploidy and the K-*ras* oncogene were much greater among those not pretreated with chemotherapy. Nonetheless, this study should help improve the treatment of patients with this deadly form of cancer.—R.C. Bone, M.D.

References

1. Martini N, Flehinger BJ: The role of surgery in N2 lung cancer. *Surg Clin North Am* 67:1037–1049, 1987.
2. Watanabe Y, Shimizu J, Oda M, et al: Aggressive surgical intervention in N2 non–small-cell cancer of the lung. *Ann Thorac Surg* 51:253–261, 1991.
3. Naruke T, Goya T, Tsuchiya R, Suemasu K: The importance of surgery to non-small-cell carcinoma of lung with mediastinal lymph node metastasis. *Ann Thorac Surg* 46:603–610, 1988.
4. Mountain CF: Expanded possibilities for surgical treatment of lung cancer: Survival in stage IIIA disease. *Chest* 97:1045–1051, 1990.

5. Skarin A, Jochelson M, Sheldon T, et al: Neoadjuvant chemotherapy in marginally resectable stage III M0 non–small-cell lung cancer: Long-term follow-up in 41 patients. *J Surg Oncol* 40:266–274, 1989.
6. Faber LP, Kittle CF, Warren WH, et al: Preoperative chemotherapy and irradiation for stage 111 non–small-cell lung cancer. *Ann Thorac Surg* 47:669–677, 1989.
7. Martini N, Kris MG, Gralla RJ, et al: The effects of preoperative chemotherapy on the resectability of non–small-cell lung carcinoma with mediastinal lymph node metastases (N2 M0). *Ann Thorac Surg* 45:370–379, 1988.
8. Martini N, Kris MG, Flehinger BJ, et al: Preoperative chemotherapy for stage IIIA (N2) lung cancer: The Sloan-Kettering experience with 136 patients. *Ann Thorac Surg* 55:1365–1374, 1993.
9. Burkes RL, Ginsberg RJ, Shepherd FA, et al: Induction chemotherapy with mitomycin, vindesine, and cisplatin for stage III unresectable non–small-cell lung cancer: Results of the Toronto Phase II Trial. *J Clin Oncol* 10:580–586, 1992.
10. Weiden PL, Piantadosi S: Preoperative chemotherapy (cisplatin and fluorouracil) and radiation therapy in stage III non–small-cell lung cancer: A phase II study of the Lung Cancer Study Group. *J Natl Cancer Inst* 83:266–273, 1991.
11. Strauss GM, Herndon JE, Sherman DD, et al: Neoadjuvant chemotherapy and radiotherapy followed by surgery in stage IIIA non–small-cell carcinoma of the lung: Report of a Cancer and Leukemia Group B phase II study. *J Clin Oncol* 10:1237–1244, 1992.

17 Pulmonary Vascular Disease

Introduction

Several noteworthy items in the field of pulmonary vascular disease have occurred during the past year:

- A high incidence of silent pulmonary embolism has long been suspected and has been confirmed in the first abstract, which discusses the clinical impact of these events.
- The role of low-molecular-weight heparin in deep venous thrombosis, the topic of the second abstract, may open the doors to new methods of dealing with embolism.
- Use of the international normalized ratio for monitoring doses of warfarin may bring improvements in anticlotting therapy, as discussed in the third abstract.

What may be the most important contribution made to the science of diagnosing and treating deep venous thrombosis and pulmonary embolism was discussed by Hull and colleagues (1, 2). They present the following guidelines to deal with suspected acute pulmonary embolism:

- When a normal lung scan is obtained, no treatment is indicated.
- When a high-probability scan is seen, the patient should be treated with anticoagulants.
- When nondiagnostic lung scans are obtained from patients with positive results from noninvasive leg tests, treatment with anticoagulants should be started.
- With a negative noninvasive leg test result, either pulmonary angiography or serial noninvasive leg studies should be performed. If these studies are positive, treatment should be started. If serial tests are negative, however, the patient should be followed but not treated.

Another advance is the use of a simple blood test to rule out venous thromboembolism (3–5). This is a test for D-dimer in the blood through the use of enzyme-linked immunosorbent assay or latex agglutination tests. The negative predictive values of these tests and of the rapid red cell agglutination assay are excellent at approximately 96%.

Roger C. Bone, M.D.

131

References

1. Stein DD, Hull RD, Saltzmann M, Pineo GF: Strategy for diagnosis of patients with suspected acute pulmonary embolism. *Chest* 103:1553–1559, 1993.
2. Hull RD, Raskob GE, Ginsberg JS, Panju AA, et al: A non-invasive strategy for the treatment of patients with suspected pulmonary embolism. *Arch Intern Med* 154:289–297, 1993.
3. Ginsberg JS, Brill-Edwards PA, Demers C, Donovan D, et al: D-dimer in patients with clinically suspected pulmonary embolism. *Chest* 104:1679–1684, 1993.
4. Harrison KA, Haire WD, Pappas M, Pumell GL, et al: Plasma D-dimer: A useful tool for evaluating suspected pulmonary embolus. *J Nucl Med* 34:896–898, 1993.
5. Wells PS, Stevens P. Massicotte P, Ginsberg JS: A rapid D-dimer (DD) assay with high sensitivity and negative predictive value (NPV) in patients with suspected deep vein thrombosis (DVT). *Blood* 82:407A, 1993.

Silent Pulmonary Embolism in Patients With Deep Venous Thrombosis: Incidence and Fate in a Randomized, Controlled Trial of Anticoagulation Versus No Anticoagulation

Nielsen HK, Husted SE, Krusell LR, Fasting H, Charles P, Hansen HH (County Hosp of Århus, Denmark; Municipal Hosp of Århus, Denmark)
J Intern Med 235:457–461, 1994   119-95-17–1

Introduction.—Patients with deep venous thrombosis (DVT) are reported to have a high incidence of clinically silent pulmonary embolism (PE). Little is known, however, about the natural history of asymptomatic PE. The occurrence of PE and the effects of anticoagulant (AC) therapy on the resolution rate of PE were evaluated.

Patients and Methods.—Eighty-seven consecutive patients (mean age, 57 years) with venographically proven DVT were followed for 3 months. Patients had symptoms of DVT for less than 6 days and a diagnosis confirmed by ascending venography within 24 hours. None of the patients had either symptoms of PE on perfusion lung scintigraphy at study entry, or severe cardiovascular disease. All patients were mobilized from the first day of admission and wore graduated compression stockings. Forty-six were randomized to AC therapy and 41 to no AC therapy. Patients in the AC group received IV heparin for at least 6 days until a therapeutic level for oral treatment with phenprocoumon was obtained. Oral AC was continued for 3 months. Each group was evaluated for improvement or the presence of new perfusion defects at 10 and 60 days. Repeat venograms were performed after 30 days to compare the effects of AC vs. non-AC treatment.

Results.—Approximately 65% of patients had possible thrombotic risk factors. The overall incidence of silent PE was 49%. Distal vein thrombosis embolized in 33% of patients and femoral vein thrombosis embolized in 53%. Progression rates after 10 days were 13% for the AC group and 8% for the non-AC group; after 60 days, both groups had a progression rate of 3%. Clinical signs of PE developed in 2 patients receiving

AC therapy and in 1 patient without AC therapy; 1 patient in the AC group died.

Conclusion.—The prognosis of patients with DVT and silent PE was good. Anticoagulation therapy had no effect on the resolution rate of PE or on the rate of clinical PE during a 3-month follow-up. Late prognosis usually depends on the presence of an underlying illness.

▶ Despite the recommended use of prophylactic AC therapy in hospitalized patients at high risk, the number of patients who have died of PE has risen (1), with more than half the deaths occurring in patients for whom the diagnosis of PE was never made and therapy was never given (2). Pulmonary embolism is a frequent complication of DVT. Many patients, however, do not exhibit the classic symptoms of erythema, pain, and swelling, possibly because phlebitis is not present or is not causing pain, or possibly because the obstruction of venous blood flow is not complete.

Pulmonary embolism occurs most often in patients who are immobilized, frequently as a result of surgery. In this study, only patients who could be ambulated from the first day after surgery and those without severe cardiovascular disease were included, so these patients already had the proverbial "leg up," even before they were given AC medication or phenylbutazone.

Silent PE occurred in 49% of these patients, and the authors found no difference in the rate of resolution after 10 and 60 days between the 2 groups. Both groups had a good prognosis, with signs of DVT and PE developing in 19 patients in each group during the 3-month study. Indeed, a high degree of resolution has been shown as early as 1–2 weeks after acute PE (2, 3), and it has been suggested that fibrinolytic mechanisms that occur naturally in the lungs may be responsible (4). In a few patients, however, resolution may be delayed up to 3 months, and in some, lung scintigraphy may reveal defects up to 1–8 years after the initial event.—R.C. Bone, M.D.

References

1. Dismuke SE, Wagner EH: Pulmonary embolism as a cause of death: The changing mortality in hospitalized patients. *JAMA* 255:2039–2042, 1986.
2. Tow DE, Wagner HN: Recovery of pulmonary arterial blood flow in patients with pulmonary embolism. *N Engl J Med* 276:1053–1059, 1967.
3. Fred HL, Axelrad MA, Lewis JM, et al: Rapid resolution of pulmonary thromboemboli in man: An angiographic study. *JAMA* 196:1137–1139, 1966.
4. Benotti JR, Dalen JE: The natural history of pulmonary embolism. *Clin Chest Med* 5:403–410, 1984.

A Comparison of Subcutaneous Low-Molecular-Weight Heparin With Warfarin Sodium for Prophylaxis Against Deep-Vein Thrombosis After Hip or Knee Implantation

Hull R, Raskob G, Pineo G, Rosenbloom D, Evans W, Mallory T, Anquist K, Smith F, Hughes G, Green D, Elliott CG, Panju A, Brant R (Univ of Calgary, Alta, Canada; Chedoke–McMaster Hosps, Hamilton, Ont, Canada; Ohio State Univ, Columbus; et al)

N Engl J Med 329:1370–1376, 1993   119-95-17-2

Introduction.—Without prophylactic anticoagulation, deep venous thrombosis may develop after surgery in as many as 60% of patients who undergo hip or knee replacement. Approaches to preventing this complication have included warfarin anticoagulation, pneumatic compression, and subcutaneous heparin, which unlike warfarin does not require frequent monitoring. Few data are available comparing less intense warfarin prophylaxis with a low-molecular-weight heparin fraction.

Study Design.—In a randomized, double-blind trial, 1,436 adult patients scheduled for total hip or total knee arthroplasty were evaluated. Either daily subcutaneous treatment with low-molecular-weight heparin (75 International Factor Xa Inhibitory Units per kilogram) or adjusted dose warfarin therapy was begun after surgery and continued for 2 weeks, when venography was done, or until discharge. The warfarin dose was adjusted each day to maintain equivalence with an international normalized ratio of 2.0 to 3.0.

Results.—Warfarin was given to 721 patients, and heparin was given to 715. Interpretable venograms were available for 617 and 590 patients, respectively. Deep venous thrombosis developed in 37% of patients given warfarin and in 31% of those given heparin, representing a 16% risk reduction. Major bleeding occurred in 1.2% of the warfarin group and in 2.8% of the heparin group (table). Wound hematomas developed more frequently in patients who received heparin. There were significant differences in the absolute rates of deep venous thrombosis between treatment groups at each of the 4 participating centers.

Discussion.—Low-molecular-weight heparin is at least as effective as warfarin in preventing venous thrombosis after hip or knee implant surgery. Venous thrombosis was less frequent in patients who received heparin, but they had more instances of wound hematoma and bleeding complications. Whether preoperative or postoperative prophylaxis is superior remains to be established.

▶ Deep vein thrombosis after hip or knee surgery is a serious complication. Of patients who do not receive prophylactic anticoagulant therapy, deep venous thrombosis occurs in 40% to 60% of those who undergo hip replacement (1) and in 60% to 70% of those who undergo knee surgery (2). Standard therapy recommended by the National Heart, Lung, and Blood Institute (3) and others is relatively less intense therapy with warfarin sodium, which has been advocated for patients undergoing hip surgery and, by inference, has been used for those undergoing knee surgery as well.

Outline Events in the 2 Treatment Groups According to Whether Surgery Involved the Hip or the Knee

Type of Event	Hip Surgery			Knee Surgery		
	Warfarin Sodium (N = 397)	Low-Molecular-Weight Heparin (N = 398)	Difference* (95% CI)	Warfarin Sodium (N = 324)	Low-Molecular-Weight Heparin (N = 317)	Difference* (95% CI)
			%			%
	no. with event/no. studied (%)			*no. with event/no. studied (%)*		
Successful venography†	335 (84.4)	330 (82.9)	—	268 (82.7)	249 (78.6)	—
Deep-vein thrombosis						
All	79/340 (23.2)	69/332 (20.8)	2.4 (−3.8 to 8.7)	152/277 (54.9)	116/258 (45.0)	9.9 (1.5 to 18.3)‡
Proximal	13/340 (3.8)	16/332 (4.8)	−1.0 (−4.1 to 2.1)	34/277 (12.3)	20/258 (7.8)	4.5 (−0.5 to 9.6)
Bleeding						
Major	6/397 (1.5)	11/398 (2.8)	−1.3 (−3.3 to 0.8)	3/324 (0.9)	9/317 (2.8)	−1.9 (−4.0 to 0.2)
Minor	9/397 (2.3)	5/398 (1.3)	—	5/324 (1.5)	5/317 (1.6)	−0.1 (−2.0 to 1.9)
Wound hematoma	10/397 (2.5)	23/398 (5.8)	−3.3 (−6.0 to −0.5)§	19/324 (5.9)	28/317 (8.8)	−2.9 (−7.0 to 1.1)
	mean ±SD			*mean ±SD*		
Postoperative blood loss (ml)	515±365	520±386	—	616±540	649±563	—
Postoperative blood replacement (ml)	197±294	275±393	—	245±331	299±456	—

* Calculated by subtracting the percentage for the low-molecular-weight heparin group from the percentage for the warfarin group. CI denotes confidence interval.
† Reasons for unsuccessful venography in patients undergoing hip surgery or knee surgery included refusal to undergo the procedure (52 and 27 patients, respectively), inability to perform the procedure (42 and 33 patients), inadequate results (20 and 45 patients), and other reasons (16 and 19 patients).
‡ P = 0.02 for the difference between treatment groups in the patients with knee surgery.
§ P = 0.03 for the difference between treatment groups in the patients with hip surgery.
(Courtesy of Hull R, Raskob G, Pineo G, et al: N Engl J Med 329:1370–1376, 1993.)

The use of warfarin requires close monitoring and must be adjusted daily to maintain equivalence with an international normalized ratio of between 2.0 and 3.0–3.5. This ratio is obtained by testing a sample with the World Health Organization reference thromboplastin, which has an international sensitivity of 1.0 (4). It has been suggested, however, that low-molecular-weight heparin (LMWH), given subcutaneously, may be equally or more effective (5). Pharmacokinetically, LMWH has high bioavailability and a long half-life, which make close monitoring of the degree of anticoagulation unnecessary.

The authors found that LMWH was as effective as warfarin sodium in preventing venous thrombosis in these patients. The overall incidence of deep venous thrombosis was 37.4% in the warfarin group and 31.4% in the LMWH group. Although this incidence is less than in other studies (6, 7), it is still quite high, emphasizing the continued need for diagnostic studies. Bilateral venography was performed in most patients in this study, and an analysis of the results revealed that failure to perform venography in the limb not undergoing surgery would have resulted in the disorder not being discovered in 20% of those with deep venous thrombosis—a substantial number. Although serious bleeding and wound hematomas were uncommon in both groups, those patients receiving LMWH had a significantly higher incidence of major bleeding complications (1.5% in the warfarin group vs. 2.8% in the LMWH group) and wound hematomas (2.5% in the warfarin group vs. 5.8% in the LMWH group).

Although these results are good news for those undergoing hip surgery, the results in patients undergoing knee surgery who received warfarin sodium are disappointing. The use of pneumatic leg compression or prophylaxis with LMWH may lessen the incidence of deep venous thrombosis in these patients (8).

Because LMWH is given subcutaneously in 1 daily dose and does not require monitoring, its administration is simpler and may require less staff time. Warfarin, on the other hand, is inexpensive, but its cost is increased greatly by the need for close monitoring. Although the rate of venous thrombosis is lowered with the use of LMWH, the incidence of bleeding complications and wound hematomas is increased. Which should we use? An editorial that appeared in the same issue of the *New England Journal of Medicine* said it best: "Once more, one is left with the conclusion that the once-daily subcutaneous administration of low-molecular-weight heparin is simpler, probably less expensive, and no less effective than a daily anticoagulant pill and periodic determinations of prothrombin time" (9).—R.C. Bone, M.D.

References

1. Harris WH, Sledge CG: Total hip and knee replacement. N *Engl J Med* 323:725–731, 801–807, 1990.
2. Stamatakis JD, Kakkar VV, Sagar S, et al: Femoral vein thrombosis and total hip replacement. *BMJ* 2:223–225, 1977.
3. National Institutes of Health: Prevention of venous thrombosis and pulmonary embolism: NIH consensus development. *JAMA* 256:744–749, 1986.

4. Hirsh J, Dalen JE, Deykin D, Poller L: Oral anticoagulants: Mechanism of action, clinical effectiveness, and optimal therapeutic range. *Chest* 102(suppl): S312–S326, 1992.
5. Leyvraz PF, Bachmann F, Hoek J, et al: Prevention of deep vein thrombosis after hip replacement: Randomised comparison between unfractionated heparin and low molecular weight heparin. *BMJ* 303:543–548, 1991.
6. Verstraete M: Pharmacotherapeutic aspects of unfractionated and low molecular weight heparins. *Drugs* 40:498–530, 1990.
7. Heit J, Kessler C, Mammen E, et al: Efficacy and safety of RD heparin (a LMWH) versus warfarin for prevention of deep-vein thrombosis after hip or knee replacement (abstract). *Blood* 78:187A, 1991.
8. Leclerc JR, Geerts WH, Desjardins L, et al: Prevention of deep vein thrombosis after major knee surgery—A randomized, double-blind trial comparing a low molecular weight heparin fragment (enoxaparin) to placebo. *Thromb Haemost* 67:417–423, 1992.
9. Verstraete M: The diagnosis and treatment of deep-vein thrombosis (editorial). *N Engl J Med* 329:1418–1420, 1993.

The International Normalized Ratio (INR) for Monitoring Warfarin Therapy: Reliability and Relation to Other Monitoring Methods

Le DT, Weibert RT, Sevilla BK, Donnelly KJ, Rapaport SI (Univ of California, San Diego, La Jolla)
Ann Intern Med 120:552–558, 1994   119-95-17–3

Introduction.—Using the international normalized ratio (INR) to monitor warfarin therapy has been proposed as a way to equalize test results. The reliability of the INR was tested by comparing it with other methods of measuring prothrombin time.

Methods.—One hundred plasma samples from 79 patients treated with warfarin were used. Prothrombin time was measured by the prothrombin-proconvertin (P&P) method, with residual native plasma prothrombin antigen, and by specific prothrombin (factor II) assay; INR was measured with a portable capillary monitor and obtained with 6 commonly used thromboplastins.

Results.—There was significant variation in INR values obtained using the different thromboplastins and the capillary monitor. High-sensitivity thromboplastins achieved the best correlations with the capillary monior. There was a nonlinear relation between INR and P&P values in the higher therapeutic range. The INR range of 2.0 to 3.0 corresponded to a P&P range of 30% to 13%, a residual native plasma prothrombin range of 40% to 20%, and a prothrombin activity range of 43% to 21%.

Discussion.—International normalized ratios are most reliable when obtained with a high-sensitivity thromboplastin. When obtained with a low-sensitivity thromboplastin, INRs are particularly unreliable at the upper limits of the therapeutic range. Capillary monitors generally provide reliable INRs except at the lower limits of the therapeutic range. Because of the effects of the underlying lupus anticoagulant of prothrombin, the

P&P test provides a more reliable measure of prothrombin time in patients with a strong lupus anticoagulant; relating P&P test results to INR values will identify the ideal INR for monitoring these patients.

▶ The use of the INR was suggested as a means to ensure that anticoagulant therapy would be reliable and that between-laboratory differences in test values would be eliminated. Unfortunately, however, that has not been the case. Differences in INR values have been attributed to the use of different automated coagulation analyzers. In this study, the same instrument was used throughout, and, even then, equivalent values could not be obtained reliably. The differences for the lower sensitivity thromboplastins can be explained at least in part by the exponential function of the International Sensitivity Index (ISI) in determining INR. These thromboplastins have higher ISI values, and errors derived from any source are magnified as the ISI value is increased. On the other hand, the authors could achieve essentially identical INR values for 2 high-sensitivity thromboplastins in which ISI values approached 1.0.

An encouraging result of this study was that all thromboplastins yielded plasma prothrombin time INRs that were acceptable in the lower portion of a recently recommended range of 2.0 to 3.0–3.5 (1). A less encouraging result was that at the higher end of the therapeutic range, 3 low-sensitivity thromboplastins produced INRs that were higher than the upper limit of the range. Furthermore, using the highest sensitivity thromboplastin to obtain an INR of 4.5, which is within the accepted therapeutic range in some European countries for arterial thromboembolism (2), these low-sensitivity thromboplastins produced results that would have prompted physicians to reduce the dose of warfarin. This, of course, could lead to disaster and is further evidence that everyone should use high-sensitivity thromboplastins (and, thus, those with low ISI values) to obtain prothrombin times. The use of low ISI thromboplastins is particularly important in patients for whom the INR must remain within the upper limit of the therapeutic range to avoid thromboembolism.

Patients who are hospitalized and those under the care of a private physician are nearly always monitored using plasma prothrombin times, whereas patients who attend outpatient anticoagulation clinics are increasingly monitored by the use of capillary blood prothrombin times. These authors found that INRs obtained with capillary blood monitors were comparable to those obtained with plasma prothrombin times produced by high-sensitivity thromboplastins, although the lower limit of the therapeutic range showed a positive bias. Other studies have also reported a positive bias (3, 4), and the physician should be aware of this bias when reporting results.

It should not be assumed that the use of the INR will yield reliable prothrombin time results when different thromboplastins are used.—R.C. Bone, M.D.

References

1. Hirsh, J, Dalen JE, Deykin D, Poller L: Oral anticoagulants: Mechanism of action, clinical effectiveness and optimal therapeutic range. *Chest* 102:S312–S326, 1992.
2. Loeliger EA: Therapeutic target values in oral coagulation—Justification of Dutch policy and a warning against the so-called moderate-intensity regimens. *Ann Hematol* 64:60–65, 1992.
3. McCurdy SA, White RH: Accuracy and precision of a portable anticoagulation monitor in a clinical setting. *Arch Intern Med* 152:589–592, 1992.
4. Becker DM, Humphries JE, Walker FB IV, et al: Standardizing the prothrombin time: Calibrating coagulation instruments as well as thromboplastin. *Arch Pathol Lab Med* 117:602–605, 1993.

Impact of the Incidental Diagnosis of Clinically Unsuspected Central Pulmonary Artery Thromboembolism in Treatment of Critically Ill Patients

Patel JJ, Chandrasekaran K, Maniet AR, Ross JJ Jr, Weiss RL, Guidotti JA (Hahnemann Univ, Philadelphia; Cooper Hosp/ Univ Med Ctr, Camden, NJ; Robert Wood Johnson Med School, Camden, NJ; et al)

Chest 105:986–990, 1994   119-95-17-4

Introduction.—The characteristic signs and symptoms of pulmonary embolism (PE) are not specific for a definite diagnosis. Without prompt treatment, however, the rate of in-hospital mortality is as high as 30%. Transesophageal echocardiography (TEE) has detected PE incidentally in patients with coexisting cardiopulmonary disorders. The records of 14 such patients were reviewed, and the impact of detecting clinically unsuspected central pulmonary artery thrombi by TEE was discussed.

Methods.—Six men and 8 women (mean age, 61 years) were examined. At the time of hospital admission, PE was not clinically suspected in these patients. Their medical records were examined for initial symptoms and signs, risk factors for PE, initial diagnosis, cardiopulmonary morbidities, and the results of other diagnostic tests.

Results.—In 8 patients, the initial diagnosis was heart failure; other diagnoses were cardiogenic shock, atrial septal defect, aortic dissection, and pneumonia. Thirteen patients had risk factors for the development of venous thromboembolism, including bed rest, preexisting congestive heart failure, major surgery, a history of deep vein thrombosis, and a history of PE. Although transthoracic echocardiography (TTE) did not visualize PE in any of the patients, it did demonstrate right heart strain in 8. With TEE, central thromboemboli were directly visualized in the main pulmonary artery in 2 patients, in the right pulmonary artery in 11, and in the left pulmonary artery in 1. The TEE findings were confirmed by positive ventilation–perfusion scans in 10 patients, pulmonary angiography in 1, and surgery in 1. Autopsy confirmed the TEE diagnosis of PE in 2 patients. Treatment was altered in all 14 patients by the diagnosis of PE.

Conclusion.—Patients who are critically ill and have acute cardiopulmonary signs and symptoms should be evaluated for PE, even though this diagnosis may not be clinically suspected. In this series, risk factors for PE were not considered during the initial diagnosis, and appropriate treatment was delayed. Right heart strain on TTE is suggestive of PE. The TEE diagnosis of central PE may avoid further, time-consuming invasive measures.

▶ It is well recognized that PE can coexist with other acute cardiopulmonary disorders, and the serious nature of these coexisting disorders often results in the diagnosis of PE being overlooked (1, 2). This can be very dangerous—the rate of mortality for patients with untreated in-hospital PE is 30%, whereas those who receive appropriate treatment for PE have a mortality rate of 8%. In this study, TEE was performed in 14 patients to evaluate other cardiopulmonary disorders, and central pulmonary artery thrombi were revealed, leading to a diagnosis of PE. Risk factors for PE were present in 13 of 14 patients; 7 patients were immobilized.

Transthoracic echocardiography, performed in these patients to evaluate other conditions, revealed right ventricular dilatation and increased right ventricular systolic pressures in 8 of 11 patients, indicating right heart strain. Although this finding is suggestive of the presence of PE, the condition was not visualized by TTE in any of the patients. A similar study by Kasper et al. found that 75% of 105 patients with confirmed PE had right heart strain on TTE (3). Because TTE does not provide good visualization beyond the main pulmonary artery, thromboemboli have seldom been detected with this method, although the presence of right heart strain should increase the index of suspicion for PE.

There has been another report of PE diagnosed after TEE was performed for other reasons (4). In that study, a patient being prepared for cardiac surgery became hypoxic and hypotensive and was shown on emergency TEE to have a mass at the junction of the main and right pulmonary arteries. The thrombus was removed surgically, and the patient underwent successful aortic valve replacement. In the current study, the diagnosis of PE resulted in a change in treatment for all 14 patients, which had a favorable effect in all cases.

Clinically unsuspected thromboembolism is somewhat common, especially in patients with acute cardiopulmonary symptoms, and clinicians should maintain a high index of suspicion for this disorder. In patients who have risk factors for PE as well as right heart strain, TEE should be performed, and an evaluation of the main pulmonary artery and its branches should be accomplished.—R.C. Bone, M.D.

References

1. Modan B, Sharon E, Jelin N: Factors contributing to the incorrect diagnosis of pulmonary embolic disease. *Chest* 62:388, 1972.
2. Dalen JE, Alpert JS: Natural history of pulmonary embolism. *Prog Cardiovasc Dis* 17:259–270, 1975.

3. Kasper W, Meinertz T, Henkel B, et al: Echocardiographic findings in patients with proved pulmonary embolism. *Am Heart J* 112:1284–1291, 1986.

4. Klein AL, Stewart WC, Cosgrove DM, et al: Visualization of acute pulmonary emboli by transesophageal echocardiography. *J Am Soc Echocardiogr* 3:412–415, 1990.

18 Respiratory Infection

Introduction

My selections for the Respiratory Infection chapter this year are varied. The first abstract attempts to revitalize a relatively old technique, transtracheal aspiration. This article is topical, based on our frustration over the difficulties of diagnosing most cases of community-acquired pneumonia by the examination of sputum. This frustration has prompted the formation of a consensus conference under the auspices of the American Thoracic Society regarding therapy for community-acquired pneumonia. That conference developed guidelines, adopted by the American Thoracic Society in July 1993 (1), that include the use of posteroanterior and lateral chest radiographs, which should be helpful in distinguishing pneumonia from similar-appearing conditions and may hint at the specific causes or conditions related to the pneumonia, such as lung abscess.

Such invasive diagnostic tests as bronchoscopy, bronchoalveolar lavage, direct needle aspiration, and various laboratory tests should be reserved for the more severely ill patient. The finding was that many of these tests are not specific enough and are not cost-effective. This is not a blanket recommendation, however, and other factors, such as underlying disease and severity of disease, certainly need to be taken into account. The use of Gram's stain early in the assessment, contrary to common practice, is not recommended because of a lack of sensitivity and specificity. The policy of selectively culturing sputum samples also comes under fire. Although the use of invasive testing is generally discouraged in this consensus statement, severe cases of pneumonia may warrant use of bronchoscopy with a protected brush catheter or bronchoalveolar lavage as methods of identifying the invading pathogen. Serologic testing and molecular testing methods were discussed as techniques that may hold promise for the future. Based on the above recommendations, it then follows that empiric treatment is the norm for cases of community-acquired pneumonia. Agents chosen for such initial treatment should be relatively broad spectrum and often include second- and third-generation cephalosporins or the β-lactam/β-lactase inhibitors. Only in severe cases of pneumonia ($PaO_2/FIO_2 < 250$) should the use of more invasive methods of diagnosis be considered, along with the possibility of admission to the ICU.

Another article reviews the treatment of an infrequent but highly lethal problem: massive hemoptysis occurring from a cavitary aspergilloma of the lung. The benefits resulting from percutaneous installation of amphotericin B are described. These results are preliminary but exciting. Because of the nature of this condition, however, there will never be a randomized, controlled study to determine the best treatment.

The last article evaluates a highly controversial and expensive technique, selective digestive decontamination. Relax! If you have not been using this technique to prevent nosocomial pneumonia, you have been right so far, because the results of the study indicate that the rate of pneumonia is no different in patients treated with selective digestive decontamination.

Roger C. Bone, M.D.

Reference

1. American Thoracic Society Board of Directors: Guidelines for the initial management of adults with community-acquired pneumonia: Diagnosis, assessment of severity, and initial antimicrobial therapy. *Am Rev Respir Dis* 148:1418–1426, 1993.

Etiology of Community-Acquired Pneumonia: Evaluation by Transtracheal Aspiration, Blood Culture, or Serology
Østergaard L, Andersen PL (Marselisborg Hosp, Aarhus, Denmark)
Chest 104:1400–1407, 1993   119-95-18-1

Background.—Because community-acquired pneumonia (CAP) is caused by a wide variety of microorganisms, different antibiotic regimens are required. Accurate etiologic diagnosis is based on the results of transtracheal aspiration (TTA), blood cultures, and serologic examinations. The diagnostic benefit of direct microscopy and culture performed on transtracheal aspirated sputum (TAS) was determined. Whether clinical or laboratory findings could predict the agent involved in the infection was also assessed.

Patients and Methods.—One hundred seventeen men and 137 women (mean age, 65 years) with CAP were enrolled during a 5-year period. All patients had infiltrates on chest radiograph and clinical signs and symptoms of pneumonia. Blood cultures were performed on 201 patients, and TTA was performed on 119. Seventy-four patients underwent serologic examinations. Patients did not undergo TTA for several reasons, including refusal, anatomical or technical difficulties, and medical problems. Blood cultures were performed if body temperature exceeded 38.5°C, and serologic investigations were obtained when no bacteria were seen in tracheal aspirate. Antibiotic treatment was based on results of TTA; when TTA findings were negative or absent, patients were treated with penicillin, ampicillin, or macrolides, according to clinical findings.

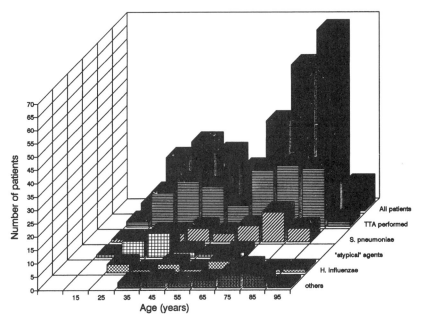

Fig 18–1.—Age distribution of different agents involved in community-acquired pneumonia. "Atypical" agents refer to: *Mycoplasma pneumoniae, Chlamydia* sp, or *Legionella pneumophila*. (Courtesy of Østergaard L, Andersen PL: *Chest* 104:1400–1407, 1993.)

Results.—An etiologic diagnosis was established in 93 patients. The most common pathogen, *Streptococcus pneumoniae*, was found in 35 patients. The mortality rate was high (27.3%) for the 11 of the 35 patients who had pneumococcemia. No patient with pneumococcal pneumonia and a negative blood culture died. In 16 patients, *Hemophilus influenzae* was the only isolated pathogen from TAS. This pathogen accounted for 17.5% of pneumonias in previously healthy individuals younger than 50 years of age. There were 10 cases of *Mycoplasma pneumonia*, 8 of *Legionella pneumophila*, and 3 of Chlamydia infections (Fig 18-1). Microscopy and culture of respiratory secretions obtained by TTA had an overall agreement of 58.8%. The mean duration of hospitalization was 15 days. Sixteen patients died, for an overall mortality rate of 6.3%.

Conclusion.—Optimal antibiotic treatment for CAP requires knowledge of the cause of the infection. Microscopic results from TAS can be used as a guide for initial antibiotic treatment. Use of antibiotics before admission does not preclude diagnosis with TTA. The procedure can be used safely when contraindications are observed.

▶ Community-acquired pneumonia, defined as pneumonia that develops in a nonhospitalized, ambulatory patient, occurs in more than 3 million individuals in the United States every year, resulting in high rates of morbidity and mortality (1). Because it is caused by a large variety of microorganisms, the treatment encompasses a wide range of antibiotic regimens, and the optimal treatment requires that the correct cause of the particular case be established. Unfortunately, no etiologic group has been found to have unique features, making it impossible to distinguish among etiologic categories on a clinical basis alone. The diagnosis, therefore, is usually made on the basis of sputum and blood culture or by serologic examination.

The process is further complicated because expectorate from coughing is contaminated by microorganisms from the upper airway. The use of TTA partially bypasses this dilemma. With this method, specimens that are suitable for microbiological and cytologic examination are directly obtained from the trachea, allowing a diagnosis to be made before antibiotic therapy is begun. The use of TAS can provide a preliminary diagnosis if bacteria are seen in sputum, but the final diagnosis depends on results of culture or serologic examination.

In 58.8% of specimens, compatibility was seen between results of microscopy and culture of TAS. Although these results are in agreement with those of Larsen and Seyer-Hansen (3), the current study found a much lesser degree of compatibility than did Ries et al. (4), who found that 92.6% of specimens were correctly identified by Gram's stain microscopy. Despite this finding, the authors of the current study still believe that direct microscopic examination of TAS is a worthwhile technique for use in obtaining an initial etiologic diagnosis. The use of TTA resulted in complications in only 1 patient in this study, leading the authors to state that this is a safe technique if contraindications for its use are respected.

I would add a word of caution, because others have found a significant rate of false positive results (indicating oropharyngeal contamination) when compared with needle aspiration of the lung. Also, even though complications are infrequent, some of these rare events are fatal. We clearly need more data.—R.C. Bone, M.D.

References

1. Fang GD, Yu VL, Vickers RM: Disease due to the Legionellaceae (other than *Legionella pneumophila*): Historical, microbiological, clinical and epidemiological review. *Medicine* (Baltimore) 68:116–132, 1989.
2. Sagel SS, Ferguson RB, Forrest JV, Roper CL, Weldon CS, Clarke RE: Percutaneous transthoracic aspiration needle biopsy. *Ann Thorac Surg* 26:399–405, 1978.
3. Larsen F, Seyer-Hansen K: Routine transtracheal aspiration in the bacteriological diagnosis of pulmonary infections. *Ugeskr Laeger* 143:1260–1262, 1981.
4. Ries K, Levison ME, Kayee D: Transtracheal aspiration in pulmonary infection. *Arch Intern Med* 133:453–458, 1974.

Guidelines for the Initial Management of Adults With Community-Acquired Pneumonia: Diagnosis, Assessment of Severity, and Initial An-

timicrobial Therapy
Niederman MS, Bass JB Jr, Campbell GD, Fein AM, Grossman RF, Mandell LA, Marrie TJ, Sarosi GA, Torres A, Yu VL (American Thoracic Society)
Am Rev Respir Dis 148:1418–1426, 1993   119-95-18-2

Objective.—Community-acquired pneumonia (CAP) is still a frequent and serious illness. Pneumonia is the sixth leading cause of death in the United States and the leading cause of death resulting from infectious illness. A conference was held to formulate an approach to the initial management of CAP, taking into account its evolving epidemiology and currently available treatments.

Patient Classification.—Four categories of patients may be distinguished on the basis of information available at initial assessment: patients 60 years or younger without comorbid conditions, who can be treated as outpatients; older patients or those with comorbidity, who also can be treated in an outpatient setting; patients who require hospitalization; and those with severe CAP who most often require intensive care.

Diagnosis.—Lateral and posteroanterior chest radiographs are obtained whenever pneumonia is a possibility. A Gram's stain of expectorated sputum may be helpful at initial assessment, but its sensitivity and specificity vary considerably with the criteria used to denote a "positive" scan. Routine sputum cultures are not sensitive or specific but may yield organisms that are never part of the normal respiratory flora. Invasive methods of sampling the lower airways are not usually warranted in patients with CAP. Patients who are admitted should have 2 sets of blood cultures. Those with pleural effusion should undergo diagnostic thoracentesis. No firm guidelines are available for admitting patients with CAP to the hospital, which may be the single most important decision made. The presence of multiple risk factors is a strong reason to admit. Social considerations may be taken into account.

General Treatment Considerations.—The advent of new drugs, such as azithromycin, may allow a shorter course of treatment. In general, oral treatment may be considered when the patient is clinically stable and afebrile. Older patients and those with more severe disease or multiple coexisting disorders generally require treatment for a longer time. Both unusual pathogens and noninfectious illness should be considered when a patient does not respond adequately to initial treatment.

▶ Community-acquired pneumonia is the sixth leading cause of death in the United States and the number 1 cause of death from infectious disease, despite the availability of effective vaccines and potent antimicrobial drugs for treatment (1, 2). As many as 4 million cases of CAP may occur each year in the United States, with as many as 20% of these patients requiring hospitalization (1). The mortality rate for CAP remains low for those who do not need hospitalization—1% to 5%—but among those who are hospitalized for CAP, the mortality rate is nearly 25% (3, 4). The mortality rate is especially high in those who are treated in the ICU (5, 6). Both the epidemiology and treatment of pneumonia have changed in recent years, with the illness increasingly striking older adults and those who are compromised because of coexisting illness. These patients are at risk to become infected with pathogens that are unrecognized or only recently identified (5). Although treatment progress has been made, with new antimicrobial agents becoming available, bacterial resistance has also evolved, and the possibility of penicillin-resistant pneumococci bacteria has become real.

The current guidelines were set forth to provide an approach for the initial treatment, including evaluation and therapy, of patients with CAP and were adopted by the American Thoracic Society in July 1993.

The authors recommend that all patients suspected of having pneumonia have posteroanterior and posterolateral chest radiographs. These tests may be helpful in distinguishing pneumonia from conditions that mimic it and may suggest specific causes or conditions related to the pneumonia, such as lung abscess. Coexisting conditions may also be identified by radiographs, and severity of illness may be indicated on radiographs by the sighting of multilobar involvement, which signifies serious illness.

In contrast to common clinical practice, these authors do not recommend the use of Gram's stain to delineate the probable causative organism and direct initial therapy. Previous studies have shown that the ability of this method to predict the recovery of pneumococcus in sputum varied widely with regard to sensitivity and specificity, depending on the criteria used to define a positive stain (7). Further, there are no large studies that show a relationship between the results of Gram's stain and cultures of alveolar material in patients with CAP, and even the policy of culturing and examining only sputum samples that have greater than 25 neutrophils and fewer than 5 squamous epithelial cells per low power field does not guarantee the usefulness of the data.

Multiple invasive diagnostic tests are not recommended by these authors. Transtracheal aspiration, bronchoscopy with a protected brush catheter, bronchoalveolar lavage with or without balloon protection, and direct needle aspiration of the lung are not indicated in most patients with CAP. In certain patients who are severely ill, bronchoscopy with a protected brush catheter or bronchoalveolar lavage can be used to provide an early, accurate diagnosis. These procedures are less risky than the others and are usually better tolerated by patients.

The authors do not recommend the use of serologic testing or cold agglutinin measurements in the initial evaluation of these patients, nor do they recommend the use of tests to measure specific microbial antigens. There is a great deal of research going on in the latter area, however, and methods using monoclonal antibodies, DNA probes, and polymerase chain reaction amplification may, in the future, allow accurate diagnostic tests on clinical specimens.

Routine laboratory tests, such as complete blood counts, serum electrolytes, hepatic enzymes, and renal function tests, are not helpful in determining the cause of pneumonia, although they may be beneficial in determining the patient's prognosis and in deciding whether to hospitalize the patient, as well as in helping the clinician choose the correct therapy in those with moderate-to-severe illness. These tests should be performed in patients who are hospitalized or being considered for hospitalization, in those who are 60 years of age or older, and in those who have a coexisting illness. Hospitalized patients should also undergo assessment of arterial oxygen saturation levels and should have 2 sets of blood cultures.

The current guidelines emphasize that it is not necessary or prudent to order extensive tests when making the initial diagnosis. Clearly, the usefulness of such testing is limited (3, 5, 7), and even after comprehensive testing, the pathogen cannot be identified in as many as half of patients. This is both frustrating for patient and physician and lacks the cost-effectiveness so important in today's health care environment. Some more advanced tests to identify the pathogens involved in pneumonia are valuable, primarily in the assessment of patients whose illness is not responding to appropriate empiric therapy and in epidemiologic studies.

Initial clinical features, including patient history, physical examination, routine laboratory tests, and radiographic evaluation, are not reliable indicators of a specific etiologic diagnosis. Whereas some signs and symptoms tend to occur more often in patients whose pneumonia is caused by *Mycoplasma* or *Legionella* species, there is too much overlap between signs and symptoms related to those pathogens and other causes of lung infiltrates, both infectious and noninfectious, and therapeutic decisions should not be made based on this information.

Because of the increased risk to patients who are hospitalized for pneumonia, this decision is perhaps the most important one to be made. Specific factors that increase the risk of a complicated course or death are well known (8), and when any of these factors are present—and especially when multiple risk factors are present—hospitalization should be seriously considered. The authors of this article point out that hospitalization does not need to be long-term, but patients should be closely observed until the physician is certain that their illness is responding to therapy.

The guidelines for treatment are based on numerous considerations, including whether there is coexisting illness, the clinical presentation of severity of illness, and whether the patient will be hospitalized or will be treated as an outpatient. In addition, these factors must also be considered when deciding on the duration of therapy (9).

Azithromycin, a new 15-member macrolide with a half-life of 11–14 hours, may make shorter treatment courses possible. Because of its exceedingly long half-life, azithromycin remains in the tissues longer than most other agents; therefore, reducing the length of treatment based on the number of days of oral administration of the drug is somewhat misleading. High serum levels are not achieved at currently approved oral doses; consequently, the drug should not be used in patients suspected of having bacteremic infection or those whose pneumonia is moderate to severe. Studies comparing 5-day treatment with azithromycin to 10-day treatment with erythromycin and cefaclor in patients with atypical pneumonia and acute bacterial pneumonia, respectively, suggest that shorter treatment courses may be used with azithromycin, but more data are needed to be certain (10,11).

Effective antimicrobial therapy should result in improvement of symptoms within 48–72 hours, although the response may be delayed with some etiologic pathogens and as a result of certain host factors. Unless the patient shows marked deterioration, therapy should not be changed within the first 72 hours. In older patients and those with more severe illness or coexisting illness, the time to resolution of symptoms will be delayed.

Finding the correct etiologic agent and choosing just the right therapy is still a guessing game in most patients with CAP. However, these guidelines provide us with the latest recommendations for this very common and very serious illness.—R.C. Bone, M.D.

References

1. Garibaldi RA: Epidemiology of community-acquired respiratory tract infections in adults: Incidence, etiology, and impact. *Am J Med* 78:S32–S37, 1985.
2. US Department of Commerce, Bureau of the Census: *Statistical Abstract of the United States* (104th ed). Washington, DC, Government Printing Office, 1984.
3. Fang GD, Fine M, Orloff J, et al: New and emerging etiologies for community-acquired pneumonia with implication for therapy: A prospective multicenter study of 359 cases. *Medicine* (Baltimore) 69:307–316, 1990.
4. Pachon J, Prados MD, Capote F, et al: Severe community-acquired pneumonia: Etiology, prognosis, and treatment. *Am Rev Respir Dis* 142:369–373, 1990.
5. Marrie TJ, Durant H, Yates L: Community-acquired pneumonia requiring hospitalization: A 5-year prospective study. *Rev Infect Dis* 11:586–599, 1989.
6. Ortqvist A, Sterner G, Nilsson JA: Severe community-acquired pneumonia: Factors influencing need of intensive care treatment and prognosis. *Scand J Infect Dis* 17:377–386, 1985.
7. Woodhead MA, Arrowsmith J, Chamberlain-Webber R, et al: The value of routine microbial investigation in community-acquired pneumonia. *Respir Med* 85:313–317, 1991.
8. Fine MJ, Smith DN, Singer DE: Hospitalization decision in patients with community-acquired pneumonia: A prospective cohort study. *Am J Med* 89:713–721, 1990.
9. McGehee JL, Podnos SD, Pierce AK, et al: Treatment of pneumonia in patients at risk of infection with gram-negative bacilli. *Am J Med* 84:597–602, 1988.
10. Schonwald S, Gunjaca M, Kolacny-Babic L, et al: Comparison of azithromycin and erythromycin in the treatment of atypical pneumonias. *J Antimicrob Chemother* 25(suppl A):123–126, 1990.
11. Kinasewitz G, Wood RG: Azithromycin versus cefaclor in the treatment of acute bacterial pneumonia. *Eur J Clin Microbiol Infect Dis* 10:872–877, 1991.

Treatment of Hemoptysis in Patients With Cavitary Aspergilloma of the Lung: Value of Percutaneous Instillation of Amphotericin B

Lee KS, Kim HT, Kim YH, Choe KO (Soonchunhyang Univ, Chunan, Korea; Yonsei Univ, Seoul, Korea)
AJR 161:727–731, 1993   119-95-18–3

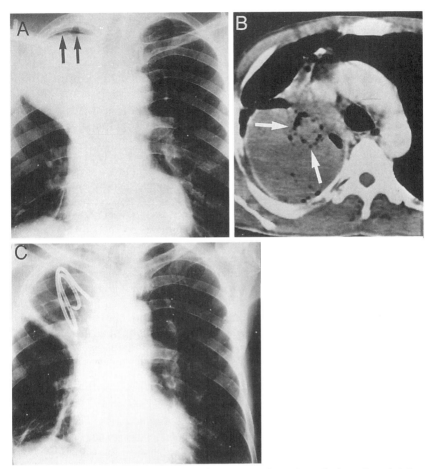

Fig 18–2.—Large aspergilloma in a man, aged 49 years. **A,** chest radiograph obtained at admission shows well-marginated lesion in the right upper lobe with air-meniscus sign (*arrows*). **B,** contrast-enhanced CT scan at level of aortic arch shows soft tissue lesion in enhancing cavity of posterior segment of the right upper lobe. Scattered multiple air densities (*arrows*) in lesion suggest a fungus ball. **C,** radiograph obtained after instillation of 750 mg of amphotericin B shows that fungus ball has completely resolved. **A** and **C** reprinted from Lee KS, Kim YH, Bae WK: AJR 154:1346, 1990. (Courtesy of Lee KS, Kim HT, Kim YH, et al: AJR 161:727–731, 1993.)

Background.—Surgery is the first-line treatment for cavitary aspergillomas of the lung, but it has high rates of morbidity and mortality. The efficacy of percutaneous intracavitary instillation of amphotericin B was evaluated in patients with hemoptysis caused by cavitary aspergilloma.

Methods.—Four patients without lung interposed between the aspergilloma and chest wall underwent intracavitary instillation of 750 mg of amphotericin B during a 15-day period. Three patients with lung interposed between the cavity and chest wall received 100 mg of amphotericin B administered in 2 three-day fine-needle instillations. The aspergilloma was monitored radiographically.

Results.—The aspergilloma disappeared at the end of treatment in 3 patients treated through a catheter (Fig 18-2) and resolved partially in the fourth. Follow-up radiographs of all 3 patients treated through fine-needle instillation revealed partial resolution of the aspergilloma.

Conclusion.—Percutaneous instillation of amphotericin B is a reliable method for treating hemoptysis caused by aspergillomas. Additional study is needed to establish the optimal dose and timing of treatment.

▶ Of all acute respiratory symptoms, massive hemoptysis is probably the most dreaded. Traditionally, massive hemoptysis has been treated with surgery; however, the surgical treatment of massive hemoptysis has been associated with a 19% mortality rate in some series and a much higher rate in others (1). Conservative "wait and see" treatment, on the other hand, has been associated with a mortality rate of 54%. I will always remember a 28-year-old woman who had fibrotic destructive sarcoidosis with aspergillomas in both upper lobes. She was admitted for hemoptysis based on history. While we were taking her to the bronchoscopy suite to determine the site of bleeding, she became cyanotic despite receiving oxygen. She arrested before we could intubate, and intubation and CPR were unsuccessful. Clearly, these patients can look good one moment and be dying of asphyxia the next. This potential should always be appreciated, even in patients with a history of nothing more than significant hemoptysis! Surgery is contraindicated in many patients with cavitary aspergilloma because of underlying pulmonary disease, and other treatments, including the use of IV amphotericin B, are ineffective.

In this study, some patients had massive hemoptysis; the rest had significant but not massive hemoptysis. Percutaneous intracavitary therapy with amphotericin B has several advantages in this patient population. Catheter insertion is not complicated; the process can be repeated in either the same or another cavity; and the patient does not lose any pulmonary function while therapy is being carried out—a very important consideration in these already compromised patients. In addition, response to therapy is rapid. These authors instilled a total of 750 mg of amphotericin B in patients with indwelling catheters and reported that hemoptysis ceased within 5 days of treatment in all patients. They also report a 57% resolution of aspergilloma (either partial or complete). In 1980, my colleagues and I used a total dose of 500 mg and found that aspergilloma was either partially or completely resolved in 66% of patients (2). Like these authors, we also found a rapid response to intracavitary amphotericin B therapy—2 to 4 weeks into our study.

As the authors of this study mention, there has been no controlled study regarding the optimal dose of amphotericin B to be instilled, and doses ranging from 500 to 800 mg have been reported. Lee et al. report that patients with indwelling catheters received a total dose of 750 mg, and those treated with fine-needle instillation received a total of 100 mg of amphotericin B.

The 100-mg dose resulted in immediate cessation of hemoptysis, suggesting that control of hemoptysis can be achieved with a low dose of this antifungal agent. These authors drew the same conclusion that my co-workers and I did: The use of intracavitary amphotericin B should be considered in patients who have symptomatic pulmonary aspergilloma.

Another treatment that is less invasive than surgery should also be considered for patients with massive hemoptysis—bronchial artery embolism. In skilled hands, this technique is highly effective (3). However, patients treated with this technique may rebleed weeks to months later.—R.C. Bone, M.D.

References

1. Crocco JA, Rooney JJ, Fankhushen DS, et al: Massive hemoptysis. *Ann Intern Med* 121:496, 1968.
2. Hargis JL, Bone RC, Stewart J, Rector N, Hiller FC: Intracavitary amphotericin B in the treatment of symptomatic pulmonary aspergillomas. *Am J Med* 68:389–394, 1980.
3. Uflocker R, Kaemmerer A, Picon PD, et al: Bronchial artery embolization in the management of hemoptysis: Technical aspects and long-term results. *Radiology* 163:361–365, 1985.

Utility of Selective Digestive Decontamination in Mechanically Ventilated Patients

Ferrer M, Torres A, González J, Puig de la Bellacasa J, El-Ebiary M, Roca M, Gatell JM, Rodriguez-Roisin R (Universitat de Barcelona)
Ann Intern Med 120:389–395, 1994   119-95-18–4

Purpose.—Nosocomial pneumonia commonly develops in patients who are mechanically ventilated, largely as a result of aspiration of oropharyngeal and gastric potential pathogens into the lower airways. This situation has led to the widespread use of selective decontamination of the digestive tract as prophylaxis against ventilator-associated nosocomial pneumonia. Although most studies have shown a reduced incidence of nosocomial pneumonia with this form of prophylaxis, methodological problems, including lack of specific diagnostic methods, have arisen. These deficiencies were addressed in a prospective, randomized, placebo-controlled, double-blind study.

Methods.—Eighty patients in a respiratory ICU who were undergoing more than 3 days of mechanical ventilation were included. They were randomized to receive either selective digestive decontamination or placebo. The active treatment group received 10 mL of an aqueous suspension of polymyxin E, 100 mg; tobramycin, 80 mg; and amphotericin B, 500 mg, through a nasogastric tube. The same drugs were also given topically for decontamination of the oropharynx. All patients received IV cefotaxime, and other systemic antibiotics were given as indicated. Quantitative culture of endotracheal aspirates, pharyngeal swabs, and gastric juice samples obtained 3 times per week was performed. Rigor-

Bronchial, Pharyngeal, and Gastric Colonization

Colonization	SDD Group*	Placebo	P Value
Bronchial			
Gram-negative bacilli (all), n/N (%)	12/39 (31)	31/40 (78)	<0.0001†
Pseudomonas aeruginosa, n/N (%)	9/39 (23)	25/40 (63)	<0.001‡
Enterobacter serratia, n/N	1/39	3/40	...
Acinetobacter species, n/N	1/39	2/40	...
Xanthomona maltophilia, n/N	1/39	2/40	...
Acinetobacter xylosoxidans, n/N	0/39	2/40	...
Other gram-negative bacilli, n/N	2/39	5/40	...
Methicillin-resistent Staphylococcus aureus, n/N (%)	14/39 (36)	12/40 (30)	P > 0.2
Candida species, n/N	8/39 (21)	16/40 (40)	P > 0.2
Pharyngeal			
Gram-negative bacilli, n/N (%)	3/39 (8)	30/40 (75)	<0.0001§
Pseudomonas aeruginosa, n/N (%)	3/39 (8)	24/40 (60)	<0.0001‖
Other gram-negative bacilli, n/N	0/39	11/40 (28)	...
Methicillin-resistent Staphylococcus aureus, n/N (%)	13/39 (33)	7/40 (18)	>0.2
Candida species, n/N (%)	3/39 (8)	15/40 (38)	<0.05¶
Gastric			
Gram-negative bacilli (all), n/N (%)	4/39 (10)	26/39 (67)	<0.0001**
Pseudomonas aeruginosa, n/N (%)	2/39 (5)	16/39 (41)	<0.0001††
Enterobacter species, n/N	1/39	8/39	...
Klebsiella species, n/N	0/39	5/39	...
Acinetobacter species, n/N	0/39	4/39	...
Other gram-negative bacilli, n/N	1/39	5/39	...
Methicillin-resistent Staphylococcus aureus, n/N (%)	6/39 (15)	3/39 (8)	>0.2
Candida species, n/N (%)	5/39 (13)	19/39 (49)	<0.001‡‡

* Abbreviations: OR, odds ratio; SDD, selective digestive decontamination; CI, confidence interval.
† OR = .13 (95% CI, .04 to .39).
‡ OR = .18 (CI, .09 to .39).
§ OR = .03 (CI, .01 to .07).
‖ OR = .06 (CI, .03 to .24).
¶ OR = .14 (CI, .03 to .59).
** OR = .06 (CI, .01 to .22).
†† OR = .04 (CI, .01 to .24).
‡‡ OR = .15 (CI, .04 to .53).
(Courtesy of Ferrer M, Torres A, González J, et al: *Ann Intern Med* 120:389–395, 1994.)

ous clinical evidence was used to define probable pneumonia, with confirmation of this diagnosis by the isolation of a potential pathogen in a protected brush specimen at a concentration of at least 10^3 colony-forming units per milliliter or in a bronchoalveolar lavage specimen at a concentration of 10^4 colony forming units per milliter or more, as well as by autopsy findings.

Results.—Bronchial colonization with gram-negative bacilli was present in 31% of the selective decontamination group vs. 78% of the placebo group. There was no significant difference in the rate of bronchial colonization with methicillin-resistant *Staphylococcus aureus*—36% and 30%, respectively—but colonization by *Candida* species was lower in the selective decontamination group, 21% vs. 40%. The findings in the oropharynx and gastric cavities were similar to those of the upper airways (table). There was no difference in the incidence of nosocomial pneumonia: 18% in the selective decontamination group vs. 24% in the placebo group. The 2 groups were not significantly different in onset of nosocomial pneumonia, duration of mechanical ventilation, length of stay in the ICU, or incidence or cause of death.

Conclusion.—Selective digestive decontamination makes no difference in the incidence of nosocomial pneumonia or other infections among patients who are mechanically ventilated. The use of systemic antibiotics in both groups precludes firm conclusions about the value of selective digestive contamination in preventing primary endogenous pneumonia; however, it does not appear to prevent secondary endogenous penumonias. The use of less complex, more economical means for the prevention of nosocomial pneumonia in this patient group is recommended.

▶ As a visiting professor, I have noticed that selective digestive decontamination is used frequently in critical care units in Europe but not in the United States. Certainly, ICU medicine in most of Europe and the United States is comparable—so why the difference? Certainly, the technique used in Europe is expensive and might lead to more resistant microorganisms in their ICUs. I think this article might help resolve this trans-Atlantic difference. Read on.

Patients who are mechanically ventilated run a well-known risk for nosocomial pneumonia. The etiology of this event often involves bacteria that colonize the oropharyngeal or gastric regions and are then aspirated into the lower airways. Recognition of this fact has led to the use of digestive decontamination through the use of topical nonabsorbable and systemic antibiotics in an effort to reduce the complication rate for these patients. Studies of such regimens have often been favorable; however, because of inconsistent techniques, definitions, and results, controversy still surrounds the issue of digestive decontamination. Thus, the authors of this study have undertaken a controlled, randomized, double-blind study with end points of nosocomial pneumonia and mortality to help resolve these issues.

Unfortunately, this study reports negative results. Selective digestive decontamination did not significantly affect either nosocomial pneumonia or mortality. Additionally, there was no significant difference between patients who received selective digestive decontamination and those who received the placebo procedure in the incidence of other infections, the length of stay at the hospital, and the duration of mechanical ventilation. There was, however, a significant decrease in the rate of gram-negative bacterial and yeast colonizations of the bronchial tree. These results agree with 2 other large, controlled, randomized studies that found no significant benefits to this procedure (1, 2). However, a number of other controlled, randomized studies have shown that selective digestive decontamination can benefit patients in the ICU. The authors point out a number of procedural differences between their study and others, such as failure to use the protected specimen brush technique for obtaining bronchial samples (see also reference 3) and failure to identify infections that resulted from exogenous sources.

The authors note that other methods such as appropriate positioning of the patient and the simple procedure of hand washing may be more cost-effective in reducing the rate of nosocomial pneumonia.—R.C. Bone, M.D.

References

1. Gastinne H, Wolff M, Delatour F, Faurisson F, Chevret S: A controlled trial in intensive care units of selective decontamination of the digestive tract with nonabsorbable antibiotics. N Engl J Med 326:594–599, 1992.
2. Hammond JM, Potgieter PD, Saunders GL, Forder AA: Double-blind study of selective decontamination of the digestive tract in intensive care. Lancet 340:5–9, 1992.
3. 1993 YEAR BOOK OF PULMONARY DISEASE, pp 280–283.

19 Pulmonary Complications in HIV

Introduction

And another year has passed without any form of breakthrough in the treatment of HIV infection. Neither have the demographics of this deadly disease changed much. The virus continues to affect largely the male homosexual and IV drug–using communities. Tuberculosis in individuals infected with HIV continues to be a deadly combination that is usually restricted to the overcrowded and poor living in the inner city.

Research is touching on the molecular control mechanisms that allow the virus to take over the cellular machinery of infected cells. Advances in the development of animal models of the disease have gained some attention, particularly in a form of simian AIDS model that closely mimics the human form of the disease. The ability of the virus to inhibit cell-mediated immunity is its hallmark; its more recently discovered ability to affect B-cell function is the subject of the selected article for this year's YEAR BOOK chapter on HIV. It is an interesting look at some of the organisms associated with bacterial pneumonia in individuals with HIV infection. An important point is that common bacterial pathogens are the most common cause of pneumonia in these patients. Encapsulated pathogens are the most frequent culprits. Bacterial pneumonia usually presents with symptoms and signs that are the same in patients with or without HIV infection. The presentation, however, can be identical to that seen in cases of *Pneumocystis carinii* pneumonia. Both polyvalent pneumococcal vaccine and influenza vaccine are recommended for patients with HIV infection and a low CD4 count.

Roger C. Bone, M.D.

Bacterial Pneumonia in HIV-Infected Patients: A Prospective Study of 68 Episodes
Falcó V, Fernández de Sevilla T, Alegre J, Barbé J, Ferrer A, Ocaña I, Ribera E, Martínez-Vázquez JM (Universidad Autónoma, Barcelona)
Eur Respir J 7:235–239, 1994   119-95-19–1

Introduction.—Although progressive deterioration of T-cell function was noted early in AIDS research, B-cell dysfunction and altered hu-

Cause of Community-Acquired Bacterial
Pneumonia (68 Episodes) in 55
HIV-Infected Patients

Streptococcus pneumoniae	22	(34%)
Haemophilus influenzae	12	(18%)
Pseudomonas aeruginosa	4	
Other Gram-negative bacilli	4	
Staphylococcus aureus	1	
Bacillus sphericus	1	
Mycoplasma pneumoniae	1	
Moraxella catarrhalis	1	
Streptococcus spp.	1	
Total	48	(71%)
Unknown	20	(29%)

(Courtesy of Falcó V, Fernández de Sevilla T, Alegre J, et al: *Eur Respir J* 7:235-239, 1994.)

moral immunity have been more recently studied in patients infected with HIV. An increasing incidence of bacterial pneumonia, an infection reflecting B-cell dysfunction, has been seen in these patients. The clinical features and outcome of pneumococcal pneumonia were compared in patients with and without HIV infection.

Methods.—Clinical and outcome data were collected for patients with HIV infection who had a total of 68 episodes of pneumonia and 69 patients without HIV infection. Clinical observations, laboratory data, and chest roentgenogram findings were compared between the 2 groups.

Results.—Of the 68 episodes of pneumococcal pneumonia occurring in the HIV group, asymptomatic patients had 41 episodes, patients with persistent generalized lymphadenopathy had 2, and patients with AIDS had 25. The pneumonia was most commonly caused by *Streptococcus pneumoniae* or *Haemophilus influenzae* (table). Using multivariate analysis, only 2 significant differences were noted in clinical comparisons of the 2 groups: radiologic signs of chest consolidation were more common in patients without HIV infection, and bacteremia was more common in patients with HIV infection. The patients with HIV infection had a higher mortality rate (19% vs. 4.3%), and 55% had recurrent episodes. In 7 of the 16 asymptomatic patients, disease progressed to AIDS within a mean of 10 months.

Discussion.—The clinical presentation of bacterial pneumonia was largely similar in patients with and without HIV infection. However, the greater prevalence of bacteremia in patients with HIV infection indicates deteriorating humoral immunity. In 27% of patients with HIV infection, bacterial pneumonia was the first sign of disease, suggesting that bacterial pneumonia may occur early in the natural history of HIV infection.

However, the rapid development of an AIDS-defining condition in nearly half of the asymptomatic patients and high recurrence rate suggest that bacterial pneumonia may be an early marker of the progression to AIDS.

▶ Although many of the effects of HIV on the immune system have been described, the topic is not exactly an open book—not a surprising assertion given the complex nature of the immune system. This article helps confirm another twist to the story's plot. The deleterious effects of HIV on cell-mediated immunity were described at about the time of the discovery of HIV, and it was generally believed that the disease had little effect on humorally mediated immune system functions. In fact, an enhanced or overreactive response of humorally mediated immunity has been described because of the large numbers of antibodies and B-cells typically found in the blood of patients with HIV.

Thus, the discovery a few years later that patients with HIV infection have significantly higher rates of pneumococcal pneumonia than the general population presented a quandary. That finding, however, was corroborated in a number of studies, and it is now considered likely that, besides the well known T-cell deficiency, HIV infection causes abnormal B-cell function. This explanation is complicated, of course, because T cells control certain aspects of B-cell function. Studies have implicated both the B cell alone and the control of the T cell of the B cell in HIV-mediated B-cell dysfunction. These authors have also observed the increasing incidence of bacterial pneumonia in patients with HIV and undertook this study to improve our understanding of the clinical and microbiological features of this phenomenon.

Most of the cases observed resulted from *S. pneumoniae* and *H. influenzae* organisms. Curiously, some organisms that were common in the general hospital population, such as *Legionella pneumophila*, were rare in individuals with HIV infection. The presence of *Pseudomonas aeruginosa* was associated with advanced-stage HIV infection, and patients harboring this organism had low lymphocyte counts and granulocytopenia.

Patients with HIV and bacterial pneumonia have clinical presentations similar to those of the general populace, although a bacteremia may be more likely to manifest. It is interesting that bacterial pneumonia was the first sign of HIV-caused immune system dysfunction in 27% of the patients examined. In 63%, pneumonia was the first opportunistic infection experienced by the patient.

Generally, these patients responded well to antimicrobial therapy, although the mortality rate was 10%. For those with HIV, the mortality rate was not significantly greater than for the general population. However, patients with HIV were likely to experience recurrent infection, particularly if advanced HIV infection manifested. The presence of bacterial pneumonia in patients with HIV is a potentially fatal complication that further signifies the profound effects of the disease on the human immune system.—R.C. Bone, M.D.

20 Tuberculosis

Introduction

Well, what's new with tuberculosis? Almost everything. We were told a few years ago that tuberculosis would be conquered. Nonsense! Since that time, there have been revolutionary changes in the presentation and treatment of tuberculosis. Almost none of the news is good. In 1984, we saw a dramatic upturn in the number of cases of tuberculosis in the United States. Additionally, we have seen the emergence of several drug-resistant forms of this disease that have become endemic in certain groups. Multidrug regimens are sometimes indicated and, in some cases, even the best combinations may not be fully effective. Tables 2 and 3, which follow Abstract 119-95-20-1, describe the initial treatment for patients with tuberculosis. The increased risk for individuals with compromised immune systems has been described. Recently, new populations at increasing risk for tuberculosis have been identified, including pregnant women in high-prevalence areas (1), airplane passengers (2), and bar patrons (3).

Is there any good news? Yes! Focal areas, particularly urban areas with large HIV-seropositive populations and immigrant populations, account for virtually all the increased numbers of cases. In fact, data recently reported from the Centers for Disease Control and Prevention indicate that the number of counties reporting no cases of tuberculosis has risen steadily since 1962. Other good news is that talk has been translated into action. Funding for local tuberculosis control programs increased from $40 million in 1992 to $104 million this year.

In the 1994 YEAR BOOK of MEDICINE , I presented a detailed argument for directly observed therapy. Dr. Michael Iseman, of the National Jewish Center for Immunology and Respiratory Medicine in Denver, states that this should be the standard of practice. In a discussion of the American Thoracic Society, he stated that observed therapy is essentially transferring responsibility from your patient to yourself. Dr. Iseman believes that directly observed therapy saves money by decreasing the need for other costly monitoring. I agree. For those patients who might have a greater risk of voluntary noncompliance, directly observed therapy should be routine. For others, one should heed the recommendations given at the end of this chapter.

Roger C. Bone, M.D.

References

1. Centers for Disease Control and Prevention: Tuberculosis among pregnant women—New York City, 1985–1992. MMWR *Morb Mortal Wkly Rep* 42:605, 611–612, 1993.
2. McFarland JW, Hickman C, Osterholm MT, MacDonald KL: Exposure to *Mycobacterium tuberculosis* during air travel. *Lancet* 342:112–113, 1993.
3. Mishu B, Gensheimeck, Bugden G, Horon JG, Andrews G, Bach A, Schaffn GW: Tuberculosis outbreak in a shipyard. 1992 Interscience Conference on Antimicrobial Agents and Chemotherapy [Abstract 554].

Nationwide Survey of Drug-Resistant Tuberculosis in the United States

Bloch AB, Cauthen GM, Onorato IM, Dansbury KG, Kelly GD, Driver CR, Snider DE Jr (Ctrs for Disease Control and Prevention, Atlanta, Ga)
JAMA 271:665–671, 1994   119-95-20-1

Background.—The recent outbreaks of multidrug-resistant (MDR) tuberculosis (TB) have raised several important questions regarding the epidemiology of drug-resistant TB in the United States. A nationwide survey of drug-resistant TB was conducted.

Methods.—The geographic distribution, demographic characteristics, and risk factors of reported cases of TB were studied to determine anti-TB drug-resistance patterns. For culture-positive cases reported to the Centers for Disease Control and Prevention (CDC), health departments

TABLE 1.—Proportion of Culture-Positive Tuberculosis Cases Resistant to Isoniazid and Rifampin, by US State, First Quarter, 1991*

State	No. Tested	No. Resistant	Percentage
New York	549	71	12.9
New Jersey	151	10	6.6
Florida	144	7	4.9
Hawaii	23	1	4.3
Alabama	91	3	3.3
Illinois	194	5	2.6
Georgia	86	2	2.3
Arizona	53	1	1.9
Washington	59	1	1.7
Virginia	63	1	1.6
Texas	326	5	1.5
California	599	6	1.0
Pennsylvania	117	1	0.9
Rest of United States	801	0	0.0
Total	**3256**	**114**	**3.5**

* Cases may be resistant to other drugs.
(Courtesy of Bloch AB, Cauthen GM, Onorato IM, et al: *JAMA* 271:665-671, 1994.)

TABLE 2.—Regimen Options for the Initial Treatment of TB Among Children and Adults

TB without HIV infection		TB with HIV infection	
Option 1	Option 2	Option 3	Option 4
Administer daily INH, RIF, and PZA for 8 weeks followed by 16 weeks of INH and RIF daily or 2-3 times/week* in areas where the INH resistance rate is not documented to be <4%. EMB or SM should be added to the initial regimen until susceptibility to INH and RIF is demonstrated. Continue treatment for at least 6 months and 3 months beyond culture conversion. Consult a TB medical expert if the patient is symptomatic or smear or culture positive After 3 months.	Administer daily INH, RIF, PZA, and SM or EMB for 2 weeks followed by 2 times/week* administration of the same drugs for 6 weeks (by DOT), and subsequently, with 2 times/week administration of INH and RIF for 16 weeks (by DOT). Consult a TB medical expert if the patient is symptomatic or smear or culture positive after 3 months.	Treat by DOT, 3 times/week* with INH, RIF, PZA, and EMB or SM for 6 months.† Consult a TB medical expert if the patient is symptomatic or smear or culture positive after 3 months.	Options 1, 2, or 3 can be used, but treatment regimens should continue for a total of 9 months and at least 6 months beyond culture conversion.

Abbreviations: INH, isoniazid; RIF, rifampin; PZA, pyrazinamide; EMB, ethambutol; SM, streptomycin; DOT, directly observed therapy.

* All regimens administered 2 times/wk or 3 times/wk should be monitored by DOT for the duration of therapy.

† The strongest evidence from clinical trials is the effectiveness of all 4 drugs administered for the full 6 months. There is weaker evidence that SM can be discontinued after 4 months if the isolate is susceptible to all drugs. The evidence for cessation of PZA before the end of 6 months is equivocal for the 3 times/wk regimen, and there is no evidence of the effectiveness of this regimen with EMB for less than the full 6 months.

(Reprinted from MMWR Recommendations and Reports 42:3, 1993.)

TABLE 3.—Dosage Recommendation for the Initial Treatment of TB Among Children and Adults

| | Dosage | | | | | |
| | Daily | | 2 times/week | | 3 times/week | |
Drugs	Children	Adults	Children	Adults	Children	Adults
Isoniazid	10–20 mg/kg Max. 300 mg	5 mg/kg Max. 300 mg	20–40 mg/kg Max. 900 mg	15 mg/kg Max. 900 mg	20–40 mg/kg Max. 900 mg	15 mg/kg Max. 900 mg
Rifampin	10–20 mg/kg Max. 600 mg	10 mg/kg Max. 600 mg	10–20 mg/kg Max. 600 mg	10 mg/kg Max. 600 mg	10–20 mg/kg Max. 600 mg	10 mg/kg Max. 600 mg
Pyrazinamide	15–30 mg/kg Max. 2 gm	15–30 mg/kg Max. 2 gm	50–70 mg/kg Max. 4 gm	50–70 mg/kg Max. 4 gm	50–70 mg/kg Max. 3 gm	50–70 mg/kg Max. 3 gm
Ethambutol*	15–25 mg/kg Max. 2.5 gm	5–25 mg/kg Max. 2.5 gm	50 mg/kg Max. 2.5 gm	50 mg/kg Max. 2.5 gm	25–30 mg/kg Max. 2.5 gm	25–30 mg/kg Max. 2.5 gm
Streptomycin	20–30 mg/kg Max. 1 gm	15 mg/kg Max. 1 gm	25–30 mg/kg Max. 1.5 gm	25–30 mg/kg Max. 1.5 gm	25–30 mg/kg Max. 1 gm	25–30 mg/kg Max. 1 gm

Note: Children ≤ 12 years of age.
* Ethambutol generally is not recommended for children whose visual acuity cannot be monitored (< 6 years of age). However, ethambutol should be considered for all children with organisms resistant to other drugs when susceptibility to ethambutol has been demonstrated or susceptibility is likely.
(Reprinted from MMWR Recommendations and Reports 42:3, 1993.)

were asked to provide results of drug susceptibility tests on initial *Myco-bacterium tuberculosis* isolates. The cases had been reported to the CDC in the first quarter of 1991.

Findings.—Fourteen percent of cases showed resistance to 1 or more anti-TB drugs. Resistance to isoniazid and/or rifampin was noted in 9.5% of the cases in which isolates were tested against 1 or both drugs. These cases occurred in 107 counties in 33 states. Resistance to isoniazid and rifampin, or MDR TB was noted in 3.5% of the cases with isolates tested against both drugs (Table 1). These cases occurred in 35 counties in 13 states. New York City had 61.4% of the MDR TB cases in the United States. The 3-month, population-based incidence rate of MDR TB in New York City was 52.4 times that of the rest of the country. Compared with the rate in non-Hispanic whites in the rest of the United States, the relative risk of MDR TB in such persons in New York City was 39.0. The relative risk was 299.3 in Hispanics, 420.9 in Asian/Pacific Islanders, and 701 in non-Hispanic blacks.

Conclusion.—With almost 10% of patients with TB resistant to isoniazid and/or rifampin, there is a need for greater use of 4-drug regimens and direct observation of therapy. Aggressive intervention to prevent the further spread of MDR TB is needed.

▶ The emergence of MDR TB poses a grave potential risk to the world's inhabitants. One does not have to look too far back in medical history to see what the effects are when an outbreak of this disease cannot be treated effectively. Thus far, most cases of MDR TB have occurred in limited localities, notably in crowded and poverty-ridden, inner-city areas. These resistant organisms probably originated through selective processes that inadvertently occurred in patients who failed to use the recommended treatment practices—namely, discontinuing the drug when the symptoms first subsided instead of taking the full course. It is interesting that however the resistant forms of the organism originated, more than 90% of cases of MDR TB are now isolated from patients with HIV infection. This fact has helped to boost the mortality rate to as high as 70% to 90%.

Despite the significance of the new forms of this old disease, little is known about the true distribution of MDR TB in the United States. This study examines critical epidemiologic questions about MDR TB in the United States. The essential finding was that some degree of drug resistance occurs in approximately 14% of cases, specific resistance to isoniazid or rifampin was seen in 9.5%, and MDR (isoniazid–rifampin) TB was seen in 3.5% of all cases tested. Although MDR TB was found in 13 states, New York City accounted for 61% of cases, and a population-based index indicated that the incidence there was 52 times that for the rest of the United States. Among those patients with recurrent TB, the rate of MDR was 26.5%, although it is unclear how many of these patients were previously treated with chemotherapy.

Unfortunately, 18% of patients with culture-positive TB were not tested for drug susceptibility. Those tested were subjected to a variety of nonstandardized testing procedures. To distance this study further from the current state of MDR TB in the United States, the data are from 1991. The lag in data collection and analysis has occurred because a large number of cultures were not initially tested for drug resistance. The data here indicate that New York City is a focal center for MDR TB; the veracity of this conclusion may be questioned by the lag in data analysis. Another key issue not identified in these numbers is the presence of concurrent HIV infection. Because of these caveats, the MDR TB problem may be considerably larger than what is pictured here.

Because of the increasing resistance to isoniazid–rifampin combinations, it is now recommended that 4-drug regimens (isoniazid, rifampin, pyrazinamide, and ethambutol; or isoniazid, rifampin, pyrazinamide, and streptomycin) be used in patients with unidentified TB, especially in areas with a high frequency of MDR TB. As the study noted, however, there was a substantial number of patients in whom even a 5-drug regimen would have been of questionable benefit. Greater efforts must be made to find and treat individuals infected with MDR TB. When patient compliance is questionable, directly observed therapy should be instituted (see the 1994 YEAR BOOK of MEDICINE for further discussion of this issue).

The treatment regimen has recently been updated by the CDC (1). The recommendations are critical to follow if we are to be successful with this disease. These guidelines were published in 1993 and were also given in the 1994 YEAR BOOK OF MEDICINE. I will repeat them again so you have access to the latest in the treatment of TB.—R.C. Bone, M.D.

Reference

1. Recommendations and Report. MMWR *Morb Mortal Wkly Rep* 42:3, 1993.

21 Interstitial Lung Disease

Introduction

Although interstitial lung disease (ILD) is a generalized category of disease, inflammation and inflammatory processes seem to be a common thread in their etiologic makeup—and various forms of fibrosis are the typical result of following that thread. Thus, the fibroproliferative diseases have received the brunt of our research attention. Unfortunately, idiopathic pulmonary fibrosis remains an unexplained disease with a poor prognosis. In ILDs, a thickening of the interstitium resulting from immune cell infiltration and edema occurs, which progresses with the proliferative and hypertrophic changes that soon follow. In patients with ILD, exertional breathlessness and a restrictive element to the respiratory function generally manifest.

The prognosis of ILD may be somewhat variable, and the first abstract in this chapter addresses the question of progression of disease. The next abstract examines the pulmonary effects of systemic sclerosis, with particular attention paid to prognostic indicators. Abstract 119-95-21-4 examines the correlation between smooth muscle proliferation in pulmonary fibrosis and digital clubbing, an as yet unexplained phenomenon.

Roger C. Bone, M.D.

Determinants of Progression in Idiopathic Pulmonary Fibrosis

Schwartz DA, Van Fossen DS, Davis CS, Helmers RA, Dayton CS, Burmeister LF, Hunninghake GW (VA Med Ctr, Iowa City, Iowa; Univ of Iowa, Iowa City)
Am J Respir Crit Care Med 149:444–449, 1994   119-95-21-1

Background.—Few researchers have tried to identify the clinical features of idiopathic pulmonary fibrosis (IPF) that independently predict progressive abnormalities in lung function. Determinants of the progressive loss of lung function in patients with IPF were identified prospectively.

Methods.—Thirty-nine patients with IPF were followed for a mean of 2 years. Lung function was determined on at least 2 occasions.

Findings.—There was an average increase of 5.3% in total lung capacity (TLC) and an increase of 9.8% in diffusing capacity of carbon monoxide (DL_{CO}) between the first and last measure of lung function. However, 25% of patients had a decrease in TLC, and 28% had a decrease in DL_{CO}. Decrements in TLC were independently associated with severe dyspnea and cyclophosphamide treatment. Decrements in DL_{CO} were significantly and independently associated with more pack-years of cigarette smoking, moderate or severe dyspnea, and cyclophosphamide therapy.

Conclusion.—Several clinical features are independently related to subsequent decreases in TLC and DL_{CO} in patients with IPF. These prognostic factors—clinical symptoms, smoking history, and need for immunosuppressive treatment—may be used to assess the risk of disease progression in patients with IPF.

▶ The diagnosis of IPF essentially sentences a patient to a median survival of less than 5 years without the benefit of a truly effective treatment. The outlook is even worse for male patients, elderly patients, those with large numbers of neutrophils or eosinophils in their bronchoalveolar lavage fluid, and those displaying "usual interstitial pneumonia" on histologic assessment. Immunosuppression is the current treatment standard, although patients with heavy neutrophilic or eosinophilic infiltrates are less likely to respond. On the other hand, those with large numbers of lymphocytes in their bronchoalveolar lavage (BAL) fluid are more likely to respond well to immunosuppression. Bearing in mind the significance of BAL cell type in diagnoses, the recent finding that cigarette smoking can alter the numbers and types of cells found in BAL (1) might be expected to have important repercussions. Although such a mechanism has not been supported in previous studies of BAL fluid and progression of fibrosis in smokers, these authors elected to perform a prospective study of the relationship between progression of fibrosis and the various clinical features that may be of prognostic usefulness.

The results of this study, which included 39 patients with IPF, indicate that a number of factors, including smoking, can be of prognostic significance. Other clinical symptoms, such as dyspnea, the presence of large numbers of eosinophils in the BAL fluid, and the need for immunosuppressive therapy, can also be used to predict progression of disease. On the other hand, radiographs of the chest were found to be relatively insensitive indicators of progression of disease. Unfortunately, the use of CT was not examined in this study, although it has been shown useful in the diagnosis of IPF. The index most strongly associated with progression of disease in this study was the clinical symptom of dyspnea. The scoring of dyspnea, however, was crude and without resolution; a more precise scoring method may improve the diagnostic power of this symptom. The deleterious effects ascribed to cigarette smoking were supported, with a decrease in diffusing capacity being associated with continued smoking. These effects may take place through the above-described mechanism of enhanced inflammation brought about by altered numbers of specific cell types in the BAL fluid or by the process of emphysema, which has been extensively described. Patients being treated with cyclophosphamide tended to have progressive disease. The authors hastened to note, however, that progression is not caused by the treatment but that progression characterizes the group requiring treatment with this anti-inflammatory agent, adding that a treatment intervention trial is needed to assess potential therapies for IPF further.

Generally, patients with more advanced cases of IPF were also more likely to have progressive disease, whereas those with mild disease tend to continue to have mild disease. Although this may not seem like a particularly applicable conclusion, it may take us closer to the point from which we can someday determine which cases are potentially reversible. Further clinical studies of this dysfunction would consider the risk categories described in this study through the use of stratification protocols.—R.C. Bone, M.D.

Reference

1. Schwartz DA, Helmers RA, Dayton CS, Merchant RK, Hunninghake GW: Determinants of bronchoalveolar lavage cellularity in idiopathic pulmonary fibrosis. *J Appl Physiol* 71:1688–1693, 1991.

Interrelationships Between Pulmonary and Extrapulmonary Involvement in Systemic Sclerosis: A Longitudinal Analysis
Tashkin DP, Clements PJ, Wright RS, Gong H Jr, Simmons MS, Lachenbruch PA, Furst DE (Univ of California, Los Angeles; Virginia Mason Research Ctr, Seattle)
Chest 105:489–495, 1994   119-95-21-2

Background.—Previous studies of lung function in patients with systemic sclerosis (SSc) have not examined the extent of involvement of pulmonary and extrapulmonary organ systems over time as a predictor of progression of disease. Whether survival could be predicted in nonsmoking patients with SSc on the basis of assessments of the degree of

Mean Annualized Rate of Change in Lung Function		
	Observed Decline	Expected Decline *
TLC, ml/yr	−41.7±45.2	−14.2
FVC, ml/yr	−52.8±37.7	−24.1
FEV$_1$, ml/yr	−36.3±21.3	−25.9
Dsb, ml/min/mm Hg/yr	−1.15±0.36	−0.17

Note: Number of patients, 47: female, 41; male, 6.
* Gender-weighted average was estimated from age-coefficients from published prediction equations for nonsmoking men and women.
(Courtesy of Tashkin DP, Clements PJ, Wright RS, et al: *Chest* 105:489–495, 1994.)

impairment of lung function at baseline or the yearly rate of change in lung function over time was determined in a longitudinal analysis.

Methods.—Sixty-three patients were selected using data collected in a prospective, randomized, double-blind trial of the effects of chlorambucil on the natural history of SSc conducted between 1974 and 1984 at the University of California, Los Angeles. Forty-seven patients were included in the nonsmoking study group; the remaining 16 were early withdrawals. Pulmonary function tests, including total lung capacity (TLC), forced vital capacity (FVC), single breath diffusing capacity (Dsb) for carbon monoxide, forced expiratory volume in 1 second (FEV_1), and the FEV_1/FVC ratio were used to assess pulmonary involvement. Radiographic evidence of interstitial pulmonary fibrosis and respiratory symptoms were also examined. The tests were done at least 6 months apart on at least 2 separate occasions.

Results.—The table shows the mean annualized rates of change in lung function, as measured by pulmonary function tests, compared with the expected rates of decline from published prediction equations for nonsmokers. Declines in TLC, FVC, and Dsb were more than the predicted declines, but declines in FEV_1 were as predicted. The extent of decline in baseline pulmonary function tests showed significant correlation to involvement of the right side of the heart but to no other extrapulmonary organ system. In addition, these declines were not significantly related to subsequent declines in lung function or expanded involvement of extrapulmonary organ systems by SSc. Declines in Dsb, TLC, and FVC were significantly correlated with survival.

Conclusion.—The extent of pulmonary involvement by SSc cannot predict the worsening of extrapulmonary involvement, except in the right side of the heart, which is consistent with cor pulmonale. The extent of extrapulmonary involvement cannot predict expanding involvement of pulmonary or extrapulmonary organ systems. An accelerated decline in lung function might predict poor survival.

▶ Systemic sclerosis is a proton disease entity with widely ranging effects in different patients. The authors of this study have taken on the difficult task of assigning characteristics to the pulmonary effects of SSc. Because the pulmonary complications can be deadly, however, it is important that this onerous task be attempted. The characteristics were assigned through assessments and comparisons of organ functions and the rates of change of organ functions. Specifically, this study examined the relationships between lung function and the degree of extrapulmonary involvement at study entry, annual rates of change in lung function and the rates of change of extrapulmonary effects, and the ability of lung function measures and their change over time to predict cumulative survival.

Previous studies have indicated that a Dsb of less than 40% of the expected value is associated with a poor prognosis (1). Patients revealing a restrictive pattern on pulmonary function tests also have a poor prognosis (2). Additionally, FVC can be used to predict survival (3).

Although this study only included nonsmoking patients, pulmonary function tests gave evidence of interstitial lung disease through variable reductions in values of Dsb and FVC. These reductions, however, did not correlate with disease duration. It may not be so surprising that the only correlation between the presence of lung involvement and other organ dysfunction was with that of the right heart—particularly when one considers the finding of pathologic changes in the precapillary blood vessels of the lung in SSc. During the study, both pulmonary function indicators and the function of other organs continued to decline, although as might be expected in cases of fibrosis, the FEV_1 did not show as great a decrement in function because of increased elastic recoil. Unfortunately, none of the pulmonary function parameters could be used to predict subsequent decline of pulmonary or extrapulmonary function, nor could any clinically significant correlations be found among the rates of change of these parameters. There was, however, a correlation between the rate of change of pulmonary function decrement and an increased rate of mortality.—R.C. Bone, M.D.

References

1. Peters-Golden M, Wise RA, Hochberg MC, Stevens MB, Wigley FM: Carbon monoxide diffusing capacity as predictor of outcome in systemic sclerosis. *Am J Med* 77:1027–1034, 1984.
2. Steen VD, Owens GR, Fino GJ, Rodnan GR, Medsger TA Jr: Pulmonary involvement in systemic sclerosis (scleroderma). *Arthritis Rheum* 28:759–767, 1985.
3. Altman RD, Medger TA Jr, Bloch DA, Michel BA: Predictors of survival in systemic sclerosis (scleroderma). *Arthritis Rheum* 34:103–113, 1991.

Clinical Relevance of Testing for Antineutrophil Cytoplasm Antibodies (ANCA) With a Standard Indirect Immunofluorescence ANCA Test in Patients With Upper or Lower Respiratory Tract Symptoms
Davenport A, Lock RJ, Wallington TB (Southmead Hosp, Bristol, England)
Thorax 49:213–217, 1994   119-95-21-3

Objective.—Wegener's granulomatosis is a necrotizing vasculitis of the upper and lower respiratory tract accompanied by glomerulonephritis. The sensitivity and specificity of the antineutrophil cytoplasm antibody (ANCA) test for this rare respiratory disease were determined.

Methods.—Three hundred thirty-five patients, aged 9–87 years, underwent the ANCA test. Wegener's granulomatosis was independently diagnosed and confirmed by biopsy. Human granulocytes were tested by direct immunofluorescence assay. Sera were categorized as c-ANCA or p-ANCA, depending on whether staining was cytoplasmic or perinuclear.

Results.—The findings of 54 c-ANCA and 52 p-ANCA tests were positive. Independent diagnoses revealed 69 cases of Wegener's granulomatosis; 35 of these patients had a positive c-ANCA, and 10 had a positive p-ANCA. Twenty-four patients with negative results had Wegener's granulomatosis. These results indicate a 65% sensitivity and a 77% specificity for a positive ANCA test. Pneumonia was diagnosed in most of the 61 patients who had a positive result but did not have Wegener's granulomatosis. Most false positive results occurred with p-ANCA tests.

Conclusion.—The sensitivity and specificity of the c-ANCA test were greater than those of the p-ANCA test, although most false positive test results became negative with time. Because there were many positive ANCA results using the indirect immunofluorescence test, it may not be as useful as previously reported. The ANCA test may be useful in confirming a diagnosis of Wegener's granulomatosis.

▶ The involvement of an IgG antibody directed against cytoplasmic components of polymorphonuclear leukocytes in glomerulonephritis was first noted in 1982 (1), and it was not much later that the significance in Wegener's granulomatosis was described (2). Although this rare disease is frequently seen with diverse symptoms, the use of antibody testing has improved the ability of clinicians to diagnose it. The antibody involved, ANCA, has been shown by various studies to have sensitivities and specificities for Wegener's disease of greater than 90%. Because most of these studies involved patients at special centers, however, there may have been a patient selection bias. The authors of this study used a patient group similar to that which would be seen everyday in a clinical practice to determine the sensitivity and specificity of 2 forms of antibodies used to detect the presence of ANCA.

In all, 335 patients with respiratory tract symptoms were examined using the criteria of Barlow and Fauci for identifying Wegener's granulomatosis (3). Diagnoses were confirmed with biopsy specimens. Samples from the patients were then subjected to the ANCA test with cytoplasmic- and perinuclear-staining anti-ANCA antibodies. In 69 patients, Wegener's disease was the final diagnosis. The sensitivity and specificity of positive ANCA tests (titer > 1/80) were 49% and 84% for the 2 antibodies combined, 36% and 79% for the c-ANCA test alone, and 13% and 77% for the p-ANCA test alone. These numbers show that the sensitivity and selectivity of these tests are much lower in patient groups exhibiting only respiratory symptoms, as opposed to those already suspected of having Wegener's disease. The authors noted that many false positive results occurred in patients with high IgG concentrations caused by a variety of conditions, suggesting the possibility of nonspecific binding by ANCA antibodies. After the first positive test, further testing was requested for 26% of patients. Eventually, negative results were obtained in all such cases. Additional conditions found in patients with Wegener's disease included upper and lower respiratory symptoms and renal involvement. Using these criteria, the clinical diagnosis of Wegener's disease should become easier and more accurate.—R.C. Bone, M.D.

References

1. Davies DJ, Moran JE, Niall JF, et al: Segmental necrotizing glomerulonephritis

with antineutrophil antibody: Possible arbor virus aetiology? *BMJ* 285:606, 1982.

2. van der Woude FJ, Rasmussen N, Lobatto S, Wiik A, Permin H, van Es LA, et al: Autoantibodies against neutrophils and monocytes: Tool for diagnosis and marker for disease activity in Wegener's granulomatosis. *Lancet* i:425–429, 1985.

3. Barlow JE, Fauci AS: Vasculitic disease of the kidney: Polyarteritis nodosa. Wegener's granulomatosis, allergic angiitis, and granulomatous and other disorders. In, Schroder RW, Gottschalk CW (eds): *Diseases of the Kidney,* ed 4. New York, Little Brown, 1988, pp 2335–2360.

Clubbing of the Fingers and Smooth-Muscle Proliferation in Fibrotic Changes in the Lung in Patients With Idiopathic Pulmonary Fibrosis
Kanematsu T, Kitaichi M, Nishimura K, Nagai S, Izumi T (Kyoto Univ, Japan)
Chest 105:339–342, 1994   119-95-21-4

Introduction.—Patients with idiopathic pulmonary fibrosis (IPF), identified pathologically as unusual interstitial pneumonia (UIP), have smooth-muscle proliferation in pulmonary fibrotic changes. To identify the relationship between pathologic and clinical findings, the extent of smooth-muscle proliferation in pulmonary fibrotic changes seen in patients with IPF was quantified, and correlations with the grade of disease and clinical characteristics were analyzed.

Methods.—Fifty-two patients with clinically diagnosed IPF underwent open lung biopsy, and the presence of UIP was established. The grade of smooth-muscle proliferation was assigned, with grade 1 representing few smooth-muscle cells in pulmonary fibrotic changes and grade 3 representing diffuse bundles or nodular growth of smooth-muscle cells in the pulmonary fibrotic changes. Clinical findings evaluated included demographic variables, smoking habits, severity of symptoms, duration of lower respiratory symptoms, the extent of chest radiographic abnormalities, clubbed fingers, and function of the lungs.

Results.—Clubbed fingers were significantly correlated with smooth-muscle proliferation in pulmonary fibrotic lesions. Clubbed fingers were found more frequently in patients with higher grades of smooth-muscle proliferation, although lower grades of honeycombing appeared in the biopsy sections of patients with clubbed fingers. The patients with extensive smooth-muscle proliferation were also more likely to have sought examination because of subjective symptoms, to have had symptoms in the lower respiratory systems of a longer duration, and to have had more pulmonary infiltrates revealed on chest radiographs.

Discussion.—There was a clear correlation between the clinical findings of clubbed fingers and the pathologic finding of smooth-muscle proliferation in pulmonary fibrotic lesions in patients with IPF. This correlation strengthened with the increasing grade of proliferation.

▶ Idiopathic pulmonary fibrosis remains a mystifying and ultimately fatal disease. In addition to dyspnea, cor pulmonale, and bibasilar end-inspiratory dry crackles, a commonly (30% to 75%) associated feature is digital clubbing. More recently, proliferative smooth-muscle changes have been associated with IPF. The authors of this study noted that smooth-muscle changes in IPF had not, however, been correlated with clinical findings common to the disease. The finding that the degree of finger clubbing was correlated with smooth-muscle proliferation in fibrotic lesions seen in open lung biopsy material is in agreement with the authors' observation that the degree of proliferation also correlates with the duration of the symptoms and the extent of pulmonary infiltration seen on radiograms.

Although this is not a particularly surprising finding, it does help us focus on the seriousness of IPF, in which the mortality rate is approximately 50% five years after diagnosis. Nor does it help us understand the pathogenesis of IPF—even the pathophysiology of digital clubbing has not been satisfactorily explained. However, the recently described association between proliferative changes in smooth muscle and IPF is a central and interesting event in this study. Further analysis of this association may someday help us understand the pathogenesis of IPF.—R.C. Bone, M.D.

22 Pleural Disease

Introduction

This year's Pleural Disease chapter contains only 1 selection, which discusses a rare, osteolytic condition known as Gorham's syndrome. Chylothorax is a complication often seen in this syndrome, and it is the opinion of the article's authors that this complication should be treated early and aggressively with surgical intervention to achieve thoracic duct ligation. If that approach is impossible, a complete pleurodesis should be performed. The most common cause of chylothorax is lymphoma (approximately 50% of all cases). Surgical trauma is the second most common cause (25%). Other, less common causes include Kaposi's sarcoma, lymphangioleiomyomatosis, and Noonan's syndrome. The pleural fluid is commonly milky but may be serous. The diagnosis can be made by a triglyceride level of greater than 110 mg/dL. A lipoprotein electrophoresis is indicated when the values fall between 50 and 110 mg/dL.

Roger C. Bone, M.D.

Chylothorax in Gorham's Syndrome: A Common Complication of a Rare Disease

Tie MLH, Poland GA, Rosenow EC III (Mayo Clinic and Found, Rochester, Minn)
Chest 105:208–213, 1994   119-95-22–1

Introduction.—Gorham's syndrome is a rare osteolytic disease, most typically involving the maxilla, shoulder girdle, or pelvis. Since 1955, there have been published reports of 146 cases. Chylothorax has been a complication in 25 of these patients. In 2 patients, this complication was addressed with aggressive surgical intervention.

Case 1.—Man, 30, had recurrent posterior thoracic pain and dyspnea. Chest radiographs revealed the absence of the left third through sixth ribs and bilateral pleural effusions. The left-sided effusion could not be medically resolved. The biopsy findings confirmed Gorham's syndrome. A left-sided thoracotomy was performed, but the effusion was not discrete enough to identify a duct for ligation; the lung was therefore decorticated with tetracycline pleurodesis. His condition deteriorated until a pericardial window was created by emergency thoracotomy. He improved after the operation but died 19 days later of adult respiratory distress syndrome.

Case 2.—Man, 18, was seen after 3 days of left-sided pleuritic chest pain and dyspnea. He had fractured his clavicle 20 months earlier. Radiographs revealed a large, left-sided pleural effusion; an absent left clavicle; and marked osteopenia in the left scapula, the first 2 ribs, and the proximal humerus. The pathologic findings were consistent with those of Gorham's syndrome. Massive chylous drainage from a chest tube could not be resolved medically. No discrete ductal structure could be ligated even after decortication of the left lung. Thoracic duct ligation was finally accomplished with a low right thoracotomy, and the patient recovered slowly; there was no recurrence of pleural effusion in 2 years of follow-up.

Discussion.—A review of the medical literature revealed that all patients with Gorham's syndrome who had reported chylothorax had rib, scapular, clavicular, or thoracic vertebral involvement. Surgical failure in these patients was caused by the inability to localize the thoracic duct. Survival was significantly improved with a right-sided approach for thoracic duct ligation (72% vs. 50% with a left-sided approach). All patients who died after a right-sided approach had undergone surgery after their condition had massively deteriorated. Prompt, aggressive surgical thoracic duct ligation using a right-sided approach is therefore recommended.

▶ The occurrence of Gorham's syndrome is rare—only 146 cases have been reported in the literature. The manifestations of the disease range from minimal disability to death, and intervention must be appropriate to the complication. For patients in whom chylothorax develops, intervention that is both timely and aggressive is required. In the current study, 17% of patients had chylothorax, a higher incidence than previously has been reported in this syndrome. In 1954, however, Gorham and co-workers reported a 25% incidence of chylothorax in patients with "bone phantom" syndrome, leading another group to suggest that the term "Gorham's syndrome" should be redefined to include the presence of chylothorax as well as the presence of skeletal abnormalities (1). Tie and colleagues recommend surgical intervention—specifically, low right-sided thoracotomy—to manage chylothorax. The authors' review of the literature revealed that only 36% of patients who did not undergo surgery survived, whereas 64% of those in whom surgery was performed did survive.

One quarter of patients with chylothorax had involvement of either rib, scapular, clavicular, or thoracic vertebral bone. These symptoms could have been reported to either their general physician or to a specialist. Gorham's syndrome may be rare, and certainly most of us will never see a case; however, the rapid and high rate of mortality in these patients with chylothorax make this syndrome something for all of us to keep in mind.—R.C. Bone, M.D.

Reference

1. Pedicelli G, Mattia P, Zorzoli AA, et al: Gorham syndrome. JAMA 252:1449–1451, 1984.

23 Occupational Lung Disease

Introduction

Although more emphasis has been placed on workplace safety, the burgeoning techniques and processes have the potential to cause various forms of pulmonary disease among workers. These conditions range from mild forms of asthma to deadly, malignant mesothelioma. In the former case, a myriad of causes may be involved, ranging from the inhalation of volatile solvents to the presence of dusts and gases generated in animal confinement buildings. The presence of inflammation appears to be particularly important in generating the various forms of asthma. Fibrosis may be directly incited by interactions between macrophages and environmental agents. For instance, in vitro experiments show that macrophages respond to the presence of silica crystals with activation and the production of growth factors that affect fibroblasts, with the likely result of fiber deposition.

It is still unclear whether the frequency of mesothelioma is decreasing, although the number of cases of asbestosis is on the decline. Both conditions are associated with breathing in the small fibers released by the various forms of asbestos used previously in the United States (and still present in far too many public and private buildings) for a variety of insulation purposes. Although 80% to 85% of these cases can be attributed to occupational exposure, the remaining cases are often unexplained. Hopefully, federal bans on the use of asbestos will reduce both occupational and unexplained cases of mesothelioma.

The first article in this chapter questions the importance of where peak flow assessment in occupational asthma should take place—at home or at work. Although the topic of the second abstract may not be interpreted by some as an occupational issue, it is an important point involving environmental toxins that needs addressing: carbon monoxide poisoning resulting from the indoor burning of charcoal briquets. This year's YEAR BOOK OF MEDICINE also includes an interesting article that examines the effect of smoking on workers exposed to asbestos and how these factors affect spirometric and radiographic assessments.

Roger C. Bone, M.D.

How Many Times Per Day Should Peak Expiratory Flow Rates Be Assessed When Investigating Occupational Asthma?

Malo J-L, Côté J, Cartier A, Boulet L-P, L'Archevêque J, Chan-Yeung M (Sacré-Coeur Hosp, Montreal; Laval Hosp, Quebec City, Canada; Vancouver Gen Hosp, BC, Canada)

Thorax 48:1211–1217, 1993   119-95-23-1

Introduction.—Serial recording of the peak expiratory flow rate (PEFR) has been proposed as a sensitive and specific means of monitoring work-related asthma. It is not clear, however, how many daily recordings are needed to ensure optimal within- and between-reader reproducibility.

Methods.—Seventy-four individuals referred with possible occupational asthma had PEFR recorded every 2 hours for at least 10 working days and for 2 weeks away from work. Graphs of PEFR were constructed at frequencies of every 2 hours, 3 and 4 times per day, and each morning and evening. Individual values of PEF taken before the use of inhaled β_2 adrenergic agents and plots of the highest, lowest, and mean daily values were graphed (Fig 23–1). Three readers at different centers examined the graphs in a blind manner. In addition, some graphs of each type were read blindly by the same reader after 1 week. Inhalation challenge testing had yielded positive results in 33 individuals.

Results.—The best sensitivity–specificity ratio with agreement of at least 2 of the 3 readers was achieved with the 2-hour graphs; sensitivity was 72%, and specificity 78%. Taking readings 4 times per day was nearly as accurate. Comparable results were obtained when participants using bronchodilators only were analyzed separately. Within-reader reproducibility ranged from 83% to 100%.

Conclusion.—Recording the PEFR 4 times per day appears to be adequate when attempting to confirm work-related asthma.

► As in the case of asthma, patients with occupational asthma may benefit from the use of peak-flow meters for disease assessment. Hourly, daily, and weekly patterns of PEFR in occupational asthma have been described (1, 2). Comparing worker at-work and away-from-work PEFRs appears to provide important data about on-the-job allergens and is simpler than the specific inhalational challenge test performed in the laboratory. This technique has not been well established, however, and questions remain regarding the optimal methods of using PEFR in occupational asthma. In particular, the appropriate timing of the measurements is not known, although most studies have used 2-hour intervals. Additionally, it has been shown that the rate of discrepancies among separate readings by different readers is high—1 study showed a 31% disagreement rate among readers, whereas discrepancies between separate readings by the same reader are less well studied but may range from 0% to 10% (3). This study compared the use of PEFR readings taken at

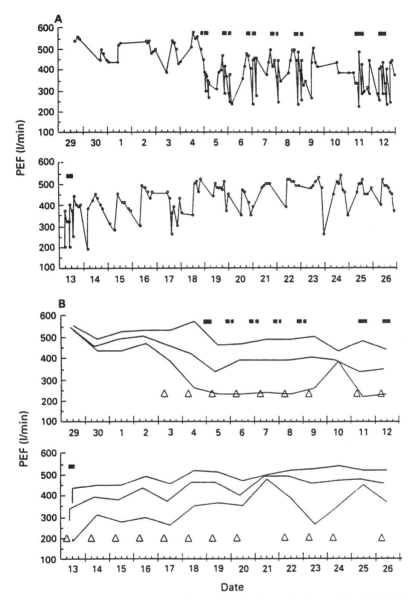

Fig 23–1.—Graphs of the same patient with occupational asthma plotted using (**A**) individual data and (**B**) daily mean, highest and lowest values. In the latter instance, *triangles* indicate days in which differences between the highest and lowest values were 20% or more. Periods at work are represented by the *horizontal bars*. (Courtesy of Malo J-L, Côté J, Cartier A, et al: *Thorax* 48:1211-1217, 1993.)

various intervals with the results of specific inhalation challenges. Between- and within-reader discrepancies were also examined.

The results indicated that visual interpretations of PEFR records taken every 2 hours provided a slightly better agreement with specific inhalation challenge testing and reduced the number of between-reader discrepancies than did readings timed at other intervals. However, these differences were not statistically significant and were very similar to those obtained when readings were taken every 6 hours. Less frequent readings provided poorer agreement with the challenge tests. The patient's use of bronchodilators or inhaled steroids affected the accuracy of PEFR readings. Within-reader agreement was good, and graph readings by the same reader 1 week apart were in 83% to 100% concordance, whereas between-reader agreement was highest at the 2- and 4-hour intervals, reaching 82% and 77%, respectively. An important factor that may affect the PEFR assessment of occupational asthma is the timing of worker exposure to the offending agent, which may only be brief or intermittent.

A number of new instruments that may be useful in assessing asthma have recently been developed. Meters that can measure and record PEFR reliably are now available, as is a meter that can measure the PEFR and forced expiratory volume in 1 second simultaneously. The latter instrument has been shown useful in identifying the late asthmatic response to asthma-causing agents. The use of these assessment methods for occupational asthma should increase the rate of diagnosis and help prevent workers at risk of more severe asthma caused by continued exposure.—R.C. Bone, M.D.

References

1. Burge P, O'Brien I, Harries M: Peak flow rate records in the diagnosis of occupational asthma due to isocyanates. *Thorax* 34:317–323, 1979.
2. Burge P, O'Brien I, Harries M: Peak flow rate records in the diagnosis of occupational asthma due ot colophony. *Thorax* 34:308–316, 1979.
3. Venables K, Burge PS, Davison A, Taylor AN: Peak flow rate records in surveys: Reproducibility of observers' reports. *Thorax* 39:828–832, 1984.

Carbon Monoxide Poisoning From Indoor Burning of Charcoal Briquets

Hampson NB, Kramer CC, Dunford RG, Norkool DM (Virginia Mason Med Ctr, Seattle)
JAMA 271:52–53, 1994   119-95-23-2

Introduction.—Carbon monoxide (CO) poisoning is the most common cause of unintentional poisoning death in the United States. Despite warnings on packaging, the indoor use of charcoal briquets may not be widely recognized as a risk for CO poisoning. Cases of CO poisoning treated at an urban tertiary care center were reviewed to gather data on the number of patients, their epidemiology, and reasons for the indoor use of charcoal briquets.

Methods.—Patients were treated in the hyperbaric department of Virginia Mason Medical Center in Seattle from October 1982 to October 1993. Hyperbaric oxygen treatment required a blood carboxyhemoglobin (COHb) level of 25% or greater, anginal pain or ischemic changes on ECG, or neurologic impairment. Treatment consisted of hyperbaric oxygen administration at 2.8–3 absolute pressure.

Results.—Seventy-nine of 509 patients treated on an emergency basis for acute unintentional CO poisoning had been exposed to the indoor burning of charcoal. Patients ranged in age from 3 months to 87 years; 48% were male, and 52% were female. Seventy-three percent of patients were from racial and ethnic minorities. A large percentage of Hispanic and Asian patients did not speak English (88% and 56%, respectively). The average level of COHb was 21.6%. Thirty-three percent of patients lost consciousness, at least transiently, and many reported headache, nausea, and dizziness. Of 32 total incidents, charcoal burned for home heating accounted for 16, and charcoal used for cooking accounted for the remaining 16. Cases of CO poisoning related to indoor use of charcoal briquets were most common during the months of October through January.

Conclusion.—An estimated 800–1,000 deaths occur in the United States annually because of unintentional CO poisoning. Individuals who burn charcoal indoors are unaware of the risk and may attribute their symptoms to food poisoning or other causes. Multilingual warnings on packages of briquets and public warnings during periods of power outages are recommended as possible solutions to the problem.

▶ To most of us, the burning of charcoal briquets heralds the beginning of summer, backyard barbecues, and, in general, good times. Unfortunately, however, CO poisoning resulting from the indoor burning of charcoal is also the most common cause of unintentional poisoning death in this country (1), with 10,000 individuals affected and 800–1,000 deaths yearly (2). Most incidents occur during the winter months, as people use charcoal to heat their homes or to cook. In this series, 73% of patients were members of a minority race. Many were first-generation immigrants who acted according to their cultural norms and were not aware of the risk involved. Even though all packages of briquets carry an explicit warning against burning indoors, many patients in this series did not understand English; therefore, the warning was useless. The death rate from unintentional CO poisoning declined during the 1980s because of increased public education about the risks involved with indoor burning of charcoal (1). Of the 32 incidents studied, 16 were associated with home heating and 16 were associated with cooking.

These authors suggest—and I agree—that the dangers of CO poisoning should be widely publicized by the media when power outages occur, and utility companies should include a warning with notices of intention to disconnect power. The United States Consumer Products Safety Commission is currently reviewing the warning carried on bags of charcoal briquets for possible clarification. It is hoped that this group will consider the number of individuals who cannot read the current warning and will make changes to correct that problem. The authors suggest printing warnings in several languages or using a nonverbal graphic warning. The nonverbal warning seems like the better idea. Let's make sure that *everyone* knows of the danger.—R.C. Bone, M.D.

References

1. Cobb N, Etzel PA: Unintentional carbon monoxide–related deaths in the United States, 1979 through 1988. *JAMA* 266:659–663, 1991.
2. Centers for Disease Control: Carbon monoxide intoxication: A preventable environmental health hazard. *MMWR Morb Mortal Wkly Rep* 31:529–531, 1982.

Spirometric Impairments in Long-Term Insulators: Relationships to Duration of Exposure, Smoking, and Radiographic Abnormalities
Miller A, Lilis R, Godbold J, Chan E, Wu X, Selikoff IJ (City Univ of New York)
Chest 105:175–182, 1994   119-95-23–3

Introduction.—A group of 2,611 insulators who had been exposed to asbestos at least 30 years ago were studied to explore the prevalence of spirometric and radiographic abnormalities, the relative effect of cigarette smoking, and the duration of asbestos exposure.

Methods.—The surviving members of the International Brotherhood of Heat, Frost and Asbestos Insulation Workers, whose exposure to asbestos began at least 30 years before the study, were examined with chest radiography and spirometry. Their smoking habits and history were recorded. The spirometry findings in nonsmokers were compared with those in a random sample of the general population of Michigan.

Results.—Of the 2,611 men, 2,096 had a smoking history: 1,221 were former smokers and 875 were current smokers. The nonsmokers had lower forced vital capacity (FVC) and forced expiratory volume in 1 second (FEV_1) and higher FEV_1/FVC findings than the same findings in the Michigan population, whereas the flow rates, forced expiratory flow (FEF) 25% to 75% and forced expiratory time (FET) 25% to 75%, were similar. Smokers had significantly more spirometric impairments than nonsmokers, with unfavorable comparisons on all of the specific tests and especially deep reductions on the FEV_1 findings. Current smokers had more significant impairments than ex-smokers, whose impairment rates were intermediate between nonsmokers and current smokers. Overt obstruction was found in 17% of current smokers and in 3% of nonsmokers. Smoking history did not affect the frequency of restrictive impairment, but combined impairment occurred in 18% of current smokers and in 3% of nonsmokers. Increasing duration of asbestos exposure correlated with increasing spirometric impairments, especially reduced FVC. The likelihood of normal spirometric findings was highest (46%) when the chest radiographs were normal and lowest (21%) when radiographs detected both parenchymal and pleural disease. Radiography failed to predict spirometric abnormalities in 27% of the population. Restrictive and combined impairments tended to be associated with both parenchymal and pleural abnormalities, and obstruction tended to be associated with parenchymal abnormalities only. Specific test associations included decreased FVC with pleural abnormality and decreased FEV_1/FVC with parenchymal abnormality.

Discussion.—Smoking significantly reduced both FVC and FEV_1/FVC, suggesting that smoking and asbestos exposure together contribute to the severe pleural involvement and airway obstruction seen in this population. Tests of lung function should be used to detect abnormalities not seen clinically or radiologically.

▶ Following a cohort of individuals for a long time provides important information about changes that occur gradually. This study examines one of the largest reported groups belonging to a single trade with heavy, long-term exposure to asbestos. Most of these men (87%) had more than 30 years of exposure—more than enough time for asbestos- and smoking-related disease to evolve. Eighty percent of these men had a history of smoking, although most were ex-smokers (56%); 34% of the total population continued to smoke, and approximately 20% were nonsmokers. The large subgroup of nonsmokers allowed the authors to analyze the relationship between inhaling asbestos fibers and pulmonary function without the confounding factor of smoking.

The use of a large, well-defined population lends itself to the analysis of independent variables, such as asbestos exposure, cigarette smoking, and radiographic abnormalities, along with the effects of these factors on spirometric lung function. Measures of FVC evaluated how much of the lung can be ventilated, with decreased FVC indicating that restriction resulted from pulmonary or pleural fibrosis and/or obstruction of the airways caused by air trapping. In this study, all significant variables of lung function, including percent of predicted FVC, measurements of $FEV_1/FVC \times 100$, and FET 25% to 75% were inversely related to FVC. The interval of exposure had the greatest effect on FVC, with the incidence of normal spirometric measures decreasing as the duration of exposure increased. The frequency of restriction and combined impairment also increased with longer exposure. Forty-five percent of those with 30 years of exposure had lower than normal levels of FVC, whereas 54% of those with 40 or more years of exposure had decreased levels. Radiographic evidence of combined pleuropulmonary involvement, smoking, and isolated pleural involvement also were inversely related to FVC.

Whereas the frequency of isolated small airways obstruction was similar for all smoking categories, the authors found that increased FET 25% to 75%, used as a measure of general airways dysfunction, varied greatly—the incidence was 34% in nonsmokers, 50% in ex-smokers, and 67% in current smokers, regardless of whether other spirometric abnormalities were present. Those with restrictive impairment showed a similar relationship between smoking and increased FET 25% to 75%. By definition, FEV_1/FVC was normal in these individuals; therefore, the relationship between smoking and increased FET 25% to 75% may be said to provide evidence of small airways dysfunction as well as restriction. Those individuals with normal findings on chest radiography were more likely to have normal measurements on spirometry, and those with radiographic evidence of parenchymal and pleural disease were least likely to have normal measurements.

The large subpopulation of nonsmokers in this study made it possible to identify patterns of pulmonary function that can be attributed only to inhalation of asbestos. Measurements of FEV_1/FVC were reduced in only 6% of this group, which is not strong evidence that impairment occurs as a result of inhalation alone. In addition, some of this nonsmoking population may have an independent cause for this obstruction, such as asthma.

Although these results demonstrate the important effect of pleural fibrosis on lung function, generalizing these results to other asbestos-exposed populations may not be possible for several reasons. Not only was this group specifically selected for the long duration and intensity of exposure but, to some extent, it is also a survivor population. It is likely that those with the most serious effects have died. In many occupations, including plumbers and shipyard workers, in which asbestos exposure is less intense than that which occurs with insulators, pleural disease is more common than interstitial fibrosis, and the serious effects that pleural disease has on lung function may be relevant to these groups as well. In addition, 13% of those with pleural disease had diffuse disease. These same authors previously reported that diffuse thickening has a greater effect on FVC and may supervene many years after first exposure (1, 2).

Finally, reductions in FVC and FEV_1/FVC occurred more frequently in insulators who smoked (49% and 34%, respectively), suggesting that an interaction between exposure to asbestos and smoking results in lowering these levels. Among nonsmokers in this group, FEV_1/FVC was reduced in only 6%, and FVC was reduced in 33%. Although educational efforts to reduce the number of insulators who smoke have been somewhat successful, it is clear that more intense efforts are warranted.—R.C. Bone, M.D.

References

1. Lilis R, Selikoff IJ, Lerman Y, et al: Pulmonary function and pleural fibrosis: Quantitative relationships with an integrative index of pleural abnormalities. *Am J Ind Med* 20:145–161, 1991.
2. Lilis R, Lerman Y, Selikoff IJ: Symptomatic benign pleural effusions among asbestos insulation workers: Residual radiographic abnormalities. *Br J Ind Med* 45:443–449, 1988.

24 Sleep Apnea

Introduction

Sleep apnea may affect as many as 2% of women and 4% of men (1, 2). The 60,000 or so patients with obstructive sleep apnea who are evaluated in the nation's sleep centers and who have a low apnea index have a 96% survival rate after 8–9 years of follow-up. In contrast, those with an elevated apnea index have a higher mortality rate.

The association between sleep apnea and other disease entities is now better understood. For instance, the presence of systemic hypertension occurs in 50% to 90% of patients with sleep apnea. Also, some studies have shown that patients with essential hypertension have a 30% incidence of obstructive sleep apnea. An increase in myocardial infarction has also been seen. Thus, the recognition of and treatment for sleep apnea becomes essential for evaluation of diseases often not thought to result from sleep apnea. Because of this, clinicians should have a high index of suspicion whenever their patients complain of the following possible signs of obstructive sleep apnea:

- Excessive daytime sleepiness
- Loud, habitual snoring
- Chronic fatigue
- Obesity
- Nocturnal choking or gasping
- Apnea witnessed by a bed partner
- Restless sleep
- Frequent nocturia
- Frequent nocturnal sweating
- Dilated cardiomyopathy or pulmonary hypertension of an obscure cause
- Personality changes
- Impotence

The 3 papers in the Sleep Apnea chapter of this year's YEAR BOOK OF MEDICINE evaluate patient compliance with continuous positive airway pressure (CPAP), the long-term survival of patients treated with either uvulopalatopharyngoplasty or nasal CPAP, and factors predictive of long-term compliance with nasal CPAP.

Roger C. Bone, M.D.

References

1. Phillips BA, Berry DTR, Schmitt FA, Magon LK, Gerhardstein DC, Cook YR: Sleep-disordered breathing in the healthy elderly: Clinically significant? *Chest* 101:345–349, 1992.
2. Young T, Palta M. Dempsey I, Skatrud J, Weber S, Badr S: The occurrence of sleep-disordered breathing among middle-aged adults. *N Engl J Med* 328:1230–1235, 1993.

Nasal CPAP: An Objective Evaluation of Patient Compliance

Reeves-Hoche MK, Meck R, Zwillich CW (Pennsylvania State Univ, Hershey; Respitech Med Services, Leola, Pa)
Am J Respir Crit Care Med 149:149–154, 1994   119-95-24-1

Objective.—Nasal continuous positive airway pressure (NCPAP) is an important treatment for obstructive sleep apnea (OSA). It not only eliminates apneas and symptoms but improves survival. The sealed nasal mask used in NCPAP treatment is uncomfortable, raising possible compliance problems, and the treatment is only effective if mask pressure is maintained at levels sufficient to prevent pharyngeal occlusion. A monitoring device was used to record NCPAP use and mask pressure over time.

Methods.—An elapsed timer and a mask pressure transducer recorder were designed and installed in the NCPAP units of 38 men and 9 women (mean age, 51 years; mean body mass index, 42) without their knowledge. All patients complained of daytime sleepiness. The mean apnea–hypopnea index (AHI) was 58, according to full-night polysomnography. The patients were seen every 2–8 weeks during a 6-month

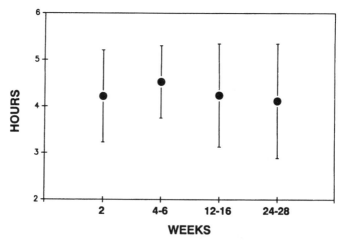

Fig 24–1.—Grouped mean hourly effective use of the NCPAP device during the 6-month evaluation period. Comparison of use during the periods of observation showed no significant differences. (Courtesy of Reeves-Hoche MK, Meck R, Zwillich CW: *Am J Respir Crit Care Med* 149:149–154, 1994.)

period. Timer data were recorded at each visit but were not used in patient care.

Results.—Thirty-eight patients completed 6 months of therapy. The mean hours of use per night in these patients was 4.7, representing 68% of reported total sleep time. All but 5 patients reported using the device for all hours of sleep. Effective use per night was 4.3 hours, representing 91% of the time that effective pressure was maintained at the mask. There was no correlation between AHI and compliance, but there was a correlation between AHI and effective use. The complaint of daytime sleepiness was correlated with compliance only during the initial visit. No factors predictive of compliance could be identified. Mean hourly effective use of the device did not change significantly during the study (Fig 24–1).

Conclusion.—Group compliance with NCPAP in patients with OSA was 68%. Considering the maintenance of adequate pressure, effective therapy is achieved for only approximately 62% of sleep time. Compliance is difficult to predict from baseline characteristics. Compliance with NCPAP is generally poor, especially considering the high discontinuation rate.

▶ With the recent discovery that serious cardiovascular complications may result from OSA, treatment modes have been receiving intense scrutiny. Although NCPAP has been shown to be an effective treatment for the condition, other studies have indicated that many patients cannot tolerate the mask and that compliance may be low. Among the complaints are nasal discomfort and dyspnea. As an additional obstacle to physicians who want to prescribe the NCPAP, there have been no studies of actual delivered pressures to determine whether therapeutic levels of pressure are achieved in home use of NCPAP.

In this 6-month study, 68% of the reported hours of sleep were accompanied by use of the machine. Therapeutic pressures were achieved during 91% of the period the machine was in use; thus, effective therapy was achieved during only 62% of the sleep time reported by the patient—an average total of 4.3 hr/night. These numbers were derived from patients who used the machine for the first 3 months of the study; however, 20% of patients had discontinued NCPAP at that point for a variety of reasons. Another study using a covert monitor found that NCPAP was used on only 66% of all nights, and the mean period of NCPAP use was 4.88 hr/night (1). The compliance rates in these 2 studies are lower than those found in many other studies. Many of those studies, however, depended on patient recall and opinion and were more likely to be biased. Although these figures are somewhat discouraging, the technique does help a substantial percentage of all patients. Treatment with NCPAP should be attempted for patients with sleep apnea and excessive daytime sleepiness, although I would recommend close follow-up to determine whether patients are complying with their treatment.

It was interesting that many patients in this study reported improvements in aspects of their lives that they previously had not considered to be impaired. This finding is an indication of the overwhelming debility that sleep apnea can have on a patient's life and makes it clear that we must do what we can for them. In patients who are compliant with NCPAP use, the therapy can greatly improve their quality of life.—R.C. Bone, M.D.

Reference

1. Kribs NB, Pach AI, Kline LR, Smith PL, Schwartz AR, Schubert NM, Redlove S, et al: Objective measurements of nasal CPAP use by patients with obstructive sleep apnea. *Am Rev Respir Dis* 147:887–895, 1993.

Predictive Factors of Long-Term Compliance With Nasal Continuous Positive Airway Pressure Treatment in Sleep Apnea Syndrome
Meurice J-C, Dore P, Paquereau J, Neau J-P, Ingrand P, Chavagnat J-J, Patte F (Centre Hospitalier Universitaire de Poitiers, France; Faculté de Médecine de Poitiers, France)
Chest 105:429–433, 1994   119-95-24–2

Introduction.—Nocturnal ventilation with nasal continuous positive airway pressure (CPAP) is the most effective treatment of sleep apnea syndrome (SAS). The factors that predicted good compliance with this treatment among patients with SAS were explored prospectively.

Methods.—Forty-four patients were initially tested for respiratory function and underwent a polysomnographic recording. During the second night of polysomnography, CPAP treatment began, and the level of effective positive airway pressure required to stop snoring, apnea, and desaturation was determined. The patients were followed after 1 week and 1 month and advised to increase daily the use of nasal CPAP. Polysomnography and physical examination was performed every 6 months, and patients were questioned about the length and frequency of nasal CPAP use and about diurnal hypersomnia.

Results.—The patients were followed a mean of 14 months. At the end of the study, 41 patients used CPAP every night, 36 used it all night, and 30 had an average time-counter measurement of more than 5 hr/night. Polysomnography during CPAP treatment revealed a reduced apnea–hypopnea index and a greater proportion of slow-wave sleep and rapid eye movement sleep. Diurnal hypersomnia was significantly reduced with CPAP treatment. The average time using the apparatus correlated positively with initial polysomnographic findings of a high apnea-hypopnea index or light sleep. Daily use of nasal CPAP was positively correlated with reductions in the apnea–hypopnea index, improvement in oxygen saturation during sleep, and reductions in hypersomnia. There was no correlation between compliance and gender or the type of mask.

Discussion.—These findings indicate that the initial gravity of the patient's condition influenced the patient's degree of compliance; those who were more severely affected used the apparatus more. Patients continued long-term compliance when they experienced recognizable improvement, especially in sleep patterns, with the therapy.

▶ The use of nasal CPAP in patients with sleep apnea has been recommended since the mid-1980s. A number of more recent studies have addressed the issues of long-term compliance and complications of nasal CPAP. These issues are important because treatment is usually expected to be lifelong and failure to treat the disease can result in serious medical complications, including heart attack. These studies, however, addressed different issues with various methodologies, making interpretation difficult. Additionally, no recommendations have been developed regarding the number of hours of daily use or complications that may accompany such long-term daily use. In this study, these issues were addressed through a prospective study of patients with SAS, which is defined as a sleeping apnea–hypopnea index of greater than 15/hr.

Compliance among this group of patients was 68%, based on a strict quota of 5 hours or more of uninterrupted use per night. The calculated compliance, however, varied dramatically when the criteria were modified. Among the patients who were compliant, 97 continued the long-term use of the system for an average of 14 months after initiation of treatment. Ninety-three percent of patients used CPAP every night, and 82% used the system throughout the night. Seventy-nine percent of patients used CPAP all night, every night. These numbers indicate relatively good compliance, which the authors state may be attributable to the manner in which patients are supervised.

Contrary to results seen in other studies, only 1 patient stopped treatment midway through the study. The event resulted from nasal obstruction and rhinorrhea, despite the use of decongestants and anti-inflammatory agents. Side effects, including cutaneous erosion of the nose bridge (52% of treated patients), rhinitis, and leakage, were seen frequently in this study. Substantial numbers of patients were bothered by the noise and/or loss of freedom. An important finding was that the degree of initial compliance was related to the seriousness of symptoms. In other words, patients most adversely affected by SAS were most likely to give CPAP a good try. Similarly, long-term compliance depended on the improvement that therapy brought. Patients who understand the possible serious consequences of SAS are most likely to comply with CPAP, even in the face of bothersome side effects.—R.C. Bone, M.D.

Long-Term Survival of Patients With Obstructive Sleep Apnea Treated by Uvulopalatopharyngoplasty or Nasal CPAP

Keenan SP, Burt H, Ryan CF, Fleetham JA (Univ of British Columbia, Vancouver, Canada)

Chest 105:155–159, 1994   119-95-24–3

Introduction.—Most studies have found that obstructive sleep apnea (OSA) is associated with decreased long-term survival. Only 1 previous

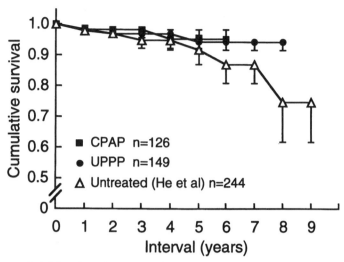

Fig 24–2.—Probability of cumulative survival for patients with obstructive sleep apnea with an apnea index ≥ 5/hr, treated with UPPP and CPAP. Data on untreated patients from He et al. (*Chest* 94:9, 1988), with permission. (Courtesy of Keenan SP, Burt H, Ryan CF, et al: *Chest* 105:155-159, 1994.)

study has compared the relative efficacy of treatment of OSA with either nasal continuous positive airway pressure (CPAP) and tracheostomy or uvulopalatopharyngoplasty (UPPP); treatment benefits were found with CPAP but not with UPPP. However, CPAP is poorly tolerated. Survival of patients with OSA treated with CPAP vs. UPPP was assessed, and other factors related to mortality and survival were examined.

Methods.—Records were reviewed for 154 patients treated with UPPP and 116 treated with long-term CPAP. Changes in the apnea index were used as indications of treatment efficacy. For those who had died, the cause of death and incidence of death during sleep were determined. The use of follow-up polysomnography after treatment and its association with survival were examined.

Results.—Treatment with nasal CPAP and UPPP produced equal increases in patient survival (Fig 24–2). The 6 deaths that occurred among patients treated with UPPP were caused by myocardial infarction (4), lung cancer (1), and accidental drowning (1). The 3 deaths that occurred among patients treated with CPAP were caused by pneumonia, prostate cancer, and postoperative respiratory arrest. Only 2 deaths occurred at night. Follow-up included polysomnography in 94% of patients treated with UPPP; 3 deaths in that group occurred in patients who did not have follow-up polysomnograms.

Discussion.—In this comparison of nasal CPAP and UPPP in patients with OSA, there were no treatment-related differences in long-term survival. There was no evidence of an increased risk of death during sleep. The most common cause of death was myocardial infarction, but it could not be attributed directly to OSA. Follow-up polysomnography should be performed after UPPP to evaluate response to treatment.

▶ Because OSA is a fairly common condition that has been associated with serious cardiovascular complications (1), it is surprising that only 1 study exists on the association between various treatment modes and mortality (2). In that study, the use of CPAP was found to decrease mortality, whereas UPPP did not have that effect. Unfortunately, other studies have shown that some patients cannot tolerate CPAP over the long term. The authors of this study opted to reexamine the long-term mortality rate of patients treated with these 2 methods. Additionally, the authors sought to determine the most common cause of death in these patients, whether patients were more likely to die at night, and whether follow-up polysomnography helped in the treatment of patients with UPPP.

This study comes to the unexpected conclusion that the 2 methods of treatment yield similar long-term survival rates. The results are surprising, because the previous study of long-term survival after CPAP and UPPP indicated that CPAP was the better treatment, whereas other studies had shown that CPAP improves a number of other outcome measures. This study also found that the most common cause of death among these patients was myocardial infarction and that death occurred most often during the day. Also, patients who had undergone UPPP but who did not return for follow-up polysomnography had a higher mortality rate than those who underwent the diagnostic procedure. All these studies are retrospective, however, and true comparisons are difficult to make because the groups do not match well. In this study, patients who received CPAP treatment tended to be more obese, whereas patients who underwent UPPP tended to have more severe OSA. Unfortunately, a true prospective study of CPAP vs. UPPP would be made difficult by the ethical problems inherent in randomization and blinding, given our current understanding of the appropriate indications for those therapeutic methods. Nonetheless, additional clinical studies should be undertaken to resolve the issue of appropriate treatment for patients with OSA.—R.C. Bone, M.D.

References

1. Partinen M, Jamieson A, Guilleminault C: Long-term outcome for obstructive sleep apnea syndrome patients: Mortality. *Chest* 94:1200–1204, 1988.
2. He J, Kryger MH, Zorick FJ, et al: Mortality and apnea index in obstructive sleep apnea: Experience in 385 male patients. *Chest* 94:9–14, 1988.

.

25 Critical Care

Introduction

The 2 leading causes of morbidity and mortality in hospital ICUs continue to be infection and sepsis. In its new guise as the systemic inflammatory response syndrome (SIRS), an endogenously mediated process, sepsis has been somewhat disconnected from its identity as a disease caused by infectious organisms. However, SIRS and infection remain related in that infection (along with a number of other conditions) can foment SIRS. Although new antibiotics are constantly being developed in the fight against infection, the struggle with SIRS has resulted in a number of apparent dead ends, such as the one hit during testing of monoclonal antibodies against endotoxin. The struggle, however, is certainly not without hope. The complexity of the inflammatory response leaves a bewildering array of doors to be tried, and a recent study of the interleukin-1 receptor antagonist may help provide some direction amid the jumble of choices in the fight against SIRS.

Topics that have been chosen for this year's YEAR BOOK OF MEDICINE include the effect of different forms of nutrition in patients who are critically ill. This subject is interesting, because the production of carbon dioxide—hence, the tendency toward hypercapnia—depends on which substrates are being used at the cellular level. The second abstract examines the risk factors for pneumonia in trauma patients. In the third study, a drug that increases oxygen delivery, dopexamine hydrochloride, was administered to patients perioperatively to determine whether it could improve the outcome of surgery. The results of that study were very good, and further clinical evaluations of the drug are eagerly awaited.

Roger C. Bone, M.D.

Ventilatory Response to High Caloric Loads in Critically Ill Patients
Liposky JM, Nelson LD (Harvard Univ, Boston; Vanderbilt Univ, Nashville, Tenn)
Crit Care Med 22:796–802, 1994   119-95-25–1

Objective.—Responses to caloric (particularly carbohydrate) loading were examined in 78 patients who were critically ill to learn whether total parenteral nutrition and/or enteral nutrition alters production and elimination of carbon dioxide. Whether patients who are overfed to the

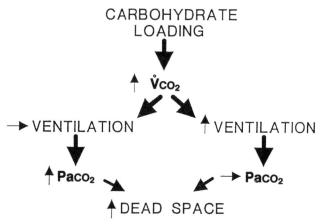

Fig 25–1.—Proposed relationship between high caloric loads and the ventilatory response. $\overset{\circ}{V}_{CO_2}$ indicates CO_2 production. (Courtesy of Liposky JM, Nelson LD: *Crit Care Med* 22:796–802, 1994.)

point of lipogenesis have an altered ventilatory response was also determined.

Methods.—A total of 129 indirect calorimetric studies were carried out, 112 in patients whose respiratory quotient was 1 or less (group 1) and 17 in patients whose quotient exceeded 1 (group 2). Parenteral nutrition only was given during 63% of the measurements, enteral nutrition only was given during 23%, and both types were given during 14%. Carbohydrate was given to provide approximately one half to two thirds the estimated caloric need.

Findings.—Intake of total calories and carbohydrate calories was approximately 20% greater in group 2. There were no significant group differences in indexed oxygen consumption, alveolar ventilation, partial pressure of carbon dioxide in arterial blood ($PaCO_2$), or measured energy expenditure. Intake of carbohydrate calories correlated with production of carbon dioxide in group 2 and with alveolar ventilation in both groups. Only patients in group 1 exhibited a correlation between production of carbon dioxide and exhaled minute ventilation (Fig 25–1). Production of carbon dioxide correlated closely with alveolar ventilation for the entire study population.

Implications.—A total caloric and carbohydrate load that exceeds energy expenditure may be associated with a respiratory quotient higher than 1, and an increased quotient may correlate with increases in both production of carbon dioxide and alveolar ventilation. A patient who can increase spontaneous ventilation may maintain a normal $PaCO_2$, whereas those who cannot augment ventilation may experience an increase in ventilation of dead space.

▶ The terms "nutritionally depleted" and "hypermetabolic" have been used to describe patients; the clinical significance of these conditions is less well understood. Several studies have indicated that parenteral nutrition high in carbohydrates causes an increase in production of carbon dioxide, with the resultant tendency to hypercapnia and increased respiratory demands (1). It has been shown that this tendency increases the difficulties faced in weaning patients from the ventilator (2). Based on those results, it was recommended that 30% to 50% of the calories administered to such patients be in the form of fat. The respiratory quotient (carbon dioxide production/oxygen consumption) can be used to determine which forms of energy a patient is metabolizing and is usually found to be 1 or less. Values of greater than 1, however, indicate that lipogenesis is taking place, a process that would tend to drive a patient toward hypercapnia. The authors of this study have chosen to investigate further the effects of feedings in patients who are critically ill. They have used calorimetry in the form of a metabolic gas monitor and have taken particular aim at determining how carbohydrate loading affects respiratory function.

The findings are in line with other studies, indicating that production of carbon dioxide correlates with consumption of carbohydrates. This fact was reflected in the increased alveolar minute ventilation. Despite similar feeding regimens, a few patients had respiratory quotients greater than 1 and were probably overfed. Although production of carbon dioxide was greater in the group with quotients greater than 1, there was no difference in consumption of oxygen between the groups. Those with the higher quotients also had the best correlation between production of carbon dioxide and consumption of carbohydrates. Curiously, the relationship between caloric load and exhaled minute ventilation is not as strong as for alveolar ventilation, possibly because increased exhaled minute ventilation may only be cycling the dead space, which was seen to increase in this study. Such an effect would adversely affect respiratory efficiency. In these patients who were mechanically ventilated, however, such an effect could also have been caused by the respiratory rate, which was higher in those with quotients over 1, probably as a response to the increased carbon dioxide load. Caloric intake also correlated with the measured energy expenditure, particularly for the group with the higher respiratory quotient. The question is: Does overfeeding somehow drive the metabolic rate to a higher level, possibly through the process of lipogenesis? Although the authors provided alternative explanations, this remains an intriguing possibility. Patients unable to respond to overfeeding with increased respiration would manifest increased $PaCO_2$ and would require increased ventilatory support.—R.C. Bone, M.D.

References

1. Askenazi J, Carpentier YA, Elwyn DH, et al: Influence of total parenteral nutrition on fuel utilization in injury and sepsis. *Ann Surg* 191:40–46, 1980.
2. Benotti PN Bistrian B: Metabolic and nutritional aspects of weaning from mechanical ventilation. *Crit Care Med* 17:181–185, 1989.

Risk Factors for Early Onset Pneumonia in Trauma Patients

Antonelli M, Moro ML, Capelli O, De Blasi RA, D'Errico RR, Conti G, Bufi M, Gasparetto A (Università "La Sapienza," Rome; Istituto Superiore di Sanità, Rome)

Chest 105:224–228, 1994   119-95-25–2

Objective.—The cases of patients who had undergone multiple trauma were reviewed to describe the incidence of early-onset pneumonia (EOP) and late-onset pneumonia (LOP) and related risk factors. Given the high incidence of pneumonia in trauma patients, identification of risk factors might lead to more effective measures of control.

Methods.—One hundred twenty-four patients were admitted to the general ICU of a university hospital from December 1990 through February 1992. One hundred patients were men, and 82 were 40 years of age or younger. Data collected included demographics, severity of trauma and coma, and the presence of pneumothorax, pulmonary contusion, rib fractures, hemothorax, and mechanical ventilation. Patients suspected of having pneumonia underwent bronchoalveolar lavage as well as blood cultures. Pneumonia occurring within the first 96 hours after trauma was considered EOP. While in the ICU, all patients were monitored daily for onset of pneumonia, sepsis syndrome, septic shock, and adult respiratory distress syndrome.

Results.—The overall mortality rate was 43.5%. The rate of mortality increased with advancing age and greater abbreviated injury scale (AIS) score. Pneumonia developed in 41 patients (33.1%) in the ICU. Twenty-six cases (63.4%) were EOP and 15 (36.6%) were LOP. Sepsis syndrome and adult respiratory distress syndrome were common in both EOP and LOP. Logistic regression analysis showed that the strongest risk factor for EOP was combined severe abdominal and thoracic trauma (table). Other independent risk factors were age older than 40 years and mechanical ventilation of less than 24 hours during the first 4 days of hospitalization. Risk factors for LOP were an AIS score of more than 4 for the abdomen and mechanical ventilation for more than 5 days.

Conclusion.—Combined abdominal and thoracic trauma is a significant risk factor, increasing the risk for EOP 11-fold. Use of mechanical ventilation during the first post-traumatic phase might improve ventilation of the lower lobes, thereby reducing the likelihood of bacterial colonization. For patients with LOP, however, mechanical ventilation has the opposite effect. Determination of the AIS score at admission is recommended for patients with abdominal and thoracic trauma.

▶ We know that pneumonia will develop in a certain percentage of trauma patients. The etiologies of these pneumonias, however, may often be considered a matter of some controversy. Fluid within the spaces of the alveoli and the airways of the lungs is often indicative of inflammatory activity in the region. One event that can cause such inflammation is the presence of bacte-

Risk Factors for EOP: Multivariate Analysis

Factors	No. of Patients	Regression Coefficient	SE	Probability Value	OR	Confidence Limit 95%
Age, yr						
>=40	82	· · ·	· · ·	· · ·	1	· · ·
>40	42	1.319	0.529	0.012	3.74	131-10.7
A/S, thorax and abdomen						
1*	57	· · ·	· · ·	· · ·	1	· · ·
2	52	1.522	0.609	0.012	4.58	1.37-15.3
3	15	2.423	0.777	0.001	11.3	2.42-52.5
Length of MV, h						
>24	61	· · ·	· · ·	· · ·	1.0	· · ·
≤24	63	1.934	0.586	0.001	6.92	2.17-22.1

* 1: thorax < 4, abdomen any score; 2: thorax > 4, abdomen < = 9; 3: thorax > 4, abdomen > 4, abdomen > 9.
(Courtesy of Antonelli M, Moro ML, Capelli O, et al: *Chest* 105:224-228, 1994.)

rial infection, which can stimulate mononuclear phagocytes to release inflammatory mediators. Although the release of inflammatory mediators brought about by pathogenic microbes is a key phase in the development of pneumonias, it is also believed to be a key starting point for the systemic inflammatory response syndrome (SIRS). In the etiology of SIRS, the origin of these mediators is less well known—in some cases, patients do not have bacteremia and appear to have no other signs of systemic or local infection. This is particularly true in SIRS associated with trauma. Pneumonias in trauma patients may be associated with the development of SIRS. In this article, it is argued that multiple trauma itself reduces the patient's immunocompetence, thus increasing his or her susceptibility to infection by pneumonia-causing organisms.

With the thought that protecting patients from possible infective sources should decrease the frequency of pneumonia in trauma patients, the authors of this study have looked at possible risk factors for pneumonia in trauma patients. In doing this, they have classified pneumonias as either EOP or LOP. Gastric aspiration, intracranial pressure monitoring, use of antacids, and mechanical ventilation have previously been associated with the occurrence of pulmonary infection in trauma patients.

The findings of this study indicate that EOP (within 4 days of the trauma) is a relatively common event in multiple trauma. Combined thoracic and abdominal trauma constitute the highest risk for the complication of pulmonary infection. The authors point out that this form of trauma may have the additional impact of diaphragmatic dysfunction. The study also found, however, that the use of mechanical ventilation within 4 days of the trauma actually decreased the incidence of EOP. Although this finding may appear to be in conflict with other findings, which suggest that the implementation of mechanical ventilation is associated with poorer outcome, the authors use the plausible argument that positive pressures in the lung improve the aeration of contused and atelectatic portions of the lung, thus reducing bacterial colonization and improving the patient's functional residual capacity. Additionally, it is easier to suction bronchial secretions with the endotracheal tube in place, which should also reduce the risk of infection.

Not surprisingly, the implementation of mechanical ventilation had the opposite effect on LOP. Mechanical ventilation lasting more than 5 days was associated with a 400% increase in LOP. The authors pointed to the usual sources of infection associated with mechanical ventilation to explain this phenomenon, e.g., oropharyngeal colonization or inoculation of the trachea by the endotracheal tube.

Because the Glasgow Coma Scale score could not be associated with either LOP or EOP, a previous finding that impaired airway reflexes can cause onset of pneumonia may be called into question. However, airway reflexes were assessed by different methods in these studies, indicating that further study would help resolve the issue.

The finding here that early mechanical ventilation decreased the rate of EOP and infection in these patients is interesting and certainly warrants further study. If the results of this study are confirmed, mechanical ventilation may become an appropriate measure for preventing pulmonary infection in patients with severe abdominal and thoracic trauma.—R.C. Bone, M.D.

A Randomized Clinical Trial of the Effect of Deliberate Perioperative Increase of Oxygen Delivery on Mortality in High-Risk Surgical Patients

Boyd O, Grounds RM, Bennett ED (St. George's Hosp, London)
JAMA 270:2699–2707, 1993   119-95-25-3

Background.—Safety concerns persist regarding perioperative hemodynamic management to increase cardiac output and oxygen delivery. The effect of goal-directed therapy on mortality and morbidity in high-risk surgical patients was evaluated prospectively.

Methods.—Fifty-three patients underwent a perioperative protocol that included deliberate increase of oxygen delivery index to exceed 600 mL/min/m² using dopexamine hydrochloride infusion. A control group of 54 patients was also included. Treatment goals for the 2 groups are presented in the table. Mortality and complications were assessed during the subsequent 28 days.

Results.—Goal-directed therapy reduced the mortality rate in the protocol group to 5.7%, which was significantly lower than the rate of 22.2% in the control group and the rates of 25% to 40% demonstrated in similar groups of high-risk patients (Fig 25–2). Patients who underwent abdominal surgery demonstrated the greatest difference in mortality rates; 0% of protocol patients vs. 25% of control patients. Ten percent of protocol patients and 21% of control patients died after vascular surgery. Protocol patients had significantly fewer complications per patient. Among survivors, there was a trend toward shorter median hospital and ICU stays in the protocol group.

Treatment Goals

Variable	Goal
For Both Study Groups	
Mean arterial pressure, mm Hg	80-110
Pulmonary arterial occlusion pressure, mm Hg	12-14
Arterial oxygen saturation, %	>94
Hemoglobin, g/L	>120
Urine output, mL/kg per h	>0.5
Additional for Protocol Patients	
Oxygen delivery index, mL/min per m²	>600

(Courtesy of Boyd O, Grounds RM, Bennett ED: JAMA 270:2699–2707, 1993.)

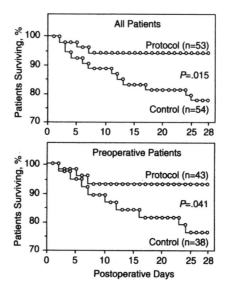

Fig 25–2.—Survival curves for protocol and control groups for all patients and for patients preoperatively allocated to the study. (Courtesy of Boyd O, Grounds RM, Bennett ED: JAMA 270:2699–2707, 1993.)

Conclusion.—Increasing perioperative oxygen delivery with dopexamine hydrochloride significantly reduces the rates of mortality and morbidity in high-risk surgical patients.

▶ It has already been proven that patients who have higher cardiac output and oxygen delivery after surgery have better recovery and lower rates of mortality and morbidity (1). The 1988 study by Shoemaker et al. (2) indicated that using the cardiac output and oxygen delivery values of previous survivors to guide therapy made it possible to improve morbidity and mortality rates in patients at high risk for both. In a pilot study, these authors found that dopexamine hydrochloride, which increases oxygen delivery, may be suitable for high-risk surgical patients (3). Dopexamine is particularly suited for this purpose, because it increases oxygen delivery without increasing oxygen demand, which is a problem with other agents (4,5).

Because of the expected vasodilatory properties of dopexamine, the protocol group received significantly more preoperative fluids than the control group; however, there was no difference in the amount of fluids given to the 2 groups during the 24 hours after surgery. The control group received more postoperative vasoactive medication than the protocol group, confirming that both groups were managed aggressively to maintain therapeutic target levels. It also suggests that the control group was less stable with regard to cardiovascular function than the protocol group during the first 24 hours after surgery.

This study found a 75% reduction in the rates of morbidity and mortality when cardiac index and oxygen delivery were increased perioperatively, and no patients who were admitted before surgery and treated entirely according to the treatment regimen died. In those patients who did die, the cause was organ failure that developed in the days after surgery rather than a catastrophic event in the immediate postoperative period.

Although these results are very similar to those of Shoemaker et al., this study had slightly different treatment goals and used dopexamine to increase oxygen delivery. The targets of Shoemaker and co-workers were a cardiac index of greater than 4.5 L/min/m², an oxygen consumption of greater than 170 mL/min/m², and an oxygen delivery of greater than 600 mL/min/m². The similarity of the results between these 2 groups suggests that oxygen delivery is a critically important factor. The benefits of deliberately increasing oxygen delivery have been reported, including a recent study in which trauma patients—most of them with gunshot wounds—had a significant reduction in rate of mortality (6, 7). Many studies have sought any link that might affect morbidity and mortality in high-risk patients, and these studies have linked higher levels of oxygen delivery with increased use of oxygen. Increasing tissue perfusion in critically ill patients may reveal a need for more oxygen, and studies have shown that in some types of critical illness, levels of oxygen consumption may be dependent on levels of oxygen delivery (8, 9). Other investigators have suggested that increases in oxygen delivery are necessary after surgery to compensate for the oxygen debt that arises during surgery, and this is the way in which increased oxygen delivery may have a beneficial effect (10).

The high-risk criteria used by these authors are broad, and refinement of the criteria, possibly combined with physiologic screening, may identify a group of patients who are particularly at risk. In addition, a general oxygen delivery target of 600 mL/min/m² may not be appropriate for all patients; some may require higher values to achieve benefit, and others may achieve benefit at lower levels. Nonetheless, the results speak for themselves: A three quarter reduction in the mortality rate is significant. Clearly, more research is needed in this area, as much of the accumulating data are negative.—R.C. Bone, M.D.

References

1. Clowes GHA Jr, Del Guercio LRM: Circulatory response to trauma of surgical operations. *Metabolism* 9:67–81, 1960.
2. Shoemaker WC, Appel PL, Kram HB, et al: Prospective trial of supranormal values of survivors as therapeutic goals in high-risk surgical patients. *Chest* 94:1176–1186, 1988.
3. Boyd OF, Grounds RM, Bennett ED: The use of dopexamine hydrochloride to increase oxygen delivery perioperatively. *Anesth Analg* 76:372–376, 1993.
4. Heistad DD, Wheeler RC, Mark AL, et al: Effects of adrenergic stimulation on ventilation in man. *J Clin Invest* 51:1469–1475, 1972.
5. Green CJ, Frazer RS, Underhill S, et al: Metabolic effects of dobutamine in normal man. *Clin Sci* 82:77–83, 1992.

6. Tuschschmidt J, Fried J, Astiz M, et al: Elevation of cardiac output and oxygen delivery improves outcome in septic shock. *Chest* 102:216–220, 1992.
7. Fleming A, Bishop M, Shoemaker WC, et al: Prospective trial of supranormal values as goals of resuscitation in severe trauma. *Arch Surg* 127:1175–1181, 1992.
8. Bihari D, Smithies M, Gimson A, Tinker J: The effects of vasodilation with prostacyclin on oxygen delivery and uptake in critically ill patients. *N Engl J Med* 317:397–403, 1987.
9. Guitierrez G, Pohil RJ: Oxygen consumption is linearly related to oxygen supply in critically ill patients. *J Crit Care* 1:45–53, 1986.
10. Hankeln KB, Gronemeyer R, Held A, et al: Use of continuous noninvasive measurement of DO_2I in patients with adult respiratory distress syndrome following shock of various etiologies. *Crit Care Med* 19:642–649, 1991.

26 Mechanical Ventilation

Introduction

The Mechanical Ventilation chapter contains 4 important studies. The first, by Neil MacIntyre et al., develops a concept that may lead to an improved ventilator technique in the future. The second, by Elpern et al., documents a surprisingly high incidence of aspiration in patients with tracheostomy who are mechanically ventilated. The third study, by Yang et al., shows that nebulized ipratropium bromide is beneficial in ventilator-assisted patients with chronic bronchitis. The fourth, by Richard et al., demonstrates the importance of cardiac function during the weaning of patients with chronic obstructive pulmonary disease.

Weaning is an enormous problem in mechanical ventilation. Current information suggests that approximately 50% of patients in an ICU require mechanical ventilation for longer than 24 hours and that weaning accounts for about 40% of total ventilatory time. In the past, Dr. Neal Beaton and I developed a mnemonic phrase, WEANS NOW, for use at the patient's bedside. The phrase is intended to help physicians remember to check each of the important variables involved with weaning: Weaning tests, Endotracheal tube, Arterial blood gas values, Nutrition, Secretions, Neuromuscular disease, Obstruction, and Wakefulness (1).

Although WEANS NOW is a useful memory check, a more specific list of criteria is necessary. The patient must be improving, alert, and responsive. I believe that the best test of weaning is the frequency to tidal volume **ratio** reviewed in the 1994 YEAR BOOK OF MEDICINE (2). A value of greater than 100 predicts the inability to wean. When lung function is judged adequate, an orderly transition to spontaneous ventilation should be initiated. If sedatives or muscle relaxants were used during the course of mechanical ventilation, their effects should be allowed to dissipate completely before weaning is begun.

When weaning is unsuccessful, a checklist may prove useful to make sure all details have been considered. Pertinent questions to consider include the following (3): Is airway obstruction present that could be reversed with bronchodilator therapy? Is the endotracheal tube too small? Are secretions a problem? Is breathing depressed by drugs? Is nutrition a problem? Is metabolic alkalemia preventing weaning? Is neuromuscular disease present? Is diaphragmatic function intact? Have psychological factors, such as adequate sleep and a calm environment, been neglected? Is the $PaCO_2$ after mechanical ventilation lower than the patient's usual $PaCO_2$? Is the PaO_2 kept in the 50–70 mm Hg range rather than the

70–100 mm Hg range to improve respiratory drive? And, would the patient benefit from a tracheostomy?

Weaning is an important aspect of mechanical ventilation that may present special difficulties. We are reminded that physicians must never take mechanical ventilation for granted and that each stage of the patient's progress should be carefully monitored.

Roger C. Bone, M.D.

References

1. Beaton N, Bone RC: Criteria for weaning your patients from respirators. *J Respir Dis* b(4): 80–83, 1985.
2. 1994 YEAR BOOK OF MEDICINE, pp 199–201.
3. Adapted from Scoggin CH: Weaning respiratory patients from mechanical support. *J Respir Dis* 1:12, 1980.

Combining Pressure-Limiting and Volume-Cycling Features in a Patient-Interactive Mechanical Breath

MacIntyre NR, Gropper C, Westfall T (Duke Univ, Durham, NC; Bear Med Systems, Riverside, Calif)
Crit Care Med 22:353–357, 1994   119-95-26-1

Background.—A patient-interactive mechanical breath, which combined the synchrony features of pressure-limited breath with the volume guarantee of volume-cycled breath, was designed and tested in an engi-

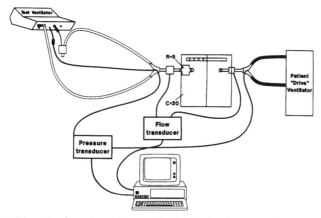

Fig 26–1.—Schematic of experimental setup. The simulated patient was a two-compartment lung model connected by a plastic strip. One compartment represented the patient's muscles and was driven by a volume-cycled ventilator. The other compartment represented the patient's lungs and was supported by the prototype ventilator using volume assist-control ventilation and pressure-support ventilation, both individually and in combination with each other (pressure augmentation). (Courtesy of MacIntyre NR, Gropper C, Westfall T: *Crit Care Med* 22:353–357, 1994.)

neering laboratory. This combined breath can be pressure-limited, as well as flow- or volume-cycled, if a target volume is not attained. Demand-valve responsiveness at breath initiation can be adjusted.

Methods.—The ventilator is microprocessor-controlled and triggered by patient effort. The simulated patient was a 2-compartment system (Fig 26–1). One compartment represented the patient's muscles, and the other represented the lungs. Patients receiving total and partial support were simulated and combined with volume assistance, pressure support, and combined pressure-limited and volume-cycled breath.

Results.—In a simulated patient receiving total support, flow dyssynchrony during fixed-flow, volume-cycled assisted breaths improved, and guaranteed tidal volume was maintained. In addition, imposed work of breathing decreased. In a simulated patient receiving partial support from pressure support, the guaranteed tidal volume could provide a volume backup.

Discussion.—This combined breath design could be used for patients receiving total support, as well as for those receiving partial support. The strategy used to combine pressure-limited breath and volume-cycled breath was to provide a volume guarantee to the pressure-limited breath. To achieve this goal, a backup minimum flow with a minimum volume was provided for several reasons: with every breath, there is support with a set pressure; air trapping is minimized because expiratory time is protected; and additional flow and volume are supplied only if required for a particular breath. Adding a minimal and maximal inspiratory time setting (eliminating separate volume or pressure modes) could enable this design to be the only positive breath system used on future ventilators.

▶ Mechanical ventilation modes have undergone an explosive diversification in the recent past. The advent of microprocessor-controlled devices has further increased the scope and function of these machines. The authors of this article have developed such a device that combines traits from the 2 forms of ventilation that are most commonly used today: the volume-assist breath, which delivers gas according to a preset flow pattern and volume but may not match patient ventilatory effort; and the pressure-limited breath, which is triggered by the patient and delivers a set pressure until it cycles off at a preset time or flow setting but does not guarantee a particular tidal volume.

The hybrid mechanical breath cycle is patient interactive and incorporates a pressure-limited flow with the ability to sense inadequate volume and adjust the breath to compensate. Thus, the ventilator provides a set pressure during every breath, has a long enough expiratory period to ensure that air trapping does not occur, and only provides the additional flow and volume to a breath if it is needed. When additional air is needed to achieve a certain tidal volume, the ventilator may provide greater pressure than the pressure setting indicates, a point that users of this ventilator should note. Such a system can provide both total and partial support. This design, with its microprocessor control system and improved responsiveness to patient demand, represents an improvement over a similar design recently reported by Amato et al. (1). Further testing is warranted to determine how this candidate for next-generation mechanical generator should best be used.

I am often on the lecture circuit with Neil MacIntyre, and he has presented this concept frequently. He is a real innovator in our approach to mechanical ventilation. So stay tuned. . .I certainly will !—R.C. Bone, M.D.

Reference

1. Amato MBP, Barbas CSV, Bonassa J, et al: Volume assured pressure support ventilation. *Chest* 102:1225–1234, 1992.

Pulmonary Aspiration in Mechanically Ventilated Patients With Tracheostomies

Elpern EH, Scott MG, Petro L, Ries MH (Rush-Presbyterian-St Luke's Med Ctr, Chicago; Suburban Hosp, Hinsdale, Ill)
Chest 105:563–566, 1994   119-95-26–2

Introduction.—Although high risk of aspiration is assumed for patients with artificial airways, the incidence and clinical significance of aspiration among these patients is not known. Many patients may have clinically silent aspiration events, and bedside assessment methods have limited value. Videofluoroscopic (VF) visualization of swallowing is a reliable but labor-intensive and time-consuming technique for demonstrating aspiration. The incidence of aspiration (demonstrated with VF examinations) and the clinical characteristics of mechanically ventilated patients with tracheostomies who are at risk were explored.

Methods.—Eighty-three ventilator-dependent adult patients, for whom oral feedings were being considered, underwent VF examination of modified barium swallow procedures. The VF tapes were reviewed, and aspiration events were counted and characterized by the co-occurrence of symptomatic distress. The associations between aspiration events and demographic or clinical variables were analyzed.

Results.—Forty-two patients (50%) had 48 aspiration events, 37 of which were silent. The patients who aspirated were significantly older and had marginally higher serum levels of albumin than those who did not aspirate. Sex, the size of the tracheostomy tube, the duration of tracheostomy, the duration of ventilator support, and the presence or type of feeding tube were all nonsignificant variables. There were no significant demographic or clinical variables that separated silent from overt aspirators. Of the swallowing disorders seen, reduced laryngeal elevation was more characteristic of patients who aspirated, occurring in 55%, than in those who did not, occurring in 5%.

Discussion.—The incidence of aspiration in this group of long-term ventilator-dependent patients was 50%. Elderly patients were at increased risk for aspiration. The high incidence of silent aspiration illustrates the difficulty of bedside identification of aspiration. The disturbances seen in laryngeal elevation and laryngeal closure are consistent with other reports of patients with tracheostomy, but the contribution of positive pressure ventilation is not clear.

▶ One of the important findings of this study was that a high percentage of the observed aspirations in these ventilated patients were asymptomatic. Although the clinical significance of that observation was not demonstrated, such small, unnoticed aspirations clearly could be the cause of various pulmonary problems. This study made use of VF imaging to assess the swallowing process carefully during a trial ingestion. These tests were performed on patients before oral feedings and provided much more detail than such standard tests as dye recovery or tracheal-secretion glucose measurements.

Of the 83 patients examined in this study, 50% aspirated swallowed substances—77% of those events were silent. Another significant finding was that increasing age correlated with the tendency to aspirate. Patients were much more likely to aspirate thin liquids than solid food, with thick liquids and pureed foods having an intermediate likelihood.

Interestingly, the investigators could observe disturbances in the ordered events of the swallowing process. Dysfunctions during the oral phase of swallowing occurred only half as often as dysfunctions during the pharyngeal phase; these dysfunctions occurred with equal frequency among patients who aspirated and those who did not, with the exception of diminished pharyngeal elevation, which was much more common among aspirators (55%) than nonaspirators (5%).

Other studies of aspiration in intubated patients have not used fluoroscopy and have obtained widely ranging rates of aspiration—from 0% to 95%. This range certainly points to the need for more studies along these lines. A better knowledge of the risk factors associated with the use of this procedure and of the clinical significance of aspiration events in various patient populations would be of benefit to us all.—R.C. Bone, M.D.

Nebulized Ipratropium Bromide in Ventilator-Assisted Patients With Chronic Bronchitis
Yang SC, Yang SP, Lee TS (Natl Taiwan Univ, Taipei, Republic of China)
Chest 105:1511–1515, 1994   119-95-26–3

Background.—The effect of nebulized ipratropium bromide solution on respiratory function in patients with chronic bronchitis who require mechanical ventilation was investigated in a randomized, double-blind, placebo-controlled trial.

Methods.—Forty-two patients with acute exacerbations of chronic bronchitis who required mechanical ventilation were evaluated. Patients were randomly assigned to receive either 500 µg of ipratropium bromide as a nebulized solution or .9% saline solution every 6 hours for 24 hours. The patients continued to use their bronchodilators and were treated

Group Mean Respiratory Mechanics and P Values Reflecting Difference in Change Between Ipratropium and Placebo Groups

| | Ipratropium | | Placebo | | |
	Baseline	After Fourth Treatment	Baseline	After Fourth Treatment	p Value*
MAP, cm H_2O	7.2 ± 2.8	4.8 ± 2.0	5.8 ± 2.5	7.1 ± 4.1	0.003
PIP, cm H_2O	33.9 ± 8.6	25.5 ± 5.3	39.9 ± 10.7	39.2 ± 8.3	0.045
PP, cm H_2O	18.8 ± 7.3	18.2 ± 7.7	23.3 ± 9.2	22.1 ± 8.1	0.642
MRaw, cm H_2O/L/s	13.2 ± 3.6	7.9 ± 2.2	12.3 ± 5.0	12.5 ± 4.2	0.043
Cst, ml/cm H_2O	25.1 ± 5.3	24.1 ± 8.5	24.9 ± 6.7	23.5 ± 5.2	0.511
Exhaled V_T, ml	532	544	546	538	0.625

* The P value reflects the difference between the 2 groups in change after fourth treatment from baseline.
(Courtesy of Yang SC, Yang SP, Lee TS: Chest 105:1511–1515, 1994.)

with antibiotics, as they would have been had they not been in the clinical trial. Respiratory mechanics, arterial blood gas analysis, and respiratory symptoms were assessed.

Results.—After 24 hours, the ipratropium group did statistically better than the placebo group in reducing mean airway pressure, peak inspiratory pressure, and mean airway resistance (table). There were no statistically significant differences between the groups in plateau pressure, static lung compliance, exhaled tidal volume, oxygenation, or arterial carbon dioxide tension. The respiratory symptom score improved to a greater extent in the ipratropium group than in the placebo group.

Conclusion.—In patients with acute exacerbations of chronic bronchitis who require mechanical ventilation, additional benefit can be obtained by adding nebulized ipratropium to the patients' usual bronchodilator regimen. The response is attributable to the bronchodilatory effect of ipratropium, which results in decreases in mean airway pressure and mean airway resistance.

▶ Although the use of anticholinergics and β-adrenergic agonists alone or in combination has been the subject of many clinical studies, clear-cut answers have been hard to come by. Perhaps the technique applied by the authors of this study will ultimately help clinicians find the answers they need. The authors narrowed the focus of their study to include only older patients with chronic bronchitis who required mechanical ventilation. Rather than comparing the effects of 2 different drugs or combinations, they simply compared the effects of nebulized ipratropium with those of a placebo. Lung mechanics, pulmonary gas exchange, and the patient's symptoms were used to assess the effects of the drug.

The authors concluded that ipratropium is beneficial under the circumstances of this study; the drug improved both the pulmonary and respiratory mechanics of these patients. Significantly decreased airway pressures and resistances were measured in patients receiving ipratropium. However, beneficial effects did not appear to be conferred on the gas exchange capabilities of the patients who were treated, as measured by the partial pressure of carbon dioxide in arterial blood/inspiratory oxygen fraction. The authors thought that this failure to show improved gas exchange may have occurred because the mechanical ventilation had already corrected ventilation–perfusion matching or because the drug had failed to improve small airway conductance in this study. This latter point has been shown possible in studies that indicate differences exist in the response to anticholinergic treatment between the small and large airways.

This study also searched for such systemic side effects as increased heart rate or blood pressure, tremor, or bronchospasm but found no significant changes. The use of nebulized ipratropium in patients with bronchitis who require mechanical ventilation is further supported by the results of this study.—R.C. Bone, M.D.

Left Ventricular Function During Weaning of Patients With Chronic Obstructive Pulmonary Disease

Richard C, Teboul J-L, Archambaud F, Hebert J-L, Michaut P, Auzepy P (Hôpital de Bicêtre, Le Kremlin-Bicêtre, France)
Intensive Care Med 20:181–186, 1994   119-95-26-4

Introduction.—Acute left ventricular dysfunction can occur in patients with chronic obstructive pulmonary disease (COPD) during weaning from mechanical ventilation. Left ventricular ejection fraction (LVEF) was monitored during the transition from mechanical to spontaneous ventilation in patients with COPD but without coronary artery disease.

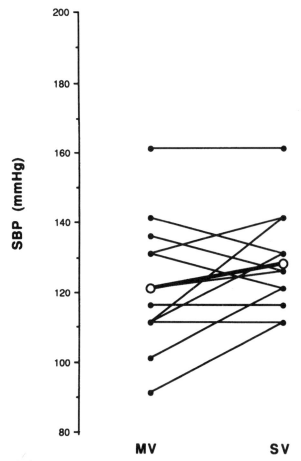

Fig 26–2.—Individual values of systolic blood pressure evolution (*SBP*) from mechanical ventilation (MV) to spontaneous ventilation (SV) in the 12 patients with COPD. (Courtesy of Richard C, Teboul J-L, Archambaud F, et al: *Intensive Care Med* 20:181-186, 1994.)

Methods.—The left ventricular ejection fraction was assessed with radionuclide angiography in 12 patients with COPD and no evidence of coronary artery disease who were capable of weaning. The data were acquired 5 times: mechanical ventilation (MV1), spontaneous ventilation (SV), mechanical ventilation (MV2), inspiratory pressure support, and mechanical ventilation (MV3).

Results.—The left ventricular ejection fraction remained consistent at an average of 55% during the 3 MV readings. It decreased significantly during the transition to spontaneous ventilation, from 54.5% at MV1 to 47% at SV. A nonsignificant decrease was observed during the transition to inspiratory pressure support, from 55% at MV2 to 50.3%. There were no signs of myocardial ischemia, and myocardial thallium 201 imaging performed 15 minutes after weaning revealed normal left ventricular perfusion. In 5 patients, systolic blood pressure increased during weaning, but for the whole population the increase was not significant (Fig 26-2).

Discussion.—During weaning, LVEF consistently decreased but was not accompanied by decreased myocardial contractility or myocardial ischemia. An increase in left ventricle afterload caused by reduced negative swings in intrathoracic pressure may be the cause of the decreasing LVEF; this hypothesis needs further study. Patients with COPD who are mechanically ventilated should be assessed for left ventricular dysfunction before weaning.

▶ The weaning of patients who have COPD can be a difficult process. This is particularly true if the patient has preexisting coronary artery disease causing ventricular dysfunction. In these patients, weaning often brings on myocardial ischemia and increased cardiac dysfunction. This effect may be enhanced by the effect of weaning on pumping dynamics—an increased left ventricular afterload caused by the negative swings in intrathoracic pressure during ventilation. To determine the relative contributions of increased afterload and myocardial ischemia to pump dysfunction during weaning, the authors have carefully examined LVEF and the left ventricular end-diastolic volume (LVED) during weaning in 12 patients with COPD but without coronary artery disease. Patients without coronary artery disease were used in this study because the focus was on cardiac dysfunction caused by processes other than myocardial ischemia. The question of the presence of coronary artery disease was specifically answered through the use of myocardial ^{201}Tl dipyridamole single-photon emission CT imaging some time after weaning was completed. The use of inspiratory pressure support was also examined, because it is supposed to decrease the negative intrathoracic pressure swings typical of other forms of ventilation. Unfortunately, the results obtained with that method were not significant.

This study found that weaning is accompanied by a decrease in the LVEF, whereas the LVED, which is a measure of the heart's preload, was not affected. Radionuclide assessments of left ventricular wall motion and coronary perfusion were used to estimate the significance of ischemic effects in cardiac function. The reduction in LVEF was uniformly distributed over the myocardium without apparent regional effects, which supports the idea that the reduced LVEF did not result from myocardial ischemia. Additionally, myocardial perfusion images did not reveal any ischemia of the heart muscle. Based on these results and the fact that these patients did not bear any signs of coronary artery disease, it may be assumed that much of the reduced LVEF results from increased afterload on the left ventricle.

The left ventricular afterload can be estimated as the systemic blood pressure (SBP) minus the intrathoracic pressure, because the SBP approximates the pressure found within the left ventricle. Thus, an increased SBP along with a decrease in intrathoracic pressures, both of which may occur with weaning, could explain the decreased LVEF. An increase in SBP may be induced by the stress of weaning or hypercapnia and was seen in 5 of the 12 patients; however, the decreased intrathoracic pressure may be the more important part of the equation, particularly for patients with COPD and exaggerated negative swings in intrathoracic pressure during inspiration.

Weaning has always been a critical period, and the results of this study do not provide us with any easy answers. They do suggest. however, that patients with left ventricle dysfunction should receive special attention during that period and that physicians should be aware that occult ventricular dysfunction could further endanger a patient during weaning. In fact, previous studies have shown that dopamine may assist in weaning. I think this is the reason. What about you?—R.C. Bone, M.D.

27 Sepsis

Introduction

The Odyssey, by Homer, dates back to the eighth century, B.C. It is an epic adventure tale of Odysseus's dramatic journey from Troy to his home in Ithaca. Odysseus survives many ordeals during his journey and returns with new powers and insights. The study of the pathogenesis and treatment of sepsis has also been an odyssey, and I believe we will return from this odyssey with new insights and treatments. As with Odysseus, however, this will occur only after considerable struggle.

In the 1980s, we had a rather simplistic view of sepsis. It was a highly lethal complication caused by infection and often characterized by shock and multiorgan failure. Our understanding of the inflammatory responses associated with sepsis was embryonic compared with what we know today. The inflammatory response was often treated with megadose corticosteroids, along with fluid resuscitation, vasopressors, and antibiotics. Because of the paucity of multicenter, controlled trials documenting the risk–benefit ratio of the treatment of sepsis with corticosteroids, 2 large, multicenter controlled trials were organized to evaluate the role of these agents (1, 2). Because animal models revealed benefits of corticosteroids only when they received pretreatment or early treatment, a definition of sepsis was used that did not require positive culture documentation or septic shock for inclusion in the study. Patients with sepsis syndrome met the following criteria in those studies: clinical evidence of infection, tachypnea, tachycardia, and hyperthermia or hypothermia. In addition, patients had evidence of altered organ perfusion, including 1 or more of the following: first, acute changes in mental status; second, PaO_2/FIO_2 less than 280 without other pulmonary or cardiovascular diseases as the cause; third, increased lactate; and finally, oliguria (3).

Sepsis syndrome had a predictable mortality rate, incidence of shock, incidence of bacteremia, and subsequent development of multiorgan failure. This definition, or a modification of it, has been used for all subsequent large sepsis trials.

Our hope of finding a "magic bullet" to treat sepsis has been frustrating. Part of this frustration emanates from our incomplete understanding of sepsis and the conduct of clinical trials. Like Odysseus, however, we now recognize that we are on an incredible journey with a destination yet to be determined. What are the bright spots?

- Our understanding of the pathogenesis of sepsis has made incredible advances in the past 2 decades.

- Our knowledge of the epidemiology of sepsis has advanced.
- Our appreciation of the complexity of the inflammatory response, with its beneficial and detrimental aspects, is greater.
- Our design and conduct of clinical trials have achieved greater scrutiny.

These advances have been achieved because of dedicated investigators who have carefully documented the results of their trials, a pharmaceutical industry that has fostered the support and leadership necessary to conduct such trials, and the Food and Drug Administration, which has worked diligently with investigators and the pharmaceutical industry to learn from our past clinical trials.

Despite this optimistic attitude, however, we have been greeted with negative results from trials searching for the magic bullet to fight sepsis. In fact, the score is currently biotechnology, 0; sepsis, 5. I think we should recognize that these trials of monoclonal antibodies to endotoxin and tumor necrosis factor and the interleukin-1 receptor antagonist have taught us much about sepsis. It was probably naive to think that a magic bullet could improve survival in such a complicated state as sepsis. We must go back to the drawing board and redesign these trials with our improved knowledge of sepsis and systemic inflammatory response syndrome (SIRS). (See the 1993 and 1994 YEAR BOOKS OF MEDICINE). For instance, blocking these mediators may actually cause harm in selected patients; thus, we need to find ways of avoiding the potentially harmful effects of these agents. I appreciate the magnificent contributions made by the pharmaceutical industry in conducting these trials that have taught us so much about sepsis, even if they have not yet produced a magic bullet.

The first study presented in this year's chapter on sepsis discusses the initial evaluation of an interleukin-1 receptor antagonist that yielded beneficial results, although that study was followed by a still unpublished study that yielded negative results. Another report informs us of the importance of the liver in endotoxemia, and the third tells us about the significance of adhesion molecules, such as E-selectin, in SIRS.

Roger C. Bone, M.D.

References

1. Bone RC, Fisher CJ Jr, Clemmer TP, Slotman GJ, Metz CA, Balk RA, and the Methylprednisolone Severe Sepsis Study Group: A controlled clinical trial of high-dose methylprednisolone in the treatment of severe sepsis and septic shock. N Engl J Med 317:653–658, 1987.
2. Hinshaw L, and the Veterans Administration Systemic Sepsis Cooperative Study Group: Effect of high-dose glucocorticoid therapy on mortality in patients with clinical signs of systemic sepsis. N Engl J Med 317:659–665, 1987.
3. Bone RC: Let's agree on terminology: Definitions of sepsis. Crit Care Med 19:973–976, 1991.

Initial Evaluation of Human Recombinant Interleukin-1 Receptor Antagonist in the Treatment of Sepsis Syndrome: A Randomized, Open-Label, Placebo-Controlled Multicenter Trial

Fisher CJ Jr, Slotman GJ, Opal SM, Pribble JP, Bone RC, Emmanuel G, Ng D, Bloedow DC, Catalano MA, and the IL-1RA Sepsis Syndrome Study Group (Cleveland Clinic Found, Ohio; Cooper Hosp, Camden, NJ; Brown Univ, Pawtucket, RI; et al)

Crit Care Med 22:12–21, 1994   119-95-27–1

Introduction.—In sepsis, the release of exogenous microbial components stimulates host inflammatory responses medicated by tumor necrosis factor-α, interleukin-1 (IL-1), and IL-6. Macrophages produce IL-1 receptor antagonist (IL-1ra), which recognizes and binds to both types of IL-1 receptors but has no IL-1 agonist activity, in response to endotoxin and other microbial products. Recombinant IL-1ra has prevented mortality in animal studies of sepsis. The safety, pharmacokinetics, and efficacy of human recombinant IL-1ra in patients with sepsis syndrome were assessed in a prospective, open-label, placebo-controlled study.

Methods.—Ninety-nine patients in the ICU at 12 academic medical centers across the United States were included. The patients had sepsis syndrome or septic shock; all received standard supportive care and antimicrobial therapy, as well as escalating doses of IL-1ra or placebo. Treatment began with an IV loading dose of IL-1ra, 100 mg, or placebo. The patients then received a 72-hour IV infusion of either IL-1ra, 17, 67, or 133 mg/hr, or placebo (Fig 27–1). Treatment groups were compared for 28-day, all-cause mortality rates.

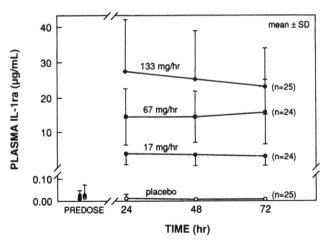

Fig 27–1.—Plasma IL-1ra concentrations at predose and during the 72-hour infusion period for each of the 4 groups. (Courtesy of Fisher CJ Jr, Slotman GJ, Opal SM, et al: *Crit Care Med* 22:12–21, 1994.)

Results.—Treatment with IL-1ra carried a dose-dependent survival benefit. Forty-four percent of placebo patients died, compared with 32% of those receiving the lowest dose of IL-1ra, 25% of those receiving the intermediate dose, and 16% of those receiving the highest dose. The survival benefit held for the 65 patients in septic shock at entry and for the 45 patients with gram-negative infection.

Treatment with IL-1ra also enhanced survival in patients with an increased circulating IL-6 concentration of greater than 100 pg/mL at entry. In this group, the magnitude of the decrease in IL-6 occurring 24 hours after therapy was correlated with an increasing dose of IL-1ra. Treatment with IL-1ra was also associated with a significant dose-related reduction in Acute Physiology and Chronic Health Evaluation score. Plasma clearance of 1L-1ra was correlated with estimated creatinine clearance, suggesting that IL-1ra was eliminated by the kidneys. The placebo and active treatment groups were no different in their incidence of adverse effects.

Conclusions.—The safety and efficacy of human recombinant IL-1ra in patients with sepsis syndrome is supported in this phase II clinical study. The dose-related survival benefit of IL-1ra, which appears to increase with increasing severity of illness, needs to be confirmed in a larger, more definitive clinical trial.

▶ The mortality associated with sepsis syndrome continues to run at a high rate, although estimates vary. This form of the systemic inflammatory response syndrome (SIRS) is most often initiated by the presence of pathogens or the mediators associated with them, such as endotoxin and exotoxins. Because the levels of circulating tumor necrosis factor-α and IL-1 have been shown to increase during SIRS, and because it is believed that these pro-inflammatory mediators are key players in the etiology of that condition, they have been the focus of many investigations.

Previous efforts have largely centered on endotoxin, a constituent of the gram-negative bacterial cell wall that has been shown to induce the release of inflammatory mediators and a pathophysiologic state resembling SIRS. Unfortunately, efforts to block the effects of endotoxin with specific antibodies have not yielded successful clinical results. It also makes sense, however, to block the inflammatory response at one of the first phases of the body's reaction, i.e., the initial release of inflammatory mediators, using IL-1ra.

Interleukin-1 receptor antagonist is a naturally occurring peptide that binds to IL-1 receptors but does not have IL-1 activity. Additionally, IL-1ra–bound receptors are unable to bind with IL-1 and are thus inactivated until they become unbound from the antagonist. The human form of this receptor blocker has been produced through recombinant DNA technology, and similar forms have been used successfully in animal models of endotoxemia and bacteremia, reducing the rate of mortality and increasing the mean arterial pressure (1–4). In vitro studies have shown that IL-1ra can reduce the production of another cytokine, IL-6, which occurs in response to the presence of endotoxin (5). This study is the first to evaluate the effects of IL-1ra on patients with sepsis syndrome in a clinical situation. Patients with sepsis syndrome were administered the blocker to determine whether it improved the rate of mortality or decreased the cytokine response.

The results of this small-scale study are encouraging. A dose-related decrease in the mortality rate of patients with septic syndrome was observed. This finding is in accord with a recently completed clinical study of IL-1ra, for which the preliminary data indicate a decreased mortality rate within the first 28 days (6). The question of dosage, however, remains to perplex some researchers: an approximate $100,000–1,000,000 \times$ molar excess of this antagonist must be used, relative to circulating IL-1$_\beta$ concentrations. Although not yet published at the time of this writing, the second phase III trial of IL-1ra has been reported to have obtained a negative result. At approximately the same time, the results from the Bradycor trial were released by Cortech and were also negative. Bradycor is a kinin antagonist, and the trial examined changes in survival over a 28-day period.

At last count, the score is sepsis, 5; biotechnology, 0. On the other hand, we have learned much from these trials. They have taught us about the pathogenesis of sepsis and SIRS. We have the pharmaceutical industry to thank for these advances. Improvement in survival may be an end point that is not attainable with a single "magic bullet." Additionally, the mortality attributable to SIRS and sepsis may not be large enough to show a statistically significant benefit. And remember, these patients often have underlying illness and are immunosuppressed, facts that may contribute to mortality. I believe the reversal of multiple organ dysfunction syndrome is an appropriate and achievable end point that should be used in these studies of SIRS and sepsis. If we can get agents approved using these end points, we can possibly use combination therapy at lower doses to block the systemic inflammatory response without so altering normal homeostasis that mortality end points can be achieved.—R.C. Bone, M.D.

References

1. Ohlsson K, Bjork P, Bergenfeldt M, et al: An interleukin-1 receptor antagonist reduces mortality from endotoxin shock. *Nature* 348:550–552, 1990.
2. Fischer E, Marano MA, VanZee KJ, et al: Interleukin-1 receptor blockade improves survival and hemodynamic performance in *E. coli* septic shock, but fails to alter host responses to sublethal endotoxemia. *J Clin Invest* 89:1551–1557, 1992.
3. Wakabayashi G, Gelfand JA, Burke JF, et al: A specific receptor antagonist for interleukin-1 prevents *Escherichia coli*–induced shock in rabbits. *FASEB J* 5:338–343, 1991.
4. Aiura K, Gelfand JA, Burke JF, et al: Interleukin-1 receptor antagonist prevents *Staphylococcus epidermis* induced hypotension and reduces circulating levels of tumor necrosis factor and IL-1 in rabbits. *Infect Immun* 61:3342–3350, 1993.
5. Granowitz EV, Porat R, Mier JW, et al: Pharmacokinetics, safety, and immunomodulatory effects of human recombinant IL-1ra in healthy humans. *Cytokine* 4:353–360, 1992.
6. Fisher CJ Jr, Dhainaut JF, Pribble JP, et al: A study to evaluate the safety and efficacy of human recombinant IL-1ra in the treatment of patients with sepsis syndrome. *Clin Intensive Care* (Abstract) 4:8S, 1993.

Liver-Lung Interactions During *E. coli* Endotoxemia: TNF-α:Leukotriene Axis

Matuschak GM, Mattingly ME, Tredway TL, Lechner AJ (St Louis Univ, Mo; Saint John's Mercy Med Ctr, St Louis, Mo)

Am J Respir Crit Care Med 149:41–49, 1994   119-95-27–2

Introduction.—During infection with *Escherichia coli*, tumor necrosis factor-α(TNF-α) and eicosanoid mediators, which are produced and cleared by the liver, are known to be involved in the development of adult respiratory distress syndrome. Because the mechanism of this involvement is not well understood, the role of the liver in modulating cytokines and eicosanoid products that promote lung injury was determined in a rat model.

Methods.—Twenty-two male Sprague-Dawley rats underwent an end-to-side portacaval shunt (PCS), and 13 underwent a sham operation. Fifteen shunted rats and 13 sham-operated rats received IV *E. coli* lipopolysaccharide (LPS), 2.5 mg/kg, and 5 rats in each group received saline. Interarterial pressure, heart rate, and serum TNF-α were measured, and blood samples were analyzed at 0, 1.5, 3.5, and 24 hours. The animals were killed, and organ weights were determined. Levels of TNF-α, leukotrienes, and polymorphonuclear neutrophils in bronchoalveolar lavage fluid were measured.

Results.—The mortality rate in the LPS-treated groups was 4 times higher, and peak serum TNF-α levels were $2\frac{1}{2}$ times higher in PCS rats than in sham-operated rats, as were wet–dry cecal, heart, and liver weight ratios. Hypotension developed in the LPS-treated PCS rats. Neutrophils in the lavage fluid for the LPS-treated PCS group were significantly higher than for their sham-operated counterparts, but recovery was markedly reduced when rats were given N,N-diethyl-4-methyl-1-piperazine carboximide (DEC). This agent also significantly reduced levels of leukotriene in bronchoalveolar lavage fluid. Clearance of infused TNF-α was unaffected in nonendotoxemic PCS rats.

Discussion.—Treatment with PCS reduces liver blood flow as much as 75%. The level of liver blood flow plays an important role in the morbidity and mortality during endotoxemia, which causes an increase in the concentration of TNF-α. Serum TNF-α was decreased by DEC before and after LPS administration by 72% and 91%, respectively. Also, DEC stabilized blood pressure and wet–dry cecal weight ratios and significantly reduced mortality, bronchoalveolar lavage fluid leukotrienes, and polymorphonucleur neutrophils.

Conclusion.—Decreases in liver blood flow increase the immunologic consequences to the lungs of patients with endotoxemia.

▶ The occurrence of acute respiratory distress syndrome (ARDS) may or may not result from intrapulmonary events. In either case, however, the presence of TNF-α and a number of secondary mediators, which include TNF-α–

induced release of leukotrienes in the lower respiratory tree, may mediate the detrimental effects. These effects include a disruption of endothelial barriers resulting in edema, along with the aggregation of polymorphonuclear leukocytes and their infiltration into the tissues. The authors point out, however, that although many of these mediators have been shown to promote inflammation on an individual basis, their interactions in vivo are poorly understood. This is particularly true with regard to the control of circulating mediator activity accomplished by other organs, especially the liver, which metabolizes these mediators. It has been shown that endotoxemia induced in animals with preexisting acute liver injury results in more damage to the lung than it does in healthy animals (1). The question of hepatic function is also crucial in this regard, because a number of conditions associated with ARDS, including endotoxemia, trauma, mechanical ventilation involving positive end-expiratory pressure, and α-adrenergic therapy, may also effect blood flow to the liver. The authors of this study have directly examined the effects of induced endotoxemia in animals that have received a PCS.

Peak circulating levels of TNF-α in the animals with shunts were significantly higher than in sham-operated animals, although there was no difference in cellular levels of the mediator. The animals with shunts also had exacerbated hypotension and capillary leakage and a higher mortality rate. Interestingly, the use of DEC, which inhibits the formation of leukotrienes, reversed these effects in shunted animals, indicating that these secondarily released mediators may be more important in causing these effects than are the increased levels of circulating TNF-α. The inhibition of leukotriene production seemed to have reciprocal effects on the levels of circulating TNF-α, an observation that needs explanation and mandates further study.

These findings signify the importance of liver clearance of inflammatory mediators in endotoxemia. The many factors that affect hepatic perfusion may also be predictors of which patients will have ARDS or other indications of systemic or localized inflammation characteristic of systemic inflammatory response syndrome or multiple organ dysfunction syndrome.—R.C. Bone, M.D.

Reference

1. Matuschak GM, Pinsky MR, Klein EC, et al: Effect of D-galactosamine-induced acute liver injury on mortality and pulmonary responses to E. *coli* lipopolysaccharide: Modulation by arachidonic acid metabolites. *Am Rev Respir Dis* 141:1296–1306, 1990.

Increased Circulating Adhesion Molecule Concentrations in Patients With the Systemic Inflammatory Response Syndrome: A Prospective Cohort Study

Cowley HC, Heney D, Gearing AJH, Hemingway I, Webster NR (St. James' Univ Hospital, Leeds, England; British Bio-Technology, Oxford, England)
Crit Care Med 22:651–657, 1994   119-95-27-3

Background.—Increased expression of endothelial adhesion substances is evidence of endothelial activation in experimental animals with systemic inflammatory response syndrome (SIRS). Extravasation of activated leukocytes is mediated by adhesion molecules on both endothelial cells and leukocytes and leads to both local tissue damage and systemic inflammatory effects culminating in organ dysfunction.

Method.—Enzyme-linked immunosorbent assays were used to relate soluble derivatives of endothelial adhesion molecules to systemic inflammation and organ dysfunction in a prospective series of 35 patients with SIRS. Fourteen of these patients had organ dysfunction. Five other patients who were severely ill and 85 healthy individuals were also studied. Levels of soluble E-selectin (sE-selectin), vascular cell adhesion molecule-1, and intercellular adhesion molecule-1 were estimated.

Findings.—Patients with organ dysfunction had significantly higher levels of sE-selectin than did those with either uncomplicated SIRS or other severe illness. All patient groups had elevated levels of both vascular cell adhesion molecule-1 and circulating intercellular adhesion molecule-1 compared with the control groups. There was no significant overall difference in mean plasma adhesion molecule levels between patients who survived and those who died, but no patient whose initial or peak level of sE-selectin exceeded 35 units/mL survived.

Conclusion.—Estimating circulating levels of adhesion molecules, particularly sE-selectin, may prove helpful in predicting which patients with SIRS will have organ dysfunction develop.

▶ The aggregation and infiltration of leukocytes in various tissues, particularly the lung, in SIRS have been well documented and described. The process of leukocytic extravasation has also been examined. Activated endothelial cells produce cell surface molecules, known as adhesion molecules, that promote the movement of activated leukocytes across the capillary wall. One such adhesion molecule, E-selectin, has been characterized as a marker of endothelial cell activation and is produced by inflammatory endothelial cells that have been activated by inflammatory mediators. E-selectin has been associated with neutrophilic, monocytic, and T-cell infiltrates. This adhesion molecule is capable of releasing the extracellular portion of its structure, which then circulates freely in the blood. The authors of this study have attempted to correlate circulating levels of sE-selectin, along with circulating levels of soluble intercellular adhesion molecule-1 and vascular cell adhesion molecule-1, with the presence and severity of SIRS and multiple-organ dysfunction syndrome. The latter 2 adhesion molecules may be less specific for endothelial cell activation, because several cell types produce them.

Increased levels of all 3 adhesion molecules examined were seen in patients with SIRS. These levels increased even further with progression of disease and with the complication of organ dysfunction. The concentrations of E-selectin were also predictive of survival: no patient with greater than 36 units/mL of E-selectin survived. Levels of vascular cell adhesion molecule-1 showed increases similar to those of E-selectin, although they were slower and somewhat less specific. Levels of intercellular adhesion molecule-1 were the least specific of these indicators and have been shown to increase in a variety of conditions. In vitro results indicate that E-selectin can reach peak expression within 4–6 hours of the exposure of endothelial cells to cytokines and that this increased expression can last for several days, a time course that corresponds with that of SIRS.

Although the predictive capability of E-selectin in SIRS is strongly supported by this study, the reason for this capability is unclear. Could this molecule be causative in severity of SIRS and progression to organ failure or is it merely a passive marker of events? Further study of this molecule is warranted, given its potential to promote leukocytic infiltration of the tissues with commensurate progression of disease.—R.C. Bone, M.D.

28 Ethics

Introduction

I have added this new chapter, Ethics, to my section of the YEAR BOOK OF MEDICINE for a number of reasons. Most important, there has been a virtual explosion of issues that are essentially ethical in nature. The whole issue of managed care, which is often couched in terms of what is right and wrong, can be further reduced to a series of smaller questions of the efficacy and cost-effectiveness of specific techniques and procedures. The issue of withdrawal of care is also critical and sometimes divisive, bringing up specific questions of the living will, patient autonomy, and do-not-resuscitate orders.

This year's YEAR BOOK OF MEDICINE includes 2 abstracts regarding issues in ethics. The first addresses the question of surrogates—usually family members—who make important care decisions for an incapacitated patient. At issue is the point that patients, who may be unable to communicate their wishes, may change their minds about the type of care they want over the course of a hospital stay. The second study questions our (by "our," I mean physician, patient, and family/surrogate) ability to make decisions regarding when to withdraw critical life support. These are very difficult questions, and I believe they should be part of the public forum afforded by publications such as this.

Roger C. Bone, M.D.

Stability of Choices About Life-Sustaining Treatments
Danis M, Garrett J, Harris R, Patrick DL (Univ of North Carolina, Chapel Hill; Univ of Washington, Seattle)
Ann Intern Med 120:567–573, 1994   119-95-28–1

Background.—Because patients are often unable to make decisions about their health care during a life-threatening illness, health care providers have come to rely on the previously expressed wishes of these patients. Many patients have a living will, assign a health care power of attorney, or have another written directive. It is usually assumed that patients' wishes are stable. The few studies examining this issue were done with small samples of patients over short periods of time. A large group of elderly patients was examined to determine the stability of their decisions about life-sustaining treatment.

Stability of Preferences at Baseline and Follow-Up

Preference	Baseline	Number	Follow-up			P Value*
		n	Yes	No	Don't know	
			%			
Hospitalization	Yes	877	38	43	19	<0.001
	No	240	19	66	15	
	Don't know	955	27	50	23	
Intensive care	Yes	1055	18	50	32	<0.001
	No	325	8	71	21	
	Don't know	688	14	58	28	
Cardiopulmonary resuscitation	Yes	1272	34	40	26	<0.001
	No	261	8	75	17	
	Don't know	540	13	58	29	
Surgery	Yes	1301	30	43	27	<0.001
	No	284	11	71	18	
	Don't know	485	13	62	25	
Artificial respiration	Yes	1459	31	42	27	0.11
	No	235	12	71	17	
	Don't know	379	16	57	27	
Tube feeding	Yes	1182	43	41	16	<0.05
	No	523	11	75	14	
	Don't know	366	19	52	29	

* The McNemar test for no association of paired data.
(Courtesy of Danis M, Garrett J, Harris R, et al: *Ann Intern Med* 120:567–573, 1994.)

Methods.—Participants were 2,536 Medicare recipients, aged 65–99 years. At an interview, they were asked about health status, well-being, depression, possession of a living will, and desire for life-sustaining treatment. Two years later, 82% of those participants responded to the same questions.

Results.—At follow-up, approximately 42% of participants desired less treatment than at the initial interview, 38% expressed no desire for change, and 20% desired more treatment (table). Participants who wanted the least treatment at the initial interview were most likely to make the same choices at follow-up. Those with a living will were more likely to maintain their wishes than those without one. Participants were more likely to desire more treatment at follow-up if they had been hospitalized, had an accident, became less mobile, became more depressed, or had less social support.

Discussion.—Wishes for life-sustaining treatment are not entirely stable and can change as the patient's health changes. Choices for treatment expressed at admission to a hospital might be influenced by feelings of vulnerability and may change at a less traumatic time. It is important to review patients' preferences for life-sustaining treatment over time, regardless of whether they have written directives.

▶ Often, by the time a decision must be made about the use of life-sustaining therapy, the patient is unable to participate in the choice. Physicians and family must then make a decision based on what the patient has previously said. Although advance directives and living wills are clear and legal documents intended to ensure that a patient's wishes will be carried out, few individuals actually have such documents written. As a result, it has become acceptable for a surrogate to make care decisions based on the patient's past wishes (1). Accepting the validity of a previous statement to direct current care assumes that a patient's decision in this difficult area does not change over time.

These authors interviewed a cohort of elderly patients (average age, 77.5 years) as they were seeing their primary care physician. Patients were interviewed twice, 2 years apart. As expected, those who had been hospitalized 1 or more times between interviews were more likely to revise their choice to more desired treatment, as did those who experienced a loss of mobility or health-related loss of social activity. The authors speculate that these vulnerability factors may heighten an individual's awareness of his or her own mortality. This result is consistent with findings in terminally ill patients, who often desire the use of vigilant life support measures. Overall, however, these patients tended to want less treatment at the follow-up interview. The authors hypothesize that their decisions may have been influenced by historical events that occurred during their lives or by the increased frequency of public discussion regarding life-sustaining treatment.

Analysis of the stability of preference scale shows that 62% of the respondents revised their wishes in some way, with only 38% of the participants having "essentially" no change during the 2-year interval. This result, combined with similar results from other trials (2, 3), indicates that instability increases as the interval between interviews lengthens. This is not good news and makes it clear that physicians must discuss the topic of life-sustaining therapy with patients, preferably during a nonstressful time, such as during a routine office visit.

A very interesting finding in this study was that patients who had written advance directives or a living will before the study began had more stable preferences (86% remained in the same treatment category). Those who had living wills at the initial interview and chose the least amount of care had the most stable preferences—96% unchanged. To me, this says that these patients gave the matter a great deal of thought, made a decision based on what they knew to be in their best interest, and were comfortable with that decision.

This study illustrates both the low number of patients who have advance directives and the importance of such directives. It could be argued that, because some patients change their minds, the use of advance directives is not valid. The authors of this study suggest that advance directives should be used as a guide, not as a prediction of future wishes, and that patients should be asked routinely how closely they want the directive followed. Or, perhaps, we should discuss the use of advance directives with our patients and encourage them to write a living will or advance directive, letting them know that if they change their mind in the future, the document can be altered. In addition, perhaps the advance directive should be updated every year to reflect changes in both the patient's thinking and health.—R.C. Bone, M.D.

References

1. Menikoff JA, Sachs GA, Siegler M: Beyond advance directives—Health care surrogate laws. N Engl J Med 327:1165–1169, 1992.
2. Everhart MA, Pearlman RA: Stability of patient preferences regarding life-sustaining treatments. *Chest* 97:159–164, 1990.
3. Silverstein MD, Stocking CB, Antel JP, et al: Amyotrophic lateral sclerosis and life-sustaining therapy: Patients' desires for more information, participation in decision making, and life-sustaining therapy. *Mayo Clin Proc* 66:906–913, 1991.

Withdrawing Care: Experience in a Medical Intensive Care Unit
Lee DKP, Swinburne AJ, Fedullo AJ, Wahl GW (Univ of Rochester, NY)
JAMA 271:1358–1361, 1994   119-95-28-2

Background.—Although ethical guidelines for withholding life-sustaining interventions and patient rights of refusal are well established, withdrawal of futile interventions has been less well described. Available studies do not distinguish between withholding and withdrawing care or provide only anecdotal reports. The process and outcomes of withdrawing life-sustaining interventions in a medical ICU were described.

Decision-Making

	Reason for Withdrawal		
Variable	**Physiological**	**Neurological**	**Functional**
No. of patients	12	11	5
APACHE II score, mean±SD*	28.5±8.9	27.5±6.7	22.6±1.3
Predicted mortality, %, mean±SD	63±25	67±16	44±15
No. of competent patients	2	0	3
No. of patients with advance directive	4	3	1
No. of patients who underwent therapeutic trial	10	7	4
Duration of discussion, d, mean±SD	4.5±3.7	2.3±2.7†	9.2±6.8

* APACHE II indicates Acute Physiology and Chronic Health Evaluation.
† One outlier was removed. P < .03.
(Courtesy of Lee DKP, Swinburne AJ, Fedullo AJ, et al: JAMA 271:1358–1361, 1994.)

Methods.—Case records of 28 consecutive patients, in whom mechanical ventilation, dialysis, and/or vasopressor therapy were withdrawn, were reviewed. Physiologic, neurologic, and functional rationales for withdrawal of care were distinguished, and duration of discussion was assessed.

Results.—Five patients participated in the decision to discontinue life-sustaining therapy; the remaining patients' interests were represented by their families or by the hospital's ethics committee. Eight patients had previously stated to physicians or family members that they did not want prolonged life support for serious illness. Physiologic futility was the reason for discontinuation of life support in 12 patients; in 11, persistent coma and unacceptable neurologic prognosis; and in 5, alleviation of suffering and unacceptable functional prognosis (table). Decision-making averaged 2.3 days in patients with unacceptable neurologic prognoses, compared with 5.9 days in patients with no irreversible brain injury.

Conclusion.—In reaching end-of-life decisions, finding an accommodation between physician judgments and patient preferences takes time, but it is an effective means of limiting ineffective life-sustaining efforts without resorting to unilateral judgments of medical futility.

▶ In principle, the withdrawal of life support measures when they are either unwanted or futile sounds like the right thing to do. Making the decision, however, is less straightforward. This article discusses both the process of withdrawing life support and the consequences—which are not always what are expected. Of the current patients, 14 died within 24 hours of discontinuing life support measures; however, 7 patients remained alive for 1–7 days after life support was withdrawn, 7 patients survived for 7 or more days, and 4 patients were discharged alive from the hospital. Withdrawal of life support therapy is a difficult decision for the patient and the patient's family. Critical illness is a stressful event for all concerned; regardless of the seriousness of the illness, the patient and the family expect, or at least hope, to see a dramatic change for the better. Discussion of withdrawal of life support not only destroys that hope, but it also forces the patient and family to think about the many possible bleak outcomes that could occur. So, what should be done? Clearly, lengthy discussion and gradual decision-making, as these authors advocate, are key factors. In this study, an average of 5.2 ± 5.5 days elapsed from the time discontinuation was first discussed and withdrawal of therapy actually began. The patient's capability to make the decision had no bearing on the time it took—some insisted that therapy be withdrawn immediately, and others considered the decision for several days. Decisions were made most quickly in patients who were considered to have a poor neurologic prognosis (2.3 ± 2.7 days) and least quickly in those who did not have irreversible brain injury (5.9 ± 5.1 days). In most cases, the final decision to withdraw therapy was made after the patient did not benefit from a specific therapeutic trial. In some cases, withdrawal of therapy was delayed by physicians after it was requested by the family. Physicians wanted to be certain that further treatment would not benefit the patient, raising the question of whether care was withdrawn only when both physician and patient or surrogate agreed that it should be withdrawn or whether the patient's right to self-determination was respected. In addition, 1 patient who was discharged from the hospital alive was an elderly woman who had an apparent stroke and had undergone prolonged mechanical ventilation. She was judged by both her children and physician to have too great an impairment to warrant further life support, and measures were withdrawn. Nonetheless, her condition stabilized. After several months in a skilled nursing facility, she required no further long-term nursing care. So, how do we decide who should be withdrawn from life support therapy? As physicians, how should we react when a patient or surrogate wishes to cease therapy that we believe may still be beneficial? And finally, how do we reconcile our duty to heal with our knowledge that we cannot always do so?—R.C. Bone, M.D.

29 Acute Respiratory Distress Syndrome

Introduction

Acute respiratory distress syndrome (ARDS) was described more than a quarter century ago (1). Although we have learned much about its pathogenesis, therapy for the condition continues to be supportive in nature, consisting largely of mechanical ventilation and treatment of the underlying disease entity. The field of mechanical ventilation, however, has undergone major advances in the past decade. We now understand the deleterious effects of the inflation volumes and distending pressures used in routine care just a few years ago. The concept of permissive hypercapnia, which is associated with decreased distending pressures, has been a major advance. In this chapter on ARDS, the use of CT as a research tool in the study of the pathophysiology of ARDS is discussed, and the use of pressure-controlled, inverse-ratio ventilation is compared with extracorporeal removal of carbon dioxide. The potential role for corticosteroids in the fibroproliferative process of late ARDS is described. The American–European Conference on ARDS has contributed an up-to-date, consensus picture of the pathophysiology of the condition. The role of inhaled nitric oxide in ARDS is further evaluated (see reference 2 for a discussion of the initial trial). Also, see my commentary in this edition for discussion of a possible dark side to nitric oxide. In fact, it was referred to as a "Jekyll and Hyde" compound at the 1994 American Thoracic Society Meeting. Finally, a possible role for surfactant merits discussion in this year's edition of the YEAR BOOK OF MEDICINE.

Roger C. Bone, M.D.

References

1. Ashbaugh DG, Bigelow DB, Petty TL: *Lancet* 2:319–323, 1967.
2. 1994 YEAR BOOK OF MEDICINE, pp 215–220.

Vertical Gradient of Regional Lung Inflation in Adult Respiratory Distress Syndrome

Pelosi P, D'Andrea L, Vitale G, Pesenti A, Gattinoni L (Istituto di Anestesia e Rianimazione dell'Universitá degli Studi di Milano–Ospedale S Gerardo, Monza, Italy)
Am J Respir Crit Care Med 149:8–13, 1994   119-95-29-1

Objective.—Patients with adult respiratory distress syndrome (ARDS) and normal adults were studied with chest CT to examine regional lung inflation. Previous studies suggest that a progressive deflation of gas-containing alveoli along the gravity gradient exists in lungs of patients with ARDS, with a quantitatively smaller deflation found in lungs of normal individuals who are awake and anesthetized-paralyzed.

Methods.—Thirteen men and 4 women had moderate-to-severe ARDS and a variety of underlying problems. Nine patients survived and were discharged from the hospital. A CT study was performed an average of 7.5 days after endotracheal intubation. The control group included 9 men and 3 women who underwent chest CT scanning to provide a reference. Basal CT sections just above the diaphragm were obtained in the supine position at 0 cm water end-expiratory pressure. After the average density and the volume of 10 lung levels from ventral to dorsal were obtained, the tissue volume, gas/tissue (g/t) ratio, and hydrostatic pressure superimposed on each level (SPL)—estimated as density × height—were computed.

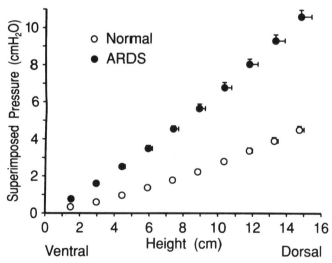

Fig 29–1.—The estimated superimposed pressure as a function of ventral-to-dorsal lung height in normal subjects (*open circles*, 24 lungs) and patients with ARDS (*filled circles*, 34 lungs). The data (mean ± SE) of both normal subjects and patients with ARDS fits the general quadratic equation: SPL = a × hL + b × hL². (Courtesy of Pelosi P, D'Andrea L, Vitale G, et al: *Am J Respir Crit Care Med* 149:8–13, 1994.)

Results.—The mean total volume of the basal CT section did not differ significantly in the control group (49 mL $\times$ m^{-2}) and the patient group (43 mL $\times$ m^{-2}). Tissue volume, however, differed significantly between the 2 groups: 16.7 mL $\times$ m^{-2} for control individuals and 31.6 mL $\times$ m^{-2} for patients with ARDS. The g/t ratio, which averaged 4.7 in control individuals and 1.2 in patients, decreased exponentially from level 1 (ventral) to level 10 (dorsal) in both groups. The SPL in level 10 was 4.5 cm water in controls and 10.5 cm water in patients (Fig 29–1).

Conclusion.—In the comparative analysis of the basal CT sections, total lung dimensions were not altered by ARDS, even though the lung in patients with ARDS is characterized by decreased gas volume and increased tissue volume. The gas space in patients is substituted by tissue volume, probably edema, at each lung level. Along a vertical gradient, gas content decreases and SPL increases at a greater rate in patients with ARDS than in normal individuals.

▶ Dr. Gattinoni has been a pioneer in our understanding of ARDS as a non-homogeneous disease. He has developed the concept of lung injury from overinflation, which then precipitated the development of permissive hypercapnia. I think that when this form of ventilation is used appropriately, survival will improve compared with conventional ventilation. Bravo, Dr. Gattinoni—keep those concepts coming!

The heterogeneity of lung density and function in ARDS has been a matter of discussion among pulmonary specialists for some time. Some believe that an understanding of the factors that determine these regional differences in the lung could be an important key to new treatments. A typical observation of patients with ARDS is that inflation decreases and density increases as one moves down the gravitational gradient. This general scheme is, of course, a natural result of hydrostatic pressure and may be observed in normal lungs; however, these differences appear to be exaggerated in the lungs of patients with ARDS. This study examined the patterns of inflation in patients with ARDS and in normal individuals at end expiration and at functional residual capacity (FRC) through the use of CT. The resolution of the machine allowed discrimination at the level of approximately half a pulmonary acinus, a unit called the voxel. Each voxel is assigned a density by the computer. In this study, only a single CT section was used—a basal section taken just above the level of the diaphragm and found to be representative of other sections. The lung was arbitrarily divided into 10 levels based on progressively changing gravitational effects. The voxel densities within a single lung level of this section were then averaged.

Total lung volume did not differ between patients with ARDS and normal individuals; however, the overall density of the section for the patient group was about 3 times greater than that of the control group. This finding indicates that gas volume has been replaced with intravascular and extravascular water, infiltrating cells, and fibrosis, to mention 3 of the more likely constituents. It is this reduced gas volume that underlies the decrease in FRC seen in patients with ARDS. At each level, the tissue volume of patients' lungs is approximately twice that of normal lungs, suggesting that excess lung fluids and tissues are uniformly distributed and not influenced by gravity. This finding is in agreement with a previous study of CT scans of lungs of patients with ARDS (1) and with animal lungs when other methods of measuring were used (2).

The mechanisms at work in the lung during ARDS appear to act equally at all lung levels, and the accumulated fluids are unable to move freely through the interstitial space. As in normal patients, the g/t ratio of lungs in patients with ARDS decreases exponentially with depth from the surface of the lung; however, the rate of decrease is much greater in ARDS lungs. In ARDS, the g/t in tissue 7–8 cm below the surface of the lung is 37% of that at the surface of the lung; this means that there is nearly total alveolar collapse in the lower half of the lung of patients not receiving positive end-expiratory pressure. Controversy regarding the cause of a level-associated pressure (PL) in normal lungs continues; it is generally agreed that the PL depends on lung weight, the shape and mechanical properties of the chest wall, and the shape and mechanical properties of the lung. For the sake of this study, the authors assumed that PL at a given site was equivalent to the hydrostatic pressure that would result from a column of water the same depth as that of the lung tissue—about .23 cm H_2O. The authors believe that a greater PL gradient occurs in patients with ARDS, which results in the increased g/t rate changes with depth. Although the exact reasons for this increased PL gradient are not known, theory indicates that they result from changes in thoracic and lung compliance, along with changes in lung weight. It may be that lung weight is the most important factor in ARDS as the tissue volume and weight above a given lung area increases.—R.C. Bone, M.D.

References

1. Gattinoni L, Pelosi P, Vitale G, Pesenti A, D'Andrea L, Mascheroni D: Body position changes redistribute lung computed tomographic density in patients with acute respiratory failure. *Anesthesiology* 74:15-23, 1991.
2. Hales CA, Devid JK, Ahlualia B, Latty A, Erdman J, Javehery S, Kazeni H: Regional edema formation in isolated perfused dog lungs. *Circ Res* 48:121-127, 1981.

Randomized Clinical Trial of Pressure-Controlled Inverse Ratio Ventilation and Extracorporeal CO_2 Removal for Adult Respiratory Distress Syndrome

Morris AH, Wallace CJ, Menlove RL, Clemmer TP, Orme JF Jr, Weaver LK, Dean NC, Thomas F, East TD, Pace NL, Suchyta MR, Beck E, Bombino M, Sittig DF, Böhm S, Hoffmann B, Becks H, Butler S, Pearl J, Rasmusson (LDS Hosp, Salt Lake City, Utah; Univ of Utah, Salt Lake City)
Am J Respir Crit Care Med 149:295–305, 1994   119-95-29-2

Introduction.—Patients with adult respiratory distress syndrome (ARDS) generally have a poor prognosis, with a mortality rate greater

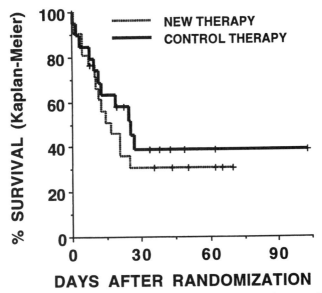

Fig 29–2.—Kaplan–Meier survival curves for the 19 control patients who underwent traditional therapy (*solid line*) and the 21 patients who had new therapy (*dotted line*). *Small vertical bars* superimposed on curves indicate censored patients. P = .47. (Courtesy of Morris AH, Wallace CJ, Menlove RL, et al: *Am J Respir Crit Care Med* 149:295–305, 1994.)

than 60%. Mechanical ventilation is currently the centerpiece of supportive therapy for these patients, but this therapy may further damage the lung. However, pressure-controlled inverse-ratio ventilation (PCIRV) followed by extracorporeal carbon dioxide removal (ECCO$_2$R) may minimize iatrogenic lung injury and promote longer survival. The rate of survival in patients with ARDS treated with PCIRV and ECCO$_2$R vs. those treated with conventional ventilator therapy was compared.

Methods.—Patients with severe ARDS who had not already undergone mechanical ventilation were stratified by age (older or younger than 40 years) and by presence or absence of trauma. The patients were then assigned randomly to receive either PCIRV with ECCO$_2$R (21 patients) or the control ventilator therapy (19 patients). Survival, physiologic data, length of hospital stay, and cost of care were compared for the 2 groups.

Results.—All deaths occurred within 30 days of the start of therapy. More patients in the control group (42%) than in the experimental group (23%) were still alive at 30 days, a difference too small for statistical significance (Fig 29–2). There were also no significant differences between the 2 groups for length of hospital or ICU stay, clinical trial duration, blood gas values, or total complications. However, non-CNS hemorrhage occurred more often in the new therapy group, which required more blood products than the control group. The cost of care was higher with PCIRV and ECCO$_2$R therapy.

Discussion.—There was no significant difference in survival rate between patients receiving PCIRV with ECCO₂ R therapy and those receiving conventional ventilator therapy. In addition, the higher incidence of non-CNS hemorrhage with the new therapy is cause for concern. Therefore, PCIRV-ECCO₂R cannot be recommended as a therapy for ARDS, and its use should be restricted to controlled clinical trials.

▶ When I was a medical student in the mid-1960s, we used intermittent–positive pressure ventilation (IPPV) with the "Bird" ventilator to ventilate patients. The tidal volumes produced were small. In Vietnam, I was an "on-the-job–trained" anesthesiologist and used volume ventilation with large tidal volumes (16–22 mL/kg) exclusively for the treatment of ARDS with mechanical ventilation. This was close to the time that ARDS was first described. Although I certainly wasn't getting *Lancet* in Vietnam, we were using positive end-expiratory pressure (PEEP), because some physicians had seen it used in the States. Our methods, however, were crude. We stuck a tube on the expiratory port of the ventilator and put it under water to the level of PEEP we desired. Now, we have come full circle to use a variation of IPPV, pressure-limited ventilation. The way we use PEEP now is also similar to the way we used it in the 1960s. Isn't it fascinating how long it takes to change and how change has led us back to doing largely what we were doing more than 20 years ago? A big change, however, is the use of small tidal volume and permissive hypercapnia.

Although the reported survival of European patients treated for severe ARDS with PCIRV, followed by low-frequency positive-pressure ventilation ECCO₂R (LFPPV-ECCO₂R), was considerably higher than has been seen in ARDS studies performed in the United States, the European studies suffer from the lack of an appropriate control (1). This difference is particularly noticeable when we consider studies of extracorporeal membrane oxygenation (ECMO) in the United States, where the reported survival rate was 9% (2). There is evidence to support belief that the high peak-airway pressures needed to maintain tidal volumes typically used in the United States may damage the lung. This damage may be particularly severe in portions of the lung that remain functional and compliant. The authors of this study have undertaken a randomized study of PCIRV followed by LFPPV-ECCO₂R in patients with severe ARDS. Continuous positive-pressure ventilation (CPPV) was used as a control in this experiment. Survival was the main outcome measure, although hospital costs and stay were examined, along with physiologic data and consumption of blood products. The inclusion criteria were essentially those of the ECMO study. To duplicate the European application of PCIRV-ECCO₂R precisely, much collaborative work was undertaken in this study.

Sixteen percent of patients identified as having ARDS had disease severe enough to match the ECMO study and to be enrolled in this study. The overall survival rate of all patients was 38%—much higher than would be expected for such a group of patients. The 42% survival rate in the control group did much to support this unexpectedly high overall survival figure. Another important consideration is the etiology of ARDS—of the many potential causes of this condition, trauma was recorded much more frequently in the European study than in this study. The survival rate in the control group was also significantly higher than that found by the same authors in a previous study of similar patients with similar etiologies. This anomalous figure could cast doubts on the validity of the study and makes the task of proving that treatment with PCIRV-ECCO$_2$R is significantly better than CPPV in patients with severe ARDS much more difficult. The reasons for this high survival rate remain unknown. Careful assessment of patient physiologic and demographic variables indicated that the control and treatment groups of this study were similar and that patients had been appropriately randomized into the treatment arms of this study.

The survival rate in the treatment arm of this study was 32%, however, which is not statistically different from the 43% to 50% survival logged by European studies of this technique. The goal of PCIRV-ECCO$_2$R is to reduce peak-airway pressures and ventilatory rates to allow the lung to rest. This did occur: average peak-airway pressures were 8.3 cm H$_2$O lower in the treatment group; however, the goal of holding peak pressures to 45 cm H$_2$O could not be achieved if minimal tidal volumes of approximately 3.5–4.5 mL/kg of predicted body weight during periods of low compliance were to be maintained.

Given the current state of our knowledge, it is very difficult to make heads or tails of the fact that there appears to be a difference between studies performed in Europe and in the United States. In the recent American–European Consensus Conference on ARDS, the committee pointed out that uniform definitions are not used in the context of ARDS (3) (see also Abstract 119-95-29-3). The consensus committee concluded that joint European–American clinical studies should be encouraged. Clearly, we still have some things to learn about the pathogenesis of ARDS and related dysfunctions. It may be that our ability to predict the severity of disease is not accurate, resulting in inappropriate patient groupings. As much good as empiric treatment can sometimes do, it may ultimately be necessary to know the disease to treat it.

I believe the improved survival rates result from Dr. Morris' skilled, highly professional ICU team. Around the world, ICUs with such expert and dedicated teams have seen an improvement in survival. This is *not* because of a major drug or a new technique. Rather, it is the result of superior training and superior medical care. Let's work for breakthroughs in our knowledge, but let's not underestimate the power of superior training and medical care. I don't think we need a randomized trial to prove that, but if so, please do not randomize me to inferior training and inferior care, even if that arm of the trial includes treatment with a "magic bullet" and the other, a placebo.—R.C. Bone, M.D.

References

1. Bone RC: Extracorporeal membrane oxygenation for acute respiratory failure. JAMA 256:910, 1986.

2. Zapol WM, Snider MT, Hill JD, et al: Extracorporeal membrane oxygenation in severe acute respiratory failure. *JAMA* 242:2193–2196, 1979.
3. Bernard GR, Artigas A, Brigham KL, and the Consensus Committee: The American–European consensus conference on ARDS. *Am J Respir Crit Care Med* 149:818–824, 1994.

The American–European Consensus Conference on ARDS: Definitions, Mechanisms, Relevant Outcomes, and Clinical Trial Coordination

Bernard GR, Artigas A, Brigham KL, Carlet J, Falke K, Hudson L, Lamy M, Legall JR, Morris A, Spragg R, and the Consensus Committee (LDS Hosp, Salt Lake City, Utah; St Joseph's Hosp, Paris; Sabadell, Spain; et al)
Am J Respir Crit Care Med 149:818–824, 1994   119-95-29-3

Introduction.—The true incidence of acute respiratory distress syndrome (ARDS) is uncertain because of a lack of uniform definitions and the heterogeneity of diseases underlying the condition. The American–European Consensus Committee on ARDS was formed to clarify issues of incidence and outcome and to investigate the pathophysiologic mechanisms of the process. Four subcommittee reports from this group were presented.

Subcommittee I: Definitions.—The original term "acute" was preferred, rather than "adult," because ARDS is not limited to adults. Acute lung injury (ALI) was applied to a wide spectrum of a pathologic process, with ARDS reserved for the most severe end of this spectrum. Both ALI and ARDS have an acute onset, with bilateral infiltrates seen on frontal chest radiograph and pulmonary artery wedge pressure of less than 18 mm Hg when measured or no clinical evidence of left atrial hypertension (table). Oxygenation is the distinguishing criterion for ARDS. A cutoff of less than 200 mm Hg was accepted with a caution that other disease processes be excluded to minimize the chance of including non–ARDS-related illnesses.

Recommended Criteria for ALI and ARDS

	Timing	Oxygenation	Chest Radiograph	Pulmonary Artery Wedge Pressure
ALI criteria	Acute onset	$Pa_{O_2}/F_{I_{O_2}} \leqslant 300$ mm Hg (regardless of PEEP level)	Bilateral infiltrates seen on frontal chest radiograph	$\leqslant 18$ mm Hg when measured or no clinical evidence of left atrial hypertension
ARDS criteria	Acute onset	$Pa_{O_2}/F_{I_{O_2}} \leqslant 200$ mm Hg (regardless of PEEP level)	Bilateral infiltrates seen on frontal chest radiograph	$\leqslant 18$ mm Hg when measured or no clinical evidence of left atrial hypertension

(Courtesy of Bernard GR, Artigas A, Brigham KL, et al: *Am J Respir Crit Care Med* 149:818–824, 1994.)

Subcommittee II: Mechanisms of Acute Lung Injury.—There are many accepted etiologies of ALI, but the pathogenesis consists of 2 pathways: the direct effect of an insult on lung cells and the indirect result of an acute systemic inflammatory response. The inflammatory response includes both cellular and humoral components. Neutrophils, macrophage–monocytes, and lymphocytes are involved in the cellular response. No consensus was reached, however, on the order of events in the pathogenesis of ALI. Many members thought that the pathogenesis might differ for different precipitating causes.

Subcommittee III: Risk Factors, Prevalence, and Relevant Outcomes.—There was a consensus that risk factors should be categorized into direct, such as infection and lung contusion, and indirect, such as sepsis syndrome and severe nonthoracic trauma. It was decided, although not unanimously, that pulmonary infections meeting physiologic criteria should be considered ALI/ARDS. A scoring system for the purpose of prognosis should include only measurements that are readily available, widely acceptable, objective, and easily quantifiable.

Subcommittee IV: Mechanisms That Promote Clinical Study Coordination.—A process of treatment standardization for conducting clinical trials should be continued in cases for which data strongly support certain clinical methods. Accepted therapies include supplemental oxygen, positive endoexpiratory pressure/continuous positive airway pressure; mechanical ventilation, if required to support gas exchange; avoidance of fluid overload; and treatment in the ICU. Stratification of patients in clinical studies by severity and mechanism of disease is desirable. A database of centers capable of performing clinical studies should be maintained, and methods of routine data collection should be established.

▶ This consensus conference was called to address many uncertainties associated with a diagnosis of ARDS. As with many other disease entities that have been recognized before their pathophysiologies were understood, the definition of ARDS has varied considerably. To complicate matters further, ARDS may be precipitated and/or accompanied by any number of underlying conditions, each with a different option for treatment and likelihood of outcome.

The situation for ARDS is much the same as that faced by the related disease entities—sepsis, sepsis syndrome, and multiple-organ dysfunction. The common thread binding these disease entities together is an inflammatory dysfunction. The differences among these conditions lie in which tissues are struck, how the tissues are affected, and with what severity. The need for consensus in this situation is strong; without such agreement, diagnosis, prognosis, and treatment must be considered imprecise. Possibly even more important is the fact that, without a consistent set of definitions for a disease, comparing clinical trials regarding the disease is very difficult.

In trying to find a unifying definition for ARDS, the committee divided the severity spectrum into a most-severe range, to be termed ARDS, and a wide range of less severe disease, to be termed ALI. Both conditions indicate the presence of inflammatory dysfunction and increased vascular permeability. Threshold values for physiologic scores are used to categorize patients into these categories: when the PaO_2/FIO_2 ratio drops to 200 mm Hg or below, and the pulmonary artery wedge pressure is 18 mm Hg or less (or there is no clinical evidence of left atrial hyptension) in an acute-onset and persistent condition that is accompanied by bilateral infiltrates seen on frontal radiographs, the criteria for ARDS have been met. Less severely deficient oxygenation ($PaO_2/FIO_2 \leq 300$ mm Hg) is used to define ALI. It must be determined that deficient oxygenation does not stem from some other disease process, such as heart failure. The committee recognized that these definitions were not perfect and that some individuals would be inappropriately included or excluded from the definition; however, these definitions were considered the best compromise that would result in the most consistent appraisals. Using these new definitions, such basic demographic particulars as the true incidence of ARDS and ALI need to be reevaluated.

The committee embraced an earlier definition, which classified ARDS as being caused by either a direct insult on the lung that ultimately foments the inflammatory response or by a secondary effect in which systemic inflammatory mediators bring about the condition. Manifestations of the inflammatory process are too numerous to list here, but they include accelerated cellular synthesis of specific proteins, altered coagulation and complement systems, and the release of additional inflammatory mediators and cellular killing agents (proteases and oxygen radicals). The net effect of these manifestations is to cause the endothelial damage characterized as the critical defect in ARDS.

A number of risk factors for ARDS were identified by the committee, including aspiration, diffuse pulmonary infection, infection, near-drowning, toxic inhalation, and lung contusion, all of which directly affect the lung. Indirect causes of ARDS include systemic inflammation, such as is seen in sepsis; severe, nonthoracic injury; hypertransfusion therapy; and cardiopulmonary bypass techniques. The use of severity-of-illness scoring systems, such as the Acute Physiology and Chronic Health Evaluation and Simplified Acute Physiology Score series may be useful for assessing patients with ARDS, although more studies are needed to determine the significance of such scores. These scores are also appropriate for stratifying patients in clinical studies.

The importance of standardized definitions cannot be understated when it comes to clinical trials involving patients with ARDS. New definitions mean that current studies can be compared and older results contrasted with newer results. The committee had an extensive list of recommendations for future studies, including the types of data that should be universally collected and the maintenance of the following goals: first, a corrected determination of the incidence of ARDS and ALI; second, the rapid evaluation and dissemination of data regarding clinical interventions; third, the development of a database containing information from large numbers of patients with ARDS; and finally, the use of controlled, prospective protocols.

Despite the fact that ARDS is a very important clinical entity, too little is known about its pathophysiology and treatment. Only through such efforts as this consensus conference can we hope to approach the important questions reasonably and scientifically. Certainly, the efforts of this conference are an important first step in the right direction.—R.C. Bone, M.D.

Cytokine, Complement, and Endotoxin Profiles Associated With the Development of the Adult Respiratory Distress Syndrome After Severe Injury
Donnelly TJ, Meade P, Jagels M, Cryer HG, Law MM, Hugli TE, Shoemaker WC, Abraham E (Univ of California, Los Angeles; King-Drew Med Ctr, Los Angeles; Scripps Research Inst, La Jolla, Calif)
Crit Care Med 22:768–776, 1994   119-95-29–4

Introduction.—Studies suggest that interleukin (IL-6), tumor necrosis factor (TNF-α), IL-1β, endotoxin, and complement fragments are involved in the development of adult respiratory distress syndrome (ARDS) in patients who are traumatically injured. The sequence and pattern of release of these components immediately after injury, however, has not been characterized. Plasma concentrations of these mediators were examined in patients who sustained traumatic injuries.

Methods.—Plasma samples were obtained every 4 hours from 15 patients with an Injury Severity Score of 25 or more. Hemodynamic and oxygen metabolism factors were measured in 7 patients with ARDS (mean age, 31 years) and 8 patients without ARDS (mean age, 27 years), without lung injury. In patients with ARDS, immunologic assays were used to determine TNF-α; IL-6, IL-8, and IL-1β; endotoxin; and complement fragments C3a and C4a.

Results.—Three patients with ARDS and 7 patients without ARDS survived. There was a significant decrease in oxygenation and PaO_2/FIO_2 and a significant increase in shunt fraction, mean pulmonary arterial pressures, and central venous pressure for patients with ARDS (Fig 29–3). Concentrations of IL-8, C3a, and C4a were significantly increased in patients with ARDS 16 hours after injury. No patients had detectable levels of circulating IL-1β, and TNF-α, or endotoxin.

Summary.—None of these mediators showed changes that would indicate the onset of ARDS. Severe oxygenation impairment appeared at 4 hours after injury, long before systemic release of inflammatory mediators. Measurement of inflammatory mediators is not predictive of the development of ARDS in patients with traumatic injury.

▶ An association between severe trauma and ARDS has been described, although the reasons for such an association are not clear. Multiple fracture, prolonged hypotension, and hypertransfusion therapy are forms of trauma that have a particularly high risk (greater than 20%) for the complication of

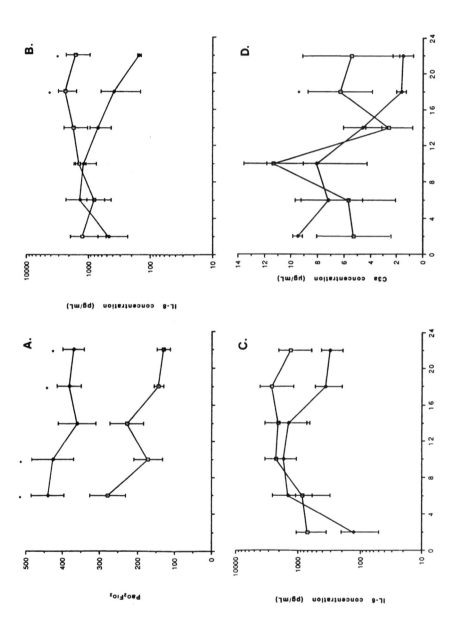

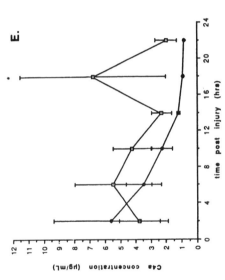

Fig 29-3.—**A,** Pao$_2$:Fio$_2$. **B,** Circulating IL-8 concentrations; **C,** circulating IL-6 concentrations; **D,** circulating complement C3a concentrations; and **E,** circulating C4a concentrations in patients with ARDS (*open squares*) and patients without ARDS (*filled diamonds*) measured at 4-hour intervals from the time of injury. The Pao$_2$/Fio$_2$ was significantly lower in patients with ARDS during the 4- to 8- ($P < .05$), 8- to 12- ($P < .001$), 16- to 20- ($P < .001$), and 20- to 24- ($P < .05$) hour time periods after injury. Interleukin 8 concentrations were significantly higher in patients with ARDS during the 16- to 20- ($P < .05$) and 20- to 24- ($P < .05$) hour time periods. There were no significant differences between the 2 groups in IL-6 concentrations. The C3a concentrations were significantly higher in patients with ARDS during the 16- to 20-hour time period ($P < .05$). The C4a concentrations were significantly higher in patients with ARDS during the 16- to 20-hour time period ($P < .05$). Results are shown as mean ± SEM. (Courtesy of Donnelly TJ, Meade P, Jagels M, et al: *Crit Care Med* 22:768–776, 1994.)

ARDS (1–3). Of the many molecular mediators associated with the induction and progression of ARDS, several, including IL-6 and IL-8, can also be associated with various forms of trauma. However, the release patterns of several other potential mediators of trauma-associated ARDS have not been described. The authors examined the role of these potential mediators more fully in trauma-associated ARDS by sequentially measuring the serum levels of the various mediators over time in patients who had experienced trauma. The mediators examined included TNF-α, IL-1β, IL-6, IL-8, endotoxin, and complement fragments C3a and C4a. Additionally, a number of hemodynamic parameters were examined. It was hoped that the measure of 1 or more of these features would be predictive of which patients would eventually have ARDS.

Unfortunately, the results of this study were negative—none of the mediators examined were capable of predicting the development of ARDS, although the levels of IL-8, C3a, and C4a were increased 16 hours after the injury in only those patients who already had ARDS or serious oxygenation defects. On the other hand, the authors found that some physiologic factors could predict a risk for ARDS. Patients in whom ARDS later developed showed significantly impaired oxygenation within 4 hours of the trauma. The cause for this impairment is unknown: it was not associated with altered levels of the mediators examined in this study and warrants further study. In essence, this finding shows that ARDS is a disease with a spectrum of severities, ranging from acute lung injury and sometimes progressing to ARDS. The more severe the hypoxemia associated with acute lung injury, the higher the incidence of ARDS.

These results generally support earlier findings. In infection-associated ARDS, the serum levels of endotoxin, TNF, and IL-1 are considered important mediators; however, this is not the case for trauma-associated ARDS, and these mediators were not elevated in this study. The possible role for complement fragments in the development of ARDS is supported in this study, because these fragments and IL-8 were increased in patients who already had ARDS.

The search for physical features predictive of ARDS and such associated illnesses as the systemic inflammatory response syndrome and multiple organ dysfunction syndrome has become one of the more frustrating tasks facing clinical researchers. The authors of this study point out what may be an important problem in this quest: The release and action of the involved mediators may be very isolated in a temporal and spatial sense, making detection difficult. The development of more sensitive techniques may be necessary before some of the more subtle effects of these mediators can be observed.—R.C. Bone, M.D.

References

1. Fowler AA, Hamman RF, Good JT, et al: Adult respiratory distress syndrome: Risk with common predispositions. *Ann Intern Med* 98:593–597, 1983.
2. Pepe PE, Potkin, RT, Reus DH, et al: Clinical predictors of the adult respiratory distress syndrome. *Ann Surg* 144:124–130, 1982.

3. Faist E, Baue AE, Dittmer H, et al: Multiple organ failure in polytrauma patients. *J Trauma* 23:775–787, 1983.

Effects of Inhaled Nitric Oxide on Pulmonary Hemodynamics and Gas Exchange in an Ovine Model of ARDS

Rovira I, Chen T-Y, Winkler M, Kawai N, Bloch KD, Zapol WM (Harvard Med School, Boston)
J Appl Physiol 76:345–355, 1994   119-95-29-5

Background.—Inhalation of nitric oxide (NO) in low concentrations leads to pulmonary vasodilation in ventilated regions of the lung. Nitric oxide activates guanylate cyclase, thereby increasing the availability of guanosine 3′,5′-cyclic monophosphate (cGMP). Inhibiting the synthesis of NO promotes hypoxic pulmonary vasoconstriction. The effects of inhaled NO and a systemic inhibitor of NO synthase N^G-nitro-L-arginine

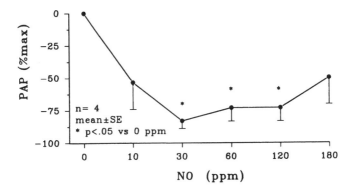

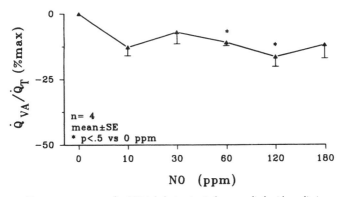

Fig 29–4.—Dose-response curve for NO inhalation in 4 sheep studied with preliminary protocol. **Top,** percent maximal change of PAP vs. NO concentration. **Bottom,** percent maximal change of venous admixture (Q̇va/Q̇T) vs. NO concentration. (Courtesy of Rovira I, Chen T-Y, Winkler M, et al: *J Appl Physiol* 76:345–355, 1994.)

Effects of Bilateral Lung Lavage and 60 ppm NO Inhalation on
Pulmonary and Systemic Hemodynamics and Gas Exchange in
Experimental Group at Baseline $\dot{Q}T$ (Condition A)

	Baseline 1	Lung Lavage	NO Inhalation
HR, beats/min	139±11	163±13*	150±12
SAP, mmHg	117±2	115±3	109±4
PAP, mmHg	17±0.5	20±0.7*	16±0.6*
PCWP, mmHg	8±0.6	9±0.7	9±0.9
CVP, mmHg	8±0.8	9±1.0	9±1
LAP, mmHg	7±0.4	8±0.5	7±0.8
$\dot{Q}T$, $l \cdot min^{-1} \cdot m^{-2}$	2.6±0.3	3.6±0.2*	3.2±0.2
SVR, $mmHg \cdot l^{-1} \cdot min$	39±4	26±2*	26±3
PVR, $mmHg \cdot l^{-1} \cdot min$	3.0±0.3	2.5±0.2*	2.1±0.1*
RVSWI, $g \cdot m \cdot m^{-2} \cdot beat^{-1}$	2.3±0.3	3.3±0.5*	2.4±0.2*
Paw, cmH_2O	20±1.0	28±0.7*	29±0.5
pH_a	7.47±0.01	7.34±0.02*	7.38±0.01*
Pa_{O_2}, Torr	484±19	68±5*	115±12*
Pa_{CO_2}, Torr	33±1	40±1*	34±1*
$P\bar{v}_{O_2}$, Torr	51±2	42±1*	44±1
$\dot{V}O_2$, $ml \cdot min^{-1} \cdot kg^{-1}$	3.2±0.1	3.6±0.2	4.2±0.3
$\dot{D}O_2$, $ml \cdot min^{-1} \cdot m^{-2}$	380±36	431±39	435±34
$\dot{Q}va/\dot{Q}T$, %	10±1	51±3*	34±2*

Abbreviations: $\dot{Q}T$, cardiac output; *HR*, heart rate; *SAP*, systemic arterial pressure; *PAP*, pulmonary arterial pressure; *PCWP*, pulmonary capillary wedge pressure; *CVP*, central venous pressure; *LAP*, left arterial pressure; *SVR*, systemic vascular resistance; *PVR*, pulmonary vascular resistance; *RVSWI*, right ventricular stroke work index; *Paw*, peak inspiratory airway pressure; pH_a, Pa_{O_2}, Pa_{CO_2}, arterial pH, PO_2, and PCO_2, respectively; $P\bar{v}_{O_2}$, mixed venous PO_2; VO_2, O_2 consumption; $\dot{D}O_2$, O_2 delivery; $\dot{Q}va/\dot{Q}T$, venous admixture.
* $P < .05$ vs. previous column.
Values are means ± SE of 9 sheep.
(Courtesy of Rovira I, Chen T-Y, Winkler M, et al: *J Appl Physiol* 76:345–355, 1994.)

methyl ester (L-NAME) on pulmonary hemodynamics and gas exchange were examined in sheep with adult respiratory distress syndrome (ARDS).

Methods.—Anesthetized, mechanically ventilated sheep had acute lung injury produced by bilateral lung lavages with .5% polyoxyethylene-sorbitan mono-oleate. Nitric oxide was inhaled at incremental concentrations of 10 to 180 parts per million (ppm) for 10-minute periods while the pulmonary vascular pressure–flow relationship, gas exchange, and plasma level of cGMP were monitored. Some animals had an IV administration of inhibitor after lavage in a dose of 30 mg/kg.

Results.—Inhaling NO at a level of 60 ppm after lung lavage reduced the pulmonary artery pressure (PAP) and resistance without altering systemic hemodynamics (Fig 29–4, table). The arterial oxygen pressure increased, and venous admixture decreased. There was no indication of a change in the extent of intrapulmonary shunting. The PAP–left atrial pressure (LAP) gradient decreased during inhalation of NO. Infusion of L-NAME led to pulmonary and systemic vasoconstriction and an increased PAP-LAP gradient, and subsequent inhalation of NO was followed by pulmonary vasodilation. The arterial plasma level of cGMP increased 80% after NO inhalation regardless of whether the inhibitor was administered.

Conclusions.—Brief inhalation of NO rapidly lowered the PAP and improved oxygen exchange in an ovine model of ARDS. It is a selective flow-independent pulmonary vasodilator.

▶ This study looks at the use of NO, a newly described vasodilator, in an animal model of ARDS. It lends additional support to the purported usefulness of NO in ARDS and other conditions in which pulmonary perfusion–ventilation mismatching may occur. In a previous, uncontrolled clinical study, Rossaint et al. showed that NO could reduce pulmonary artery pressure and increase arterial oxygenation in patients with ARDS (1). The explanation for this effect was that inhaled NO selectively vasodilated ventilated portions of the lung. In the current study, NO was used in combination with systemically administered L-NAME, an inhibitor of NO synthase that decreases levels of NO. This treatment was expected to enhance the hypoxic vasoconstriction of pulmonary vessels in atelectatic regions of the lung, a response that should bring about a decrease in ventilation–perfusion mismatching. It was hoped that the 2 substances would work synergistically: as the NO synthase decreased circulation in nonventilated regions of the lung, ventilated regions of the lung would receive increased circulation through the effects of inhaled NO. If this process occurs, the effect should be to improve oxygenation dramatically, increase compliance, decrease right-to-left shunting, and relieve pulmonary hypertension.

In general, the hoped-for effects were seen in this study: inhaled NO at 60 ppm improves oxygen exchange and decreases right-circuit pressure, as has previously been shown. However, it also improved the venous admixture ($\dot{Q}va/\dot{Q}T$) through a range of experimentally manipulated cardiac outputs ($\dot{Q}s$). Unfortunately, the $\dot{Q}va/\dot{Q}T$ was not improved by the administration of NO combined with L-NAME. Although pulmonary artery pressure increased in response to L-NAME, oxygen exchange did not improve. This could be explained by the failure of shunted vessels in the pulmonary circuit to express NO synthase. This may not occur in human ARDS, however, and it was believed that this did not rule out the potential usefulness of L-NAME in such illnesses as sepsis, even though the initial animal studies have not been promising.

This study also helped elucidate the mechanisms by which NO acts to improve pulmonary vascular function. Because NO works through a cGMP-mediated mechanism involving cGMP-activated smooth muscle relaxation, the levels of systemic arterial and mixed venous plasma cGMP were measured. The difference between these 2 measures increased in response to administration of NO, indicating that release of cGMP into the pulmonary circuit had increased. However, there was no systemic vasodilation resulting from these increased levels of circulating cGMP.

The only qualifying point to this study was that their animal model does not reflect the vascular injury seen in human ARDS accurately. Damage in the model is restricted largely to the epithelial, rather than the endothelial, layers of the lung, which could decrease the relevance of these results to human ARDS. It is clear that inhaled NO has dramatic effects on the pulmonary circulation. Further studies are needed immediately to define its use in the clinical setting better. This drug continues to hold great potential for treating patients with a variety of lung dysfunctions. See Abstract 119-95-29–6 for more interesting findings on this substance.—R.C. Bone, M.D.

Reference

1. Rossaint R, Falke KJ, Lopez F, et al: Inhaled nitric oxide for the adult respiratory distress syndrome. N Engl J Med 328:399–405, 1993.

Long-Term Inhalation With Evaluated Low Doses of Nitric Oxide for Selective Improvement of Oxygenation in Patients With Adult Respiratory Distress Syndrome

Gerlach H, Pappert D, Lewandowski K, Rossaint R, Falke KJ (Free Univ, Berlin)

Intensive Care Med 19:443–449, 1993   119-95-29–6

Background—Nitric oxide (NO) is equivalent to endothelium-derived relaxing factor in reducing pulmonary vascular resistance. At doses of 5–80 ppm, inhaled NO reduced pulmonary hypertension in sheep, adults, and newborns; by reducing intrapulmonary right-to-left shunt, doses of 18–36 ppm improved arterial oxygenation in patients with severe adult respiratory distress syndrome (ARDS). The lowest effective dose of inhaled NO for patients with ARDS was evaluated.

Methods.—Three patients with severe ARDS were mechanically ventilated to achieve positive end-expiratory pressure of 8–12 cm H_2O. Nitric oxide was delivered through a blender system and Servo 300 ventilator and titrated to achieve 30% improvement of PaO_2/FIO_2. This dose was used for continuous, long-term NO inhalation. Hemodynamic values and blood gas exchange were measured initially and at 3 and 6 days.

Results.—The 30% increase in PaO_2 at FIO_2 1.0 from baseline was achieved with 250 parts per billion (ppb) NO in patient 1, 100 in patient 2, and 50 in patient 3 (Fig 29–5). The lowest effective NO dose for long-term inhalation was 230 ppb NO for patient 1, 100 for patient 2, and 60 for patient 3. During inhalation at the lowest effective dose, arterial-alveolar oxygen ratio increased significantly from baseline, associated with a reduction of venous admixture (Fig 29–6). Oxygenation appeared to be enhanced throughout the NO inhalation treatment, indicated by increased differences of arterial–alveolar oxygen ratio and venous admixture between NO and control periods. Mean systemic arterial pressure, mean pulmonary artery pressure, cardiac output, and heart rate did not

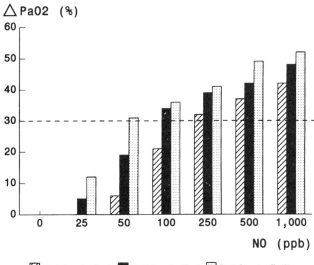

△ Pao2 (%)

NO (ppb)

⊠ Patient # 1 ■ Patient # 2 ☐ Patient # 3

Fig 29–5.—Effect of inhaled NO (x-axis: NO dose in ppb according to the blender position of the ventilator after the initial calibration) on arterial oxygenation (y-axis: relative increase of Pao₂, measured at Fio₂ = 1.0, expressed as percent increase compared with the value at 0 ppb NO) during the initial NO dose evaluation in 3 patients with severe ARDS. The *horizontal line* marks the arbitrary limit of 30% increase. As demonstrated, the 3 patients present an increase of Pao₂/Fio₂ of more than 30% at blender positions of 50 (patient #3), 100 (patient #2), and 250 ppb NO (patient #1), corresponding to measured inspiratory NO concentrations of 60, 100, and 230 ppb, respectively, which were defined as lowest effective NO dose for the following long-term inhalation therapy. (Courtesy of Gerlach H, Pappert D, Lewandowski K, et al: *Intensive Care Med* 19:443-449, 1993.)

change significantly, despite a decrease in mean pulmonary artery pressure when baseline data exceeded 45 mm Hg (Fig 29-7). Blood gas exchange calculation revealed a significant increase in oxygen delivery but increased consumption only when control data were low.

Conclusion.—Inhalation of NO improves arterial oxygenation in patients with ARDS at nontoxic ppb concentrations. Individual dose-response studies should be performed before implementation.

▶ Nitric oxide has been touted as a possible miracle treatment for ARDS through its ability to improve ventilation–perfusion mismatches when inhaled. This benefit is believed to result from its highly localized vasodilating effect. When inhaled, this gas acts selectively on the capillaries of ventilated alveoli to improve ventilation–perfusion matching and blood oxygen levels. So far, the facts have borne out this theory: NO has been shown to reduce pulmonary hypertension in animal models (1) and human patients (2, 3). Additionally, the arterial oxygenation of patients with ARDS improved with the inhalation of 18–36 ppm NO (4). However, most other studies of NO have used doses in the range of 20–80 ppm. In a previous study, Rossaint et al. noted that there was no difference between the effects of the 18 and 36 ppm treatments, which would be typical of the maximal response region on the

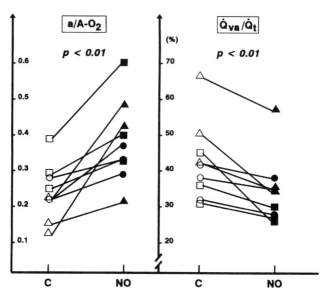

Fig 29–6.—Arterial/alveolar-oxygen ratio (a/A-0₂, *left side*) and venous admixture ($\dot{Q}_{va}/\dot{Q}_t$, *right side*) in the 3 patients with ARDS during inhalation of NO (*closed symbols*) in a dose of 230 (patient 1, *circle*), 100 (patient 2, *square*), and 60 ppb (patient 3, *triangle*), measured in the inspiratory limb of the breathing circuit, near to the patient, compared with baseline data (control = C, *open symbol*) during noninhalation periods. Each point represents 1 determination, 3 determinations per patient. (Courtesy of Gerlach H, Pappert D, Lewandowski K, et al: *Intensive Care Med* 19:443-449, 1993.)

dose-response curve (4). These authors have now gone on to perform this study of the minimum effective dose of NO in patients with ARDS.

The surprising finding of these authors is that significant improvements in PaO_2 occur when NO concentrations of 60–230 ppb are respirated, a range that covered a large portion of the dose-response curve. When one realizes that room air contains 2–130 ppb NO, this finding becomes downright perplexing: If most of the dose-response curve takes place in the ambient atmosphere, how can this agent be an effective treatment? The authors propose the following scenario: measurements of the compressed gases used in ventilators shows only small amounts of NO—none in compressed oxygen supplies and only 4 ppb in compressed air supplies. Thus, the shocking conclusion drawn is that mechanical ventilation may actually be depriving patients of a vital environmental constituent, NO. The authors point out that this could revise our understanding of the pathophysiology of ARDS.

They conclude that increased pulmonary artery pressure in ARDS is, at least in part, caused by active restriction of the pulmonary vasculature rather than an irreversible circulatory restriction. This was shown when the decrease in pulmonary artery pressure caused by NO was not associated with a decrease in cardiac output. The authors believe that in patients respiring adequate NO, levels of NO synthetase may be decreased by feed-back inhibition. In that case, a sudden decrease in respirated levels of NO, as may happen

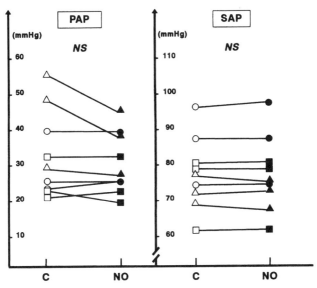

Fig 29–7.—*Abbreviations:* PAP, pulmonary artery pressure; SAP, systemic artery pressure; NS, not significant. Mean PAP (*left side*) and mean SAP (*right side*) during NO-inhalation and control periods. (Courtesy of Gerlach H, Pappert D, Lewandowski K, et al: *Intensive Care Med* 19:443–449, 1993.)

during intubation, could cause sudden vasoconstriction in ventilated regions of the lung, with the commensurate decrease in PaO₂.

These are important findings that have immediate clinical impact. Just as urgently, they call for further study of dose-related aspects of NO treatment. We need to know the optimal levels of NO for increasing PaO₂ or for decreasing pulmonary artery pressure. Certainly, the use of levels of NO in the ppb range could be regarded as nontoxic; however, even patients receiving such low levels should be weaned rather than suddenly withdrawn from this environmental inhibitor of pulmonary vasoconstriction.

At the 1994 American Thoracic Society Meeting, a symposium on NO made some important points yet to be extensively reviewed in the literature:

- The beneficial effects of NO were reviewed; however, it may be a "Jekyll and Hyde" compound. In high levels, it can be a powerful pro-oxidant, causing lipid peroxidation and facilitating free-radical injury by other mechanisms. For this reason, the recommended treatment doses are less than 20 ppm.

- Nitric oxide is rapidly becoming the treatment of choice in persistent pulmonary hypertension in the newborn. In fact, it is rapidly replacing extracorporeal membrane oxygenation in most infants with this condition.

- For ARDS, the findings, although impressive, are equivocal. Nitric oxide does decrease pulmonary artery pressure and improve gas exchange. However, because the underlying cause of ARDS may be untreatable, the benefits in some patients may last only as long as NO is given. It is important not to forget that other interventions are required to reverse the underlying disorder.

- In addition to its vasodilatory action, NO also acts as a mild bronchodilator, furthering its potential to act beneficially in ARDS.

So, the first evidence is in. Nitric oxide may not be the completely benevolent substance we first imagined it to be. However, it is still in its infancy as a treatment. Many more studies of its actions will be needed before its true potential for good and bad will be known.—R.C. Bone, M.D.

References

1. Frostel C, Fratacci MD, Wain JC, Jones R, Zapol WM: Inhaled nitric oxide: A selective pulmonary vasodilator reversing hypoxic pulmonary vasoconstriction. *Circulation* 83:2038–2047, 1991.
2. Zepke-Zaba J, Higenbottam TW, Dinh-Xuan AT, Stone D, Wallwork J: Inhaled nitric oxide as a cause of selective pulmonary vasodilation in pulmonary hypertension. *Lancet* 338:1173–1174, 1991.
3. Roberts JD Jr, Polaner DM, Lang P, Zapol WM: Inhaled nitric oxide in persistent pulmonary hypertension of the newborn. *Lancet* 340:818–819, 1992.
4. Rossaint R, Falke KJ, Lopez F, Slama K, Pison U, Zapol WM: Inhaled nitric oxide for the adult respiratory distress syndrome. *N Engl J Med* 328:399–405, 1993.

Corticosteroid Rescue Treatment of Progressive Fibroproliferation in Late ARDS: Patterns of Response and Predictors of Outcome
Meduri GU, Chinn AJ, Leeper KV, Wunderink RG, Tolley E, Winer-Muram HT, Khare V, Eltorky M (Univ of Tennessee, Memphis)
Chest 105:1516–1527, 1994   119-95-29–7

Introduction.—Pulmonary fibroproliferation is fatal in 15% to 40% of patients with late-onset ARDS. Use of IV corticosteroids in such patients led to significant improvement in lung injury score. How IV corticosteroid treatment acts and which factors determine the response to and result of treatment for late-onset ARDS were investigated.

Methods.—Twenty-five patients with ARDS and progressive respiratory failure had diagnostic bronchoscopic evaluations. Thirteen underwent open lung biopsy. Corticosteroid treatment was begun an average of 15 days after mechanical ventilation became necessary. Respiratory and cardiovascular parameters, multiple organ failure, systemic inflammatory response syndrome, and type of infection were monitored.

Results.—Nineteen of 25 patients survived. Within 7 days, significant increases were seen in PaO_2/FIO_2. Significant decreases were observed in positive end-expiratory pressure (PEEP), lung injury score and minute ventilation (V_E) (table). Patients were classified on the basis of their responses to treatment as rapid, delayed, or nonresponders. The 15 rapid responders improved by day 7, 6 delayed responders improved by day 14, and 4 nonresponders did not improve by day 14 (Fig 29-8). The inci-

Physiologic Findings Before and After Treatment With Corticosteroids

Day of ARDS and Treatment	$PaO_2:FIo_2$	PEEP, cm H_2O	Lung Injury Score	Minute Ventilation
1	205±15	6.1±.8	2.3±.1	14.2±.8
7	151±14	11.6±.7	2.9±.1	14.1±.9
−5	158±14	9.6±.8	2.8±.1	14.8±.8
−3	159±14	10.1±.7	2.9±.1	15.1±.8
0	162±14	11.2±.7	3.0±.1	16.1±.8
+3	200±14	9.8±.7	2.6±0.1 (p=0.04)	14.2±.7
+5	212±14 (p=0.01)	8.9±0.7 (p=0.02)	2.3±0.1 (p=0.001)	13.2±0.7 (p=0.01)
+7	234±14 (p=0.0004)	6.8±0.7 (p=0.001)	2.1±0.1 (p=0.001)	13.6±0.8 (p=0.01)
+10	246±16 (p=0.0001)	6.4±0.8 (p=0.001)	1.9±0.1 (p=0.001)	13.8±0.8 (p=0.01)
+14	258±17 (p=0.0001)	4.4±0.9 (p=0.001)	1.7±0.1 (p=0.001)	13.3±0.1 (p=0.01)

Note: Day of initiation of corticosteroid treatment is day 0. Statistical comparison is made with day 0. (Courtesy of Meduri GU, Chinn AJ, Leeper KV, et al: *Chest* 105:1516–1527, 1994.)

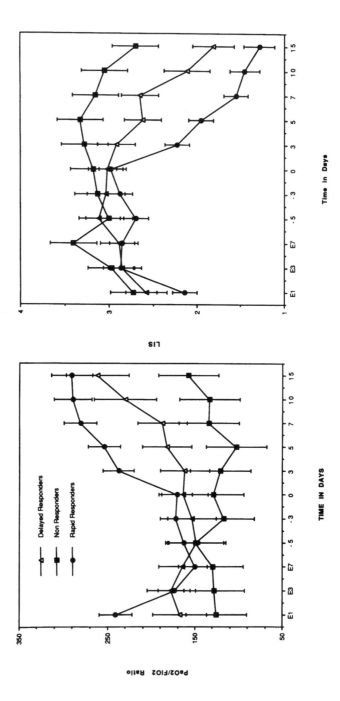

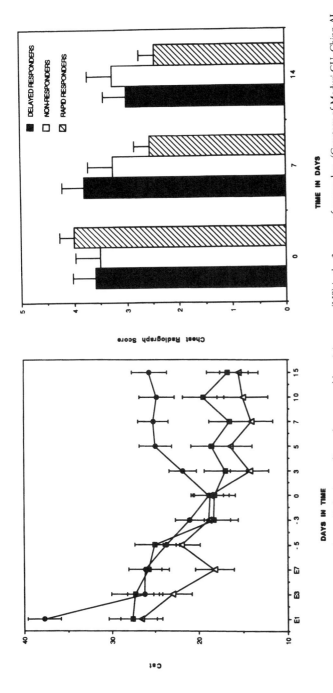

Fig 29–8.—Pao$_2$/Fio$_2$, static compliance (Cst), chest radiograph score, and lung injury score (LIS) in the 3 groups of responders. (Courtesy of Meduri GU, Chinn AJ, Leeper KV, et al: *Chest* 105:1516–1527, 1994.)

dence of pneumonia was related to responder type. Histologic differences between survivors and nonsurvivors were significant and included alveolar structure, myxoid type alveolar and interstitial fibrosis, intraluminal bronchiolar fibrosis, and absence of arteriolar subintimal fibroproliferation. Other indicators that differed significantly between survivors and nonsurvivors were presence of liver failure and pattern of physiologic response.

Conclusion.—Early corticosteroid treatment of pulmonary fibroproliferation can be effective. Outcome depends on type of response.

▶ In ARDS, lung endothelial and epithelial cells respond to injury with the production of fibrillar proteins in a process probably mediated by cytokines and other molecular messengers. Although this is generally thought of as a repair process, the response may become excessive or maladaptive, resulting in fibrosis. This production of extracellular fibers is a leading cause of death in late ARDS. Because this fiber production is part of an inflammatory process, anti-inflammatory drugs may be used to treat patients with such fibroproliferation. The authors of this study have already used IV corticosteroids in patients with biopsy-proven pulmonary fibroproliferation with apparent success; lung injury scores were improved, and 7 of 8 patients survived their ICU stay (1). Other authors have reported similar results (2–4). To examine the use of corticosteroids in fibroproliferative disease further, the authors of this study used corticosteroids to treat 25 patients who had ARDS.

The production of fibers during ARDS can be broken down into 2 stages: the proliferative stage, characterized by the production of easily degraded type III collagen, followed by the fibrotic phase, associated with the production and deposition of thick type I collagen fibers. Patients who die of ARDS-associated fibrosis generally have a twofold increase in collagen content of the lung within 2 weeks of the development of ARDS. By modulating the activity of fibroblasts and macrophages, corticosteroids should arrest this activity, thus promoting the resorption of fibers during the normal metabolic turnover of extracellular matrix components. This concept has been supported by work with animal models of ARDS, in which the administration of corticosteroids late in ARDS protects against excessive collagen deposition (5).

The findings of this study support the use of corticosteroids in patients who survive the early phase of ARDS. The patients in this study could be categorized as those that have a rapid response (15), a delayed response (6), or no response (4) to the anti-inflammatory treatment. Of the patients who responded to the methylprednisolone treatment 2–3 mg/kg/day, 86% survived, whereas only 25% of the nonresponders survived. All patients in this study were severely ill and had features typical of nonsurvivors, including a neutrophilic bronchoalveolar lavage fluid and inability to improve gas exchange and static compliance. Responders quickly evidenced reduced inflammation with reduced neutrophilia and fever.

Patients whose fibroproliferation had advanced to form a dense acellular fibrosis involving type I collagen were not likely to improve with this treatment; however, this was a histologic criterion rather than a clinical one, making it difficult to define in the patient population. On the other hand, intervention earlier in the fibroproliferative stage yielded better results with better physiologic improvements and reduced infectious complications. In this study, the optimal treatment time coincided with approximately the seventh day of mechanical ventilation.

Side effects are frequently associated with corticosteroid treatments, and this study provided no exception: pneumonia developed in 11 patients, and several other infectious complications were noted. These findings are exciting and should stimulate a large-scale study of corticosteroid treatment for ARDS. That study should be a double-blind, placebo-controlled trial to avoid the possibility of selection bias that might blemish this study. We need to find out whether such treatment is warranted and what the risk–benefit ratio is. As an additional critique, any study that separates patients after treatment into responders and nonresponders has a basic defect. The data, when compiled for all patients, might *not* be impressive or significant and pose considerable risk. I repeat again, these data may be exciting, but a controlled study should be done to validate or refute these findings.—R.C. Bone, M.D.

References

1. Meduri GU, Belenchia JM, Estes RJ, et al: Fibroproliferative phase of ARDS: Clinical findings and effects of corticosteroids. *Chest* 100:943–952, 1991.
2. Ashbaugh DG, Maier RF: Idiopathic pulmonary fibrosis in adult respiratory distress syndrome. *Arch Surg* 20:530–535, 1985.
3. Hooper RG, Kearl RA: Established ARDS treated with a sustained course of adrenocortical steroids. *Chest* 97:138–143, 1990.
4. Hooper RG, Kearl RA: Treatment of established ARDS—steroids, antibiotics, and antifungal therapy. *Chest* 100:S137, 1991.
5. Jones RL, King EG: The effects of methylprednisolone on oxygenation in experimental hypoxemic respiratory failure. *J Trauma* 15:297–303, 1975.

Acute Effects of a Single Dose of Porcine Surfactant on Patients With the Adult Respiratory Distress Syndrome

Spragg RG, Gilliard N, Richman P, Smith RM, Hite RD, Pappert D, Robertson B, Curstedt T, Strayer D (Univ of California, San Diego; Centre Hospitalier Universitaire Vaudois, Lausanne, Switzerland; Emek Hosp, Afula, Israel; et al)
Chest 105:195–202, 1994   119-95-29-8

Objective.—Six patients with adult respiratory distress syndrome (ARDS) were treated with a single dose of porcine surfactant to restore surfactant activity to the alveolar lining fluid. Although surfactant recovered from patients just before the onset of ARDS appears to have normal phospholipid composition, surfactant dysfunction may develop in the acute stage of the disorder.

Methods.—Adult respiratory distress syndrome had been diagnosed in all patients within the 48 hours preceding study entry. Patients were randomized in a crossover design to either surfactant (4 g in 50 mL) or placebo. One fifth the treatment dose was administered through a flexible fiberoptic bronchoscope to a lower lobe after bronchoalveolar lavage (BAL). The remainder was given 15 minutes later to the remaining lobes. The alternative treatment was given after BAL was repeated 3.5–4 hours later. A third BAL was performed after another 3 hours, and a final BAL 24–30 hours after the initial treatment.

Results.—The administration of exogenous surfactant was well tolerated in these patients and caused a modest, generally transient improvement in gas exchange. No patient showed significant changes in chest radiograph or lung compliance. Analyses of BAL fluids showed no alteration in the inflammatory process resulting from the surfactant. One patient with prolonged improvement in gas exchange also provided evidence through BAL analysis that surfactant inhibitor function was overcome for 24 hours. Phospholipid concentrations in BAL were elevated 3 hours after surfactant administration relative to pretreatment levels and fell by 24 hours.

Conclusion.—There is a fairly clear relationship between the deficiency of surfactant in the bronchial wash of infants with respiratory distress syndrome. It is not yet known, however, whether the lungs of patients with ARDS have a quantitative deficiency of surfactant. A small dose of surfactant, however, did improve gas exchange in these patients, and more significant benefits may be provided with repeated dosing or alternative methods of delivery.

▶ Although we don't know what causes abnormalities to occur in the surfactant of patients with ARDS, it seems rational that replacing abnormal surfactant with intact surfactant would reestablish surfactant activity to the alveolar lining fluid—at least for awhile. These authors administered a total dose of 4 g of surfactant in 50 mL of vehicle, or approximately 50–60 mg/kg of body weight. This is a relatively small dose and resulted in only transient improvement in gas exchange. The average change in PaO_2 was 49 mm Hg, which occurred from 5 minutes to 2 hours after treatment. Phospholipid concentrations in BAL were elevated 3 hours after surfactant was given but fell to preadministration levels by 24 hours. Phospholipids account for 90% of pulmonary surfactant, with the other 10% comprised of apoproteins. Other studies, including one of neonates, found that 100 mg of phospholipid per kg in a bolus dose administered through an endotracheal tube was needed to improve pulmonary function (1). Another study of neonatal respiratory distress syndrome found that an initial dose of 200 mg/kg divided in 2 portions and instilled into each main bronchus usually resulted in a sustained therapeutic response, whereas the administration of 100 mg/kg usually resulted in a pattern of relapse (2). The aerosol administration of much smaller quantities of surfactant (2–5 mg of phospholipid per kg) to surfactant-deficient sheep (3) and to rabbits with lung injury (4) produced beneficial effects, suggesting that this method of drug delivery may be useful. Clearly, this issue deserves further study.—R.C. Bone, M.D.

References

1. Jobe A, Ikegami M: Surfactant for the treatment of respiratory distress syndrome. *Am Rev Respir Dis* 136:1256–1275, 1987.
2. Speer C, Robertson B, Curstedt T, et al: Randomized European multicenter trial of surfactant replacement therapy for severe neonatal respiratory distress syndrome: Single versus multiple doses of Curosurf. *Pediatrics* 89:13–20, 1992.
3. Lewis J, Tabor B, Ikegami M, Jobe A: Physiological response to aerosolized surfactant in lung-lavaged sheep. Abstract. *Am Rev Respir Dis* 143:A769, 1991.
4. Lewis J, Ikegami M, Higuchi R, Jobe A, Absolom D: Nebulized vs. instilled exogenous surfactant in an adult lung injury model. *J Appl Physiol* 71:1270–1276, 1991.

30 Transplantation

Introduction

The new era of lung transplantation has been with us for approximately 10 years now, and its benefits are multiple. Antirejection drugs may largely be responsible for these recent successes, although various forms of rejection and infection continue as the most important problems with the procedure. Single-lung transplants are indicated for patients with restrictive, obstructive, or pulmonary vascular problems, whereas the double-lung procedure is reserved for those with infective pulmonary disease. The sequential–double-lung procedure is a recent advance that alleviates the need for cardiopulmonary bypass during surgery and reduces the number of complications. The 1-year survival rate for single-lung transplant has approached 90% in some series, and 80% survival has been recorded for the double-lung procedure. This certainly is an optimistic account; however, obtaining donor lungs continues to be an important problem that will grow as success with the procedures improves and transplant is used as therapy for a broader range of conditions.

This year's YEAR BOOK OF MEDICINE has 1 selection for the chapter on transplantation. This is an important, large-scale study of the long-term results obtained from transplants over the past 10 years. The authors show that survival has grown considerably since then and estimate that current, 5-year survival will be 50% to 60%. I predict that survival will continue to grow as antirejection and anti-infective therapies improve.

Roger C. Bone, M.D.

Results of Single and Bilateral Lung Transplantation in 131 Consecutive Recipients
Cooper JD, Patterson GA, Trulock EP, and the Washington University Lung Transplant Group (Washington Univ, St Louis, Mo)
J Thorac Cardiovasc Surg 107:460–471, 1994   119-95-30–1

Introduction.—The techniques involved in lung transplantation have developed quickly; success rates now approach those achieved with other organ transplants. Survival rates and the predictors of long-term outcome were explored.

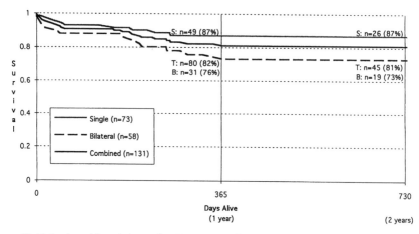

Fig 30–1.—Actuarial survival curve for 131 recipients of single or bilateral lung transplant. (Courtesy of Cooper JD, Patterson GA, Trulock EP, and the Washington University Lung Transplant Group: *J Thorac Cardiovasc Surg* 107:460–471, 1994.)

Methods.—From July 1988 to July 1992, 134 single or bilateral lung transplantations were performed in 131 patients at Barnes Hospital, St. Louis, Mo. The effect of several variables on long-term outcome was assessed.

Results.—The hospital survival rate was 92%, and the overall survival rate is 81.6% to date, with a median follow-up of 19 months. Overall, the 1-year and 2-year actuarial survival rates were 82% and 81%, respec-

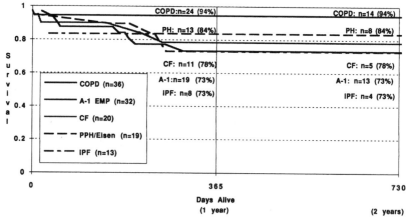

Fig 30–2.—Actuarial survival curve for major diagnostic groups receiving single or bilateral lung transplants between July 1, 1988 and July 31, 1992. *Abbreviations:* COPD, chronic obstructive pulmonary disease; *A-1 EMP*, α_1-antitrypsin emphysema; *CF*, cystic fibrosis; *PPH*, primary pulmonary hypertension; *IPF*, idiopathic pulmonary fibrosis; *PH*, pulmonary hypertension; *Eisen*, Eisenmenger's syndrome. (Courtesy of Cooper JD, Patterson GA, Trulock EP, and the Washington University Lung Transplant Group: *J Thorac Cardiovasc Surg* 107:460–471, 1994.)

tively. Survival was higher among patients receiving single-lung transplants, mainly because patients who underwent bilateral transplantation had a higher hospital mortality rate (Fig 30–1). Chronic rejection was the most frequent cause of death. Survival also varied by diagnostic findings, with patients who had α_1-antitrypsin emphysema having the lowest mortality rate and those who had idiopathic pulmonary fibrosis having the highest mortality rate (Fig 30–2). Some functional deterioration was experienced by 27% of patients, with subsequent improvement in 29% of these patients. Long-term lung function was not significantly correlated with early rejection episodes, type of transplantation, diagnostic findings, or cytomegalovirus antibody status matching. The hemodynamic improvements remained stable.

Discussion.—Approximately 75% of the patients had no or only slight lung function impairment after transplantation. The greatest threats to long-term survival appear to be the poor availability of donor organs and chronic rejection. A longer period of follow-up is required to confirm the validity of these findings.

▶ The technique of lung transplant is being used with increasing frequency—fully 66% of the procedures reported to the St. Louis International Lung Transplant Registry have taken place in the past 2 years. Yet, over the past 10 years, numerous changes have taken place in the way this procedure is performed. This has resulted in a knowledge gap: the long-term effects of the current standards need solid retrospective scrutiny to ensure their efficacy and safety. This study attempts to do that by examining patients who recently underwent lung transplant and have had at least 5 months of follow-up. This is particularly important because of the poor outcome logged for patients who received transplants before approximately 1983.

The results of this study are generally quite optimistic: The authors predict that current 5-year survival will be between 50% and 60%. This is a dramatic improvement from the pre-1983 era, when the 5-year survival in pulmonary transplant was nil. On their way to arriving at this new figure, the authors make a number of interesting observations.

Probably the most important tool to be used in patients who undergo transplant is immunosuppression. Advances in that field have provided physicians with numerous immunosuppressive drugs, along with the hope that new and better drugs will be developed. The development of bronchiolitis obliterans, which can occur at any time after transplant, is an ominous event and is probably related to chronic rejection. At present, approximately 25% of patients who receive pulmonary transplants subsequently have bronchiolitis obliterans. Fortunately, a number of these patients respond to increased immunosuppressive treatment. Nonetheless, bronchiolitis obliterans may currently be the most important obstacle to success in lung transplant, with most morbidities and mortalities being associated with the process.

The presence of infections in pulmonary grafts may enhance the rejection process. Prophylaxis against infection is always improving, and there is cause to hope that this problem will diminish. The presence of cytomegalovirus has been shown to predispose patients to bronchiolitis obliterans and, in a portion of this study, it was found that matching cytomegalovirus-negative patients with donors reduced the incidence of this infection. Curiously, however, this appears to have no effect on the subsequent development of bronchiolitis obliterans. Additionally, the number of early rejections and the type of transplant (single or bilateral) appear to have no significant effect on graft dysfunction or the development of bronchiolitis obliterans.

The waiting period for donor organs is becoming longer, although the increased use of single-lung transplants should help to reduce that constraint. This is particularly critical for patients with pulmonary hypertension. This group currently has a high mortality rate during the waiting period, and that rate is expected to increase. Currently, pulmonary hypertension is not cause for special consideration in the allocation of lungs, a strategy that may require modification.

The best bet for improving the success of pulmonary transplant probably lies in improved methods of inhibiting the rejection process. By improving the tolerance of the immune system to grafted tissue, it may someday be possible to perform transplant routinely between unmatched donors and recipients. This would have the additional benefit of greatly increasing the number of available donor lungs.—R.C. Bone, M.D.

PART THREE

HEMATOLOGY AND ONCOLOGY

MARTIN J. CLINE, M.D.

Introduction

Basic molecular biology continues to make enormous contributions to our understanding of the mechanisms of human diseases, and, as observed in the 1994 YEAR BOOK OF MEDICINE, this new biology is sometimes translated to the clinic in a remarkably short period. In this YEAR BOOK, we note that the genetic mechanisms of paroxysmal nocturnal hemoglobinuria have been elucidated; that 1, and perhaps 2, of the genes for familial forms of breast cancer have been identified; and that there is a new method for detection of the gene abnormality in familial adenomatous polyposis. In 1994, a new clotting abnormality resulting in a hypercoagulable state also was described. What follows is a brief summary of these important observations.

Paroxysmal nocturnal hemoglobinuria is a disorder with an acquired defect in the red cell membrane that increases the sensitivity of the cell to complement-mediated lysis. The cause, identified in 1994, is an abnormality of a gene for a protein that serves as an "anchor" that attaches certain proteins to the red cell membrane. An abnormality in the anchor protein results in the accumulation of complement on the surface of the red blood cell and cell lyses.

Two genes, the BRCA1 gene, on the long arm of chromosome 17, and the gene BRCA2 on the long arm of chromosome 13, have been identified as being associated with familial breast cancer. It is estimated that the lifetime risk for breast cancer in American women is between 1 in 8 and 1 in 10, and that between 5% and 10% of breast cancers are associated with an inherited susceptibility. The estimated incidence of germline mutations is about 1 in 200 women for the BRCA1 gene and about the same for the BRCA2 gene. These are, therefore, very important observations.

There are 3 types of colorectal cancer. The first type is associated with familial adenomatous polyposis, which accounts for about 1% of the cases of colon cancer in the Western world; second, the "sporadic" type, which accounts for the bulk of the cases of colon cancer; and finally, hereditary nonpolyposis form of colorectal cancer, which accounts for 4% to 13% of cases in the West. A gene for type 1 and multiple genes for type 3 colon cancer have now been identified, and a screening test for type 1 is just about in place.

A newly defined genetic hypercoagulable syndrome leading to thrombosis at a young age is hereditary resistance to activated protein C. It is caused by a mutation in the gene for factor V. This abnormality may be 10 times more common in thrombosis-prone young individuals than any other known deficiency of anticoagulant proteins.

In addition to these topics in the 1995 YEAR BOOK OF MEDICINE, I have emphasized novel attempts at treating chronic lymphocytic leukemia, multiple myeloma, breast cancer, and the use of Taxol in several different tumor types. The efficacy of screening for breast cancer is also analyzed in an important article.

Martin J. Cline, M.D.

31 Red Cells, White Cells, and Platelets

Introduction

The chosen emphasis in this year's chapter devoted to classical hematology is aplastic anemia and heparin-induced thrombocytopenia, but the really important article is on protein C. The article on resistance to activated protein C (Abstract 119-95-31–11) has been called "the coagulation discovery of the decade."

Martin J. Cline, M.D.

Malignant Tumors Occurring After Treatment of Aplastic Anemia
Socié G, for the European Bone Marrow Transplantation–Severe Aplastic Anaemia Working Party (Hôpital Saint Louis, Paris)
N Engl J Med 329:1152–1157, 1993   119-95-31–1

Background.—The proportion of long-term survivors of aplastic anemia is expected to increase, making treatment complications an important issue. Research suggests that long-term survivors of aplastic anemia treated with immunosuppressive therapy are at risk for hematologic cancers. The incidence of solid cancers after bone marrow transplantation for aplastic anemia also appears to be increased. These complications were explored further in a large cohort.

Methods.—Eight hundred sixty patients treated by immunosuppression and 748 treated with bone marrow transplantation were included in the study (table). The cancer risk was analyzed overall and by treatment and compared with the risk in the general population.

Findings.—The 42 malignant conditions among patients given immunosuppressive therapy included 19 cases of myelodysplastic syndrome, 15 of acute leukemia, 1 of non-Hodgkin's lymphoma, and 7 solid tumors. Among the patients receiving bone marrow transplantation, the 9 cases of malignant disease included 2 cases of acute leukemia and 7 solid tumors. The overall risk was 5.5 compared with the general population. The immunosuppression and transplantation groups had cancer risks of 5.15 and 6.67, respectively. The 10-year cumulative incidence rates were 18.8% and 3.1% after immunosuppression and transplantation, respectively. Risk factors for myelodysplastic syndrome or acute leukemia after

Type of Initial Treatment According to Treatment Group

VARIABLE	IMMUNO-SUPPRESSIVE THERAPY (N = 860)	BONE MARROW TRANSPLAN-TATION (N = 748)
	no. of patients (%)	
Previous therapy*	413 (48)	476 (64)
First-line therapy		
Antithymocyte globulin + methyl-prednisolone†	437 (51)	—
Antithymocyte globulin + methyl-prednisolone + androgens	273 (32)	—
High-dose methylprednisolone	79 (9)	—
Other	69 (8)‡	—
Conditioning regimen before BMT§		
Cyclophosphamide ‖	—	406 (54)
Cyclophosphamide + total-body irradiation	—	62 (8)
Cyclophosphamide + limited-field irradiation ¶	—	260 (35)
None or other	—	20 (3)

* Previous therapy consisted mainly of androgens before immunosuppressive therapy and of antithymocyte globulin, androgens, or both before bone marrow transplantation.
† With or without androgens.
‡ Including 25 patients who received cyclosporine as first-line immunosuppressive therapy.
§ BMT denotes bone marrow transplantation.
‖ With or without other drugs.
¶ Total lymphoid irradiation or thoracoabdominal irradiation.
(Courtesy of Socié G, for the European Bone Marrow Transplantation-Severe Aplastic, Anaemia Working Party: N Engl J Med 329:1152-1157, 1993.)

immunosuppression were the addition of androgens to the immunosuppressive regimen, older age, treatment in 1982 or later, splenectomy, and treatment with multiple courses of immunosuppression. The risk factors for solid tumors after marrow transplantation were age and the use of pretransplantation radiation. In addition, solid tumors occurred only in male patients.

Conclusion.—Survivors of aplastic anemia have an increased risk of malignant diseases. In this series, myelodysplastic syndrome and acute leukemia tended to follow immunosuppression. The incidences of solid tumors were similar in the immunosuppression and bone marrow transplantation groups.

▶ Patients with aplastic anemia have reticulocytopenia and pancytopenia in the peripheral blood as well as bone marrow that is empty of hematopoietic cells or is severely hypocellular. The clinical manifestations are those of anemia, increased susceptibility to infection as a result of granulocytopenia, and bleeding from thrombocytopenia. Idiopathic aplastic anemia with an empty marrow, severe granulocytopenia, and thrombocytopenia have a poor prognosis, and unless there is a response to treatment, most patients die within 18 months of the diagnosis.

In severe aplastic anemia, the treatment options are immunosuppressives, such as antithymocyte globulin, or bone marrow transplantation, which have about a 50% and a 70% response rate, respectively. As this article indicates, a late complication of the disease and its treatment is the development of malignancy in 3% to 18% of patients. No doubt some of the responsibility for cancer development lies with the therapy, as both immunosuppression and genetic damage by cytotoxic drugs and irradiation increase the frequency of cancer development.—M.J. Cline, M.D.

Aplastic Anemia and Pesticides: An Etiologic Association?
Fleming LE, Timmeny W (Univ of Miami, Fla)
J Occup Med 35:1106–1116, 1993   119-95-31–2

Background.—Relatively little is known about the causes of and risk factors for aplastic anemia. However, during the past 3 decades, case reports have suggested an etiologic association between this disease and pesticide exposure. The medical literature pointing to this association was reviewed, and the types of pesticides implicated, the exposure scenario, and the latency period were examined.

Method.—The medical literature of the past 30 years was searched for articles relating to aplastic anemia and pesticide exposure, as well as for any studies relevant to the etiologic association of pesticides with aplas-

---

Aplastic Anemia: Incidence and Mortality Rates

Location	Incidence	Citation
United States	2–5/1,000,000	Custer, 1946; Smick, 1964; Wallerstein, 1969
Israel	7.8/1,000,000	Modan, 1975
China	18.7–21/1,000,000	Wang, 1981
Sweden	13.2–24.6/1,000,000	Bottiger, 1981
Baltimore	6.2/1,000,000	Szklo, 1985
Europe/Israel	20.5/1,000,000	IAAAS, 1987
France	1.5/1,000,000	Mary, 1990
Age Adjusted Mortality		
California	4–6/1,000,000	
United States	4.0–5.4/1,000,000	
Canada	3.5–5.3/1,000,000	Smick, 1964
Japan	9/1,000,000	
United States	4.8/1,000,000	
Europe	3/1,000,000	Aoki, 1978

(Courtesy of Fleming LE, Timmeny W: *J Occup Med* 35:1106–1116, 1993.)

tic anemia. Reports were studied to identify the age and sex of patients, the exposure circumstances, and the time lapse between exposure and onset of disease. Reports from several large case series or registries were also reviewed for numbers of individuals believed to have aplastic anemia of unknown cause, as those cases might be linked to pesticides. Finally, a study was made of the available basic science literature relating pesticides to aplastic anemia and/or blood disorders.

Results.—A total of 280 reports of aplastic anemia associated with pesticide exposure were identified (table). The mean patient age was 34 years, and the ratio of women to men was 1:2. The average latency period was 5 months from time of exposure to onset of disease. Apart from the therapeutic use of lindane, 62% of cases of pesticide exposures were occupational. Sixty-six percent involved the use of organochlorine pesticides, although more recent cases were associated with the new organophosphate pesticides. Formal epidemiologic studies gave limited information; none reported an association between pesticides and aplastic anemia. However, a study of farmers in British Columbia found a significant increase in the proportional mortality rate for aplastic anemia from 1950 to 1959, with a subsequent decline. Several studies have also shown high rates of leukemia in farmers. Within the basic science literature, 1 study of commonly used organophosphate pesticides found that their primary metabolites inhibit in vitro human bone marrow stem cell colony formation. The compounds were seen to produce significant dose-dependent depression of colony formation of erythrocyte and granulocyte-macrophage progenitors at doses of 10^{-8} mol/L. Rats injected with lindane had depressed mitotic rates in the bone marrow preparations for up to 6 weeks after injection. An inhibitory effect on leukocyte migration after administration of DDT, DDE, lindane, and methoxychlor in human lymphocyte culture has also been noted. Significant numbers of sister chromatic exchanges and chromosomal aberrations were also seen in cultured human lymphocytes exposed to malathion, methyl bromide, and chlorpicrin.

Conclusion.—From this review, it is concluded that there is an etiologic association between cases of aplastic anemia and a history of pesticide exposure. The majority of patients were young, with predominantly occupational exposures to a variety of pesticides. Organochlorines, the oldest group of pesticides, were most often implicated; they can remain in adipose tissue for a lifetime. However, aplastic anemia after exposure to some of the newer pesticides such as organophosphates was also reported. Suggestive evidence shows that these compounds can cause dose-response depression of human bone marrow stem cell colony formation, including erythrocyte precursors.

▶ In urbanized societies, the most common identifiable cause of stem cell injury at this time is drugs that are used either in cancer chemotherapy or for other purposes such as treatment of infection or the suppression of inflammatory disease. More often than not, suppression of erythropoiesis is part of a global injury of hematopoietic stem cells, so anemia is accompanied by varying degrees of granulocytopenia, thrombocytopenia, and lymphopenia. When several cell lineages are affected and the bone marrow is hypocellular, the disorder is called aplastic anemia. Most cases of aplastic anemia are unknown or are presumed to result from an autoimmune disorder; however, many classes of drugs can potentially injure hematopoietic cells. Some of the drugs and chemicals that have been associated with multilineage stem cell injury include:

- anticancer: many different drugs
- anti-inflammatory: gold, phenylbutazone, Clinoril®
- anticonvulsants: phenytoin, Mesantoin®, Tridione®
- psychoactive: carbamazepine [Tegretol®]
- antibiotics: chloramphenicol
- chemical toxins: benzene derivatives, petrochemicals, insecticides

In addition to drugs and chemicals, a variety of viral infections have been associated with stem cell injury. There are a number of reports of aplastic anemia after hepatitis and rare instances in which aplasia occurs in the setting of infectious mononucleosis. Human parvovirus can produce a transient red cell aplasia. However, deranged immune function with T-cell cytotoxicity to stem cells is presumed to be the mechanism involved in many cases of the common variety of idiopathic aplastic anemia, as about one half of patients respond to immunosuppression with agents such as antithymocyte globulin.—M.J. Cline, M.D.

Gamma-Interferon Gene Expression in the Bone Marrow of Patients With Aplastic Anemia

Nisticò A, Young NS (Natl Heart, Lung, and Blood Inst, Bethesda, Md)
Ann Intern Med 120:463–469, 1994   119-95-31–3

Introduction.—Although aplastic anemia has been thought to have a heterogeneous group of causes, the response of patients to immunosuppressive therapy suggests the possibility of a common immune pathophysiologic origin. A recent study found γ-interferon gene expression in the bone marrow of patients with aplastic anemia to be highly predictive of a response to cyclosporine therapy. Patients with aplastic anemia and control subjects were evaluated for γ-interferon gene expression in the bone marrow.

Methods.—Study participants were 43 patients with aplastic anemia (25 newly diagnosed and 18 who were previously treated), 39 patients with other hematologic syndromes, and 20 normal controls. Approximately .5 mL of marrow was withdrawn for analysis, and γ-interferon was detected by the reverse polymerase chain reaction method. Additionally, serum γ-interferon, soluble CD8, and soluble interleukin-2 receptor levels were determined.

Results.—γ-Interferon signal was observed in most samples from patients with newly diagnosed aplastic anemia and was present in 14 of 18 patients with severe aplasia at diagnosis, 4 of 7 patients with moderate aplastic anemia, and 1 of 2 patients with the paroxysmal nocturnal hemoglobinuria–aplasia syndrome. The marrow from 20 normal controls and from patients who had received many transfusions for chronic anemia showed no expression of the γ-interferon gene. Similarly, there was no expression of the gene in patients with pancytopenia after chemotherapy or in those with marrow failure of other types. The γ-interferon gene was present in 3 of 4 previously treated patients who had a relapse of aplastic anemia but not in those who were in recovery after treatment. Peripheral blood cells showed γ-interferon gene expression in a few normal controls but not in all patients with gene expression in marrow.

Conclusion.—The prevalence of γ-interferon expression in acquired aplastic anemia suggests that this finding is a marker for the disease and may distinguish it from other forms of bone marrow failure. Analysis of marrow is more specific and sensitive than analysis of peripheral blood cells. Data indicate a pathophysiologic role for γ-interferon in aplastic anemia.

▶ For several years, the senior author of this article has espoused the idea that γ-interferon is the mediator of idiopathic aplastic anemia. This concept is based on several observations: first, that γ-interferon is produced by activated T lymphocytes; second, that γ-interferon can suppress hematopoiesis in tissue culture and in patients treated with γ-interferon in vivo; and finally, that peripheral blood lymphocytes from patients with aplastic anemia have been reported to make excessive amounts of γ-interferon. In this report, the investigators show that γ-interferon gene expression is correlated with idiopathic aplastic anemia. It makes an interesting story, but proving the concept will require demonstration that a specific inhibitor of γ-interferon can stop the progress or reverse the course of aplastic anemia.—M.J. Cline, M.D.

Cost Implications to Medicare of Recombinant Erythropoietin Therapy for the Anemia of End-Stage Renal Disease
Powe NR, Griffiths RI, Bass EB (Johns Hopkins Univ, Baltimore, Md)
J Am Soc Nephrol 3:1660–1671, 1993   119-95-31-4

Background.—The use of recombinant human erythropoietin (EPO) in place of red blood cell transfusion or androgens in the management of anemia in patients undergoing hemodialysis is now a realistic option for patients with end-stage renal disease. Because 93% of these patients are entitled to Medicare benefits, the net cost to the Medicare program of EPO treatment was estimated and the effectiveness and side effects of the alternative therapies were considered.

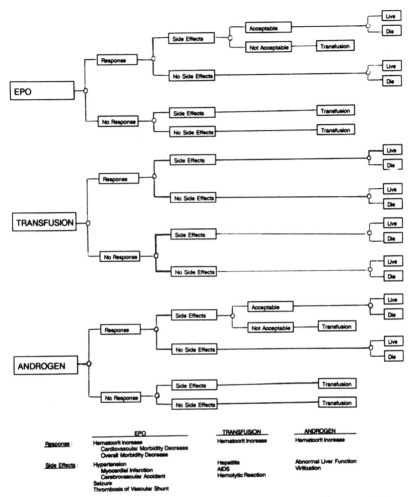

Fig 31–1.—Decision model for the treatment of anemia in patients with end-stage renal disease. (Courtesy of Powe NR, Griffiths RI, Bass EB: *J Am Soc Nephrol* 3:1660-1671, 1993.)

Method.—A decision model was designed to assess the clinical paths that Medicare hemodialysis patients traverse and the associated costs that they incur when treated for anemia by 1 of 3 alternative therapies (EPO, androgens, and transfusions) over a period of 1-5 years (Fig 31-1). After the initiation of treatment, the model accounted for patients' response (increase in hematocrit) or lack of response on a monthly basis. The model also evaluated the possible benefits of therapy to cardiovascular and overall morbidity and assessed the probable side effects. Estimates of the direct Medicare cost were assigned to each of the 3 alternative anemia therapies and to each of the potential clinical events.

Results.—The 1-year net cost to Medicare of treating anemia with EPO was significantly greater than the cost incurred by treatment with infusion or androgens. Treatment with EPO during 1 year was estimated at $4,428 (including treatment and related services and the cost of treating potential side effects) compared with $175 for transfusion therapy and $185 for androgens. The 5-year net cost for EPO was estimated at $12,327 compared with $522 for transfusion and $490 for androgens. The 1-year incremental net cost per 10,000 patients of EPO relative to transfusion was $42,530,000, and the 5-year incremental cost was $118,050,000. The incremental cost of EPO relative to androgen therapy was slightly greater. Cost differences among the different therapies were seen to be highly sensitive to changes in the dose of EPO. They were moderately sensitive to changes in estimated anemia response rates for EPO, frequency of EPO-induced vascular access clotting, and reduction in cardiovascular or overall morbidity. They were slightly sensitive to transfusion rates; estimated anemia response rates for androgens; frequency of EPO-induced seizure or hypertensive complications such as stroke or myocardial infarction; frequency of transfusion-related viral infection; and frequency of androgen-induced virilization.

Conclusion.—When both the effectiveness and side effects of alternative treatments for anemia in patients receiving hemodialysis were considered, it was projected that the increasing use of EPO therapy will lead to a significant increase in Medicare costs for these patients.

▶ Sensors in the kidney detect the available O_2 concentration and direct the production of appropriate amounts of EPO. The erythropoietic hormone is then carried by the blood back to the sites of red blood cell production in the bone marrow, where it interacts with EPO receptors on the surface of red blood cell precursors.

Normally, this system is finely tuned, and the concentration of red blood cells in our blood demonstrates little fluctuation. However, chronic kidney disease can interfere with the production of EPO and cause anemia. In this situation, the logical choices are EPO or red blood cell transfusion.

I was surprised by the information in this article. I had not realized just how much more expensive EPO therapy was than transfusion management of anemia of chronic renal disease—an excess cost of over $4,000 per year per patient. One wonders whether our society can really afford this kind of medical bill for EPO when there are so many other demands for medical care.—M.J. Cline, M.D.

Abnormalities of *PIG-A* Transcripts in Granulocytes From Patients With Paroxysmal Nocturnal Hemoglobinuria
Miyata T, Yamada N, Iida Y, Nishimura J, Takeda J, Kitani T, Kinoshita T

(Osaka Univ, Japan; Nagoya Univ, Japan)
N Engl J Med 330:249–255, 1994

119-95-31–5

Background.—Paroxysmal nocturnal hemoglobinuria (PNH) is an acquired blood cell disorder caused by the deficient synthesis—by hematopoietic cells deriving from an abnormal stem cell—of the glycosyl-phosphatidylinositol molecules that serve to anchor proteins to the cell membrane. A previous study of 2 patients with PNH showed that the disease was caused by the gene *PIG-A*, for phosphatidylinositol glycan class A, a component of glycosyl-phosphatidylinositol synthesis.

Objective and Methods.—An attempt was made to characterize the somatically acquired abnormalities of *PIG-A* by examining granulocytes from 15 patients with PNH. The cellular contents of CD55 and CD59 were determined by fluorescence-activated flow cytometry. Gene transcripts were reverse-transcribed, amplified by the polymerase chain reaction technique, and closed into plasmids. The structure of the cloned complementary DNA was analyzed by nucleotide sequencing, and it was tested for its ability to restore the abnormal phenotype of a gene-deficient cell line after transfection.

Findings.—Three of the 15 patients had varying patterns of abnormal-sized *PIG-A* transcripts, and 1 had a very low level of transcript. In each of the 11 patients with normal-sized transcripts, the transfection assay showed that some of the transcripts were nonfunctional. The proportion of nonfunctional gene transcripts correlated with that of affected granulocytes. Sequencing demonstrated somatic mutations in 2 instances.

Conclusion.—It appears that *PIG-A* is responsible for somatic mutation, causing most if not all cases of PNH.

▶ Paroxysmal nocturnal hemoglobinuria is a disorder with an acquired defect in the red blood cell membrane that increases the sensitivity of the cell to complement mediated lysis. The clinical consequence is a hemolytic anemia of an intermittent or "paroxysmal" nature. Dark urine is sometimes seen as a consequence of nocturnal hemolysis. This phenomenon, which gives its name to the disorder, is thought to be the result of a slight nocturnal fall in blood pH with secondary complement activation.

The basic defect in PNH arises in a multipotent stem cell, as abnormalities are seen in leukocytes and platelets as well as red blood cells. The cause was identified in 1994 as an abnormality of the so-called *PIG-A* gene. The defect results in incomplete synthesis of glycosyl-phosphatidylinositol, which serves as an "anchor" that attaches certain proteins to the red blood cell membrane. Associated with this is deficient anchoring of a protein called "decay accelerating factor," or DAF. Decay accelerating factor functions to accelerate the inactivation of C3b, a key intermediate in the complement activation cascade. A deficiency of DAF results in the accumulation of C3b on the surface of the PNH red blood cell. This leads to further activation of the cascade and accumulation of the "membrane attack complex" of C5b, 6, 7, 8, and 9. When sufficient attack complex accumulates, it bores holes in the cell membrane and the cell lyses.

The defective stem cell that gives rise to the complement lysis-sensitive red cells is monoclonal. It may exist side by side with normal erythropoietic stem cells so that in the peripheral blood, there is a mixed population of normal and abnormal red cells. There may even be several monoclonal populations differing in complement sensitivity and derived from different abnormal stem cells.

Defective stem cell proliferation in PNH is common, and the marrow, instead of showing the erythroid hyperplasia one expects in hemolytic anemia, may sometimes be hypocellular with variable degrees of hypoplasia of the erythroid, granulocytic, and megakaryocytic series.

Paroxysmal nocturnal hemoglobinuria usually begins insidiously. Its onset occasionally follows drug-induced or idiopathic aplasia, but more often there is no recognized antecedent event. The initial symptoms are usually those of anemia, and the patient may or may not notice dark morning urine. The anemia is usually intermittent in nature but may be continuous. It may be complicated by the development of iron deficiency as iron is lost in the urine as hemosiderin.

Thrombosis is a major complication of PNH. Venous thromboses may occur anywhere in the body, and bowel infarction or occlusion of hepatic veins may be fatal. The mechanism of the thrombotic tendency is not known but is probably linked to the abnormal platelet surface.

Infections are also common in PNH, and these may trigger hemolytic or thrombotic episodes. The affected patient may die of these complications, or the disease may progress to aplasia or acute leukemia—a course that is consistent with the notion that this is a disease of acquired injury to stem cells.

The diagnosis of PNH should be considered in any anemia that does not have an obvious cause. The diagnosis is made by the sucrose hemolysis test, in which a 10% sucrose solution is added to anticoagulated blood in the ratio of 9:1. This low ionic strength isotonic solution activates complement, and within 30 minutes, the PNH cells lyse. Ethylenediaminetetraacetic acid should not be used as anticoagulant as it blocks complement activation.—M.J. Cline, M.D.

Recombinant Human Granulocyte Colony-Stimulating Factor (rhG-CSF; Filgrastim) Treatment of Clozapine-Induced Agranulocytosis
Nielsen H (Hvidovre Univ, Denmark)
J Intern Med 234:529–531, 1993   119-95-31–6

Background.—Drug-induced agranulocytosis is a potential side effect of medical therapy, in particular after treatment with the atypical neuroleptic drug, clozapine. Granulocyte colony-stimulating factor (G-CSF), a glycoprotein that is produced by bone marrow stromal cells and various immunologic cells, has been shown to stimulate the proliferation and differentiation of myeloid precursor cells in the bone marrow. The use of recombinant human G-CSF in the treatment of clozapine-induced granulocytosis was demonstrated.

Case Report.—Woman, 33, with a chronic psychiatric disorder that was unresponsive to usual antipsychotic preparations, was given clozapine, 200 mg/day. Her psychiatric condition improved considerably and the dosage was raised to 250 mg/day after 8 weeks. After 9 weeks of therapy, neutrophil counts were 6.305×10^9/L and after 10 weeks dropped to .234 × 10^9/L. The patient was subsequently admitted to the ICU and clozapine treatment was stopped. Stimulation of myelopoiesis was induced by filgrastim, 5 µg/kg per day. The patient was also given ceftazidime, 6 g; gentamycin, 600 mg; and nystatin, 6 MIE daily. Her skin was decontaminated with daily washings with chlorhexidine. Three days later, clinical pharyngitis with fever and difficulty in swallowing developed. The patient responded clinically to ampicillin and gentamycin for 5 days. Daily measurements of neutrophil granulocytes showed a complete agranulocytosis for 10 days. After 8 days of filgrastim treatment, the dosage was increased to 10 µg/kg per day. A rapid neutrophil response was seen, including circulation of immature myeloid cells. After 11 days, treatment was stopped and the patient was discharged with no further symptoms. Her leukocyte count returned to normal within 2 weeks.

Conclusion.—Early treatment with filgrastim is required in severe cases of clozapine-induced agranulocytosis. A dose of 10 µg/kg per day is recommended.

▶ The mature polymorphonuclear leukocyte is resident in the circulation for only a few hours, and most of its life span of a few days is spent in the tissues where it dies. It never returns to the blood or bone marrow. The whole process from birth to death of the cell takes about 2 weeks. The impressive thing is that the granulocyte turnover rate is between 50 and 350 × 10^7 cells/kg per day. This means that about 50 billion neutrophils are made per day under normal circumstances, and more are made in inflammatory conditions. Combined with a marrow reserve of about 700 billion neutrophils, this adds up to an impressive array of cells.

Normally, the neutrophils in the circulation are about equally divided between those in the freely flowing blood and those marginated along the walls of small vessels and in the sinusoids of the spleen. With increased demand in inflammation, the marginated pool is quickly mobilized into the flowing blood. This also happens with administration of glucocorticoids.

"Neutropenia" is defined as a blood neutrophil count below the normal range, and "agranulocytosis" as an absence of blood neutrophils. In general, when the count falls below 500/µL, the frequency of infections increases. Neutropenia is more often caused by underproduction of neutrophils than by excessive destruction. Unfortunately, neutrophil kinetic tests to determine rates of cell production are too cumbersome for routine use, so one must often rely on the rather imprecise morphologic assessment of the bone marrow to determine whether neutrophils are being produced. Sometimes the mobilization of cells into the blood by administration of glucocorticoids is used to gauge neutrophil reserves, but the results are too haphazard for easy interpretation. The best test may be a trial of administered G-CSF with follow-up of the blood neutrophil count over several days.

In developed countries, the most common causes of neutropenias are probably stem cell injury from anticancer and other myelosuppressive drugs, but neutropenia from underproduction of cells can also be caused by marrow replacement by tumor or granulomata; extreme deficiency of nutrients, often in association with alcoholism; and by a variety of congenital defects.

Accelerated neutrophil destruction that results in neutropenia is less common, but one should think of drug-induced agranulocytosis, systemic lupus, Felty's syndrome, and hypersplenism.

A number of drugs are frequently associated with neutropenia, and these are listed below. In some cases, the neutropenia is mediated by drug–antibody interactions, but more often than not, we do not know the mechanism of the decrease in neutrophils.

Drugs Frequently Associated with Neutropenia
- Anti-Inflammatory: indomethacin, gold, phenylbutazone
- Anticonvulsants: phenytoin
- Antidepressants: various hypnotics
- Antithyroid: propylthiouracil
- Cardiovascular: hydralazine, procainamide, quinidine

In drug-induced agranulocytosis, withdrawal of the offending drug and supportive therapy with antibiotics are usually sufficient until the bone marrow recovers. If granulocytopenia is severe, then G-CSF is sometimes administered.—M.J. Cline, M.D.

α-Interferon Treatment for Idiopathic Hypereosinophilic Syndrome
Bockenstedt PL, Santinga JT, Bolling SF (Univ of Michigan, Ann Arbor; Ann Arbor VA Med Ctr, Mich)
Am J Hematol 45:248–251, 1994   119-95-31-7

Background.—The often fatal disorder termed idiopathic hypereosinophilic syndrome (HES) is characterized by a marked elevation of eosinophils in the absence of any known cause. It can result in end-organ damage of the heart, lungs, gastrointestinal tract, and CNS. Known causes of hypereosinophilia include some parasitic infections (*Toxocara canis, Trichinella spirella, Ascaris*) and selected autoimmune disorders such as eosinophilic fasciitis, vasculitis, and the L-tryptophan syndrome. The most marked eosinophil elevations are seen in HES and with malignancies such as acute lymphocytic leukemia, eosinophilic leukemia, myeloproliferative disorders, and lung cancer. Treatment focuses on eosinophilic reduction, which should minimize damage from tissue infiltration.

Steroids, hydroxyurea, vincristine, etoposide, 6-mercaptopurine, and other antitumor agents have been used.

Case Report.—Man, 28, had abdominal pain, nausea, and vomiting, especially after alcohol consumption. There was a 3-month history of a 10-pound weight loss and easy fatigability but no L-tryptophan exposure. Vital signs were normal, the chest was clear, no murmurs were detected, the liver span was normal, and the spleen was not palpable. The patient was mildly anemic, with a hematocrit of 38.5% and normal indices. The white blood cell count was 16,400/mm³ with 60% eosinophils, whereas other laboratory results were normal, except for lactic dehydrogenase of 362. A biopsy specimen of the small bowel showed eosinophil infiltration throughout the jejunum and proximal ileum. Bone marrow, stool parasite, and allergy tests; chest x-ray studies; ECG, echocardiogram, and abdominal CT scan all gave normal results. Prednisone, 60 mg/day, decreased eosinophils, but after 3 months, white blood cells were difficult to control and hydroxyurea was added. Five months after treatment was sought, bilateral hilar adenopathy, splenomegaly, and intra-abdominal lymphadenopathy were found, and a splenectomy was performed.

The patient was followed for 1 year, during which a cyclic rise in eosinophils was accompanied by a fall in platelets. After a bout with monocular blindness, a grade 4 holosystolic murmur was found. Intracardiac studies showed a 4+ mitral regurgitation with blood flowing back into the pulmonary veins. On surgery, the posterior mitral leaflet and annulus were destroyed; the anterior leaflet was less affected, although papillary muscle showed fibrotic granular debris. A porcine value was inserted. Bone marrow biopsy specimens showed eosinophilia, and the patient was cross-matched for bone marrow transplantation. A course of α-interferon (6 million units 3 times per week) controlled the eosinophilia, and the patient was clinically improved. The dosage was halved after 3 weeks because of fatigue. The white blood cell count was 8,500/mm³ with 10% eosinophils and normal platelets and hemoglobin. Cardiopulmonary tests showed no sign of disease progression.

Conclusion.—If a patient with HES does not respond to hydroxyurea and prednisone, α-interferon should be considered. Valvular thrombosis is a complication of valve replacement, and interferon's control of eosinophilia may have played a role in avoiding thrombosis in this patient.

▶ The normal eosinophil count is less than 400 cells/μL. Eosinopenia is found in conditions of glucocorticoid excess, but this is not a particularly useful clinical sign. Significant elevations of blood eosinophils are often a sign of allergic reactions or parasitic diseases. Tumors of lung or pancreas or Hodgkin's disease may rarely be associated with eosinophilia. Other causes include sensitivity to drugs such as phenytoin and penicillin, hay fever, asthma, serum sickness, urticaria, hypersensitivity pneumonitides, tryptophan sensitivity, eczema, dermatitis herpetiformis, pityriasis rubra, and pemphigus.

Hypereosinophilic syndromes may be defined as disorders in which the concentration of blood eosinophils is greater than 1,500/μL for more than 6 months without evidence of parasitism or allergy and in which there is evidence of organ injury. In most cases, the cause is unknown. In a few cases, the eosinophilia is associated with lymphoma, with a clonal expansion of helper T cells, eosinophilic leukemia, or other myeloproliferative disorder. Below is a list of the organs involved in HES. Involvement of the heart or lungs is most ominous.

Hypereosinophilic Syndromes

ORGAN INVOLVED	% OF CASES
Blood	100
Heart	50–70
Skin	50–70
Nervous System	35–70
Lungs	40–60
Spleen	30–60

Glucocorticoids or myelosuppressive anticancer drugs such as hydroxyurea have often been used, but treatment is generally not very satisfactory. This article suggests that α-interferon may be a useful treatment in some cases.—M.J. Cline, M.D.

Heparin-Induced Thrombocytopenia (HIT): An Overview of 230 Patients Treated With Orgaran (Org 10172)
Magnani HN (Organon Internatl BV, Oss, The Netherlands)
Thromb Haemost 70:554–561, 1993   119-95-31–8

Background.—Heparin-induced thrombocytopenia (HIT) with thrombosis affects 1 in 2,000 patients treated with heparin. Because the arterial or venous thromboses can be life threatening, an alternative anticoagulation is required. The treatment of patients with HIT with Orgaran, a low-molecular-weight heparinoid, was reviewed.

Method.—The outcome of 230 patients with HIT treated with Orgaran was analyzed during the treatment period plus 2 days. The dosage was dependent on the clinical status of the patient. The criteria for judging the success or failure of Orgaran included an increase of platelet count in a thrombocytopenic patient or lack of clinically significant change in a nonthrombocytopenic patient, control of the hemostatic process, stabilization or improvement in ischemia, and no development of cross-reactivity of Orgaran with the antibody in patients with HIT.

Results.—The majority of patients responded well to Orgaran. The overall mortality was 59 of 250 patients treated. Thirty-two of these deaths occurred during Orgaran therapy or within 48 hours of treatment; the remainder occurred in the follow-up period. Mortality was highest in patients undergoing hemofiltration, resulting particularly from multiple organ failure. The mortality from bleeding (1 patient), thrombosis (5 patients), or septic shock (1 patient) which could be attributed to Orgaran was 3%. The other deaths were attributed to the poor underlying clinical status of the patients. The mortality in patients with an acute thrombo-embolic event before and/or secondary to their HIT episode was 19.7%. Nonfatal effects of treatment included 40 patients with bleeding, none of whom were considered treatment failures. Finally, a lower cross-reactivity rate (approximately 10%) was seen with the heparin-induced antibody compared with that of the low-molecular-weight heparin.

Conclusion.—The efficacy and safety of Orgaran seen here, together with evidence of its low cross-reactivity with the heparin-induced antibody, indicate that it is a viable alternative to heparin in the treatment of prophylaxis of both arterial and venous thrombosis in patients with HIT.

▶ Heparin-induced thrombocytopenia is an important clinical problem. Withdrawal of heparin may result in a recovery of the platelet count, but if the underlying thrombotic problem persists, there may be serious clinical problems. The incidence of HIT with thrombotic complications may be as high as 1 in 400 heparin-treated patients, and the mortality rate may be as high as 25%. Poor prognostic factors in HIT include failure of the platelet count to increase with heparin withdrawal or a recurrence of the thrombocytopenia. The presumed mechanism of HIT is interaction of antibodies to heparin with heparin at the platelet surface; however, there are no reliable routine laboratory tests that can predict the occurrence of HIT. This paper examines the use of a low-molecular-weight heparinoid (Orgaran) in treating patients with HIT. The authors believe that the treatment may be effective. I am not so sure. The theme of HIT and low-molecular-weight heparinoids continues in Abstract 119-95-31–9, which examines the safety of these compounds as deduced by in vitro testing.—M.J. Cline, M.D.

Can Low Molecular Weight Heparins and Heparinoids Be Safely Given to Patients With Heparin-Induced Thrombocytopenia Syndrome?
Kikta MJ, Keller MP, Humphrey PW, Silver D (Univ of Missouri, Columbia)
Surgery 114:705–710, 1993   119-95-31–9

Background.—Heparin-induced thrombocytopenia syndrome (HIT) is an immune-mediated disorder that develops in .9% to 31% of patients receiving heparin. It occurs when heparin-induced antibodies (usually IgG) that are responsible for platelet activation and aggregation develop. A large number of patients who take heparin become sensitized and have heparin-associated antiplatelet antibodies (HAAb). Reanticoagulation of these patients with heparin should be avoided. Low-molecular-weight heparins (LMWHs) and heparinoids have been used to anticoagulate small groups of patients with HIT with mixed results. Some of the patients had HIT in the presence of the unfractionated heparin (UH) substitutes. Knowing whether the heparin substitute is likely to cause patients' platelets to aggregate before administering the substitute to patients with HAAb would be valuable.

Method.—The HAAb were identified in 51 patients with HIT by positive platelet aggregometry testing with commercial UH. Plasma from the patients with HAAb was tested for the ability to aggregate platelets in the presence of 2 LMWHs—Mono-Embolex NM and Fragmin—and 1 heparinoid, Org 10172.

Results.—Fragmin and Org 10172 aggregated platelets in the presence of HAAb significantly less often than Mono-Embolex NM. The proportion of plasma reacting to UH substitutes was 60.8% for Mono-Embolex NM, 25.5% for Fragmin, and 19.6% for Org 10172.

Conclusion.—The HAAb that cause platelet aggregation with UH have a substantial likelihood of causing platelet aggregation with a heparinoid or the LMWHs. Fragmin, an LMWH, and Org 10172, a heparinoid, aggregated platelets in the presence of HAAb significantly less often than the LMWH Mono-Embolex NM. In vitro testing of the patient's HAAb should be conducted before administering LMWHs or heparinoid to ensure that a patient's HAAb will not cause platelet aggregation in the presence of a heparin substitute.

▶ Patients with HAAb frequently require repeated anticoagulation because of recurrent thrombotic events. The authors examined platelet aggregation with LMWH and a heparinoid. They found that in 20% to 60% of the patients, sera reacted with these compounds in inducing platelet aggregation. It is assumed that these positive reactors will have thrombocytopenia when the compounds are given in vivo. However, as mentioned in Abstract 119-95-31–8, the laboratory tests for HIT are not completely reliable. In the clinic, the results of using LMWH and heparinoids have beeen mixed—some treated patients have no recurrent thrombocytopenia and in some, thrombocytopenia occurs or persists. One can conclude that the routine use of these heparin substitutes is not recommended unless there is no alternative and the situation is desperate. The usual alternatives in such cases are nonheparin anticoagulants or antiplatelet drugs.—M.J. Cline, M.D.

Establishing a Therapeutic Range for Heparin Therapy
Brill-Edwards P, Ginsberg JS, Johnston M, Hirsh J (McMaster Univ, Hamilton, Ont, Canada; Hamilton Civic Hosps Research Centre, Ont, Canada)
Ann Intern Med 119:104–109, 1993   119-95-31–10

Background.—The responsiveness of different activated partial thromboplastin time (aPTT) reagents to heparin varies greatly. Thus, the use of the same fixed therapeutic range for all aPTT reagents is problematic. Two methods of determining a therapeutic range of aPTT results were compared.

Methods.—Inpatients receiving unfractionated IV heparin for venous thromboembolic disease were studied. Two methods were compared for determination of the therapeutic range of aPTT results—aPTT ratios of

1.5 to 2.5 times the control value and protamine titration heparin levels of .2 to .4 units/mL.

Results.—A ratio of 1.5 times the control value was much less than a minimum protamine titration heparin level of .2 units/mL for all aPTT reagents studied. Various manufacturers' aPTT reagents and reagent lots from the same manufacturer showed substantial variation in response to heparin and, thus, had different therapeutic ranges.

Conclusion.—Depending on the reagent used, a different dose of heparin would be needed to produce an aPTT ratio of 1.5 times the control value. A practical way to compensate for the variable response of aPTT reagents to heparin is to establish a therapeutic range for aPTT results by using protamine titration heparin levels of .2 to .4 units/mL as a reference standard.

▶ The anticoagulant effect of heparin is usually measured by the aPTT, and the dose of heparin is usually adjusted to keep the aPTT in the range of 1.5 to 2.5 times the control value. However, the response of different aPTT reagents to heparin is quite variable, and a value of 1.5 times control may have different meanings in different laboratories. This failure to use absolute standards of heparinization may be one of the many factors that make the frequency of bleeding complications so high with heparin anticoagulation.

In an attempt to develop better standards, the authors used the protamine titration assay to measure heparin levels in blood. It is known that a heparin level of .2–.4 units/mL with this assay correlates with clinical efficacy and safety. Not surprisingly, the authors found that different lots of aPTT reagents show considerable variation in defining the therapeutic range for heparin and that an aPTT of 1.5 times the control value is frequently below the therapeutic range. They suggest that clinical laboratories establish an appropriate therapeutic range for heparin by comparing the aPTT with protamine titration for each batch of aPTT reagents. Does your clinical laboratory do this?—M.J. Cline, M.D.

Resistance to Activated Protein C as a Basis for Venous Thrombosis
Svensson PJ, Dahlbäck B (Univ of Lund, Malmö, Sweden)
N Engl J Med 330:517–522, 1994   119-95-31–11

Background.—Protein C is a vitamin K–dependent plasma protein that is key to the anticoagulant system. An apparently inherited poor response to the anticoagulant activated protein C (APC) was described.

Methods.—One hundred four consecutive patients with venous thrombosis were compared with 130 control subjects to determine the prevalence of APC resistance in patients with venous thrombosis. Two hundred eleven members of 34 families of individuals with APC resistance were also assessed.

Findings.—A positive family history of thrombosis was noted in 45% of the patients. Patients with thrombosis and control subjects differed significantly in APC ratios. In 33% of patients, the APC ratio was below the fifth percentile of control values. However, the results of the family assessments suggested that the prevalence of APC resistance may be even higher in patients with thrombosis. In most cases, the inherited nature of the defect was confirmed. The family studies suggested that the mode of inheritance was autosomal dominant. The thrombosis-free survival of APC-resistant family members was significantly lower than in family members without APC resistance.

Conclusion.—A high prevalence of APC resistance among young persons with a history of venous thrombosis was found. This resistance was apparently inherited as an autosomal dominant trait.

▶ Under normal conditions, the procoagulant and anticoagulant mechanisms in blood are in neat balance, and neither spontaneous bleeding nor thrombosis occurs in blood vessels.

One of the key players in the anticoagulant system is protein C, a vitamin K–dependent plasma protein. Another is protein S, also a vitamin K–dependent protein, which is thought to function as a cofactor of APC.

Protein C is activated on the surface of endothelial cells by a combination of thrombin and thrombomodulin and exerts its anticoagulant effect by selectively degrading clotting factors Va and VIIIa.

It is well known that homozygous or heterozygous deficiency of protein C or protein S is associated with increased risk of thrombosis. This study provides good evidence that an inherited resistance to APC is common among young individuals with a history of venous thrombosis. The authors initially based their investigation on the observation that there is frequently a positive family history of thrombosis among young patients with thrombosis, but only a minority of these individuals have deficiency of protein C, protein S, or antithrombin III, suggesting that another genetic defect was involved in the predisposition to thrombosis. They then found a relationship between familial thrombosis and resistance to the anticoagulant activity of APC and postulated a defect in a previously unknown anticoagulant cofactor of protein C. They have now found that the defective cofactor may be an abnormal factor V, which has normal procoagulant activity but fails to function normally with protein C. This abnormality may be 10 times more common in thrombosis-prone young individuals than any other known deficiency of anticoagulant proteins.

This is one more step—and an important one—in understanding why thromboembolic disease develops in some young individuals.—M.J. Cline, M.D.

Platelet Dysfunction Associated With Clozapine Therapy
Durst R, Dorevitch A, Fraenkel Y (Talbieh Mental Health Ctr, Jerusalem; He-

brew Univ-Hadassah Med School Hosp, Jerusalem)
South Med J 86:1170–1172, 1993   119-95-31–12

Background.—Clozapine, an atypical antipsychotic agent used in patients with treatment-resistant schizophrenia, is thought to be relatively free of adverse extrapyramidal effects. Its potentially hazardous effects on white blood cell function have been reported. A patient with clozapine-associated epistaxis and platelet count reduction was described.

Case Report.—Man, 45, with a 23-year history of paranoid schizophrenia had been treated unsuccessfully through the years with various antipsychotic drugs. Dosages reached an equivalent of 3,000 mg of chlorpromazine. Attempts at ambulatory treatment and rehabilitation in the community failed; the patient needed continued treatment in the closed ward. Subsequently, he was selected for a trial of clozapine therapy. All psychotropic drugs were gradually discontinued, and clozapine treatment was begun at 25 mg/day and increased to 100 mg/day over 6 days. Epistaxis developed on day 7, and a subsequent blood screen showed a 50% decline in platelet count to 140,000 µL. Clozapine was stopped. The epistaxis resolved after 1 day, and the platelet count rebounded to 250,000 µL. Treatment with other psychotropic drugs was reinitiated, and the patient's psychiatric status remained unchanged.

Conclusion.—Epistaxis and platelet count reductions resulted from clozapine treatment in this patient. Cessation of treatment eliminated epistaxis and normalized the platelet count. The routine monitoring of platelet count and function in clozapine-treated patients is recommended.

▶ In the clinical evaluation of thrombocytopenia, it is often necessary to determine whether the low platelet count is the result of inadequate production, accelerated destruction, or pooling of platelets in an enlarged spleen. Although this evaluation can be done with radioisotopes, this is rarely practical, and one generally relies on morphology of platelets and megakaryocytes and assessment of the size of the spleen. A key component of the evaluation is an examination of the blood film to detect spurious levels of platelets because of erroneous electronic counting of cellular fragments or in vitro agglutinated platelets or very large platelets. Next is the evaluation of the bone marrow smear for estimation of megakaryocyte number. This is at best a semiquantitative assessment, but you can use 2 megakaryocytes per low-power field as a reasonable average. Almost always, there is accelerated destruction of platelets if megakaryocytes are abundant in the bone marrow when, at the same time, there is thrombocytopenia in the blood.

Unfortunately, this simple but systematic evaluation is often not possible because of a rapidly deteriorating clinical situation with bleeding. In the case presented in this article, we know there was a decrease in the platelet count and epistaxis when the patient received clozapine. It is known that exposure to the drug can be associated with agranulocytosis (see Abstract

119-95-31–6 in the section on granulocytes). As the authors say, monitoring the platelet count of patients taking clozapine may be a good idea.—M.J. Cline, M.D.

Cocaine-Induced Platelet Defects

Jennings LK, White MM, Sauer CM, Mauer AM, Robertson JT (Univ of Tennessee, Memphis; Baptist Health Care System, Memphis, Tenn)
Stroke 24:1352–1359, 1993   119-95-31–13

Background.—Cocaine use has been associated with strokes and acute cardiac events, but its role in coagulation disorders has not been extensively studied. Research has demonstrated that local anesthetics inhibit platelet adhesion to foreign surfaces, platelet aggregation initiated by adenosine diphosphate (ADP) and thrombin, and platelet activation. Conflicting evidence from various in vitro models has shown that cocaine, up to or greater than an order of magnitude of the lethal dose, has either an inhibitory or pro-aggregatory effect on platelet function. The effect of cocaine and its carrier on the activation and aggregation of human platelets in vitro was investigated.

Method.—Platelets from 4 medication-free donors were preincubated with increasing concentrations of cocaine or carrier and challenged with the agonists ADP or collagen in the aggregometer.

Results.—Cocaine inhibited platelet aggregation response to challenge with ADP, collagen, or arachidonic acid. Cocaine had a direct effect on fibrinogen binding to the activated platelet and also dissociated preformed platelet aggregates. Cocaine's effect appears selective because there was no evidence of inhibition of agonist-mediated increases in cytosolic calcium or change in platelet shape. Cocaine did disrupt the organization of the cytoskeleton of activated platelets, a secondary event critical to cell receptor clustering and clot retraction. Preincubation of platelets with cocaine produced alterations in platelet protein electrophoretic patterns.

Conclusion.—These in vitro data suggest that cocaine has an effect on mechanisms mediating both adhesive and cohesive properties of platelets. Cocaine had a direct effect on fibrinogen binding to the activated platelet. It also dissociated preformed platelet aggregates and disrupted the organization of the cytoskeleton of activated platelets. It did not inhibit agonist-mediated increases in platelet cytosolic calcium. Cocaine may have a direct inhibitory effect on the ability of platelets to participate in thrombus formation. The contribution of this inhibitory effect on sudden death in cocaine abusers is still unclear.

▶ Within seconds of cutting a blood vessel, platelets adhere to the disrupted connective tissue at the edges of the wound. Over the next few minutes, they form a plug made up almost entirely of platelets, which may occlude the wound entirely or, at the least, slow the leakage of blood. Initially, most of the platelets remain intact, but many discharge the contents of their granules within the plug. Within a minute of disruption of the vessel, the coagulation process is activated locally, and fibrin strands begin to surround the plug. Over the next few hours, fibrin forms an increasing component of the occluding mass and may ultimately form the entire mass. The functions of platelets in this process can be divided into 4 phases: *adhesion, aggregation, secretion,* and the production of *procoagulant activity.*

When the endothelial lining of a blood vessel is disrupted, platelets adhere to and spread out on the subendothelial matrix. Components of the matrix such as fibronectin and collagen, together with divalent cations, may interact with glycoproteins on the platelet surface to stimulate the adhesion process. The adhesion of platelets to the subendothelium requires another factor— von Willebrand factor, a glycoprotein that is synthesized both by endothelial cells and by megakaryocytes.

Platelet aggregation requires active platelet metabolism and is stimulated by "agonists," including strong agonists such as thrombin and collagen and weaker agonists such as ADP, serotonin, and platelet-activating factor. Fibrinogen is also a necessary cofactor in the aggregation process. Platelet aggregation by agonists and cofactors is measured in the laboratory with an instrument appropriately called an *aggregometer.* Some of the substances that regulate platelet adhesion and aggregation in vivo include positive regulators such as collagen, thrombin, ADP, serotonin, fibrinogen, and von Willebrand factor, and negative regulators such as prostaglandins including TXA_2 and prostacyclin, bradykinin, and histamine.

In vitro cocaine behaves as a negative regulator or inhibitor of aggregation. One wonders whether this phenomenon relates to the association of strokes with cocaine use.—M.J. Cline, M.D.

Transfusion-Associated Graft-Versus-Host Disease in Immunocompetent Patients: Report of a Fatal Case Associated With Transfusion of Blood From a Second-Degree Relative, and a Survey of Predisposing Factors

Petz LD, Calhoun L, Yam P, Cecka M, Schiller G, Faitlowicz AR, Herron R, Sayah D, Wallace RB, Belldegrun A (Univ of California, Los Angeles; City of Hope Med Ctr, Duarte, Calif)
Transfusion 33:742–750, 1993   119-95-31–14

Background.—Graft-versus-host disease (GVHD) associated with transfusion is now known to occur in patients without evident immune deficiency. It is associated with cases in which the blood donor is homozygous for an HLA haplotype for which the recipient is heterozygous (a 1-way HLA match). To prevent transfusion-associated GVHD in this setting, the American Association of Blood Banks established a policy of irradiating blood from first-degree family members. The first known occurrence of transfusion-associated GVHD in a patient without evident immune deficiency who received blood from a donor who represented a 1-way HLA match, but who was a second-degree family member, was described.

Case Report.—Man, 73, underwent a radical retropubic prostatectomy with bilateral pelvic lymph node dissection for a stage B2 prostate adenocarcinoma. Blood was provided by his grandson, and the patient received 4 units of autologous red cells perioperatively and an additional unit postoperatively. None of the blood was irradiated. Twelve days after the transfusion, a generalized erythematous maculopapular rash developed. It was later followed by lethargy, confusion, anorexia, and scleral icterus. The patient had a white blood cell count of .5 × 10^9/L, hemoglobin of 110 g/L, platelet count of 208 × 10^9/L, lactate dehydrogenase level of 328 units/L, total bilirubin of 9.9 mg/dL, aspartate aminotransferase of 183 units/L, and alanine aminotransferase of 350 units/L. Over the next 10 days, a high fever, oral mucosal ulcerations, and hemoccult-positive diarrhea developed. Skin punch biopsy results were consistent with cutaneous GVHD.

The patient died 32 days after transfusion despite treatment with high-dose corticosteroids, IV immunoglobulin, antithymocyte globulin, granulocyte colony-stimulating factor, and transfusion support. To document the engraftment of the donor's lymphohematopoietic cells, DNA probes were used to highly polymorphic tandem-repeat sequences that are independent of HLA. This determined the patient's genotype and made it possible to compare it with the genotypes obtained by using DNA from the peripheral blood of the donor and the patient during the GVHD reaction. The results showed that the patient's circulating lymphohematopoietic cells were derived from both the donor and the recipient, although most of the DNA was of donor origin.

Conclusion.—The view that cellular blood components should be irradiated when the blood donor and transfusion recipient are blood relatives, because of the increased likelihood of a 1-way HLA match, is supported in the literature.

▶ Until recently, transfusion-associated GVHD was only thought to be a potential complication of blood transfusion in a severely immunocompromised patient, such as a patient with AIDS or one receiving immunosuppressive treatment. However, in the 1994 YEAR BOOK OF MEDICINE, I included 2 reports that demonstrated that the disorder can also rarely occur in presumably immunologically intact patients. This is another such report.

Transfusion-associated GVHD in immunologically intact individuals probably occurs because the HLA antigens of the transfused blood do not differ sufficiently from those of the blood recipient, with the consequence that the transfused T lymphocytes that cause GVHD are not recognized as foreign and are not eliminated by the host's immune system. If the HLA antigens of blood donor and recipient match, the potential for development of GVHD exists. Matches are more likely to occur among closely related individuals. Consequently, blood obtained from a first-degree family member should be irradiated before it is transfused. In this report, fatal transfusion-associated GVHD occurred in an immunologically intact individual who received blood from a second-degree relative.

If you are considering the possibility of transfusion-associated GVHD, look for the appearance of skin rash, fever, profuse diarrhea, jaundice and, ultimately, of bone marrow failure with onset usually within 30 days of transfusion. Infection may further complicate the clinical picture.—M.J. Cline, M.D.

32 Leukemia, Lymphoma, and Myeloma

Introduction

This has been a year for reevaluating the "best" therapies for non-Hodgkin's lymphomas, chronic lymphocytic leukemia, chronic myelocytic leukemia, and multiple myeloma. Once again, the role of the new agents such as deoxycoformycin, 2-chlorodeoxyadenosine, and fludarabine has been examined.

Martin J. Cline, M.D.

Treatment of Acute Lymphoblastic Leukemia: 30 Years' Experience at St. Jude Children's Research Hospital

Rivera GK, Pinkel D, Simone JV, Hancock ML, Crist WM (St Jude Children's Research Hosp, Memphis, Tenn; Univ of Tennessee, Memphis; M.D. Anderson Cancer Ctr, Houston)
N Engl J Med 329:1289–1295, 1993
119-95-32–1

Background.—The treatment of childhood lymphoblastic leukemia has progressed during the past 3 decades, but it is still unclear which form of therapy is the most effective and least toxic. The long-term outcomes of treatment were studied by comparing 4 consecutive eras of clinical trials of treatment for childhood acute lymphoblastic leukemia.

Method.—Between 1962 and 1988, 1,702 patients with lymphoblastic or undifferentiated leukemia were enrolled in 11 treatment studies typical of 4 eras: exploratory combination chemotherapy (era 1, 1962 to 1966; 91 patients); regimens for the control of meningeal leukemia (era 2, 1967 to 1979; 825 patients); limited intensification of therapy (era 3, 1979 to 1983; 428 patients); and extended intensification of therapy, which incorporated strategies of systemic chemotherapy that are more aggressive than conventional ones (era 4, 1984 to 1988; 358 patients). The end points studied were survival and event-free survival. The relative risk for treatment failure and the rate of relapse or death after treatment ended were also calculated.

Results.—Event-free survival improved progressively through each successive era, reaching 71% in era 4. A decrease of approximately 50% was seen in the risk for treatment failure from one era to the next in each subgroup of patients defined according to different combinations of the leukocyte count, race, age, and sex. Changes in treatment within the program also influenced the pattern, as did the frequency of treatment failure. Early advances in prophylactic therapy for meningeal leukemia led to a decrease in the rate of meningeal relapse, although the frequency of hematologic relapse remained high. With limited intensification of therapy in era 3, the proportion of patient with hematologic relapses decreased to 23%. This decrease continued in era 4, when only 12% of patients had a hematologic relapse as their first adverse event. An estimated 765 patients (45%) are considered long-term survivors, and most of them (80%) have no health problems related to leukemia or its treatment.

Conclusion.—Thanks to the advances of modern clinical hematology, acute lymphoblastic leukemia is highly curable today. However, infants younger than 1 year and patients with leukocyte counts greater than 100,000 cells/mm³ continue to fare poorly. New approaches that may help these subgroups include strategies that specifically target recurring genetic lesions, earlier therapeutic interventions when minimal residual disease is found in patients with apparently complete responses, and modification of treatment on the basis of a better understanding of variables that affect cytotoxicity.

▶ This article documents the steady progress that has occurred in the treatment of childhood acute lymphoblastic (ALL) leukemia from 1962 to the present.

Acute lymphoblastic leukemia is heterogeneous, with some cases arising in very early B cells, others in more differentiated B cells, and still others in T cells. Not surprisingly, prognosis worsens with increasing age beyond childhood and certainly after 30 years of age. A white blood cell count of greater than 30,000/µL, certain cytogenetic abnormalities including the Philadelphia 1 (Ph1) chromosome and t(4;11) translocation, disease outside the bone marrow at clinical presentation, disease evolving from chronic myelocytic leukemia, mixed lineage leukemia, and more than 4–5 weeks of therapy to achieve a remission are other negative factors.

Although these distinctions are clinically important in childhood disease, it is not so clear that they are important in adults, for whom all forms of ALL have a poor prognosis and may require aggressive treatment. Here, adulthood is defined as greater than 15 years of age. Although everyone agrees that negative prognostic factors—such as delayed response to therapy—are important, there is an increasing consensus that even in their absence, ALL in adults requires an extreme therapeutic approach if cure is the objective. This simplifies the selection of treatment strategy and dictates that the only variables of significance are advanced age, the presence of comorbid disease, and the availability of a suitable marrow donor. Patients older than 60 years of age do very poorly, and it is doubtful whether aggressive therapy should be used in this group.

Chemotherapy of ALL is generally divided into sequential phases of induction, consolidation intensification, and maintenance, usually in conjunction with a separate phase of CNS prophylaxis. Mediastinal irradiation is also frequently given in patients with T-cell ALL and a mediastinal mass. Prednisone, vincristine, and an anthracycline are the stable elements in chemotherapy programs, to which are added—in varying combinations—methotrexate, cyclophosphamide, asparaginase, etoposide, and ara-C—often with the addition of hematopoietic growth factors. Some studies suggest that the inclusion of cyclophosphamide and high-dose methotrexate in programs for adult T-cell and B-cell ALL are responsible for improved remission and survival statistics in these disorders.

There are surprising unknowns in the best management of adult ALL. Maintenance chemotherapy is standard in childhood ALL, but the role of maintenance therapy in adults is unclear, as is that of intensive consolidation therapy. The role of CNS irradiation in adults over the age of 25 years is controversial and has not been unequivocally established.

Although intensive chemotherapy has been associated with high rates of remission (> 95%) and cure (65% to 75%) in childhood ALL, this has unfortunately not been the case in adult disease, in which cure is relatively uncommon, except with bone marrow transplantation.—M.J. Cline, M.D.

A Double-Blind Controlled Study of Granulocyte Colony-Stimulating Factor Started Two Days Before Induction Chemotherapy in Refractory Acute Myeloid Leukemia

Ohno R, Naoe T, Kanamaru A, Yoshida M, Hiraoka A, Kobayashi T, Ueda T, Minami S, Morishima Y, Saito Y, Furusawa S, Imai K, Takemoto Y, Miura Y, Teshima H, Hamajima N, and the Kohseisho Leukemia Study Group (Nagoya Univ, Japan; Hyogo College of Med, Nishinomiya, Japan; Jichi Med School, Tochigi, Japan; et al)
Blood 83:2086–2092, 1994   119-95-32–2

Introduction.—Intensive chemotherapy and bone marrow transplantation (BMT) offer a cure to patients with acute myeloid leukemia (AML), although not without risk of myelosuppression and resultant infectious complications. Granulocyte colony-stimulating factor (G-CSF), used for the recovery of severe neutropenia after chemotherapy and BMT, is reported to accelerate the regrowth of AML cells. The consequences of G-CSF treatment in patients with relapsed or refractory AML were evaluated in a double-blind controlled study.

Patients and Methods.—The multicenter study enrolled 50 patients with AML and 8 with proven myelodysplastic syndromes that had given rise to AML. All received chemotherapy and either G-CSF or placebo. Recombinant human G-CSF (200 μg/m²) was administered 2 days before the start of induction therapy and continued until the neutrophil count recovered to greater than 1,500/μL or until 35 days after the start of induction therapy. After complete remission was obtained, therapy with the same drugs was repeated until relapse.

Results.—Recovery of the neutrophil count was significantly faster in the G-CSF group than in the placebo group. Among the 28 patients in the G-CSF group, neutrophil counts in 24 patients recovered to more than 1,000/μL within a median of 25 days; this level of recovery was achieved by 15 of 30 patients in the placebo group within a median of 32 days. Recovery of platelet counts and the incidence of febrile episodes and documented infections were similar in the 2 groups. Treatment with G-CSF did not stimulate the growth of AML cells in the bone marrow during the 2 days before the start of chemotherapy, nor did it accelerate regrowth of AML cells during the 5-week period after the therapy. The rate of complete remission was higher in the G-CSF group (50%) than in the placebo group (37%), but the difference was not statistically significant. Rates of event-free survival and disease-free survival were similar in the 2 groups. The only adverse effect of G-CSF was bone pain, reported by a single patient.

Conclusion.—The clinical application of G-CSF in leukemia has been controversial. This study of patients with a poor prognosis revealed no differences between G-CSF and placebo groups in the regrowth of leukemia cells or in the occurrence of relapse. Until the question is resolved, however, G-CSF administration should be limited in AML to high-risk patients and to standard-risk patients with life-threatening or uncontrollable infections.

▶ The median duration of initial remission in AML is generally less than 18 months. Once disease relapses, almost all patients are dead within 1 year unless some other form of therapy, such as BMT, is undertaken. So-called "salvage" chemotherapy of relapsed or refractory AML only works for short periods, if it is effective at all. A variety of salvage programs have been used involving standard- and high-dose cytarabine, mitoxantrone, oral idarubicin, amscarine, or a combination of mitoxantrone–etoposide–ara-C (MEC). The percentage of complete remissions with these programs may be 25% to 50%; however, such remissions generally endure 3 months or less, and the drug combinations are often very toxic. In the MEC program, major hemorrhage was observed in 39% of patients and infection in 100%.

This article examines the use of G-CSF together with induction therapy in refractory AML. As with many other studies, the use of G-CSF is associated with a faster recovery of granulocyte levels in the peripheral blood, but there is little evidence that the hemopoietin either reduces the levels of infections or improves survival.—M.J. Cline, M.D.

Myelodysplastic Syndrome and Acute Myeloid Leukemia After Treatment for Solid Tumors of Childhood
Farhi DC, Odell CA, Shurin SB (Emory Univ, Atlanta, Ga; Case Western Re-

serve Univ, Cleveland, Ohio)
Am J Clin Pathol 100:270–275, 1993   119-95-32–3

Background.—Acute myeloid leukemia (AML) and myelodysplastic syndrome (MDS) can be caused by treatment given for other malignancies. Most research on secondary AML and MDS has focused on their occurrence in adults. The occurrence of treatment-related AML and MDS in children was investigated.

Patients and Findings.—The cases of 95 children as old as 18 years of age were reviewed. Three cases of secondary hematologic malignancies were identified in this group. The affected patients, diagnosed between 1984 and 1990, were 2 boys and 1 girl, aged 10, 18, and 4 years, respectively. Acute lymphoblastic leukemia, AML, and MDS were the respective diagnoses. These cases represented 10% of all new cases of AML and MDS seen at 1 center during this period. They were unrelated to congenital factors. The 3 patients' primary tumors were an Askin tumor, neuroblastoma, and Burkitt's lymphoma, respectively. The secondary malignancies had a prominent monocytic component: acute monocytic leukemia, MDS evolving to acute myelomonocytic leukemia, and chronic myelomonocytic leukemia. The average interval between primary malignancy treatment and the onset of the new disease was 36 months. All patients had been given cyclophosphamide and an epipodophyllotoxin for the primary tumor, and 2 patients were given radiation therapy. The cytogenetic abnormalities included del(5), del(13), t(1;6), and t(9;11). After the onset of the secondary malignancy, survival time was only 5 days in the 2 younger children and 6 months in the oldest.

Conclusion.—Ten percent of new childhood cases of MDS and AML not associated with congenital disorders occurred after treatment for primary tumors that had been diagnosed 19–68 months previously. Thus, secondary MDS and AML represent a significant percentage of all MDS and AML cases in children. As the number of survivors of childhood malignancies increases, secondary hematologic disorders in children and young adults will become more important, especially as survival after the diagnosis of treatment-related MDS and AML is so short.

▶ This article describes a greatly increased incidence of myelodysplasia and AML in survivors of childhood cancer treatment.

Myelodysplasia or myelodysplastic syndrome (MDS) is the name given to a group of disorders characterized by morphologically abnormal and often ineffective hematopoiesis. Myelodysplastic syndrome usually occurs in older individuals and is characterized by anemia refractory to therapy and a variable decrease in other cells in the peripheral blood. The disorders have diverse clinical manifestations and are probably of diverse etiologies. Some cases of MDS progress to AML. In most cases, the molecular defect causing the abnormal hematopoiesis has not been identified, although chromosomal abnormalities are common, including loss of all or parts of chromosomes 5q, 7q, 12q, and 21q and translocations involving chromosomes 1 and 3.

Five groups of MDS cases are recognized in the French–American–British classification. Although this classification is obviously not very logical, as it combines malignant and nonmalignant diseases, for the moment it is the standard:

I. Refractory anemia (RA)

II. Refractory anemia with ring sideroblasts (> 15%) (RARS)

III. Refractory anemia with excess blasts (5% to 20%) (RAEB)

IV. Chronic myelomonocytic leukemia (CMML)

V. Refractory anemia with excess blasts in transformation (20% to 30% blasts)

Clinically, most patients with MDS have anemia, usually associated with some other evidence of bone marrow failure such as frequent infections and/or bleeding. In all types of MDS, abnormal red cells with marked anisocytosis and poikilocytosis, frequently with nucleated red cells, are seen in the blood. Giant platelets and abnormal monocytes and granulocytes are also frequent in some types. The bone marrow is typically hypercellular with grossly abnormal erythropoiesis. Abnormal small mononuclear and binuclear megakaryocytes occur in types III–V MDS.

Refractory anemia and refractory anemia with ring sideroblasts have anemia as their most prominent manifestation, have few myeloblasts in the bone marrow, and rarely progress to acute leukemia. On the other hand, refractory anemia with excess blasts frequently evolves into AML, and refractory anemia with excess blasts in transformation represents an early AML. Chronic myelomonocytic leukemia generally has a blood monocytosis in excess of 1 $\times$ 10^9/L. Treatment is not very satisfactory and consists mainly of transfusion support, antibiotics for infection, and iron chelation therapy for transfusion hemosiderosis. Attempts at preventing the evolution of leukemia by mild or intensive chemotherapy usually fail. Allogeneic bone marrow transplantation may be considered in younger individuals with types III, IV, or V disease who have a matched donor.

Acute myeloid leukemia developing after anticancer treatment also has a poor prognosis and responds poorly to conventional chemotherapy. Bone marrow transplantation may be considered as an alternative if a matched donor is available.—M.J. Cline, M.D.

Diagnostic Assessment of Enlarged Superficial Lymph Nodes by Fine Needle Aspiration

Pilotti S, Di Palma S, Alasio L, Bartoli C, Rilke F (Istituto Nazionale per lo Studio e la Cura dei Tumori, Milan, Italy)

Acta Cytol 37:853–866, 1993   119-95-32-4

Background.—Although fine-needle aspiration (FNA) of superficial lymph nodes is currently accepted as a reliable means of detecting metastatic diseases, its value in the diagnosis of lymphoproliferative disorders—in particular non-Hodgkin's lymphoma (NHL)—is still controver-

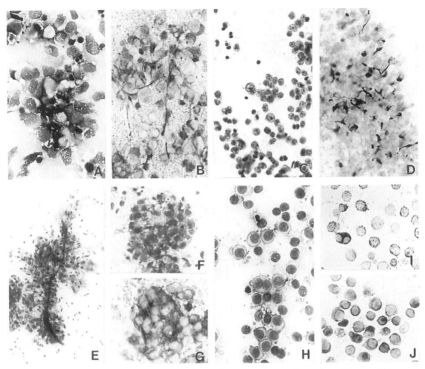

Fig 32–1.—A, B, inguinal lymph node. Metastasis from a dysgerminoma in a 15-year-old woman with a large intra-abdominal mass. Subsequent surgery revealed a tumor of the right ovary and histology a dysgerminoma. **A,** large, undifferentiated cells with delicate cytoplasm show immunoreactivity for (**B**) placental alkaline-phosphatase (**A,** May-Grünwald-Giemsa stain, ×250; **B,** immunoperoxidase, ×250). **C, D,** inguinal lymph node. Metastasis of a peripheral neuroepithelioma in a 21-year-old woman. The patient had been treated for neuroepithelioma of the abductor region of the left thigh 6 months before. **C,** small, noncohesive cells with prominent nucleoli and scanty cytoplasm were immunoreactive for (**D**) NF68Kd (**C,** May-Grünewald-Giemsa stain, ×315; **D,** immunoperoxidase on a cryopreserved smear, ×315). **E, G,** cervical lymph node. Metastasis from an endodermal sinus tumor in a 28-year-old man. The diagnosis was confirmed on a cervical nodal biopsy. The patient had advanced disease and revealed a testicular mass and multivisceral metastases. **E,** trabecular cluster of epitheliumlike cells show, at higher power; **F,** vacuolated cytoplasm that is immunoreactive for (**G**) α-fetoprotein (**E,** May-Grünewald-Giemsa stain, ×80; **F,** May-Grünewald-Giemsa stain, ×180; **G,** immunoperoxidase, ×180). **H–J,** cervical lymph node from a 38-year-old man showing metastatic malignant melanoma. The primary was removed 8 months before from the trunk at another hospital. **H,** round, occasionally binucleate tumor cells immunoreactive for (**I**) HMB45 and (**J**) S-100 protein (May-Grünewald-Giemsa stain, ×315; immunoperoxidase, ×315). The diagnoses given are the final histologic diagnoses. (Courtesy of Pilotti S, Di Palma S, Alasio L, et al: *Acta Cytol* 37:853–866, 1993.)

sial. The effectiveness of FNA in the assessment of unselected nodal enlargement suspicious for malignancy was evaluated with an emphasis on primary and recurrent low-grade NHLs.

Method.—A total of 285 outpatients with enlarged superficial lymph nodes that were either clinically suspicious (152) or had a previous diagnosis of malignant tumor (133) underwent FNA followed by excisional biopsy. Cytologic and/or cytologic-immunophenotypic diagnoses made on direct smears were compared with subsequent histologic findings.

Results.—Three groups of diseases were identified on the basis of the histologic diagnoses: 128 metastases; 88 malignant lymphomas, and 69 non-neoplastic lymphadenopathies. Within the 128 cases of metastatic tumors, involvement of the lymph nodes was obtained for 54 new cases and 62 with known primary tumors. In 11 cases, the aspirate was unsatisfactory. With the exclusion of 11 unsatisfactory aspirates, the cytologic accuracy rate of malignancy was 99.1%. Immunophenotyping aided in the final diagnosis of 27 of the 128 cases of metastatic tumors (Fig 32–1). A high rate of conclusive diagnoses were also made in the detection of high-grade non-Hodgkin's lymphomas and Hodgkin's disease, the latter with the exclusion of the lymphocytic predominance variant. In contrast, the procedure was seen to be of limited value in the assessment of low-grade malignant lymphomas. A high rate of false negative diagnoses was made for centroblastic-centrocytic follicular lymphomas, emphasizing the difficulty in differentiating this type of NHL from reactive processes. Immunocytochemistry also appeared to be of limited value in the differentiation of centroblastic-centrocytic follicular lymphomas and reactive follicular hyperplasia.

Conclusion.—The diagnostic value of FNA as the initial step in the workup of patients with clinically suspicious enlarged superficial lymph nodes was confirmed. However the procedure is of limited value in the diagnosis of low-grade malignant lymphomas characterized by a substantial nonmalignant component and, in particular, centroblastic-centrocytic follicular lymphoma. Only the application of molecular techniques will provide conclusive information in most of these cases and will, thus, enhance the efficacy of FNA in NHLs.

▶ Fine-needle aspiration is a good place to start in the evaluation of lymphadenopathy. The accuracy of diagnosis of most malignancies is very high, but the procedure is of limited value in lymphomas and leukemias in which there are a predominance of mature-appearing small lymphocytes.—M.J. Cline, M.D.

Randomized Comparison of MACOP-B With CHOP in Patients With Intermediate-Grade Non-Hodgkin's Lymphoma
Cooper IA, for the Australian and New Zealand Lymphoma Group (Peter MacCallum Cancer Inst, Melbourne, Australia)
J Clin Oncol 12:769–778, 1994   119-95-32–5

Background.—In several prospective randomized, controlled trials conducted by the Australian and New Zealand Lymphoma Group (ANZLG), complete response rates in patients with non-Hodgkin's lymphoma (NHL) have remained between 50% and 60%, with no advantage associated with regimens more intensive than cyclophosphamide, doxorubicin, vincristine, and prednisolone (CHOP) therapy. Initial encouraging results from a study of a regimen of methotrexate, doxorubicin, cyclophosphamide, vincristine, prednisolone, and bleomycin (MACOP-B) prompted a new ANZLG study comparing MACOP-B with CHOP chemotherapy in patients with NHL.

Methods.—A total of 304 patients were enrolled in the study between October 1986 and June 1991. To be eligible for randomization, patients had to have diffuse small cleaved-cell, diffuse mixed small- and large-cell, follicular large-cell, diffuse large-cell, or large-cell immunoblastic stages I bulky or II to IV disease. Application of criteria left 236 patients eligible for analysis.

Findings.—Patients in the MACOP-B and CHOP treatment arms did not differ in complete response rates, failure-free survival, or overall survival. When patients were stratified by prognostic group, the death rate of patients in the MACOP-B group compared with the CHOP group was estimated to be .91. None of the prognostic subgroups in the 2 regimens differed significantly. The MACOP-B treatment was associated with significantly more severe toxicity, especially cutaneous toxicity, stomatitis, and gastrointestinal ulceration. The mean relative dose-intensities of MACOP-B and CHOP were .91 and .90, respectively, indicating good dose delivery.

Conclusion.—In these patients with intermediate-grade NHL, CHOP chemotherapy yielded results comparable to those of MACOP-B, with significantly fewer toxic complications. Although results in some subgroups are relatively poor with CHOP, this treatment remains the standard chemotherapy for NHL.

▶ Non-Hodgkin's lymphomas are a heterogeneous group of diseases. They are monoclonal malignancies that arise from cells of the lymphoid system. Approximately 85% arise from B cells and about 15% from T-cell precursors. Rare lymphomas arise from other cell types such as dendritic cells. The B-cell lymphomas fall into the 7 main categories. About 40% are follicular and another 40% are diffuse. A follicular pattern means that there is some preservation of nodal architecture; a diffuse pattern means it is destroyed. In addition to distinctive cell surface markers for each category of lymphoma, for some there are identified chromosomal or molecular abnormalities. For example, the great majority of follicular lymphomas have an abnormality of the *bcl*-2 gene, which is involved in lymphoid cell apoptosis, and nearly 100% of Burkitt's lymphomas have an *myc* gene translocation.

The T-cell lymphomas are even less well defined by phenotypic and molecular markers than the B-cell disorders. Certain points are clear, however. Acute T-cell leukemia/lymphoma is a well-defined entity, and those lymphomas with a predilection for skin involvement are usually of T–helper-cell phenotype. Some of the diffuse large cell lymphomas are of T phenotype.

The main features to be ascertained about a lymphoma are: whether it is follicular or diffuse, and whether it contains small, well-differentiated cells or large, poorly differentiated cells. From this information, one can generally conclude whether the tumor is of high, low, or intermediate grade and can make certain limited predictions about clinical behavior. Those with a follicular pattern and those with relatively small uniform lymphoid cells generally have a more favorable natural history but rarely enter complete remission with chemotherapy.

In general, the objective of treatment of the low-grade lymphomas is palliation rather than cure of disease. One reason for this is the extreme difficulty of achieving a complete remission of disease short of using life-endangering levels of chemotherapy or radiation therapy. Paradoxically, high-grade lymphomas, such as those discussed in this article, which have a more aggressive natural history, may be brought into remission in as many as 50% to 70% of cases, and nearly 40% may be cured by intensive therapy. Many types of drugs are effective against lymphomas including alkylating agents, vinca alkaloids, corticosteroids, anthracycline antibiotics, nitrosoureas, and etoposides. In addition, radiation therapy is used to treat symptomatic local disease, or more extensively in programs aimed at disease eradication. As discussed in previous YEAR BOOKS, there has been a recent tendency to return to CHOP chemotherapy as the standard in the NHLs. Additionally, intensive multimodality therapy combined with autologous bone marrow transplantation is being used increasingly in high-grade lymphomas, as discussed in the next chapter.—M.J. Cline, M.D.

Recombinant Interferon Alfa-2b Combined With A Regimen Containing Doxorubicin in Patients With Advanced Follicular Lymphoma

Solal-Celigny P, for the Groupe d'Etude des Lymphomes de l'Adulte (Hôpital Saint-Louis, Paris)
N Engl J Med 329:1608–1614, 1993　　　　　　　119-95-32-6

Objective.—Because interferon alfa and cytotoxic drugs act synergistically against non-Hodgkin's lymphoma (NHL), an open phase III trial was planned at 31 medical centers to determine the value of combining a chemotherapy regimen including doxorubicin with recombinant interferon-α to treat patients with follicular NHL.

Study Plan.—A total of 242 patients with advanced low-grade disease were studied. They were previously untreated and had small-cell or mixed-cell follicular NHL at Ann Arbor stages II through IV. Each patient had a large tumor burden. All received cyclophosphamide, doxorubicin, teniposide, and prednisone (CHVP) treatment at monthly intervals for 6 cycles, and then every other month for 1 year. In addition, 123 patients were randomly selected to receive 5 million units of interferon-α-2b, 3 times a week for 18 months.

Results.—After 6 cycles of chemotherapy, 58% of patients given CHVP alone and 76% of those also given, interferon had responded. The rates of complete remission were 13% and 20%, respectively, which was not a significant difference. The final response rates were 69% with chemotherapy alone and 85% with combined treatment. Event-free sur-

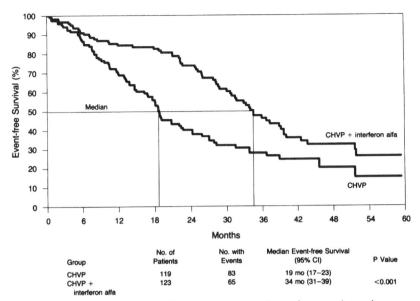

Group	No. of Patients	No. with Events	Median Event-free Survival (95% CI)	P Value
CHVP	119	83	19 mo (17–23)	
CHVP + interferon alfa	123	65	34 mo (31–39)	<0.001

Fig 32–2.—*Abbreviation: CI,* confidence interval. Estimated event-free survival according to treatment group. (Courtesy of Solal-Celigny P, for the Groupe d'Etude des Lymphomes de l'Adulte: *N Engl J Med* 329:1608–1614, 1993.)

vival was significantly longer in patients given interferon during a median follow-up of nearly 3 years (Fig 32–2).

Safety.—Both neutropenia and associated infection were more frequent in interferon-treated patients. One patient in each treatment group had significant cardiotoxicity from doxorubicin. Interferon therapy was withdrawn in 11% of patients because of adverse reactions.

Conclusion.—Adding interferon-α to doxorubicin-based chemotherapy significantly prolongs event-free survival in patients with advanced low-grade follicular NHL.

▶ Follicular lymphomas are the most common type of NHL. Most are low grade and have an indolent course that may last 7–10 years. Some patients, usually those with a larger tumor burden, may have a more aggressive course, with death occurring within 3–5 years of diagnosis. The great majority are not cured by modern aggressive chemotherapy and are consequently treated by simple minimal chemotherapy such as alkylating agents. However, because most patients die of lymphoma, investigators have constantly explored new treatment protocols. This study explores the use of interferon-α in combination with a multiagent, moderately aggressive chemotherapy program similar to that used in high-grade lymphomas. Interferon added benefit to the anticancer drugs in terms of response, survival, and event-free survival, but it was toxic and had to be stopped in 11% of treated patients.

The longest experience with interferon for the treatment of a hematologic malignancy is in hairy cell leukemia, where it was first used in 1984. For several years thereafter, it remained an important therapy for this disease, until it was replaced by nucleoside analogue drugs. As noted in the 1994 YEAR BOOK OF MEDICINE, second malignancies were a surprisingly common cause of death in patients with hairy cell leukemia treated with interferon (1).—M.J. Cline, M.D.

Reference

1. 1994 YEAR BOOK OF MEDICINE, pp 264–265.

Interferon Alfa-2a as Compared With Conventional Chemotherapy for the Treatment of Chronic Myeloid Leukemia

Baccarani M, for The Italian Cooperative Study Group on Chronic Myeloid Leukemia (Udine Univ, Italy)
N Engl J Med 330:820–825, 1994   119-95-32–7

Objective.—Indications that interferon-α is an effective treatment for chronic myeloid leukemia (CML) and prolongs survival prompted a prospective study comparing this agent with conventional chemotherapy.

Study Plan.—A total of 322 patients with Philadelphia (Ph^1) chromosome–positive CML, who had received minimal or no treatment, were randomly assigned to receive interferon-α-2a or conventional chemotherapy. All 218 patients in the interferon group received a daily dose of 3 million IU for 2 weeks, 6 million IU for 2 weeks, and then 9 million IU. After 8 months, the dose was increased according to the karyotypic response. The 104 patients given conventional chemotherapy received hydroxyurea as the first-line agent. Ten patients later received busulfan in place of hydroxyurea.

Results.—A karyotypic response, defined as a lack of the Ph^1 chromosome in at least one third of metaphases, was observed in 30% of interferon-treated patients and 5% of those given conventional chemotherapy. The median interval to an accelerated or blastic phase was longer in the interferon group (72 vs. 45 months). Median survival also was greater in the interferon group (72 vs. 52 months). Half the interferon-treated patients and 29% of those treated conventionally lived 6 years. One treatment-related death occurred in each group. Interferon therapy was withdrawn because of side effects in 16% of cases. The cost of interferon treatment was 200 times more than conventional chemotherapy.

Conclusion.—Interferon-α should be first-line treatment for CML. It may be even more effective in delaying the progression of disease and prolonging survival than was apparent in this study.

▶ Chronic myeloid leukemia is classified among the myeloproliferative disorders, which include acute myeloid leukemia, polycythemia rubra vera, myeloid metaplasia, and essential thrombocytosis. It is a monoclonal disease that arises from an abnormality in a hemopoietic stem cell that can differentiate into several different lineages: granulocyte, macrophage, basophil, erythroid, and megakaryocyte; however, the predominant manifestation is in the granulocyte lineage.

Even before the modern era of therapy, CML usually evolved relatively slowly over months or even years, hence the designation of *chronic*. With modern treatment, the white blood cell count and splenomegaly are kept suppressed, and there may be little external manifestation of disease. Eventually, but usually within a period of 3–5 years, the course of the disease changes. The white cell count rises, more primitive cells appear in the marrow and blood, anemia and thrombocytopenia may become prominent, and therapy is less effective—in short, the picture of an acute leukemia. The disease is said to have entered the *blast crisis* phase. Life expectancy is now usually less than 18 months. Between the chronic and blast crisis phases of CML, there may be an intermediate *accelerated* phase of increasing white cell count, increasing splenomegaly, and drug resistance.

The fusion of *c-ABL* with another gene, called *BCR,* results in a characteristic chromosomal translocation called the Ph[1] chromosome, t(9;22). The Ph[1] chromosome was identified in 1960 and was the first consistent chromosomal anomaly in a cancer. It is detected in virtually all cases of CML. It is formed by a reciprocal translocation that fuses part of the *BCR* gene on chromosome 9 with sequences upstream of exon 2 of the *c-ABL* proto-oncogene on chromosome 22. This fusion produces a protein of 210 kd that is larger than the normal ABL protein. Its tyrosine kinase activity is expressed inappropriately, sending an unregulated proliferation signal to the nucleus of the cell.

Although fusion of the *c-ABL* and *BCR* genes is the pathogenetic lesion in the chronic phase of CML, other molecular changes are necessary for progression to the blast crisis phase. The genes most often implicated in this progression are *p53* and *Rb1*. Their structures are almost always normal in the chronic phase but are frequently deranged in blast crisis.

For many years, busulfan and hydroxyurea have been the staples of therapy of CML. They are used to suppress the elevated white cell count and other manifestations of disease without attempting to eliminate the Ph[1] positive cell clone from the bone marrow. Recently, interferon-α has been used in treatment. Although it is a more difficult drug to use, it may produce longer remissions of disease and occasionally suppresses the Ph[1] clone in the marrow, as shown in this article.

The authors of this article conclude that interferon is superior to drug therapy despite its higher costs, greater difficulty in administration, and more side effects. They believe it should be used as standard therapy. I am not so certain that there is enough information to make that judgment.

In younger patients, intensive treatment followed by allogeneic bone marrow transplantation is often used in an attempt to cure disease. The success rate is greater than 50%. In allogeneic bone marrow transplantation, the induction of graft-versus-host disease may have an antileukemic effect.—M.J. Cline, M.D.

Chronic Lymphocytic Leukemia: A Retrospective Study of 122 Cases
Erlanson M, Osterman B, Jonsson H, Lenner P (Umeå Univ, Sweden)
Eur J Haematol 52:108–114, 1994   119-95-32-8

Introduction.—Chronic lymphocytic leukemia may have a benign course with minimal symptoms or it may be highly malignant and difficult to treat. Current data on the natural history are based on a young population because older patients may not have been referred. Older patients from northern Sweden were examined retrospectively. Symptoms, disease staging, and prognosis were reported.

Methods.—All patients in whom the diagnosis of chronic lymphocytic leukemia was made and recorded in the regional cancer registry were reviewed. Of the 143 patients registered, 122 met the criteria for review. Patients were grouped according to Binet state with 61 stage A, 29 stage B, and 32 stage C patients. The median follow-up was 105 months. Survival curves were determined from diagnosis to end of follow-up or death.

Results.—The overall incidence was 4.7 of 100,000 males and 2.7 of 100,000 females. The 2.2:1 male-to-female ratio was higher than expected. The majority of diagnoses were made when the patient saw a physician for other reasons or during a periodic health examination. This was most frequent for Binet stage A patients. Treatment was administered to 48 patients immediately and to 32 after a range of 1–81 months; the remaining 42 received no treatment. The therapy included 15 patients receiving steroids only, 43 receiving monochemotherapy, 17 receiving combination chemotherapy, and 5 receiving radiotherapy. Complete remission was seen in 12 patients (all receiving combination chemotherapy). Survival was not statistically longer for patients who had delayed treatment vs. those who had immediate treatment (64 vs. 51 months). Patients who had no treatment survived a median of 35 months, which was not statistically different from the 51 months for those who received treatment. Crude survival for all patients was 51 months with no difference between stages. However, when cause-specific mortality was determined, Binet stages A, B, and C survived 102, 80, and 63 months, respectively with age (older than 70 years) and sex (male) increasing the risk of cause-specific death. Of the 90 patients in stages A and B, 34 progressed to stage C in about 26 to 27 months. During the examination period, 102 patients died, 43 from reasons unrelated to chronic lymphocytic leukemia, with unrelated deaths occurring most commonly in stage A patients. Of these 43 patients, 30 showed underlying disease related to the leukemia. Other malignancies were found in 16 patients.

Discussion.—In this population of patients, the staging systems were not pertinent because so many of the patients had no symptoms and diagnosis was made in passing during clinic visits for other reasons. An advanced stage of the disease, however, was associated with a high risk of death, whereas death resulting from unrelated causes was frequent for early stages of disease, resulting in a crude survival rate that was not different between these 2 groups.

▶ Chronic lymphocytic leukemia (CLL) is by far the most common of the chronic lymphoid leukemias. It is almost always a malignancy of B cells. Cases of T-cell origin are rare, and some cases of typical CLL make a transition to prolymphocytic leukemia with the passage of time. Chronic lymphocytic leukemia is usually a disease of the elderly, and cases before the age of 40 years are rare. The onset is often insidious, with a gradually increasing blood lymphocytosis followed after months or years by increasing generalized lymphadenopathy and splenomegaly. At presentation, many patients are asymptomatic, and the diagnosis is often made at the time of a routine blood count that reveals lymphocytosis. If the disease is left untreated, the white blood cell count may eventually exceed 500×10^9/L, and the lymph nodes and spleen may be massively enlarged. With time, manifestations of both immunodeficiency and autoimmune phenomena frequently develop. Bacterial, fungal, and viral infections; autoimmune hemolytic anemia; and immune thrombocytopenic purpura may follow.

The blood count invariably reveals a lymphocytosis, usually with typical, mature-appearing small lymphocytes. The cells have low-density surface immunoglobulin. Anemia may be present and have the characteristics either of a normochromic, normocytic anemia of chronic disease or of a Coombs' positive hemolytic anemia. The platelet count may be normal or low. With advanced disease, the bone marrow and lymph nodes are densely infiltrated by a uniform population of small lymphocytes. The morphology of the nodes may be indistinguishable from that of small-cell, well-differentiated lymphoma, which is probably a variant of the same disease as CLL.

The commonly used clinical staging system for CLL is that described by Rai in 1975, although other classification schemes—such as the one used in this article—simply divide patients into good, intermediate, and poor prognosis categories. The good prognosis category has no significant anemia or thrombocytopenia and less than 3 sites of palpable organ enlargement. The molecular defect in B-cell CLL is not known, although there are some frequent sites of chromosomal abnormality.

Patients in the earlier stages of CLL often do not require any therapy. Increasing lymphocytosis, lymphadenopathy, and splenomegaly are often treated with an alkylating drug given by mouth. Patients with autoimmune manifestations of disease and those with marked suppression of normal hematopoiesis often receive adrenocorticosteroids as well. Because of the advanced age of most of the patients, few are candidates for bone marrow transplantation.

This article describes the natural history of CLL, and I have chosen it as the introduction to the following articles, which describe new directions in therapy. Note that many patients with CLL require no therapy for long periods. The median survival for those with early-stage disease is about 9 years, and many patients with CLL die of other diseases.—M.J. Cline, M.D.

Results of Fludarabine and Prednisone Therapy in 264 Patients With Chronic Lymphocytic Leukemia With Multivariate Analysis-Derived Prognostic Model for Response to Treatment

O'Brien S, Kantarjian H, Beran M, Smith T, Koller C, Estey E, Robertson LE, Lerner S, Keating M (M.D. Anderson Cancer Ctr, Houston)

Blood 82:1695–1700, 1993   119-95-32–9

Background.—Prednisone is often used together with chlorambucil in the treatment of chronic lymphocytic leukemia (CLL). In an attempt to improve the remission rates and duration of remission in CLL, a trial of prednisone and fludarabine was initiated.

Methods.—A total of 264 patients with CLL were given IV fludarabine, 30 mg/m², for 30 minutes each day for 5 days and oral prednisone, 30 mg/m², each day for 5 days. This course was repeated every month.

Findings.—Overall response (OR) and complete response (CR) rates were 52% and 37%, respectively, in 169 previously treated patients. In this patient group, the respective OR and CR rates were 74% and 63% in patients with Rai stage 0–II disease and 64% and 46% in patients with Rai stage III–IV disease. Among previously untreated patients, OR and CR rates were 79% and 63%, respectively. The respective OR and CR rates in this group were 85% and 70% in Rai 0–II patients and 64% and 46% in Rai III–IV patients. The incidence of minor infections or fever of unknown origin, occurring in 22% of the courses, was similar in all patient groups. The incidences of sepsis and pneumonia were significantly associated with the extent of previous treatment and Rai stage, ranging from 3% of courses in previously untreated patients with Rai stage 0–II disease to 13% in previously treated patients with Rai stage III–IV disease. Fourteen patients had *Listeria* sepsis or *Pneumocystis carinii* pneumonia. Response and infection rates were identical to those occurring in 110 patients treated with the same dose schedule of fludarabine alone. Factors significantly associated with poorer response were Rai stages III–IV, previous treatment, older age, and low albumin levels.

Conclusion.—The combination of fludarabine and prednisone is an effective regimen for treating patients with CLL. However, adding prednisone did not increase the response rate vs. that achieved with fludarabine alone.

▶ There has been some progress in the treatment of CLL in the past few years with the introduction of new agents such as fludarabine and 2-chloro-deoxyadenosine. Fludarabine was first introduced in 1986. In a study of 236 patients treated according to a National Cancer Institute protocol, 2% achieved a complete remission and 35% achieved a partial remission with the drug. It is often effective in disease that has become resistant to alkylating agents, such as chlorambucil, and may produce response rates of about 50% in previously treated patients. For the moment, chlorambucil with or without pulse prednisone is still the standard treatment for CLL, and fludarabine is reserved for resistant/refractory disease. In previously reviewed studies, fludarabine appeared to be quite good in low-grade follicular lymphomas, with response rates of about 60%.

Like most chemotherapeutic agents, fludarabine does have some undesirable side effects. It suppresses normal hematopoiesis in the bone marrow, and it is toxic to CD4-positive lymphocytes. The resultant immunosuppression sets the stage for opportunistic infection. Because immunodeficiency is often a feature of CLL—particularly in advanced disease—the additional immunosuppression of fludarabine is a problem.

This article examined whether the combination of prednisone with fludarabine is better than fludarabine alone. Answer: *It is not.*—M.J. Cline, M.D.

Lack of Effect of 2-Chlorodeoxyadenosine Therapy in Patients With Chronic Lymphocytic Leukemia Refractory to Fludarabine Therapy
O'Brien S, Kantarjian H, Estey E, Koller C, Robertson B, Beran M, Andreeff M, Pierce S, Keating M (M.D. Anderson Cancer Ctr, Houston)
N Engl J Med 330:319–322, 1994   119-95-32–10

Background.—Fludarabine and 2-chlorodeoxyadenosine (2-CdA) are nucleoside analogues that have proven effective in treatment of patients with chronic lymphocytic leukemia (CLL). The drugs are believed to have similar mechanisms of action, but a small number of patients who fail to respond to fludarabine have responded to 2-CdA.

Objective.—The efficacy of 2-CdA was examined in 28 patients with CLL that had proven refractory to fludarabine treatment. The patients had a median age of 63 years. A large majority had advanced disease with anemia and/or thrombocytopenia.

Treatment.—All the patients had received alkylating agents before fludarabine, and two thirds received other treatment after a trial of fludarabine—most often an anthracycline-based regimen or etoposide with or without mitoxantrone. The median interval from fludarabine treatment and the use of 2-CdA was 1 month. A dose of 4 mg/m^2 of 2-CdA daily was given by continuous infusion for 1 week. Treatment could be repeated at monthly intervals.

Results.—Two of the 28 patients had a partial response to 2-CdA treatment. Minor antitumor activity was noted in some other patients who failed to meet criteria for remission. Only 1 patient with anemia or thrombocytopenia improved appreciably. Ten patients died during the first 2 monthly courses of 2-CdA. Myelosuppression was frequent; a majority of patients sustained neutropenia and thrombocytopenia. Non-hematologic toxicity was minimal.

Conclusion.—Patients with CLL who fail to respond to fludarabine and who have poor marrow reserve are not likely to enter remission if given 2-CdA, which itself induces substantial myelosuppression.

▶ 2-Chlorodeoxyadenosine is another interesting new addition to our therapeutic armamentarium. It is one of the few new treatments for Waldenstrom's macroglobulinemia to be introduced in the past 2 decades. Fludarabine and 2-CdA are now widely used in many B-cell malignancies including CLL, hairy cell leukemia, and indolent lymphomas. They are thought to have the same or a similar mechanism of action. It is not surprising, therefore, as this article shows, that only very rare patients with CLL previously treated with fludarabine can be expected to respond to 2-CdA.—M.J. Cline, M.D.

Complete Remissions in Hairy Cell Leukemia With 2-Chlorodeoxyadenosine After Failure With 2′-Deoxycoformycin
Saven A, Piro LD (Scripps Clinic and Research Found, La Jolla, Calif)
Ann Intern Med 119:278–283, 1993   119-95-32–11

Background.—Hairy cell leukemia, or leukemic reticuloendotheliosis, is an uncommon, chronic B-cell lymphoproliferative disorder primarily affecting elderly men. Both 2-chlorodeoxyadenosine (2-CdA) and 2′-deoxycoformycin (DCF) are active agents in the treatment of this disease. These 2 agents are similar structurally and affect the same enzyme pathway. Thus, a group of patients with hairy cell leukemia resistant to or intolerant of DCF were treated with 2-CdA to determine the cross-resistance and safety of such therapy.

Methods.—Five patients were studied in a phase II clinical trial. Three were resistant to DCF, and 2 had experienced life-threatening toxic reactions to it. A single course of 2-CdA was given at .1 mg/kg per day for 7 days by continuous IV infusion.

Outcomes.—A complete response was achieved in 4 patients, with a median follow-up of more than 11 months. A partial response was noted in the fifth patient in whom splenectomy, interferon, and DCF treatment had been unsuccessful. This partial response lasted 2 months. The patient subsequently died of *Streptococcus pneumoniae* bacteremia. Three of the complete responders continued in unmaintained remission, and the fourth had progressive splenic enlargement with stable hematologic parameters. The median leukocyte count rose from 2×10^9/L to 3.8×10^9/L, and the median absolute neutrophil count increased from .56 $\times 10^9$/L to 2.73 $\times 10^9$/L. Increases also occurred in the median hemoglobin level, from 112 g/L to 140 g/L, and in the median platelet count, from 55 $\times 10^9$/L to 123 $\times 10^9$/L. Treatment was associated with culture-negative neutropenic fever in 2 patients.

Conclusion.—There is a lack of cross-resistance between DCF and 2-CdA in patients with hairy cell leukemia. Furthermore, 2-CdA is not prohibitively toxic in patients who cannot tolerate DCF, suggesting that the therapeutic-to-toxic ratio for 2-CdA is superior to that of DCF in this patient population. Further research, involving larger numbers of patients, is needed to study the immunosuppressive effects and their clinical consequences in patients treated with multiple nucleoside agents.

▶ Hairy cell leukemia (HCL) is an indolent B-cell malignancy, although very rare T-cell variants have been reported. First described in 1958, its original name was leukemic reticuloendotheliosis. Patients with HCL are typically middle-aged men whose disease presents with pancytopenia and marked splenomegaly without much lymphadenopathy. Susceptibility to infection with opportunistic pathogens is prominent and is often the principal clinical feature of the disease. The marrow, which is usually packed with lymphoid cells and reticulin fibers, is difficult to aspirate. The hairy cells in the marrow have abundant pale cytoplasm, giving them the appearance of a fried egg. The blood smear contains lymphoid cells with fine hairlike projections of the cytoplasm. The cells stain strongly for tartrate-resistant acid phosphatase and often show perinuclear staining with a naphthyl butyrate esterase. Finding these cells in the appropriate clinical setting makes the diagnosis.

Therapy is often instituted when the patient has severe neutropenia, thrombocytopenia, or recurrent infections. In recent years, nucleotide analogues such as 2-deoxycoformycin, 2-CdA, and fludarabine have largely replaced interferon-α and early splenectomy in treatment, although splenectomy is sometimes still used later in the disease. 2-Chlorodeoxyadenosine is emerging as the treatment of choice because there is minimal toxicity associated with induction of durable remissions after a single course of treatment. This article demonstrates that complete remissions can be achieved with this drug. Corticosteroids should be avoided. The disease process often goes on for years if therapy is mishandled.—M.J. Cline, M.D.

High-Dose Sequential Chemoradiotherapy, a Widely Applicable Regimen, Confers Survival Benefit to Patients With High-Risk Multiple Myeloma

Gianni AM, Tarella C, Bregni M, Siena S, Lombardi F, Gandola L, Caracciolo D, Stern A, Bonadonna G, Boccadoro M, Pileri A (Istituto Nazionale, Tumori, Milan, Italy; Univ of Milan, Italy; Univ of Turin, Italy; et al)
J Clin Oncol 12:503–509, 1994   119-95-32–12

Background.—Despite recent advances in standard-dose chemotherapy, the prognosis for multiple myeloma has not appreciably changed. The toxicity, efficacy, and applicability of high-dose treatment with bone marrow and/or peripheral-blood autotransplantation were assessed in high-risk, previously untreated patients with multiple myeloma.

Methods.—Thirteen patients with high-labeling index (LI) multiple myeloma were treated with a novel high-dose sequential (HDS) regimen: cyclophosphamide (7 g/m²), followed by vincristine (1.4 mg/m²), methotrexate (8 g/m²) with leukovorin rescue, etoposide (2 g/m²), total body irradiation (10 Gy), and melphalan (120 mg/m²), with autografting of peripheral blood hematopoietic progenitor cells. Recombinant human granulocyte-macrophage colony-stimulating factor was infused continuously after cyclophosphamide and etoposide to accelerate hematopoietic recovery and expand the hematopoietic progenitor-cell pool.

Findings.—Twelve patients completed treatment. Seventy-seven percent responded completely. Five are alive without disease after a median follow-up of 36 months. The length of freedom from disease progression and overall survival were significantly better in the HDS-treated patients than in 19 well-matched historical control patients.

Conclusion.—High-dose sequential therapy is an effective, well-tolerated, widely accessible regimen that can increase survival in patients with high-LI multiple myeloma. Studies of larger numbers of patients using this or a similar protocol in standard-risk myeloma are now warranted.

▶ Multiple myeloma is typically a disease of the middle-aged or elderly, and cases are rare before the fourth decade of life. This age distribution often influences how aggressive one can be in therapy.

The well-known clinical manifestations of multiple myeloma are produced by: first, loss of normal hematopoietic cells from the bone marrow; second, osteolysis by products of the neoplastic cells; and finally, the effects of high concentrations of paraprotein.

Loss of normal hematopoietic cells results in a variable degree of anemia, leukopenia, and thrombocytopenia. Defects in normal immune function contribute to increased susceptibility to infection, and *Streptococcus pneumoniae* infection is particularly common. Thrombocytopenia, plus coating of the remaining platelets with paraprotein, contributes to a bleeding diathesis.

Lytic lesions of bone may be the result of production of osteoclast activating factor by plasma cells. The lesions may be localized, widespread, or manifest as generalized osteoporosis. Lytic lesions of the skull are typical, but any bone may be involved. Lesions are usually painful and often result in fractures of weight-bearing bones. Vertebral collapse with damage to the spinal cord is a dreaded complication.

The paraprotein produced by the myeloma cells is excreted by the kidneys and may cause damage to the tubules. This may be exacerbated by nephrocalcinosis produced by high concentrations of calcium mobilized from bone and by pyelonephritis. With all these assaults on the kidney, it is not surprising that renal failure is a common complication. Some cases of multiple myeloma also have amyloid deposition in the tissues, with resultant hepatosplenomegaly, macroglossia, and cardiac and renal damage.

Typically, in multiple myeloma the paraprotein does not reach high enough levels in blood to produce a hyperviscosity syndrome, except in the IgA variant where multimers of the immunoglobulin can increase serum viscosity to the dangerous levels frequently encountered in macroglobulinemia (IgM paraproteinemia). Cerebral and sometimes pulmonary manifestations of impaired blood flow result.

Death in multiple myeloma usually occurs from renal failure or infection, usually within 3–5 years of diagnosis. One gauges the results of therapy in multiple myeloma by following the level of paraprotein in blood and urine and by repeated aspirations of bone marrow for evaluating plasma cell number. For decades, the standard treatment of multiple myeloma has been a combination of an alkylating agent, such as melphalan or cyclophosphamide, with corticosteroid. The combination often reduces the body burden of plasma cells and occasionally improves azotemia but rarely produces complete remission of disease. There have been many attempts, such as the one described in this article, at more aggressive therapy, but generally they have contributed little. Recently, there has been a vogue for intensive therapy and autologous bone marrow transplantation in younger patients. Its benefits are still uncertain.—M.J. Cline, M.D.

High-Dose Melphalan for Multiple Myeloma: Long-Term Follow-Up Data
Cunningham D, Paz-Ares L, Gore ME, Malpas J, Hickish T, Nicolson M, Meldrum M, Viner C, Milan S, Selby PJ, Norman A, Raymond J, Powles R (Royal Marsden Hosp, Sutton, England; St Bartholomew's Hosp, London)
J Clin Oncol 12:764–768, 1994   119-95-32-13

Introduction.—Long-term survival is uncommon in patients with multiple myeloma, despite efforts to increase the intensity of standard chemotherapy regimens. There have been some encouraging results, however, with the use of single-agent high-dose melphalan (HDM). Sixty-three previously untreated patients with multiple myeloma were followed for a median of 74 months to assess the long-term results of HDM.

Patients and Methods.—Patients were enrolled in the prospective study between November 1981 and April 1986. The group included 43 men and 20 women and had a median age of 48 years. Fifty-one had stage III myeloma. All patients received a priming dose of cyclophosphamide (400 mg/m² as an IV bolus), followed in 7 days by melphalan (140 mg/m² as an IV bolus). Complete remission (CR) was defined as normal bone marrow morphology and no measurable serum or urine paraprotein for at least 3 months. Patients in partial remission (PR) showed a 50% or greater reduction in serum and urine myeloma protein and improvement in all other clinical features sustained for more than 1 month. Relapse was treated with second-line chemotherapy when clinically indicated.

Results.—Nine patients died within 2 months after the first course of HDM. The overall response rate was 82%, with 32% of patients achieving CR. The median duration of response in the 52 patients who entered CR or PR was 18 months. Of these patients, 41 received additional therapy at relapse. Three patients have remained in CR and 3 in PR for periods ranging from 60+ to 84+ months. For the group as a whole, the median survival is 47 months and estimated survival at 9 years is 34.5%. There have been no second malignancies or other late side effects from treatment. Both male sex and early-stage disease were associated in univariate analysis with significantly longer survival.

Conclusion.—If the 9 early deaths are excluded, only 2 patients did not respond and 32% entered CR. Patients who achieved CR were similar in duration of response and survival to patients who achieved PR. The quality of life was improved, especially in terms of pain control and performance status. High-dose melphalan improved response rates and survival duration relative to other therapies and is a valuable first-line treatment in patients with myeloma.

▶ This article explores the use of high-dose intensive therapy of multiple myeloma. The standard treatment of this disease against which other programs are judged consists of prednisone in combination with melphalan, an alkylating agent. Physicians, dissatisfied with the limited achievements of this program, have explored progressively more aggressive and more toxic combinations of drugs to treat multiple myeloma. Most of these combinations of drugs have proven to be no better, and many were worse, than melphalan and prednisone. One drug combination called VAD (vincristine-Adriamycin-dexamethasone) is useful and is widely used in patients with poor prognostic markers or whose disease is resistant to melphalan and prednisone. However, there are other options in treatment. In the 1994 YEAR BOOK OF MEDICINE (1), we reviewed dexamethasone as a single agent for the treatment of multiple myeloma, and we also reviewed the "minimalist" approach of watchful waiting, which has something to recommend it for those patients with minimal disease.

Most students of this disease agree that HDM and other more aggressive approaches should be reserved for cases with indicators of poor prognosis, including a short interval between asymptomatic illness and progressive disease, multiple bone lesions identifiable by conventional radiographs, peak serum proteins of greater than 30 g/L, or Bence Jones proteinuria or other evidence of renal involvement.—M.J. Cline, M.D.

Reference

1. 1994 YEAR BOOK OF MEDICINE, pp 257–259.

Peripheral Neuropathy in IgM Monoclonal Gammopathy and Wäldenstrom's Macroglobulinemia: A Frequent Complication in Elderly Males With Low MAG-Reactive Serum Monoclonal Component

Baldini L, Nobile-Orazio E, Guffanti A, Barbieri S, Carpo M, Cro L, Cesana B, Damilano I, Maiolo AT (G Marcora Centre for Blood Diseases, Milan, Italy; Dino Ferrari Centre for Neuromuscular Diseases, Milan, Italy; Univ of Milan,

Italy; et al)
Am J Hematol 45:25–31, 1994   119-95-32–14

Purpose.—Among patients with IgM monoclonal gammopathy or primary macroglobulinemia (PM), peripheral neuropathy (PN) is a common complication. Neuropathologic studies of this complication suggest an immunologic cause. However, there are few data on the associations between PN and the clinicopathologic aspects of the hematologic disease responsible for the IgM monoclonal gammopathy. The incidence of peripheral nervous system involvement in 65 consecutive patients with PM of varying severity was examined.

Methods.—The patients were 44 men and 21 women with a mean age of 62 years. Thirty-one were classified as having monoclonal gammopathies of undetermined significance (MGUS), 24 as having indolent Waldenström's macroglobulinemia (IWM), and 10 as having symptomatic Waldenström's macroglobulinemia. A full neurologic examination was performed in all patients, including electrodiagnostic studies and measurement of serum antimyelin-associated glycoprotein (MAG) titer.

Findings.—The overall prevalence of PN was 32%. Seventy-three percent of the patients with PN had both clinical and electrophysiologic signs of the complication, mainly of the demyelinating type. The PN was significantly correlated with male sex, older age, low monoclonal component levels, high anti-MAG titers, and high hemoglobin. Although most of the patients with PN, especially demyelinating PN, had MGUS or IWM, the correlation was not significant. After multivariate analysis, the correlations of PN with sex and anti-MAG titer remained significant; MAG reactivity was absent in 38% of patients with PN.

Conclusion.—These findings add to the evidence for an antibody-mediated origin of PN in many cases. The development of PN appears to rely more on the characteristics of the proliferating pathologic B clone than on the tumor burden or the type of macroglobulinemia. A number of simple variables to select patients at risk of PN were identified.

▶ A variety of diseases are associated with an abnormal paraprotein in the blood. They may be divided into diseases routinely associated with paraproteinemia—multiple myeloma, Waldenström's macroglobulinemia (WM), heavy chain diseases, and benign monoclonal gammopathy—and diseases sometimes associated with paraproteins—non-Hodgkin's lymphoma, amyloidosis, dermatopathies, and chronic cold agglutinin disease.

Waldenström's macroglobulinemia is a lymphoproliferative disease whose hallmarks are a proliferation of characteristic "lymphoplasmacytoid" cells in the bone marrow and a high concentration of a monoclonal IgM in the serum. The cells are intermediate in morphology between lymphocytes and plasma cells. They express cytoplasmic and surface IgM and secrete large amounts, resulting in a monoclonal peak in serum. They have typical B-lymphocyte markers.

Generally, WM is a disease of the elderly with a chronic indolent course. Neither lymphadenopathy nor splenomegaly is particularly prominent, except late in disease, and lytic bone lesions are rare. Infiltration of the bone marrow may produce a moderate anemia, and coating of platelets with IgM may cause bleeding problems. However, the major clinical manifestation of disease in advanced cases is a hyperviscosity syndrome characterized by various combinations of visual and CNS disturbances and pulmonary and cardiac symptoms. The cause is the high intravascular concentrations of IgM protein. The normal serum concentration of IgM is .5–3.7 g/L, but in WM it may reach 20 or more times that level.

Benign monoclonal gammopathy is probably the most frequent cause of an elevated serum paraprotein (also called an M protein). It is quite common in elderly individuals who have no abnormal symptoms related either to the paraprotein or to any lymphoproliferative disease. It is distinguished from multiple myeloma, WM, and the rare cases of non-Hodgkin's lymphoma with paraprotein by: the fact that the concentration of M protein is relatively low (< 20 g/L) and is stable for long periods; by the absence of significant infiltration of the marrow by lymphocytes or plasma cells; and finally, by the absence of Bence Jones protein.

In general, treatment is not required. Occasional cases, as noted in this article, have peripheral neuropathy or acquired von Willebrand's disease, and in about 1 in 5, myeloma or lymphoma may eventually develop after many years.

Peripheral neuropathy also occurs in other paraproteinemias, including WM and that associated with amyloidosis and some lymphomas. There are probably diverse mechanisms of impaired peripheral nerve function, as outlined in this article. Treatment is not usually very satisfactory.—M.J. Cline, M.D.

33 Bone Marrow Transplantation and Gene Therapy

Introduction

The role of autologous bone marrow transplantation in selected disease is examined, and the now extensive experience with transplantation in thalassemia is reviewed.

Martin J. Cline, M.D.

The U.S. National Marrow Donor Program

Perkins HA, Hansen JA (Irwin Memorial Blood Centers, San Francisco, Fred Hutchinson Cancer Research Inst, Seattle)
Am J Pediatr Hematol Oncol 16:30–34, 1994   119-95-33–1

Background.—Bone marrow transplants are denied for two thirds to three quarters of potential patients because they lack a compatible donor in the family. The United States Congress has approved and funded a program to provide a national registry of bone marrow donors. In the United States, nearly 1 million donors are registered with the National Marrow Donor Program and over 2,000 transplants have been performed. About 70 transplants are performed each month, with patients with myeloid leukemia making up over 40% of the transplant recipients.

Methods.—Nearly half of the search requests found identical human leukocytic antigen–compatible donors. Preliminary searches are free, and coded lists of matches are completed within 24 hours for the requesting physician. A formal search, for an activation fee, is conducted if the patient decides to proceed. Donors who match the patient profile are contacted and typed for HLA-DR. The need for a mixed lymphocyte culture has been replaced with typing for class II DNA alleles. The eligible donor is interviewed and submits to a complete history and physical examination. The donor may withdraw at any time but is informed that the patient may die once the rigorous preparation program is begun.

Results.—The time required from beginning the search to transplant is a median of 163 days, ranging from 16 to 1,324 days. Transplants may be delayed because of problems with the recipient or the donor. The patient may not be medically ready or may be indecisive. An analysis several years ago showed that more than 5% of donors had changed their minds and nearly as many had moved without leaving a forwarding address. Another 5% were temporarily unavailable and 2% were ineligible. Searches are also slowed because less than 20% have been HLA-DR typed. Over 20% are incompletely typed. Despite these limitations, fully 43% of searches have resulted in at least one 6-antigen (complete A,B,DR identity) match. In a 5-year period, nearly 10,000 preliminary searches were initiated. During the same period, nearly 5,700 formal searches resulted in 1,223 transplants, 2,808 searches had been halted and 1,638 were in various stages of the process.

Problems.—Finding a donor is best within one's own ethnic group. To date, 67% of the registered donors are white, 3.8% are black, 3% are Asian, 3.9% are Hispanic, and .8% are Native American. The low numbers of nonwhite patient recipients is reflected in the racial mix of the donor pool. To extend the donor pool, the United States has reciprocal agreements with Canada, Great Britain, and France, for an added 200,000 donors. Transplant centers are found in the Netherlands, Israel, Germany, Italy, and Australia, with Japan and Hong Kong applying for inclusion. There is not much hope for an African center in the near future. The speed of searches still needs to be increased by focusing on prospective typing, more participating laboratories, and minimization of redundancies. More sophisticated techniques will allow the cell repository of donor and recipient cells to be used for matching to ensure optimal results.

▶ This is an excellent article summarizing the United States National Marrow Donor Program.

Last year, we reviewed a series of bone marrow transplants in chronic myelocytic leukemia using matched marrow from unrelated donors. Survival in these transplants was considerably less than in transplants from a matched family member (36% to 45% vs. 50% to 65%). The main problems were graft-versus-host disease (GVHD) and bone marrow failure, with a 54% incidence of grade III or grade IV acute GVHD and a 52% incidence of extensive chronic GVHD.

Although these results for bone marrow transplantation from an unrelated donor were not nearly as good as those with a family member donor, it must be recalled that only about 1 patient in 3 or 4 in the United States has a matched potential family donor. Consequently, one must consider using unrelated matched donors in the appropriate circumstances. This article summarizes the progress that has been made and continues to be made in finding unrelated matched donors.—M.J. Cline, M.D.

Preliminary Results of Treatment With Filgrastim for Relapse of Leukemia and Myelodysplasia After Allogeneic Bone Marrow Transplan-

tation
Giralt S, Escudier S, Kantarjian H, Deisseroth A, Freireich EJ, Andersson BS, O'Brien S, Andreeff M, Fisher H, Cork A, Hirsch-Ginsberg C, Trujillo J, Stass S, Champlin RE (M.D. Anderson Cancer Ctr, Houston)
N Engl J Med 329:757–761, 1993   119-95-33–2

Background.—Patients with leukemia who relapse after allogeneic bone marrow transplantation (BMT) have a poor prognosis. Few such patients respond to additional chemotherapy. Almost none survive in the long term. Preliminary observations on the use of filgrastim, or granulocyte colony–stimulating factor, for post-transplantation relapse were reported.

Methods.—Seven female patients with leukemia, aged 16–50 years, were included in the study. The diagnosis was chronic myelogenous leukemia in 1 case, acute myelogenous leukemia in 5, and myelodysplastic syndrome transformed to acute myelogenous leukemia in 1. In all cases, disease relapsed within 360 days after allogeneic BMT. Filgrastim, 5 µg/kg per day in a subcutaneous injection, was given to reinduce remission by stimulating residual donor mast cells.

Findings.—Three patients had a complete hematologic and cytogenetic remission. Hematopoiesis of donor origin was reestablished in these cases. In 1 patient, mild chronic graft-versus-host disease developed. One patient had a relapse 1 year after therapy. Two remained in remission at 10 and 11 months, respectively. In 2 responders, fluorescence in situ hybridization revealed donor cell stimulation without leukemic clone differentiation.

Conclusion.—Filgrastim treatment can reestablish normal donor hematopoiesis in selected patients with leukemic relapse after allogeneic BMT. This treatment offers a new potential for reinducing remission and, possibly, for preventing relapse in such cases. Further research is needed to elucidate the mechanisms involved in remission maintenance after allogeneic BMT.

▶ When leukemia relapses after BMT, the outlook is grim. Although additional chemotherapy or even a second bone marrow transplant is sometimes used, almost invariably these efforts fail, and the patient dies of disease within a few months. This article describes the unexpected observation that some patients with relapsed leukemia after BMT benefit from filgrastim, or granulocyte colony-stimulating factor (G-CSF). It is not entirely clear why the investigators undertook the experiment in the first place, but the results were impressive—3 of 7 patients had a complete hematologic remission with restoration of donor hematopoiesis. The mechanism is uncertain, but one can speculate that the normal bone marrow stem cells derived from the donor are responsive to pharmacologic doses of G-CSF, whereas the leukemic clone is not. When large doses of G-CSF are given, the normal population expands and, at least temporarily, overwhelms the leukemic stem cells.

So much for explanations; now let us see whether the strategy works in the hands of other leukemia doctors.—M.J. Cline, M.D.

High-Dose Chemotherapy and Autologous Hematopoietic Stem-Cell Transplantation for Aggressive Non-Hodgkin's Lymphoma

Vose JM, Anderson JR, Kessinger A, Bierman PJ, Coccia P, Reed EC, Gordon B, Armitage JO (Univ of Nebraska, Omaha)
J Clin Oncol 11:1846–1851, 1993   119-95-33–3

Background.—Previous studies have shown high-dose chemotherapy combined with stem cell transplantation to be a successful treatment modality for patients with recurrent non-Hodgkin's lymphomas (NHLs). The impact of this treatment combination on clinical and tumor progression in patients with intermediate-grade recurrent NHL was assessed.

Methods.—During an 8-year period at a single center, 158 patients with intermediate-grade, relapsed, or primary refractory NHL received high-dose chemotherapy and either autologous bone marrow transplan-

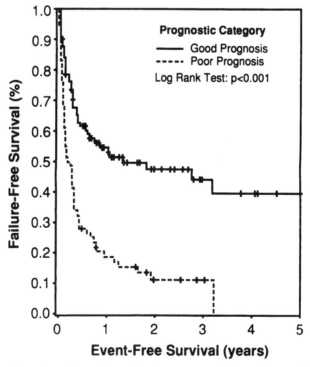

Fig 33–1.—Comparison of survival for good and poor prognosis groups. (Courtesy of Vose JM, Anderson JR, Kessinger A, et al: *J Clin Oncol* 11:1846–1851, 1993.)

tation (ABMT) or peripheral stem cell transplantation (PSCT). A prognostic model was developed, and the cohort was divided into good and poor prognosis groups, based on tumor size and the presence of 1 (good prognosis) or more (poor prognosis) of the following adverse conditions: 3 or more prior chemotherapy regimens, an above normal lactate dehydrogenase level, or chemoresistance. The effects of each transplantation type on failure-free survival (FFS) were assessed with each group. The immunophenotype was analyzed in 138 of the patients.

Results.—Patients with a B-cell immunophenotype had a lower FFS rate than did those with a T-cell immunophenotype. Of the 158 patients, 51 had achieved FFS at 21 months (compared with a 29% actuarial FFS rate). The 3-year FFS was 10% in the poor prognosis group and 45% in the good prognosis group (Fig 33-1). The effects of the transplantation types were differential. There was no difference between ABMT and PSCT effects in the poor prognosis group, whereas in the good prognosis group, the 3-year FFS rate was more than twice as high for those who received PSCT as for those who received ABMT (70% vs. 32%).

Discussion.—The success of this treatment regimen in the good prognosis group suggests that patients should not be denied transplantation based on the presence of only 1 adverse indication. The data further suggest that chemoresistance, although important, may be related to other prognostic factors. The comparatively high success rate with PSCT over ABMT in the good prognosis group is important and may indicate that the timing of treatment correlates with maximal peripheral stem cell effectiveness.

▶ This study examined high-dose chemotherapy combined with either ABMT or PSCT in 158 patients with refractory NHL of intermediate histologic grade. About one third of the patients were alive and in remission at 21 months after treatment. The authors identified a subgroup of patients with a good prognosis for response to this therapy. Interestingly, in this group, disease-free survival at 3 years was twice as high when PSCT rather than ABMT was used. Does this mean that the marrow may have harbored malignant cells?

Last year, I reviewed an important study comparing ABMT with allogeneic bone marrow transplantation in patients with advanced NHL (1). Approximately 100 patients received an ABMT, and about the same number received an allogeneic transplant. Survival without recurrent disease was nearly 50% in both treatment groups over the period of observation. There was a tendency for more frequent relapses in the patients who received their own bone marrow than in patients who received allogeneic bone marrow, but this effect was offset by the decreased frequency of graft-versus-host disease and death resulting from the transplantation procedure in the autologous group. Autologous bone marrow transplantation has a low mortality rate of about 10%.

The basic question is: Is high-dose chemotherapy combined with autologous stem cell rescue a valid treatment for resistant intermediate-grade NHL? The answer is *"Perhaps."*—M.J. Cline, M.D.

Reference

1. 1994 YEAR BOOK OF MEDICINE, pp 281–282.

Induction of Graft-Versus-Host Disease as Immunotherapy for Relapsed Chronic Myeloid Leukemia

Porter DL, Roth MS, McGarigle C, Ferrara JLM, Antin JH (Brigham and Women's Hosp, Boston; Harvard Med School, Boston; Univ of Michigan, Ann Arbor)
N Engl J Med 330:100–106, 1994   119-95-33–4

Background.—Allogeneic bone marrow transplantation (BMT) cures chronic myeloid leukemia (CML) both through the effects of conditioning and the antileukemic action of lymphocytes in the transplanted marrow. Graft-vs.-leukemia effects have been documented in animal models of BMT, but their significance in the clinical setting remains uncertain.

Objective.—Treatment of CML in relapse after BMT was attempted by administering interferon-α-2b and infusing mononuclear cells from the bone marrow donor.

Patients.—Eleven consecutive patients with CML who had relapsed after allogeneic BMT entered the study. All had a hematologic relapse necessitating cytoreductive treatment. No patient required immunosup-

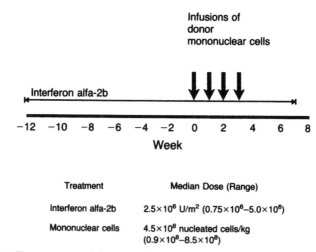

Fig 33–2.—Treatment protocol. (Courtesy of Porter DL, Roth MS, McGarigle C, et al: *N Engl J Med* 330:100–106, 1994.)

pression for chronic graft-versus-host disease. Most of the patients had received marrow grafts depleted of T cells. The median interval between BMT and relapse was 13 months, and from relapse to cell infusion treatment it was 22 months.

Treatment.—Patients injected themselves subcutaneously with interferon-α-2b in a planned daily dose of 5 million units/m². After 6–12 weeks of interferon therapy, 9 of the patients received 4 weekly infusions of mononuclear cells freshly harvested by leukapheresis from the bone marrow donor (Fig 33-2). One other patient received a single infusion, and 1 withdrew from the study.

Results.—Ten patients were controlled hematologically at the outset, but none had cytogenetic or molecular genetic remission before donor cells were infused. After 4–10 weeks of interferon treatment, marrow hypercellularity had developed, and at least three fourths of metaphases contained the Ph¹ chromosome. All 8 patients with stable CML had a complete hematologic response. One patient sustained acute graft-versus-host disease and died of aspergillus infection. Bone marrow aplasia developed in another 6 of the 8 patients who responded hematologically also had a complete cytogenetic remission and a complete molecular genetic remission. Acute graft-versus-host disease developed in 9 patients, and limited chronic disease developed in 5 of 8 who were followed for longer than 100 days. Three patients had life-threatening opportunistic infections.

Conclusion.—Treatment with interferon-α-2b and infused donor mononuclear cells can be effective in patients with CML who are in relapse after BMT, but the long-term effects on survival remain to be established.

▶ This article summarizes another (desperate?) attempt to rescue leukemic patients whose disease has relapsed after BMT. It is known that graft-versus-host disease (GVHD) has an antileukemic effect, and this was the rationale for its purposeful induction in the patients with relapsed disease. It is also known that GVHD is a serious physician-induced illness. The target organs include skin, gut, liver, and bone marrow. Graft-versus-host disease can also be immunosuppressive with secondary viral, bacterial, and fungal infections. In standard bone marrow transplantation (where one is trying to avoid GVHD), the mortality rate of this complication may approach 25% in some conditions. Therefore, the intentional induction of GVHD takes some courage (if that is the correct word).

In this study, induction of GVHD was combined with interferon-α, so it is a bit difficult to sort out the contribution of each component of the program. Nevertheless, it was impressive that 6 of 8 patients with stable chronic-phase leukemia entered a disease remission. Not unexpectedly, myelosuppression was prominent in 8 of 11 patients, and some died of treatment plus disease. My conclusion is the same as in the Abstract 119-95-33-3: Let us see if the strategy works in the hands of other leukemia doctors.—M.J. Cline, M.D.

Bone Marrow Transplantation for Sickle Cell Disease: The United States Experience

Johnson FL, Mentzer WC, Kalinyak KA, Sullivan KM, Abboud MR (Univ of Chicago; Univ of California, San Francisco; Children's Hosp, Medical Ctr, Cincinnati, Ohio; et al)
Am J Pediatr Hematol Oncol 16:22–26, 1994   119-95-33–5

Introduction.—The sickle cell trait is carried by about 30 million individuals worldwide. Screening, prophylactic care, pain management, transfusions, and antibiotics have improved life quality and length to the point where patients live into their sixth decade. Mortality has dropped from 15% to 1% in centers providing comprehensive care. Vaso-occlusive crises and damage to the CNS, kidneys, and lungs are seen in early adulthood From 5% to 18% of children show proof of organ failure, which accounts for the majority of clinic appointments and hospital admissions. Although some medication has been helpful, allogeneic bone marrow transplantation (BMT) is currently the only curative therapy. This carries a significant risk of graft-vs.-host disease and is effective only in patients with a suitably matched donor.

Patients and Methods.—Five patients (4 girls) between 3 and 10 years of age with sickle cell disease have undergone sibling BMTs in the United States. Two patients had previous cerebrovascular accidents, 1 had severe vaso-occlusive crises, 1 had acute myeloid leukemia, and 1 had Morquio's disease. Donors (4 boys) ranged in age from 4 to 13 years. To prevent graft-vs.-host disease, a regimen of cyclosporine A, methotrexate, and prednisone was administered.

Results.—The graft failed in the patient with Morquio's disease, but retransplantation was successful. Moderate graft-vs.-host disease of the skin and gastrointestinal tract was seen in 2 patients. Resolution was achieved with prednisone therapy; however, 1 of these patients had transient chronic graft-vs.-host disease of the skin. Other acute problems included mild hepatic veno-occlusive disease, infection with bacteremias, uterine hemorrhage, and pseudomonas sepsis.

Conclusion.—After a follow-up of 8 months to more than 9 years, all patients were in good-to-excellent clinical condition. Both patients who previously had cerebrovascular accidents have had further neurologic events. Graft-vs.-host disease is related to age, but performing BMTs in infants is not realistic considering that as many as half the infants with the trait never experience life-threatening events.

▶ No specific treatment has been found to be effective in preventing the sickling process, although many have been tried over the years. Consequently, standard treatment consists of supportive measures and exchange transfusion under some circumstances. Supportive measures include adequate hydration, oxygen, antibiotics for infection, and analgesics including narcotics for pain. Transfusions for support of the hematocrit are not usually given, unless one is dealing with an aplastic crisis. Exchange transfusions in which more than 50% of the patient's red blood cells are replaced by normal cells may be indicated in a variety of circumstances: first, in pregnancy; second, to break a cycle of continuous vascular occlusive episodes; third, in the treatment of indolent nonhealing skin ulceration; and finally, in relieving priapism. Some physicians also use exchange transfusion after a stroke, but that is a bit like locking the barn, etc. One should not use exchange transfusion without a justifiable reason, as there is always the danger of transmitting infectious agents, of sensitizing the patient to erythrocyte antigens, and of transfusion hemosiderosis.

In recent years, BMT has become a therapeutic option. It should be reserved for young children in whom severe organ damage has not yet occurred. Even in this setting, the mortality of the procedure probably exceeds 30%.

This article reviews a small experience with BMT in sickle cell disease. A much larger experience has recently been reported from Europe (1). Of 41 patients who underwent transplantation, 38 are alive and cured of their disease and 6 have chronic graft-vs.-host disease. It is still too early to tell whether this approach can be generally recommended.—M.J. Cline, M.D.

Reference

1. Vermylen C, Cornu G: Bone marrow transplantation for sickle cell disease. *Am J Pediatr Hematol Oncol* 16:18–21, 1994.

Bone Marrow Transplantation for Thalassemia
Giardini C, Angelucci E, Lucarelli G, Galimberti M, Polchi P, Baronciani D, Bechelli G (Ospedale di Pesaro, Italy; Ospedale San Salvatore di Pesaro, Italy)
Am J Pediatr Hematol Oncol 16:6–10, 1994   119-95-33–6

Introduction.—The defective or absent production of the β-globin chain in thalassemia major results in intramedullary destruction, hemolytic anemia, and inadequate erythropoiesis. This disease, which used to be fatal in infancy, is treated with hypertransfusion and chelation with deferoxamine, resulting in prolonged survival. The only curative regimen is bone marrow transplantation (BMT) in patients who have an identically matched donor.

Methods.—Over a 10-year period, 484 patients ranging in age from 1 to 32 years underwent BMT. Donors for 16 of the patients were identically matched parents, and the remaining donors were matched siblings. Preconditioning, in all but the first 11 patients, was a combination of oral busulfan, for 4 days at 16 mg/kg in 440 patients and 14 mg/kg in 33 patients, plus 4 days of IV cyclophosphamide at 200 mg/kg in 413 patients and 120 mg/kg for 2 days in 71 patients. Transplantation occurred 36 hours after the final dose of cyclophosphamide. A variety of protocols were used to prevent graft-vs.-host disease, the severity of which was graded according to the Seattle criteria.

Results.—Of the 484 patients, 88 died, 41 rejected the graft, and the remaining 355 were cured. Survival probability was estimated at 82% with event-free survival at 75% and a 12% chance of rejection. Risk factors identified included hepatomegaly, portal fibrosis, and a history of chelation treatment. Patients with no risk factors (class 1) had a survival probability of 97%. Those with 1 or 2 risk factors (class 2) had a survival probability of 84%, whereas patients with all 3 risk factors (class 3) had a survival probability of 54%.

Conclusion.—There is no reason to delay BMT because conventional treatment has failed and the patient deteriorates to a higher class. Class 1 patients show less graft rejection and high survival probability.

▶ The thalassemias arise from genetic abnormalities in the synthesis of the α- or β-globin chains. Unbalanced globin chain production leads to unstable hemoglobin molecules, premature destruction of the developing red blood cell with ineffective erythropoiesis in the bone marrow, and hemolytic anemia.

A variety of molecular defects can cause thalassemia disorders: gene deletions, mutations at sites controlling production of globin messenger RNA or protein, and, rarely, gene fusion. More than 40 genetic lesions have been described, so the situation is complex. The overall pattern, however, is relatively simple.

The clinical manifestations of the thalassemias vary from none to a severe fatal anemia with intrauterine death. In thalassemia major, all the characteristics of a chronic severe hemolytic anemia are present. Because the disorder begins early in life, bony abnormalities occur from the intense erythropoietic activity, unless transfusion therapy is given to maintain the blood count. Bone fractures and a characteristic facial appearance are frequent. Hepatosplenomegaly is usual, both from iron overload and extramedullary hematopoiesis. With the passage of time, iron overload is inevitable; if untreated, it leads to skin pigmentation, endocrine gland dysfunction, delayed puberty, diabetes mellitus, and, eventually, cardiomyopathy. Heart failure or arrhythmia is a frequent cause of death in the natural history of thalassemia major, usually in the third or fourth decade of life.

To prevent the bone abnormalities of thalassemia major, blood transfusions to support the hemoglobin concentration above 9–10 g/dL are indicated from about 6 months of age. This, of course, contributes to the development of iron overload, and it is necessary to administer chronic subcutaneous deferoxamine therapy to mobilize excess iron. Splenectomy is used to reduce the transfusion requirement in patients in whom hypersplenism develops. This, of course, increases the risk of serious infections in young children. Increasingly, BMT is being used in developed countries with large populations of patients with thalassemia major.

This article describes one of the largest experiences with BMT in thalasse-mia. The important results are that 75% of patients are cured of their disease by transplantation and that 25% die of the procedure or have chronic problems. The authors make the valid point that if bone marrow transplantation is done at all, it should be done early, when the risks are lowest and the chances of success are highest.—M.J. Cline, M.D.

Correction of the Enzyme Deficiency in Hematopoietic Cells of Gaucher Patients Using a Clinically Acceptable Retroviral Supernatant Transduction Protocol

Xu L, Stahl SK, Dave HPG, Schiffmann R, Correll PH, Kessler S, Karlsson S (Developmental and Metabolic Neurology Branch, NINDS, Bethesda, Md; Naval Medical Research Inst, Bethesda, Md)

Exp Hematol 22:223–230, 1994   119-95-33–7

Background.—Gaucher's disease, a lysosomal storage disorder caused by a deficiency of the enzyme glucocerebrosidase (GC), is particularly well suited for gene replacement therapy. Two amplified retroviral producer cells—A-LG4 and A-LGSN—with multiple vector copies to produce high-titer virus supernatant were used in the development of a clinically acceptable protocol for efficient transfer of a therapeutic gene into primitive hematopoietic progenitor cells.

Methods and Findings.—Both A-LGSN and A-LG4, containing multiple proviral copies, produced about tenfold higher titers on 3T3 cells compared with their unamplified counterparts. These vectors were packaged in GP+envAml2 cells because vectors generated in this cell line transduce hematopoietic cells more efficiently than the other packaging cells tested. During 96 hours, bone marrow mononuclear cells and purified CD34+ cells were infected with virus supernatants 4 times in the presence of interleukin (IL)-3, IL-6, and stem cell factor in culture. Cells were then plated in semisolid cultures. Using polymerase chain reaction, colony-forming unit–granulocyte/macrophage (CFU-GM) colonies were scored for vector presence. The transduction efficiency of CFU-GM colonies derived from CD34+ cells were markedly improved by the amplified vectors in the GP+envAml2 packaging line. Transduction efficiencies were 41% for A-LGSN, 42% for A-LG4, and 25% for unamplified LGSN. Hematopoietic cells from patients with Gaucher's disease were transduced and put into long-term bone marrow culture. Viral supernatant from the amplified producer lines transduced long-term culture initiating cells (LTCIC) efficiently—30% to 50%—with this protocol.

Conclusion.—High-titer amphotropic retroviral producer cell lines were created using coculture or repetitive supernatant infection. Supernatants from these amplified producer cell lines efficiently transduced LTCIC from the bone marrow of patients with Gaucher's disease. Potentially therapeutic levels of GC enzyme production were achieved in their progeny cells.

▶ Gaucher's disease is the result of deficiency of the enzyme GC. This enzyme is involved in the degradation of complex carbohydrate and lipid structures, called globosides and gangliosides, found in cell membranes. As macrophages ingest senescent red cells, they normally digest these compounds; in Gaucher's disease, these materials accumulate and fill the cell, giving it a characteristic wrinkled appearance. Gaucher's cells are found in the bone marrow, liver, spleen, and lymph nodes. Discharge of their granules often results in elevated levels of acid phosphatase in the serum.

Gaucher's disease is an autosomal recessive disorder found mainly among Ashkenazic Jews. Heterozygotes are asymptomatic but can be identified by finding reduced levels of the enzyme in white cells. There are 2 forms of the disease, which are transmitted independently. The severe infantile form has serious neurologic impairment with death in early childhood. The chronic form of Gaucher's disease persists throughout life and is characterized by hepatosplenomegaly and bony defects and fractures, particularly in the extremities. These result from proliferation of macrophages and expansion of the medullary cavity, with thinning of cortical bone producing a characteristic "Erlenmeyer flask" deformity of the distal femur. Hypersplenism is common with mild-to-moderate anemia, moderate thrombocytopenia, and a variable degree of leukopenia. Therapy is rather difficult, and splenectomy must be used with caution as macrophages tend to accumulate in other sites when the spleen is removed. Enzyme replacement is now frequently used in treatment, and bone marrow transplantation may be used in the severe form of this disorder. Gene therapy with replacement of the missing gene is the next logical evolution.

This article describes a step forward in the treatment of Gaucher's disease with gene therapy.—M.J. Cline, M.D.

34 Basic Oncology and Epidemiology

Introduction

Last year I said, "I anticipate reviewing the news of genes that predispose to breast cancer within the next year or 2." It was one of my few accurate predictions. The exciting news in oncology this year is once again in the basic sciences, with identification of genes that predispose to familial colon cancer and breast cancers.

Martin J. Cline, M.D.

Molecular Diagnosis of Familial Adenomatous Polyposis

Powell SM, Petersen GM, Krush AJ, Booker S, Jen J, Giardiello FM, Hamilton SR, Vogelstein B, Kinzler KW (Johns Hopkins Univ, Baltimore, Md)
N Engl J Med 329:1982–1987, 1993   119-95-34–1

Background.—Familial adenomatous polyposis, a dominantly inherited syndrome, is characterized by the progressive development of hundreds of adenomatous colorectal polyps. Some of these inevitably progress to cancer. Presymptomatic molecular diagnosis has been made possible by the recent identification of germline mutations of the APC gene in patients with familial adenomatous polyposis, but the wide distribution of the many mutations in this very large gene have made the search for mutations impractical. A novel approach to molecular genetic diagnosis was described.

Methods.—Sixty-two unrelated patients with the disease were screened. The primary screening involved analysis of protein synthesized in vitro from surrogate APC genes. An allele-specific expression assay was used to determine the relative amount of transcript from each APC allele (Fig 34–1).

Findings.—The protein assay showed that 82% of the patients had truncated protein. In 3 of the 11 patients without this protein assay finding, the allele-specific expression assay demonstrated decreased expression of 1 allele of the APC gene. The combined use of the 2 assays identified germline APC mutations in 87% of the patients.

Conclusion.—The use of the protein and allele-specific expression assays in combination is a practical, sensitive technique for the molecular

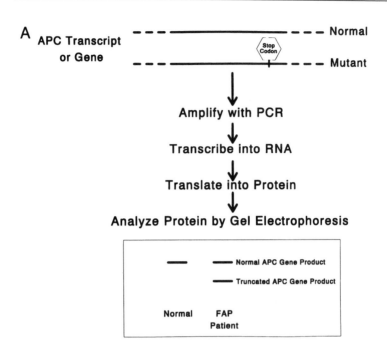

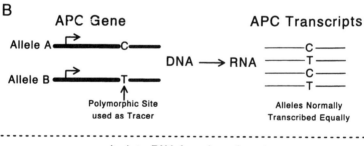

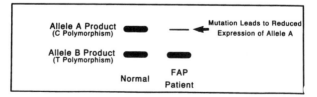

(continued)

diagnosis of familial adenomatous polyposis. This novel approach enables routine testing of individuals at risk and genetic confirmation of spontaneous mutations as well as better patient care.

▶ The gene responsible for the familial adenomatous polyposis form of carcinoma of the colon was identified in 1991. This gene, the *APC* gene, is located on the long arm of chromosome 5. A variety of germline mutations in the *APC* gene result in inactivation and loss of its gene product. The multiplicity of mutation sites made screening for affected individuals difficult. The authors devised a novel screening procedure that allowed detection of mutations in 87% of affected individuals. They estimate that there are 50,000 individuals in the United States whose families could benefit from genetic testing and that the new test can be used for prenatal diagnosis.—M.J. Cline, M.D.

Mutation of a *mutL* Homolog in Hereditary Colon Cancer

Papadopoulos N, Nicolaides NC, Wei Y-F, Ruben SM, Carter KC, Rosen CA, Haseltine WA, Fleischmann RD, Fraser CM, Adams MD, Venter JC, Hamilton SR, Petersen GM, Watson P, Lynch HT, Peltomäki P, Mecklin J-P, de la Chapelle A, Kinzler KW, Vogelstein B (Johns Hopkins Oncology Ctr, Baltimore, Md; Human Genome Sciences Inc, Rockville, Md; Inst for Genomic Research, Gaithersburg, Md; et al)
Science 263:1625–1629, 1994   119-95-34–2

Background.—Hereditary nonpolyposis colorectal cancer (HNPCC) is one of the most prevalent genetic disorders; as many as 1 in 200 individuals are affected. Mendelian inheritance is inferred from the finding

---

Fig 34–1 (cont).

Fig 34–1.—Principles of the in vitro synthesized-protein assay (**A**) and the allele-specific-expression assay (**B**). **A,** the APC gene is divided into 5 overlapping segments encompassing the entire coding region of the gene. These regions are amplified with specially designed polymerase chain reaction (PCR) primers that place the necessary transcriptional and translational regulatory sequences at the 5' end of the PCR product. Radiolabeled protein is synthesized in vitro from these surrogate genes in a simple 1-step coupled transcription-translation reaction. Truncating mutations can be identified as smaller protein products after gel electrophoresis and autoradiography. The stop codon represents a typical truncating APC mutation—for example, a change in a single base pair that creates a premature translation—termination codon. **B,** for the allele-specific-expression assay, every normal cell has 2 copies of the APC gene that are identical except for occasional polymorphisms of a single base pair (cytosine [C] or thymidine [T] in this example). Normally, both alleles of the APC gene are equally represented in the RNA fraction of the cell. However, some cases of familial adenomatous polyposis are caused by mutations that lead to reduced levels of normal APC transcript from 1 allele, resulting in an imbalance in the representation of the transcripts from the 2 alleles. This altered allele ratio in RNA can be detected with the allele-specific-expression assay (below the dotted line). First, RNA is isolated from peripheral blood mononuclear cells. Then, APC transcripts are converted to complementary DNA and amplified by reverse transcriptase PCR. The PCR products are then annealed with a common 9-bp oligomer and 2 different-sized allele-specific oligomers (8 and 10 bp). After ligation, these oligomers will yield 17-bp and 19-bp products corresponding to alleles A and B, which can be distinguished with gel electrophoresis. The box shows the expected results from a normal subject and from a patient with familial adenomatous polyposis who had a mutation that led to the reduced expression of the normal transcripts of allele A. (Courtesy of Powell SM, Petersen GM, Krush AJ, et al: *N Engl J Med* 329:1982–1987, 1993.)

that markers on chromsome 2p segregated with disease in large kindreds with HNPCC. Some cases of HNPCC are related to alterations in a *mutS*-related mismatch repair gene.

Objective.—To learn whether mutations of other mismatch repair genes might cause HNPCC, a large database of expressed sequence tags derived from random complementary DNA (cDNA) clones was searched.

Findings.—Three genes not previously described were found to bear significant resemblance to the bacterial *mutL* genes at their 5' ends. The gene most similar to the yeast *mutL* gene *MLH1*, termed *hMLH1*, was found to reside on chromosome 3p21 within 1 centimorgan of markers that have been linked with susceptibility to cancer in kindreds with HNPCC. Affected individuals from 7 Finnish kindreds all had a heterozygous deletion of codons 578 to 632 of *hMLH1*, and 5 of the 7 kindreds could be traced to a common ancestor. When HNPCC kindreds not suitable for linkage studies were evaluated by a random cDNA sequencing approach, a complex 371-nt deletion was found, starting at the first position of codon 347. This alteration was present in heterozygous form.

Implications.—It seems very likely that HNPCC is associated with heritable defects in any of several mismatch repair genes. Studies using the H6 tumor cell line are consistent with a model of HNPCC in which a second mutation is required for tumorigenesis.

▶ There are 3 types of colorectal cancer. The first type is associated with familial adenomatous polyposis described in Abstract 119-95-34-1. It accounts for about 1% of the cases of colon cancer in the Western world. The second is the "sporadic" type, which accounts for the bulk of the cases of colon cancer. The third is a hereditary nonpolyposis form of colorectal cancer that accounts for 4% to 13% of cases in the West. This form is not associated with familial adenomatous polyposis but also occurs in multiple generations of the same family and also is frequently responsible for an onset of colon cancer before the age of 50 years. This form of colon cancer is often called hereditary nonpolyposis colorectal cancer.

It is one of the most common genetic diseases in human beings and may affect as many as one in 200 individuals. In 1993, a gene responsible for some cases of HNPCC was identified on the short arm of chromosome 2. It is a human gene similar to genes found in yeast and bacteria, respectively called *mutS* and *mutL*, whose purpose is to correct mistakes in DNA bases that are generated when DNA replicates. In this investigation, the authors searched for other DNA mismatch repair genes that might be abnormal in some cases of the hereditary nonpolyposis form of colorectal cancer. They found another gene, also similar to *mutL* on the short arm of chromosome 3. This observation indicates that defects of any of several mismatch repair genes can cause the hereditary nonpolyposis form of colorectal cancer. This is another important basic science observation that will have implications for the clinic in the near future.—M.J. Cline, M.D.

A Large Kindred With 17q-Linked Breast and Ovarian Cancer: Genetic, Phenotypic, and Genealogical Analysis

Goldgar DE, Fields P, Lewis CM, Tran TD, Cannon-Albright LA, Ward JH, Swensen J, Skolnick MH (Univ of Utah, Salt Lake City)

J Natl Cancer Inst 86:200–209, 1994   119-95-34-3

Objective.—Mutation of a gene on chromosome 17q, *BRCA1*, appears to increase susceptibility to both breast and ovarian cancers. The effects of these mutations were characterized by analyzing a large multi-generation kindred known to have 17q-linked breast and ovarian cancers.

Methods.—A survey of the Utah Population Database was used to identify a family in which premenopausal breast cancers and ovarian cancers were clustered at any age level. Blood samples from 195 members of the chosen family were genotyped for 4 polymorphic markers of chromosome 17q. A reproductive history and information on lifestyle and the incidence and treatment of cancer were available for 72 women in the family.

Findings.—The odds favoring linkage of breast and ovarian cancer in this family to the *BRCA1* region of 17q exceeded 10^8 to 1. The estimated risk of breast or ovarian cancer secondary to a *BRCA1* mutation was 40% by the age of 50 years and 90% by 70 years of age. Epidemiologic risk factors for breast and ovarian cancer did not differ between older *BRCA1* carriers affected and those who were not affected. The frequency of paternal origin of the *BRCA1* allele was 69% in women with ovarian cancer, 41% in those with breast cancer only, and 26% in unaffected women more than 40 years of age.

Conclusion.—Women with the *BRCA1* mutation of chromosome 17q are at increased risk of having both breast and ovarian cancers develop. In this family, the mutation confers a lower risk of cancer at younger ages than has been found in past studies.

▶ This article describes the linkage of familial breast and ovarian cancers to a region of the long arm of chromosome 17. I selected this article relatively early in 1994. By September of 1994, this report was superseded by another article from the same group of investigators in Utah. By then, they had identified the familial breast cancer–associated gene, named the *BRCA1* gene, in the affected region of the long arm of chromosome 17 described in this abstract. Within weeks of publication, a second gene on the long arm of chromosome 13, dubbed *BRCA2*, was identified (1). It, too, is associated with familial breast cancer. It is hard to overestimate the importance of these articles. They are the first definitive steps in defining the genes responsible for familial breast cancer.

It is estimated that the lifetime risk for breast cancer in American women is between 1 in 8 and 1 in 10 and that between 5% and 10% of breast cancers are associated with an inherited susceptibility. The estimated incidence of germline mutations is about 1 in 200 women for the *BRCA1* gene and about the same for the *BRCA2* gene.

It is not yet known how these genes work, although it is known that they encode DNA-binding proteins. It was hoped that *BRCA1* would be involved in the 90% to 95% of breast cancers that are not familial. Unfortunately, this does not seem to be the case. Nevertheless, these discoveries will have important clinical implications. It has been estimated that a diagnostic test for *BRCA1* will be available within a year or 2. But the story will not end there. There is already evidence that there are familial breast cancer–related genes in addition to *BRCA1* and *BRCA2*. Note how similar the stories are for familial breast cancer and for familial colon cancer described in Abstract 119-95-34-2. Perhaps this will be the pattern for other familial cancers.—M.J. Cline, M.D.

Reference

1. Nowak R, et al: Breast cancer gene offers surprise. *Science* 265:1796–1799, 1994.

Estimates of the Worldwide Mortality From Eighteen Major Cancers in 1985. Implications for Prevention and Projections of Future Burden

Pisani P, Parkin DM, Ferlay J (Internatl Agency for Research on Cancer, Lyon, France)
Int J Cancer 55:891–903, 1993   119-95-34–4

Objective.—Mortality rates can be an important guide to the development of public health policies. Worldwide estimates of annual mortality from all cancers and for 18 specific cancers were obtained using site-specific statistics on cancer mortality from the World Health Organization database for 1985 from 71 countries (42% of the world population) and other existing data from cancer registries or population surveys.

Methods.—Crude and age-standardized mortality rates and numbers of deaths were computed for 24 geographic areas for 18 cancer sites: mouth and pharynx, esophagus, stomach, colon plus rectum, liver, pancreas, larynx, lung, melanoma of skin, female breast, cervix uteri, corpus uteri, ovary, prostate, bladder, kidney and urinary tract, lymphatic tissue, and leukemia.

Results.—Of the 5 million deaths resulting from cancer (excluding nonmelanoma skin cancer), 56% occurred in developing countries. Overall, lung cancer was the most frequent cause of cancer deaths, followed by cancers of the stomach, colorectal area, liver, breast, esophagus, and oral cavity and pharynx. In men, lung cancer was also the most common cause of cancer deaths, accounting for 22% of all cancer deaths, followed by stomach cancer and liver cancer. In women, breast cancer was the most frequent malignancy and the leading cause of death from cancer, accounting for 16% of all cancer deaths in developed countries and 11% of cancer deaths in developing countries. In developing countries, cancer of the cervix was the leading cause of cancer mortality in women, followed by breast cancer. In developed countries, the number of deaths from cancers of the colon/rectum and prostate remained high in men, whereas cancers from the lung, ovary, and pancreas were high in women. Deaths resulting from cancers of the liver, esophagus, and mouth and/or pharynx were predominant in developing countries.

Implications.—The steady increase in the world's population and its progressive aging indicate that cancer will become increasingly important as a cause of mortality and morbidity. If these estimated rates continue to prevail, the numbers of deaths from cancer will increase to 20.4% in developed countries and 18.1% in developing countries by the year 2000. These data provide an indication of the potential impact of preventive practices. It is estimated that 1 million deaths, representing 20% of all cancer deaths, could be prevented by eliminating tobacco smoking. Cancers of the liver and uterine cervix are both major problems in developing countries. Mortality from liver cancer could be substantially reduced by immunization against hepatitis B virus infection, and deaths from cancer of the cervix could be prevented by early detection through Papanicolaou smears.

▶ The abstract says it all.—M.J. Cline, M.D.

Decreasing Cardiovascular Disease and Increasing Cancer Among Whites in the United States From 1973 Through 1987: Good News and Bad News

Davis DL, Dinse GE, Hoel DG (Dept of Health and Human Services, Washington, DC; Natl Inst of Environmental Health Sciences, Research Triangle Park, NC; Med Univ of South Carolina, Charleston)
JAMA 271:431–437, 1994   119-95-34–5

Background.—At a time of spiraling health costs, methods to reduce the demand for health care by preventing costly chronic diseases are becoming a critical part of a national health strategy. The past trends in cardiovascular- and cancer-related mortality for age-specific groups of white individuals in the United States between 1973 and 1987 were explored.

Method.—Age-specific mortality rates were estimated. Population size estimates and numbers of deaths resulting from cancer, cardiovascular disease, and all causes for the years 1973 and 1987 were obtained from the United States National Center for Health Statistics. Within an individual age group or within a combination of age groups, the percentage change was obtained by taking the difference between the 1973 rate and the 1987 rate, dividing by the 1973 rate, and multiplying by 100%.

Results.—Between 1973 and 1987, cardiovascular-related mortality decreased in almost every age group, whereas cancer-related mortality decreased in the younger groups but increased in the older groups. In the age groups 0 to 54 years and 55 to 84 years, cardiovascular-related mortality decreased 42% and 33%, respectively. During the same period, cancer-related mortality decreased 17% in the younger group but increased 12% in the older group. By 1987, even though proportionally fewer people in the older age groups died, relatively more deaths were caused by cancer. Men born in the 1940s were seen to have twice as much cancer as those born between 1888 and 1897. They also showed more than twice as much non–smoking-related cancer. Women born during the same period had 50% and 30% more of these cancers, respectively. Rates of smoking-related cancers were 5 to 6 times greater in recent cohorts of women than in those of women born between 1888 and 1897, although rates in men decreased. Recent cohorts of women also showed double the rate of breast cancer compared with those born between 1888 and 1897.

Conclusion.—The good news about cancer is that impressive decreases in mortality rates have been seen in individuals younger than 55 years and in smoking-related risks for men of most ages. The bad news seen in this model is that recent birth cohorts of Americans aged 20 years and older are developing higher rates of all forms of cancer than individuals born before the turn of the century. Moreover, the incidence of smoking-related cancer in recent generations of women is about 5 times higher than it was in their 19th-century counterparts. The results of this study, together with similar findings from Sweden, indicate that the increases in cancer incidences are not solely linked to an aging population or smoking patterns. Changes in carcinogenic hazards in addition to smoking have probably occurred that require further investigation.

▶ This is an interesting article describing trends in cancer-related mortality between 1973 and 1987 and comparing these with cancer incidence at the beginning of the century. It makes the following points: first, that there is a decreasing cancer-related mortality in individuals younger than 55 years; second, that there is a decreasing smoking-related cancer mortality in men; third, that there is, not surprisingly, an increasing smoking-related cancer mortality in women relative to that early in the century; and finally, that cancer mortality in men, unrelated to smoking, is about twice as high now as it was at the beginning of the century. The authors suggest that there has been a substantial increase in carcinogenic hazards other than smoking.—M.J. Cline, M.D.

35 Clinical Oncology

Introduction

In the clinical treatment of solid tumors, I have concentrated on new combinations of agents for diverse tumors and on the use of the new drug, Taxol.

Martin J. Cline, M.D.

Report of the International Workshop on Screening for Breast Cancer
Fletcher SW, Black W, Harris R, Rimer BK, Shapiro S (American College of Physicians, Philadelphia; Dartmouth-Hitchcock Med Ctr, Lebanon, NH; Univ of North Carolina, Chapel Hill; et al)
J Natl Cancer Inst 85:1644–1656, 1993   119-95-35-1

Background.—Eight major randomized, controlled trials of breast cancer screening, including mammography and/or clinical breast examination, have been conducted during the past 30 years. Findings from several trials have been updated, and initial results from 3 other trials have been reported. In February 1993, The National Cancer Institute conducted an International Workshop on Screening for Breast Cancer to provide a thorough and objective critical review of the world's most current clinical trial data on breast cancer screening, to consider new evidence, to evaluate the present state of knowledge, and to identify areas requiring further investigation.

Methods.—Researchers representing the 8 randomized, controlled breast cancer screening trials in women aged 40–74 years reported both published and unpublished data. Evidence concerning the usefulness of screening in different age groups was also introduced.

Results.—Randomized controlled trials showed no benefit for women aged 40–49 years during the first 5 to 7 years after study entry. After performing a meta-analysis of 6 trials, a relative risk of 1.08 was noted after 7 years of follow-up. After 10–12 years of follow-up, none of 4 trials reached a statistically significant benefit in mortality, although a combined analysis of Swedish studies revealed a statistically insignificant 13% reduction in mortality at 12 years. One trial only—the Health Insurance Plan—had data beyond 12 years of follow-up. Results of this trial showed a 25% decrease in mortality at 10–18 years, although the statistical significance of this finding is controversial. All studies of women aged 50–69 years revealed mortality reductions, with 3 of 4 showing reductions of approximately 30% at 10–12 years after study entry. Of these, results from 2 trials were statistically significant. Adequate analysis has not been available for women older than 70 years of age because too few patients in this age group have been included in screening investigations.

Conclusion.—Randomized trials have yielded stronger evidence concerning the usefulness of breast cancer screening than for any other cancer, although much remains to be learned. Occasional gatherings of scientists in the field should facilitate this process.

▶ This is an important publication evaluating 8 major randomized, controlled trials of screening for breast cancer. Screening involved mammography and/or self-examination. The results, unfortunately, were disappointing with regard to the effectiveness of breast cancer screening in younger women. Screening did not reduce breast cancer mortality in women aged 40–49 years in a follow-up that has extended to 10–12 years from study entry. On the other hand, screening was associated with an apparent reduction of about one third in breast cancer mortality in women aged 50–69 years. This reduction was probably statistically significant at 10–12 years of follow-up.

Based on this information, one cannot recommend routine mammography in women under the age of 50 years. However, women with a family history of breast cancer are at higher risk of having breast cancer themselves and need frequent and attentive examinations.—M.J. Cline, M.D.

Risk Factors in Breast-Conservation Therapy
Borger J, Kemperman H, Hart A, Peterse H, van Dongen J, Bartelink H (Netherlands Cancer Inst/Antoni van Leeuwenhoek Huis, Amsterdam)
J Clin Oncol 12:653–660, 1994   119-95-35-2

Background.—Reported series of breast conservation therapy (BCT) have yielded 5-year breast recurrence rates of 1% to 13%. However, some investigators have found recurrence rates to be much higher in certain patient subgroups defined by such factors as young age, extensive intraductal component, margin involvement, and vascular invasion. There is debate about the significance of these factors, however. The clinical and pathologic factors associated with an increased risk of local recurrence after BCT were examined.

Methods.—A series of 1,026 patients with stage I or II breast cancer who were treated at a Dutch cancer center from 1979 to 1988 was analyzed. Management was with BCT, consisting of local excision and axillary lymph node dissection, followed by up to 50 Gy of irradiation to the whole breast and 15–25 Gy of boost irradiation. The median follow-up was 66 months.

Findings.—On univariate analysis, the significant risk factors of local recurrence were age, residual tumor at re-excision, histologic tumor type, any carcinoma in situ component, vascular invasion, microscopic margin involvement, and whole-breast radiation dose. On proportional-hazard regression analysis, the independent risk factors were age, margin involvement, and vascular invasion. A second analysis including only recurrences occurring before regional or distant failure found that only young age and vascular invasion were significant predictors. In a third analysis to predict the necessity of local salvage, the same 2 predictors remained significant. For patients without these risk factors, the 5-year breast recurrence rate was just 1%, compared with 6% for patients less than 40 years of age and 8% for patients with vascular invasion.

Conclusion.—This study identified 3 independent predictors for local recurrence after BCT: incomplete excision, vascular invasion, and age less than 40 years. Marginal involvement was less important when analyzing only breast recurrences as the first site of failure. On their own, the other 2 risk factors were not strong enough to affect patient selection for BCT.

▶ Evidence of tinkering with the data to the contrary, most randomized trials comparing mastectomy and BCT in stages I and II breast cancer have shown equal survival rates for the 2 types of therapy.

Studies of breast cancer recurrence rates after BCT have varied between 1% and 13% at 5 years. Some groups of patients have had higher reported recurrence rates than others. Negative prognostic factors in these groups have included younger age (< 40 years), tumor at the excision margin, vascular spread of tumor, and an extensive intraductal component of the cancer.

This study examined risk factors for local recurrence of cancer in over 1,000 patients with stage I or II disease. The identified risk factors were similar to those reported previously: age less than 40 years, involvement of the excised margins by tumor, and vascular invasion.

A recent article in *JAMA* (1) examined the effects of hospital type and treatment on outcome in breast cancer. The use of BCT was greatest at teaching hospitals, where between 40% and 50% of patients with localized or regional disease received this therapy between 1984 and 1990. At non-teaching hospitals, 30% or less of patients received BCT. Survival was at least as good with BCT as with mastectomy. Survival decreased progressively from large community hospitals to small hospitals to HMO hospitals. Interesting.—M.J. Cline, M.D.

Reference

1. Lee-Feldstein A, et al: *JAMA* 271:1163–1168, 1994.

Breast Cancer in the Elderly

Singletary SE, Shallenberger R, Guinee VF (M.D. Anderson Cancer Ctr, Houston)

Ann Surg 218:667–671, 1993   119-95-35–3

Background.—It has been shown that in women 80–84 years of age, breast cancer incidence can be as high as 435 per 100,000 patients. The selection of optimal management in this patient population may be confounded by several long-held beliefs regarding the natural history of the disease among the elderly. It has been suggested that elderly patients have more locally advanced disease at initial examination, more indolent cancer, limited life expectancies because of comorbid conditions other than breast cancer, and an intolerance for standard treatment. The clinical course and outcome of breast cancer in elderly patients were evaluated to determine whether these beliefs are indeed accurate.

Patients and Methods.—The medical records of 184 women older than 69 years were reviewed. All women underwent treatment for locoregional breast cancer between 1976 and 1985 at the M.D. Anderson Cancer Center. The median interval between diagnosis and last contact or death was 80 months.

Results.—It was found that elderly patients can tolerate standard surgical surgery and survive disease-free for many years. In this series, the breast cancer–specific survival rate was 79% at 7 years. Stage I disease was noted in 33% of the patients, of which only 10% underwent breast conservation surgery. Stage II and III disease was noted in 46% and 21% of the patients, respectively, although fewer than 13% underwent systemic adjuvant therapy. Only 3% of the patients had tumors detected by screening mammograms and only 12% by routine physical examinations, indicating a noncompliance with breast screening guidelines.

Conclusion.—All patients should be advised of treatment options for breast cancer and the benefits and drawbacks of each option based on physiologic, as opposed to chronological, age.

▶ Several observations are of interest in this article:

• Self-discovery was the most common method of initial detection (85% of patients).

• About one third of patients had significant comorbid conditions, including cardiovascular disease, hypertension, and arthritis.

• 64% of patients had large (T2 or greater) tumors.

• About one third of patients had relapse of disease within the period of observation.

• 80% of tumors were estrogen receptor–positive.

• With a median follow-up of 9 years, 101 of the 184 patients died, 40% of breast cancer and 60% of other causes.

The authors suggest that, in the light of these observations, treatment should be based on "physiologic as opposed to chronologic age." Unfortunately, they neglect to mention how one measures physiologic age. Most of us are pretty clear on how to measure chronological age.—M.J. Cline, M.D.

Sensitive Detection of Occult Breast Cancer by the Reverse-Transcriptase Polymerase Chain Reaction
Datta YH, Adams PT, Drobyski WR, Ethier SP, Terry VH, Roth MS (Univ of Michigan, Ann Arbor; Med College of Wisconsin, Milwaukee)
J Clin Oncol 12:475–482, 1994   119-95-35-4

Background.—The management and prognosis of patients with breast cancer may be greatly affected by the detection of occult carcinoma in the bone marrow and peripheral blood. Newer methods of detection—such as MRI, bone scintigraphy, flow cytometry, and immunohistochemistry—are better than conventional light microscopy but still have low sensitivity and specificity. Use of a reverse-transcriptase polymerase chain reaction (RT-PCR) to identify breast cancer patients with occult carcinoma was evaluated.

Methods.—The RT-PCR assay developed by the authors screened for keratin 19 (K19) transcripts to identify mammary carcinoma cells in the peripheral blood and bone marrow. Specimens from 34 patients with stage I to IV breast cancer and from 39 healthy controls were studied.

Results.—Initial reconstitution studies showed that the RT-PCR could detect 10 mammary carcinoma cells in 1 million normal peripheral

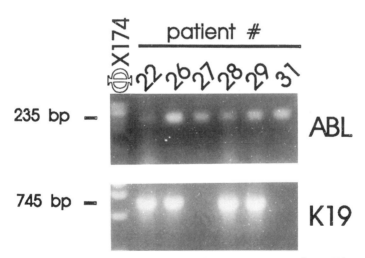

Fig 35–1.—Detection of occult breast cancer cells in bone marrow aspirates of stage IV breast cancer patients. A detectable *ABL* signal (235 bp) is evident in all patient samples (**top**), and a positive K19 signal (745 bp) (**bottom**) is evident for 4 patients. (Courtesy of Datta YH, Adams PT, Drobyski WR, et al: *J Clin Oncol* 12:475–482, 1994.)

blood mononuclear cells. The assay detected K19 transcript in the peripheral blood of 4 of 19 patients with stage IV breast cancer (Fig 35-1). The assay results were also positive in 5 of 6 patients whose bone marrow was histologically negative at evaluation of biopsy specimens obtained after preablative chemotherapy and before autologous bone marrow transplantation. The assay was negative in stem cell apheresis harvests from 1 of these patients and from 3 additional patients immediately before BMT. In 1 case, CSF from a patient with known carcinomatous meningitis tested positive. All but 1 of the control patients tested negative on the RT-PCR assay, the exception being a patient with chronic myelogenous leukemia.

Conclusion.—The K19 RT-PCR assay appears to be a sensitive, specific, and quick test for occult carcinoma in the peripheral blood and bone marrow of patients with breast cancer. These patients will commonly have residual breast cancer cells in histologically normal bone marrow but not in stem cell apheresis harvests. The new PCR will be helpful in the diagnosis of metastatic disease and the monitoring of systemic therapy.

▶ The PCR has been used during the past 3 years to detect "minimal residual disease" remaining after intensive therapy of various types of acute leukemia. Polymerase chain reaction techniques can be exquisitely sensitive and can detect 1 leukemic cell among 100,000 or 1,000,000 normal marrow cells. This article describes application of a PCR technique to the detection of occult breast cancer. The authors used the PCR reaction to detect keratin messenger RNA in blood or bone marrow, a clever choice as keratin is not normally present in these sites. Again, the sensitivity of the assay was 1 cancer cell in 100,000 normal cells. Now we must wait and see whether the technique can be used to detect occult metastases in regional lymph nodes and whether it has clinical utility in predicting recurrence of cancer.—M.J. Cline, M.D.

Vinorelbine as First-Line Chemotherapy for Metastatic Breast Carcinoma

Romero A, Rabinovich MG, Vallejo CT, Perez JE, Rodriguez R, Cuevas MA, Machiavelli M, Lacava JA, Langhi M, Acuña LR, Amato S, Barbieri R, Sabatini C, Leone BA (Grupo Oncológico Cooperativo del Sur, Bahía Blanca, República Argentina)
J Clin Oncol 12:336–341, 1994   119-95-35-5

Introduction.—A new semisynthetic vinca alkaloid, vinorelbine (VNB), has been developed that inhibits microtubule assembly and has demonstrated antitumor activity in in vitro studies using breast tumor cell lines. The usefulness of VNB as a first-line chemotherapeutic agent in patients with metastatic breast cancer was evaluated in a prospective phase II study.

Methods.—Women who had not undergone prior systemic chemotherapy for treatment of metastatic breast cancer received weekly administrations of VNB, 30 mg/m² diluted in 500 mL of normal saline, via IV infusion over 1 hour. Forty-four patients received a mean of 12.1 cycles and were followed for a mean of 9 months.

Results.—Three of the 44 patients (7%) achieved a complete response and 15 (34%) achieved a partial response; there was no change in 14 patients (32%), and there was disease progression in 12 (27%). For the entire group, the median duration of the treatment response was 9 months, and the median time to treatment failure was 6 months. The median duration of survival has not yet been reached. There were no clear clinical predictors of treatment response.

Myelosuppression was the dose-limiting toxic side effect. Leukopenia occurred in 78% of the patients, but usually it resolved within 7 days. Thrombocytopenia occurred in 13% of the patients and was usually mild. The hemoglobin level decreased progressively, and 33% of the patients had grade 2 or 3 anemia. Nineteen of the 29 patients without central implantable venous systems had phlebitis. Peripheral neurotoxicity was observed in 15 patients (33%), and 8 patients (18%) had elevated levels of liver enzymes.

Discussion.—Vinorelbine has significant antitumor activity in patients with metastatic breast cancer and produces moderate toxicity. These findings justify future trials of VNB, including investigations of the optimal dosing schedule and its efficacy in combination with other drugs.

▶ Abstracts 119-95-35–5 and 119-95-35–6 explore new drugs and new drug combinations in the initial treatment of metastatic breast cancer.

Vinorelbine is a synthetic vinca alkaloid. It produced complete or partial responses in 40% of breast cancers. Its toxicities were hematopoietic suppression, neurotoxicity, and phlebitis. In this regard, it looks much like vinblastine, 1 of the 2 vinca alkaloids introduced into medicine more than 2 decades ago. Parenthetically, none of the many synthetic vinca alkaloids that have been tried over the years have had sufficient advantages over the native vinca alkaloids, vincristine and vinblastine, to win a permanent place on the chemotherapist's medicine shelf. What I find intriguing about this article is that the authors tried a new therapy early in the course of metastatic cancer rather than late, when conventional therapies had failed.—M.J. Cline, M.D.

Paclitaxel and Recombinant Human Granulocyte Colony-Stimulating Factor as Initial Chemotherapy for Metastatic Breast Cancer

Reichman BS, Seidman AD, Crown JPA, Heelan R, Hakes TB, Lebwohl DE, Gilewski TA, Surbone A, Currie V, Hudis CA, Yao TJ, Klecker R, Jamis-Dow C, Collins J, Quinlivan S, Berkery R, Toomasi F, Canetta R, Fisherman J, Arbuck S, Norton L (Mem Sloan-Kettering Cancer Ctr, New York; Food and Drug Administration, Rockville, Md; Natl Cancer Inst, Bethesda, Md; et al)
J Clin Oncol 11:1943–1951, 1993   119-95-35–6

Background.—Previous studies of Taxol have demonstrated its activity in breast cancer, but profound myelosuppression, specifically noncumulative reversible neutropenia, was dose-limiting. In this phase II study, Taxol as initial chemotherapy for metastatic breast cancer was assessed using recombinant human granulocyte colony-stimulating factor (G-CSF) to ameliorate myelosuppression.

Patients and Methods.—Twenty-eight patients with clinically evident bidimensional breast cancer who had not previously undergone chemotherapy for metastatic disease were studied. The initial dose of Taxol was 250 mg/m² given as a continuous IV infusion over 24 hours. Treatment was repeated every 21 days with modifications in dose amount in response to toxicity. The patients also received 5 µg/kg per day of G-CSF subcutaneously from day 3 through day 10. Taxol treatments were continued for a maximum of 10 cycles, unless continued tumor regression was evident, or for 2 courses beyond the best response.

Results.—All patients were evaluated for toxicity and 26 of the 28 patients were assessable for tumor response. Patients were excluded from assessment as the result of unreported, previous hormone therapy in 1 patient and radiation therapy necessitated by spinal fracture in another patient. Objective responses were found in 16 patients. Neither hormone receptor status nor prior adjuvant therapy affected response. All metastatic sites were responsive. A median time of 5 weeks to the first observed partial response was noted. Overall, the treatment was well tolerated, with no significant hypersensitivity reactions and no cardiac toxicity noted. Generalized alopecia was found in all patients. Additionally, more than 50% of the patients experienced profound neutropenia, and only 8 received multiple courses without dose reduction. A total of 178 cycles of therapy were given, resulting in 8 hospital admissions for 6 patients because of febrile neutropenia.

Conclusion.—Taxol appears to be a very active chemotherapeutic agent for metastatic breast cancer. Further preclinical trials, including combinations with other drugs, are necessary to optimize its effectiveness.

▶ Taxol (paclitaxel) is derived from the western yew tree (*Taxus brevifolia*). It is a microtubule poison; however, unlike the vinca alkaloids it promotes formation of tubulin dimers and, thus, stabilizes the tubules against depolymerization, thus impeding cellular mitosis. Clinical trials with Taxol were initiated in the early 1980s, and activity was found against breast, ovarian, and non-small-cell lung cancers and melanoma. The drug came into widespread use about 2 years ago.

Myelosuppression and, especially, neutropenia is generally the dose-limiting toxicity of Taxol; hence, this study in which the drug was given in combination with G-CSF was done. Objective responses were observed in 62% of patients with advanced breast cancer. It took between 1 and 14 weeks for tumor responses. Administration of G-CSF reduced the severity and duration of the neutropenia. Total alopecia was a common complication of treatment.—M.J. Cline, M.D.

Phase I Trial of 3-Hour Infusion of Paclitaxel With or Without Granulocyte Colony-Stimulating Factor in Patients With Advanced Cancer
Schiller JH, Storer B, Tutsch K, Arzoomanian R, Alberti D, Feierabend C, Spriggs D (Univ of Wisconsin, Madison)
J Clin Oncol 12:241–248, 1994   119-95-35–7

Background.—Taxol (paclitaxel), a novel antitubular agent derived from the bark of the Pacific yew tree, has been found to be 1 of the most active single agents among the chemotherapy drugs. The toxicities of Taxol, which include myelosuppression, neuropathy, cardiac arrhythmias, and hypersensitivity reactions, have prompted the use of 24-hour infusions and prophylactic antiallergic regimens, which generally require hospital admission. Whether higher doses of Taxol could be administered over a shorter period, thus alleviating the need for inpatient hospital admission, was determined.

Method.—A total of 35 patients with advanced, untreatable malignancies were treated with a 3-hour infusion of Taxol every 3 weeks. Groups of 3 patients were entered at escalating dose levels of Taxol in a traditional phase I study in each of 2 parallel arms—arm A without granulocyte colony-stimulating factor (G-CSF) and arm B with G-CSF. All patients were initially given 210 mg/m² of Taxol, and dose escalations in each arm continued until 2 of 6 patients had an absolute neutrophil count of less than 500/µL for more than 5 days, febrile neutropenia, failure to recover counts in time for the next cycle of chemotherapy to be administered on time, and other grade 3 or 4 toxicities. Both groups were pretreated with dexamethasone, diphenhydramine, and ranitidine, and were continuously monitored for cardiac arrhythmias during the first treatment.

Results.—The group without G-CSF experienced dose-limiting myelosuppression with Taxol at the 250 mg/m² dose level. The dose-limiting toxicity for Taxol with G-CSF was peripheral neuropathy at doses of 300 mg/m². One of 35 patients experienced a grade 3 anaphylactic reaction at 250 mg/m². There was no significant incidence of cardiac arrhythmias. Twenty-seven of 111 courses were associated with grade 3 arthralgias or myalgias, which required narcotic pain control. Taxol plasma concentrations were seen to decline in a triexponential fashion, with a final elimination half-life of 10–12 hours. The peak Taxol plasma concentrations and total area under the curve increased as the Taxol dosage went up, although this appeared to be in a nonlinear fashion.

Conclusion.—The recommended maximum doses of Taxol for phase II and III studies when administered as a 3-hour dose alone and with G-CSF support are 210 mg/m² and 250 mg/m², respectively. There were no signs of hypersensitivity reactions or other side effects, except for arthralgias and myalgias. If ongoing trials continue to support this evidence, it seems likely that, with proper monitoring and premedication, high doses of Taxol could be safely administered in the outpatient setting.

▶ Taxol has generally been administered by 24-hour infusion in an effort to reduce the incidence of serious hypersensitivity reaction, neuropathy, and cardiac arrhythmias. This article examined the efficacy of a 3-hour drug infusion, with the obvious objective of eliminating the necessity for hospital admission for drug administration. The authors used an escalating schedule of drug administration to define dose-limiting toxicity and examined the efficacy of concomitant administration of G-CSF. They defined the upper dose that can be used (relatively) safely with a 3-hour infusion and showed that G-CSF administration allowed a higher dose of Taxol to be used.—M.J. Cline, M.D.

Dose-Intense Taxol: High Response Rate in Patients With Platinum-Resistant Recurrent Ovarian Cancer

Kohn EC, Sarosy G, Bicher A, Link C, Christian M, Steinberg SM, Rothenberg M, Adamo DO, Davis P, Ognibene FP, Cunnion RE, Reed E (Natl Insts of Health, Bethesda, Md)
J Natl Cancer Inst 86:18–24, 1994   119-95-35–8

Background.—Paclitaxel (Taxol), a diterpene plant product from the bark of the Pacific yew tree, promotes and stabilizes premature microtubule assembly. Phase I trials identified effective administration schedules, and phase I and II clinical trials without bone marrow support suggested paclitaxel's efficacy in ovarian and breast cancer, melanoma, and leukemia. Patients with previously treated breast and ovarian cancers had response rates greater than 20% in disease-specific phase I and II studies of paclitaxel. A prospective, phase II clinical trial of patients with advanced-stage, platinum-refractory, recurrent ovarian cancer was undertaken to investigate patient response to high-dose paclitaxel combined with granulocyte colony-stimulating factor (G-CSF).

Method.—Forty-seven women in the prospective phase II study were given 250 mg/m² of paclitaxel every 21 days on a rigid schedule to maintain dose intensity. A dose of 10 µg/kg of G-CSF per day was given to ameliorate myelosuppression. The G-CSF dose was escalated if a patient had fever or neutropenia so that the paclitaxel dose intensity could be maintained. The dose intensity or paclitaxel was maintained for up to 14 consecutive cycles of therapy. Patient response was assessed every 2 cycles. The patients with a complete radiographic resolution of disease underwent peritoneoscopy.

Results.—Forty-four women were assessable for response. Twenty-one achieved objective responses to therapy with paclitaxel for a response rate of 48%. Six patients had a complete response documented by physical examination, radiographs, and CA-125; 15 patients had a partial response to therapy. Neither the response rate nor the ability to maintain dose intensity was influenced by patient age, number of prior regimens, or clinical platinum resistance.

Conclusion.—Women with advanced-stage, platinum-resistant, recurrent ovarian cancer had a 48% response rate to dose-intense paclitaxel combined with G-CSF to ameliorate myelosuppression. This response rate is higher than in previous studies of lower doses of paclitaxel without G-CSF. A comparison of results of phase II studies of paclitaxel suggests a dose-response relationship seemingly independent of patient age and degree of prior therapy. Dose-intense paclitaxel and G-CSF should be considered in patients with advanced, platinum-refractory ovarian cancer.

▶ This article continues the theme of microtubule poisons in general and Taxol in particular. It examines the effect of the drug in a phase II trial in advanced platinum-resistant ovarian cancer. About one half of the patients had a response to the drug, and 6 of 44 (14%) had complete remission of disease. Unfortunately, the authors do not tell us the duration of these responses. In this study, neurotoxicity was the predominant undesirable side effect.

Taxol appears to be a useful agent in treating advanced ovarian cancer. Soon this drug will be tested as first-line therapy in this cancer.—M.J. Cline, M.D.

Ifosfamide, Carboplatin, and Etoposide: A New Regimen With a Broad Spectrum of Activity
Fields KK, Zorsky PE, Hiemenz JW, Kronish LE, Elfenbein GJ (Univ of South Florida, Tampa)
J Clin Oncol 12:544–552, 1994   119-95-35–9

Background.—Existing treatments for refractory solid tumors and lymphomas with salvage chemotherapy are frequently inadequate. Overall response rates and evidence of improved survival are minimal. For the past 5 years, the combination of ifosfamide, carboplatin, and etoposide (ICE) has been used at 1 center in patients with a variety of refractory or recurrent cancers. After 2 treatment courses, response rates and toxicity were assessed, and responders were considered for high-dose chemotherapy followed by autologous hematopoietic stem cell rescue. The outcome of this novel induction regimen was analyzed.

Methods.—Two hundred four patients 13 to 64 years of age were included in the study. The patients had a variety of malignancies, including refractory breast cancer and Hodgkin's and non-Hodgkin's lymphoma. Treatment consisted of 2 cycles of ICE, with IV ifosfamide, 2 g/m²; carboplatin, 400 mg/m²; and continuous infusion of etoposide, 600 mg/m², given in divided doses for 2 days. This regimen was repeated at intervals of about 28 days.

Findings.—Ninety-four percent of the patients received 2 cycles at full doses and were evaluable for response and toxicity. Complete and partial responses occurred in 20% of the patients with breast cancer, 30% with non-Hodgkin's lymphoma, 60% with Hodgkin's disease, 9% with melanoma, 20% with various sarcomas, and 43% with other malignancies. Myelosuppression was prominent. Significant neutropenia required frequent hospitalization for neutropenic fever, and thrombocytopenia and anemia necessitated frequent platelet and red blood cell transfusions. The overall treatment-associated mortality rate, however, was only 3%. No other moderate-to-severe organ toxicities occurred at a frequency of more than 1%.

Conclusion.—The regimen described proved to be active in patients with a variety of refractory malignancies. Hematologic toxicity was significant but tolerable. Adding hematopoietic growth factors may permit dose escalations.

▶ This article examines a multiagent "salvage" protocol for advanced cancers. It uses 3 agents, each of which has a wide spectrum of antitumor activity. The program was tested in 204 patients. Hematopoietic toxicity was prominent but was generally tolerable. Complete and partial responses occurred in about 20% of tumors.

This program can be compared with other "shotgun" chemotherapy programs that combine marrow-suppressive drugs with drugs with other toxicities; for example, the combination of cyclophosphamide and adriamycin ± etoposide ± cisplatin. All of these programs have antitumor effects in some patients, but the anticancer effects are generally of short duration, and the drugs have serious toxicities that have a markedly negative effect on the quality of life. I was struck recently by a line in an article in the lay press describing a beloved wife's death of cancer: "It doesn't take long for me to come to believe that the terrible wild power of the chemo ruthlessly destroys what the tumor itself shuns." I am not certain that this truth is widely understood by physicians who use these agents. I think this article should be mandatory reading for all those who treat patients with cancer (1).—M.J. Cline, M.D.

Reference

1. Kotlowitz R: "From my wife's room." *The New York Times Magazine*, December 4, 1994, p 84.

Metastatic Carcinoma of Uncertain Primary Site: A Retrospective Review of 57 Patients Treated With Vincristine, Doxorubicin, Cyclophosphamide (VAC) or VAC Alternating With Cisplatin and Etoposide (VAC/PE)

de Campos ES, Menasce LP, Radford J, Harris M, Thatcher N (Christie Hosp NHS Trust, Manchester, England)
Cancer 73:470–475, 1994   119-95-35–10

Background.—As many as 15% of patients in medical oncology units have metastatic carcinoma of uncertain primary site (CUPS). The prognosis in such cases is poor. The efficacy of vincristine, doxorubicin, and cyclophosphamide (VAC) given alone or alternated with cisplatin and etoposide (VAC/PE) in patients with CUPS and normal serum tumor markers was investigated.

Methods.—Fifty-seven patients were studied in the retrospective review. The first 40 patients were given 6 or 10 cycles of VAC, and 17 patients received VAC/PE for 6 cycles. The median age in the first group was 56 years, and in the second it was 47 years. Fifty percent of the first group were men, compared with 59% in the second group. When appropriate, histologic findings were reviewed using immunohistochemical methods.

Findings.—The histologic review led to reclassification of 6 tumors as non-Hodgkin's lymphoma (NHL), 1 as hepatocarcinoma, and 1 as adenocarcinoma. Six of the 11 treatment responders had a review diagnosis of NHL. When the cases of NHL and the case of hepatocarcinoma were excluded, patient survival between the VAC and VAC/PE groups was comparable. Five patients with true CUPS who responded to VAC or VAC/PE had poorly differentiated histology. Patients with poorly differentiated disease also had a significantly longer survival.

Conclusion.—Some patients with a previous diagnosis of CUPS actually have NHL. These patients respond well to chemotherapy. Patients with true CUPS respond to chemotherapy only if the tumor is differentiated poorly. In this subgroup, survival is significantly longer. There appears to be no advantage of VAC/PE vs. VAC chemotherapy.

▶ This article looks at "shotgun" chemotherapy in carcinoma of unknown primary site. Such articles appear regularly in the oncology literature. The response to treatment is almost always marginal (and probably not worth the effort), unless the patient has a lymphoma that was misdiagnosed as a carcinoma. Indeed, there are valid arguments for using antilymphoma treatment as the first line of therapy in such patients.—M.J. Cline, M.D.

Management of Terminal Cancer Pain in Sweden: A Nationwide Survey

Rawal N, Hylander J, Arnér S (Örebro Med Ctr Hosp, Sweden; Karolinska Hosp, Stockholm)
Pain 54:169–179, 1993   119-95-35-11

Introduction.—A nationwide survey was used in Sweden to study the extent of pain in patients with terminal cancer, assess management and treatment, and evaluate physician and nurse knowledge to determine educational needs.

Methods.—A survey was sent to all 228 chairmen and 228 chief nurses of the 6 major cancer treatment specialties. The physician and nurse most qualified in cancer pain management were asked to answer questions reflecting the general departmental consensus, based on the 3,767 patients admitted in 1989 with a chief complaint of severe cancer pain.

Results.—The response rate was high for physicians and nurses. Although pain assessment tools were available, 97% of physicians relied on patient history and clinical findings to assess pain levels. Physicians often stopped using peripherally acting analgesics at the onset of opioid therapy, seemingly unaware of their combined potentiating effects. Most used the World Health Organization "ladder" of pain management. Oral administration of opioids was the preferred route, and 86% of departments gave opioids "by-the-clock." Patient-controlled analgesia was used infrequently, and daily maximum opioid doses, although unrestricted, were underused. Severe pain was indicated to be common by 78% of physicians and nurses, yet 35% of nurses needed a physician's order to give additional opioid doses. The use of antidepressive agents, antinauseant agents, and prophylactic laxatives varied, despite recurrent anxiety, depression, nausea, and constipation. Physicians and nurses reported a low knowledge level of pain management. Pain management information was infrequently provided for patients or family members. According to 12% of nurses, stoic acceptance of pain resulted in underreporting.

Conclusion.—Inadequate treatment of severe cancer pain may be more the result of improper application of knowledge rather than lack of knowledge. There is a need for ongoing education of physicians, nurses, and patients.

▶ It has been estimated that one third of cancer patients in active therapy and about two thirds of patients with advanced cancers have significant pain. In the terminal stages of disease, 80% to 90% of patients may have pain. In spite of increasing attention to the management of terminal cancers, the management of pain is often inadequate. This abstract documents some of the problems of management that, in my experience, are as frequent in Los Angeles as they are in Sweden. There is a lack of a uniform approach to pain management. A frequent deficiency is the use of repeated IM injections rather than continuous IV or subcutaneous infusions. Laxatives are not routinely prescribed with narcotics. Neuropathic pain, which may not respond well to opioids, is still frequently treated with morphine rather than alternative pain control measures.

I agree with the conclusion of this article that there is a greater need for education of health care professionals in pain management.—M.J. Cline, M.D.

Infectious Morbidity Associated With Long-Term Use of Venous Access Devices in Patients With Cancer
Groeger JS, Lucas AB, Thaler HT, Friedlander-Klar H, Brown AE, Kiehn TE, Armstrong D (Mem Sloan-Kettering Cancer Ctr, New York; Cornell Univ, New York)
Ann Intern Med 119:1168–1174, 1993   119-95-35–12

Background.—Infection is a common and potentially fatal complication associated with the use of venous access devices. Recent research suggests that cancer patients with completely implanted port devices may be less vulnerable to such infections. Infectious morbidity associated with Hickman-type Silastic tunneled catheters and completely implanted subcutaneous ports was prospectively evaluated.

Methods.—Data were obtained for 1,630 venous access devices used in 1,431 consecutive patients with cancer between June 1987 and May 1989. All devices were inserted for long-term use.

Findings.—At least 1 device-related infection occurred with 43% of the catheters, compared with 8% of the ports. The most common infection associated with catheters was bacteremia or fungemia. Port use was associated with a more equal distribution of pocket, site, and device-related bacteremia. The organisms isolated were gram-negative bacilli in 55% of catheter-related bacteremia and gram-positive cocci in 65.5% of port-related bacteremia. The numbers of infections per 1,000 device days were 2.77 and .21 for catheters and ports, respectively. In a parametric model of time to first infection, devices were found to last longer in patients with solid tumors than in those with hematopoietic tumors. In all patient groups, ports lasted longer than catheters.

Conclusion.—Catheters were associated with an incidence of infections per device-day that was 12 times higher than with ports. The differences found in infectious complications may be caused by type of disease, intensity of treatment, frequency with which the devices are accessed, or duration of neutropenia.

▶ This article documents what has long been an impression in oncology services: that infections with in-dwelling Silastic venous catheters are much more common than those with subcutaneous ports. I had not realized, however, that the differences in infection frequency were quite so great—12-fold.—M.J. Cline, M.D.

PART FOUR

THE HEART AND CARDIOVASCULAR DISEASE

———————

ROBERT A. O'ROURKE, M.D.

Introduction

During the past year, many noteworthy basic and clinical research studies have been reported that will have a favorable influence on the prevention, diagnosis, and treatment of cardiovascular disease. Many of these reports are described and discussed in the Heart and Cardiovascular Disease Section of this YEAR BOOK OF MEDICINE.

The Heart and Cardiovascular Disease section of the 1995 YEAR BOOK OF MEDICINE includes 9 chapters, for a total of 56 abstracted publications with editorial comments based on these and additional references. The contents of Chapter 36, Risk Factors for Coronary Artery Disease, emphasize the success of intensive multifactor risk reduction in decreasing the rate of progression of coronary atherosclerosis and clinical cardiac events. The ability of 3-hydroxy-3-methylglutaryl coenzyme A (HMG-CoA) reductase inhibitors to prevent the progression of coronary atherosclerosis is discussed. Data concerning the inverse relationship between conditioning physical activity and the risk of acute myocardial infarction among men with abnormal resting or exercise ECGs are presented. A prospective study of the effects of alcohol consumption on cardiovascular events in middle-aged and elderly men is discussed, as is the inverse relationship between serum dehydroepiandrosterone sulfate levels and premature myocardial infarction in men.

Chapter 37, Acute Coronary Syndromes, is extensive. It presents data concerning the significance of anterior ST-depression in inferior-wall acute myocardial infarction. Data concerning the prognostic value of ambulatory ST-segment monitoring compared with exercise testing several months after acute myocardial infarction are also presented. Several articles concern the relative usefulness of serial blood levels of creatine kinase-MB (CK-MB), myoglobin, troponin T, and subforms of CK-MB and MM for the early and accurate detection of myocardial infarction and for documenting successful reperfusion in patients undergoing thrombolytic therapy or primary coronary angioplasty. Two disparate reports concerning the additive efficacy of heparin therapy along with aspirin in patients with unstable angina are discussed. The results of the Thrombosis in Myocardial Ischemia (TIMI IIIB) trial concerning the effects of tissue plasminogen activator and comparing early invasive and conservative strategies in patients with unstable angina or non–Q-wave myocardial infarction are detailed.

Further follow-up data are presented concerning the effects of primary coronary angioplasty vs. thrombolytic therapy in patients with acute myocardial infarction, and information is provided concerning the lower mortality rate in patients who undergo prehospital thrombolytic therapy at an earlier point than those who receive the same therapy after hospitalization. Several studies concern the safety and improved efficacy of direct thrombin inhibitors as adjunctive therapy to thrombolytic agents in the treatment of acute myocardial infarction. The clinical importance of thrombocytopenia early after the administration of thrombolytic therapy for acute myocardial infarction is discussed, as are the benefits of the early administration of the angiotensin-converting enzyme inhibitor captopril during thrombolysis in patients with a first anterior myocardial infarction. The Gruppo Italiano per lo Studio della Supravvivenza nell'Infarto Miocardico (GISSI-3) report concerning the favorable effect of lisinopril on overall mortality in patients with acute infarction is discussed, as is a report concerning an improved long-term survival in patients with acute infarction who were treated early with IV magnesium sulfate.

Practice guidelines for reducing the duration of hospital stay for patients with chest pain but at low risk for complications are discussed in Chapter 38, Chronic Coronary Heart Disease. Depressed left ventricular systolic function and moderate-to-severe mitral regurgitation are presented as echocardiographic findings that indicate an adverse prognosis in patients with chest pain. Evidence concerning the importance of physical activity as a determinant of the morning increase in ambulatory myocardial ischemia in patients with stable coronary artery disease is discussed. An important study reporting no relationship between myocardial blood flow, chest pain, and ECG changes during stress in patients with syndrome X is included. Pharmacologic tolerance and rebound angina pectoris during noncontinuous nitrate therapy is discussed in this chapter, as is a perspective comparison of coronary angioplasty, coronary bypass surgery, and medical therapy on employment in patients with coronary heart disease.

Chapter 39 is entitled Coronary Angioplasty, Atherectomy, and Stents. It contains a discussion of the randomized studies of coronary angioplasty compared with bypass graft surgery in patients with symptomatic multivessel coronary artery disease. The similar results of coronary angioplasty for women and men with postmyocardial infarction ischemia are detailed. Results from the first consecutive 3,000 patients undergoing excimer laser coronary angioplasty are presented. The application of newer coronary interventional techniques in patients with stenotic or occluded vein bypass grafts is discussed. Evidence indicating a lower re-stenosis rate in patients treated with coronary artery stent placement, as compared with those undergoing balloon angioplasty alone, for the treatment of coronary artery disease is discussed, as are the several limitations of stent placement.

The first 3 abstracts in Chapter 40, Valvular Heart Disease, concern the usefulness of percutaneous balloon mitral valve commissurotomy in patients with mitral stenosis. These studies in large numbers of patients followed for at least several years after the procedure indicate that balloon commissurotomy is safe and effective for many patients with rheumatic mitral stenosis. The results compare favorably with open mitral-valve commissurotomy, and moderate-to-severe preprocedure tricuspid regurgitation is a marker for adverse outcomes in patients undergoing balloon mitral commissurotomy alone. A more favorable effect on left ventricular function at rest and during exercise in patients undergoing mitral valve repair with chordal preservation, as compared with mitral valve replacement, is discussed, as are the clinical and echocardiographic predictors of long-term survival in patients undergoing surgical correction of moderate-to-severe mitral regurgitation. A meta-analysis concerning the thromboembolic and bleeding complications in patients with mechanical heart valve prostheses is reviewed, and a comparison of the effects of vasodilator therapy with enalapril vs. hydralazine in elderly patients with mild-to-severe chronic asymptomatic aortic regurgitation is analyzed.

Cardiomyopathy and heart failure are the subjects of Chapter 41. This chapter contains important information concerning the relationship of alcoholic myopathy to cardiomyopathy and provides strong evidence for an association between these 2 pathologic manifestations of disease in the setting of chronic alcoholism. An important report concerning the exercise capacity and left ventricular function in patients after recovery from acute dilated cardiomyopathy is included in this chapter, as are several studies evaluating the usefulness of therapy with conventional β-blocking drugs or with β-blocking drugs that also have a mild vasodilatory effect on rest and exercise hemodynamics, measurements of left ventricular systolic function, myocardial metabolic measurements, and clinical characteristics in patients with moderate-to-severe heart failure. A prospective, multicenter trial showing favorable effects of low-dose amiodarone on mortality in patients with severe congestive heart failure is discussed. A report concerning a decrease in the frequency of ventricular arrhythmias in patients with heart failure who received acute IV magnesium is also included.

In Chapter 42, Noninvasive Testing, the important prognostic value of thallium-201 single-photon emission CT (SPECT) myocardial perfusion imaging is discussed in patients with suspected or definite angina pectoris. Data against the routine use of dipyridamole thallium scintigraphy and gated radionuclide angiography for assessing cardiac risk before abdominal aortic surgery also are reported. The use of dobutamine stress echocardiography for predicting future cardiac events in patients with coronary artery disease is discussed, as is the role of various noninvasive techniques, such as dobutamine echocardiography, SPECT imaging with thallium and sestamibi, and metabolic and perfusion imaging with positron emission tomography for the assessment of viable myocardium in patients with depressed left ventricular systolic function. The diagnostic role of Doppler echocardiography in patients with constrictive pericarditis is also detailed in this chapter.

Chapter 43 on arrhythmias includes information concerning the increasing frequency of atrial fibrillation, the use of warfarin vs. aspirin for prevention of thromboembolism in patients with atrial fibrillation, the combination of other drugs with digoxin to slow the ventricular response during exercise in chronic atrial fibrillation, and a new technique of radiofrequency catheter modification of atrioventricular conduction for controlling the ventricular rate during atrial fibrillation. Other important studies in this chapter concern the use of the signal-averaged ECG for predicting inducible ventricular tachycardia in patients with unexplained syncope and electrical alternation of the ST segment or T wave as an independent marker of vulnerability to inducible ventricular arrhythmias and clinical arrhythmic events. Finally, this chapter includes a discussion of the efficacy and safety of multiprogrammable pacemaker-cardioverter-defibrillator devices in the treatment of patients with malignant ventricular tachyarrhythmias.

In the last chapter in this section, Other Topics, the usefulness of long-term therapy with β-blocking drugs for decreasing the rate of aortic dilatation and its consequences in patients with Marfan's syndrome are discussed. In addition, the favorable impact of the regression of left ventricular hypertrophy on systolic function and on left and right ventricular diastolic function is reported in patients undergoing successful treatment of systemic hypertension.

Robert A. O'Rourke, M.D.

36 Risk Factors for Coronary Artery Disease

Effects of Intensive Multiple Risk Factor Reduction on Coronary Atherosclerosis and Clinical Cardiac Events in Men and Women With Coronary Artery Disease: The Stanford Coronary Risk Intervention Project (SCRIP)
Haskell WL, Alderman EL, Fair JM, Maron DJ, Mackey SF, Superko HR, Williams PT, Johnstone IM, Champagne MA, Krauss RM, Farquhar JW (Stanford Univ, Palo Alto, Calif; Univ of California, Berkeley)
Circulation 89:975–990, 1994   119-95-36–1

Background.—Modifying plasma levels of lipoprotein has recently been found to alter the progression of coronary atherosclerosis favorably. There are no data, however, on the effects of a comprehensive program of risk reduction involving changes in life-style as well as medications. Whether intensive multiple risk factor reduction over 4 years would significantly decrease the rate of progression of atherosclerosis in the coronary arteries of men and women, compared with patients assigned randomly to usual physician care, was investigated.

Methods.—Two hundred fifty-nine men and 41 women (mean age, 56 years) were randomly assigned to usual care or multifactor risk reduction. All patients had angiographically determined coronary atherosclerosis. Those in the risk-reduction group were enrolled in individualized programs, including a low-fat and low-cholesterol diet, exercise, weight loss, smoking cessation, and medications to favorably affect lipoprotein profiles.

Findings.—Ninety-one percent of the randomized patients had a follow-up arteriogram, and 82% had comparative measures of segments with visible disease at baseline and follow-up. Intensive risk reduction significantly improved various risk factors, including low-density lipoprotein cholesterol and apolipoprotein B, high-density lipoprotein cholesterol, plasma triglycerides, body weight, exercise capacity, and dietary fat and cholesterol intake. The usual-care group showed relatively small changes. In both groups, lipoprotein(a) was unchanged. The rate of narrowing of diseased coronary artery segments in the risk-reduction group was 47% less than in patients receiving usual care. Three patients in each group died. Clinical cardiac events necessitated 25 hospitalizations in the risk-reduction group and 44 in the usual-care group.

Conclusions.—Combining lifestyle changes and lipid-changing medications individualized to each patient's needs resulted in a very significant improvement in the overall risk profile compared with that for usual physician care. This reduction in the risk factor significantly reduced angiographically defined progression of coronary atherosclerosis and the need for hospitalizations because of clinical cardiac events.

▶ This study contributes important new information on the success of intensive, multifactor risk reduction in decreasing the rate of progression of coronary atherosclerosis and clinical cardiac events in men and women with coronary artery disease. Coronary arteriographic benefits occurred even in individuals with a relatively low-risk profile. These data support the hypothesis that patients with coronary artery disease who sustain a substantial and permanent decrease in risk factors reduce the rate of progression of coronary atherosclerosis and the number of hospitalizations for cardiac events.

In a later report by the same investigators (1), multifactor risk reduction tended to decrease the incidence of new coronary artery lesion formation on serial arteriograms, with a mean of .47 new lesions per patient in the usual-care group and a mean of .3 in the risk-reduction group. Multiple regression analysis identified dietary fat intake as the best correlate with new lesion formation. These results indicate that intensive, multifactor risk reduction tends to diminish the frequency of new coronary artery lesion formation.—R.A. O'Rourke, M.D.

Reference

1. Quinn TG, Alderman EL, McMillan A, Haskell W: Development of new coronary atherosclerotic lesions during a 4-year multifactor risk reduction program: The Stanford Coronary Risk Intervention Project (SCRIP). *J Am Coll Cardiol* 24:900–908, 1994.

Effects of Monotherapy With an HMG-CoA Reductase Inhibitor on the Progression of Coronary Atherosclerosis as Assessed by Serial Quantitative Arteriography: The Canadian Coronary Artherosclerosis Intervention Trial
Waters D, Higginson L, Gladstone P, Kimball B, Le May M, Boccuzzi SJ, Lespérance J, and the CCAIT Study Group (Hartford Hosp, Conn)
Circulation 89:959–968, 1994   1 19-95-36–2

Background.—Patients with hyperlipidemia are often given 3-hydroxy-3-methylglutaryl coenzyme A (HMG-CoA) reductase inhibitors. However, the effect of these agents on the evolution of coronary atherosclerosis has not been established. Whether HMG-CoA reductase inhibi-

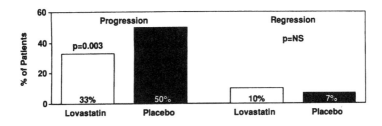

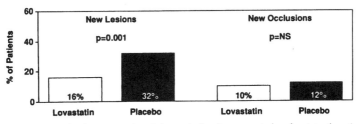

Fig 36–1.—Bar graphs showing results of the study for the categorical end points. A patient was classified as having progression if the minimum lumen diameter of at least one coronary lesion worsened by ≥ .4 mm, with no regression at other sites. Regression was defined as improvement by ≥ .4 mm of at least one lesion, with no progression at other sites. A new lesion was defined as a stenosis that was not apparent on the first film or was < 25% in diameter stenosis but that narrowed by ≥ .4 mm in minimum lumen diameter at the second angiogram. (Courtesy of Waters D, Higginson L, Gladstone P, et al: *Circulation* 89:959–968, 1994.)

tor lovastatin retards the progression or facilitates the regression of coronary atherosclerosis was investigated.

Methods.—Three hundred thirty-one patients with diffuse but not necessarily severe coronary atherosclerosis, as shown on a recent arteriogram, were enrolled in the randomized, double-blind, placebo-controlled trial. All had fasting serum cholesterol ranging from 220 to 300 mg/dL. All patients underwent intensive dietary counseling before administration of lovastatin or placebo. The active agent was begun at 20 mg/day and titrated to 40 and 80 mg during the first 16 weeks to reach a fasting low-density-lipoprotein (LDL) cholesterol level of 130 mg/dL or less. The average dose was 36 mg/day. After 2 years, a repeat coronary arteriogram was obtained.

Findings.—A total of 3,858 coronary segments containing 2,309 stenoses were blindly measured in 299 patients on pairs of films with an automated computerized quantitative system. In patients receiving lovastatin, the total cholesterol declined by 21%, and LDL cholesterol declined by 29%. In the placebo group, these values changed by less than 2%. The coronary change score, defined as the per-patient mean of the minimum lumen diameter changes for all lesions measured excluding those of less than 25% on both films, worsened by .09 mm in the placebo group and by .05 mm in the lovastatin group. Thirty-three percent of patients receiving lovastatin and 50% of those receiving placebo had a worsening in minimum diameter of 1 or more stenoses by .4 mm or greater with no regression at other sites. Twenty-three patients given lovastatin and 49 given placebo had new coronary lesions. Treatment benefits were most marked in patients with more numerous, milder lesions and in those whose baseline total or LDL cholesterol exceeded the group median (Fig 36-1).

Conclusions.—Monotherapy with the HMG-CoA reductase inhibitor lovastatin in a diverse population of patients with coronary disease retards the progression of coronary atherosclerosis and decreases the development of new coronary lesions. Patients did not commonly have regression or recanalization. Stenoses of 50% or more represented less than 15% of lesions and changed very infrequently, with no between-group differences. Therapeutic benefits were most marked in patients with more numerous, milder lesions and in patients whose baseline total or LDL cholesterol levels were above the group median.

▶ The ability of HMG-CoA reductase inhibitors to prevent the formation of new coronary artery lesions may be more important than their effect on established lesions. Because the risk of a coronary event increases with the number of coronary artery lesions demonstrated by arteriography, the lesion causing an acute coronary syndrome is usually mild until it undergoes plaque rupture. An early coronary artery lesion with a high lipid content and a thin fibrous cap is more likely to become an infarct-related coronary artery occlusion.

A report from the Monitored Atherosclerosis Regression Study (MARS) investigators (1) indicates that triglyceride-rich lipoproteins play an important role in the progression of lesions, causing less than 50% diameter stenosis in patients treated with aggressive LDL cholesterol. Thus, the triglyceride-rich lipoproteins need attention, in addition to LDL cholesterol, in the treatment of coronary atherosclerosis.

In a large, randomized, single-center study designed to assess the effects of simvastatin on blood lipids (2), this HMG-CoA reductase inhibitor effectively reduced total cholesterol and LDL cholesterol without any serious side effects during more than 3 years of follow-up. In another randomized, multicenter trial (3), the efficacy of low-dose combinations of cholestyramine and fluvastatin in lowering LDL cholesterol were compared. Reductions in LDL cholesterol of 25% to 30% were achieved with low-dose combination therapy with fluvastatin and cholestyramine. The addition of the low-dose resin produced a greater overall cholesterol reduction than did a simple doubling of the fluvastatin dosage. In another study (4), immediate-release (IR) niacin increased high-density-lipoprotein (HDL) cholesterol levels more than sustained-relief (SR) niacin, while producing a similar reduction in triglyceride levels. None of the patients taking IR niacin had liver toxicity, whereas 52% of the patients taking SR niacin did. Thus, the SR form of niacin should be restricted from use.

In another study of interest (5), the administration of antioxidant vitamin supplements (β-carotene, ascorbic acid, and vitamin E) for 1 month to patients with hypercholesterolemia reduced the susceptibility of LDL to oxidation but failed to improve the impaired endothelial-dependent vasodilation.

In the Caerphilly and Speedwell Collaborative Heart Disease Studies (6), HDL subclasses were evaluated as predictors of the risk for ischemic heart disease. In British men, both HDL_2 and HDL_3 cholesterol were inversely associated with the incidence of ischemic heart disease. However, the prediction of the risk of ischemic heart disease from total HDL cholesterol alone was not improved on by measurement of the 2 HDL subfractions.—R.A. O'Rourke, M.D.

References

1. Hodis HN, Mack WJ, Azen SP, Alaupovic P, Pogoda JM, LaBree L, Hemphill LC, Kramsch DM, Blankenhorn DH: Triglyceride- and cholesterol-rich lipoproteins have a differential effect on mild/moderate and severe lesion progression as assessed by quantitative coronary angiography in a controlled trial of lovastatin. *Circulation* 90:42–49, 1994.
2. Keech A, Collins R, MacMahon S, Armitage J, Lawson A, Wallendszus K, et al: Three-year follow-up of the Oxford cholesterol study: Assessment of the efficacy and safety of simvastatin in preparation for a large mortality study. *Eur Heart J* 15:255–269, 1994.
3. Sprecher DL, Abrams J, Allen JW, Keane WF, Chrysant SG, Ginsberg H, et al: Low-dose combined therapy with fluvastatin and cholestyramine in hyperlipidemic patients. *Ann Intern Med* 120:537–543, 1994.
4. McKenney JM, Proctor JD, Harris S, Chinchili VM: A comparison of the efficacy and toxic effects of sustained- vs immediate-release niacin in hypercholesterolemic patients. *JAMA* 271:672–677, 1994.
5. Gilligan DM, Sack MN, Guetta V, Casino PR, Quyyumi AA, Rader DJ, et al: Effect of antioxidant vitamins on low density lipoprotein oxidation and impaired endothelium-dependent vasodilation in patients with hypercholesterolemia. *J Am Coll Cardiol* 24:1611–1617, 1994.
6. Sweetnam PM, Bolton CH, Yarnell JWG, Bainton D, Baker IA, Elwood PC, Miller NE: Associations of the HDL_2 and HDL_3 cholesterol subfractions with the development of ischemic heart disease in British men: The Caerphilly and Speedwell collaborative heart disease studies. *Circulation* 90:769–774, 1994.

Relation of Leisure-Time Physical Activity and Cardiorespiratory Fitness to the Risk of Acute Myocardial Infarction in Men

Lakka TA, Venäläinen JM, Rauramaa R, Salonen R, Tuomilehto J, Salonen JT (Univ of Kuopio, Finland; Kuopio Research Inst of Exercise Medicine, Finland; Natl Public Health Inst, Helsinki)
N Engl J Med 330:1549–1554, 1994   119-95-36-3

Background.—The risk of coronary heart disease is reduced in individuals who have higher levels of regular physical activity and cardiorespiratory fitness. Most studies of this issue, however, have failed to use truly quantitative assessments of physical activity or direct measurements of maximal oxygen uptake, the most accurate method of assessing cardiorespiratory fitness.

Methods.—A detailed questionnaire was used to measure physical activity during leisure time and exercise testing to determine maximal oxygen uptake in 1,453 men. The men, aged 42–60 years at baseline examination, had no reported cardiovascular disease or cancer. Of the group, 1,166 participants were followed an average of 5 years, during which time 42 of those with initially normal ECGs sustained a first acute myocardial infarction. Independent associations were sought among physical activity, maximal oxygen uptake, and risk of acute myocardial infarction.

Results.—The relative risk of myocardial infarction was .31 in men with the highest level of physical activity—more than 2.2 hr/wk—compared with those with the lowest level, after adjustment for age and year of examination. After adjustment for age, year and season of examination, weight, height, and type of respiratory gas analyzer used, the relative hazard in patients with the highest maximal oxygen uptake—more than 2.7 L/min—was .26. Even after adjustment for as many as 17 confounding variables, the third of men with the highest level of physical activity and maximal oxygen uptake continued to have relative hazards significantly less than 1, compared with men in the lowest third of each category.

Conclusion.—A strong, graded, inverse association was found between high levels of leisure-time physical activity and cardiorespiratory fitness and risk of acute myocardial infarction in men. Low levels of physical activity and cardiorespiratory fitness are independent risk factors for coronary heart disease. Physical activity must be of moderate-to-high intensity to decrease coronary risk.

▶ Previous studies have demonstrated that leisure-time physical activity or cardiorespiratory fitness alone has an inverse and significant relationship to the risk of coronary artery disease. Also, patients with stable coronary artery disease who devote leisure time to intensive physical exercise experience a favorable upward shift of their anaerobic threshold during submaximal exercise (1). Importantly, leisure-time physical activity has been shown to be an independent predictor of change in cardiac coronary artery morphology; an inverse relationship between the amount of physical activity and the progression of coronary artery disease has been documented.

In this study, conditioning physical activity and maximal oxygen uptake were inversely associated with the risk of acute myocardial infarction among men with abnormal resting or exercise ECGs. The data suggest that physical activity with a mean intensity of 6 metabolic units (6 times higher than resting metabolic requirements) may be required to decrease the risk. Inconsistency among previous studies concerning the levels of physical activity necessary to reduce risk probably result from differences in the classification of physical activity.—R.A. O'Rourke, M.D.

Reference

1. 1994 Year Book of Medicine, p 319.

A Prospective Study of the Health Effects of Alcohol Consumption in Middle-Aged and Elderly Men: The Honolulu Heart Program

Goldberg RJ, Burchfiel CM, Reed DM, Wergowske G, Chiu D (Honolulu Heart Program, Hawaii; Natl Heart, Lung, and Blood Inst, Honolulu, Hawaii; Univ of Massachusetts, Worcester)

Circulation 89:651–659, 1994   119-95-36–4

Objective.—Although several studies have suggested that drinking a moderate amount of alcohol gives some protection against coronary heart disease, several others have shown that heavy drinkers have increased mortality from all causes, and from cardiovascular disease in particular. Data from the Honolulu Heart Program were analyzed in a prospective epidemiologic study to clarify the relationship between reported alcohol consumption and both mortality and incident nonfatal chronic disease in middle-aged (51–64 years of age) and elderly (65–75 years of age) men. Participants were followed approximately 15 years.

Study Population.—A total of 6,069 Japanese-American men who were free of coronary heart disease, cerebrovascular disease, and cancer when entered into the study and also 6 years later were enrolled. Mortality was monitored in abstainers; light drinkers, imbibing as much as 14 mL of alcohol daily; moderate drinkers, imbibing 15–39 mL/day; and heavy drinkers, imbibing 40 mL/day or more. The mortality analyses focused on 2,946 men whose alcohol intake had remained stable with time.

Observations.—Moderate drinking conferred a reduced risk of all-cause mortality and coronary heart disease in elderly men (Fig 36-2). Heavy drinkers were at the highest risk for most end points, except for an apparent beneficial effect of heavy drinking on coronary heart disease in middle-aged men. The risk of both fatal and nonfatal stroke increased with increasing alcohol consumption in middle-aged men. Elderly men who drank lightly or moderately were also at increased risk of fatal and nonfatal stroke. Heavy drinkers, whether middle-aged or elderly, were at increased risk of fatal and nonfatal malignant disease.

Implications.—These findings do not warrant a recommendation that the general population increase its alcohol intake. Men who are currently imbibing a light-to-moderate amount of alcohol, and who are not at particular risk of addiction or abuse, may continue to drink at their present level. This advice assumes that no other factors place these individuals at increased risk of chronic diseases other than coronary heart disease.

▶ Consistent with most previously published reports, this study demonstrated a protective effect on total mortality of light alcohol consumption in middle-aged men and of moderate drinking in elderly men, as well as the harmful effects of heavy alcohol consumption. As the authors note, "The finding of a beneficial effect of alcohol consumption on the occurrence of

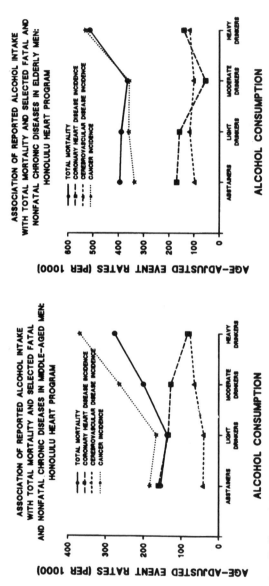

Fig 36-2.—Overall effects of alcohol intake on health-related outcomes in this cohort. (Courtesy of Goldberg RJ, Burchfiel CM, Reed DM, et al: *Circulation* 89:651–659, 1994.)

coronary heart disease, with a significant curvilinear dose-response relation observed in middle-aged men, is also consistent with the majority of [clinical] published investigations examining this issue."—R.A. O'Rourke, M.D.

Evidence for an Association Between Dehydroepiandrosterone Sulfate and Nonfatal, Premature Myocardial Infarction in Males
Mitchell LE, Sprecher DL, Borecki IB, Rice T, Laskarzewski PM, Rao DC
(Washington Univ, St Louis; Univ of Cincinnati, Ohio)
Circulation 89:89–93, 1994   119-95-36–5

Introduction.—There is considerable evidence that endogenous hormones have a causative role in coronary artery disease. Disease appears to relate inversely to serum levels of androgen and positively to serum levels of estrogen. A significant inverse relationship between coronary artery disease and the serum level of dehydroepiandrosterone sulfate (DHEAS) was described in men.

Methods.—Forty-nine men who had survived premature myocardial infarction before the age of 56 years and 49 age-matched control individuals were assessed retrospectively. The patients had a mean of 1.4 myocardial infarctions, with the most recent one an average of 3½ years before the study.

Findings.—The only endogenous hormone that correlated significantly with case-control status was DHEAS; patients had lower levels than controls. The association remained significant after controlling for total cholesterol and high-density-lipoprotein cholesterol, triglycerides, apolipoprotein fractions, and body mass index. The association between premature infarction and serum testosterone was of borderline significance. The patient and control groups did not differ significantly with respect to free testosterone or estradiol levels or the ratio of estradiol to testosterone.

Conclusion.—There is an inverse relationship between the serum level of DHEAS and premature myocardial infarction in men.

▶ In this study, "the effects of a large number of heart disease risk factors, which may confound the relation between endogenous hormones and myocardial infarction, were evaluated." Also, individuals using medications that had the potential to alter lipid, lipoprotein, or endogenous hormone levels were excluded.

This investigation "provides further evidence for an inverse association between DHEAS and myocardial infarction and confirms previous reports of an inverse association between apo A-I and myocardial infarction." The basis for the association between DHEAS and coronary artery disease is unclear.

In another study concerned with risk factors for cardiovascular disease, male Swedish construction workers were followed for 12 years during a study of cause-specific mortality (1). The age-adjusted relative risk of dying of cardiovascular disease was 1.4 for smokeless tobacco users ($n = 6,297$) and 1.9 for smokers of 15 or more cigarettes per day ($n = 13,518$) compared with nonsmokers ($n = 32,546$). Among men aged 35–54 years at the start of follow-up, the relative risk was 2.1 for smokeless tobacco users and 3.2 for smokers. Thus, both smokeless tobacco users and smokers have a significantly higher risk of dying of cardiovascular disease than do nonusers.

In a report from the Corpus Christi Heart Project (2), the overall 28-day case-fatality rate among 1,228 patients hospitalized for myocardial infarction during a 24-month period was 7.3%. The risk of 28-day case-fatality for Mexican-Americans in relation to non-Hispanic whites was 1.49. The corresponding risk for women in relation to men was 1.8. In this analysis of acute mortality after myocardial infarction, worse prognoses were observed for Mexican-Americans than for non-Hispanic whites and for women than for men. Adjustment for confounding variables, including age, diabetes, severity of myocardial infarction, and treatment, did not change the observed ethnic and sex differences in case fatality.—R.A. O'Rourke, M.D.

References

1. Bolinder G, Alfredsson L, Englund A, de Faire U: Smokeless tobacco use and increased cardiovascular mortality among Swedish construction workers. *Am J Public Health* 84:339–404, 1994.
2. Goff DC, Ramsey DJ, Labarthe DR, Nichaman MZ: Greater case-fatality after myocardial infarction among Mexican-Americans and women than among non-hispanic whites and men: Corpus Christi Heart Project. *Am J Epidemiol* 139:474–483, 1994.

37 Acute Coronary Syndromes

Significance of Anterior ST Depression in Inferior Wall Acute Myocardial Infarction
Edmunds JJ, Gibbons RJ, Bresnahan JF, Clements IP (Mayo Clinic and Found, Rochester, Minn)
Am J Cardiol 73:143–148, 1994   119-95-37–1

Background.—The mechanism of reciprocal ST depression during inferior-wall acute myocardial infarction (AMI) remains unclear. Injection of the myocardial perfusion agent technetium-99m sestamibi can be performed within a short time of the initial ECG and provides an accurate reflection of myocardial perfusion at the time of injection. Myocardial perfusion studies using this agent were performed during inferior-wall AMI to determine the relationship between the extent and location of

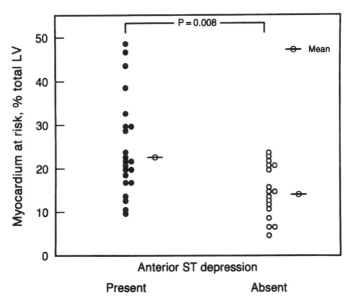

Fig 37–1.—Comparison of groups with and without ST depression during inferior infarction with respect to left ventricular (*LV*) myocardium at risk. The group with anterior ST depression has significantly more myocardium at risk. (Courtesy of Edmunds JJ, Gibbons RJ, Bresnahan JF, et al: *Am J Cardiol* 73:143–148, 1994.)

at-risk myocardium and the presence or absence of reciprocal ST depression.

Methods.—Thirty-nine consecutive patients admitted with greater than 30 minutes of chest pain and ECG evidence of inferior-wall AMI were included. Twenty-two patients had anterior ST depression on their initial ECG (median, 5.5 mm) and 17 did not. All patients underwent early tomographic myocardial perfusion imaging with technetium-99m sestamibi, with measurement of the total size of the acute perfusion defect and its lateral and septal borders.

Findings.—The patients with anterior ST depression had a mean of 23% of left ventricular myocardium at risk, significantly more than the 15% in patients without this ECG finding (Fig 37–1). Eight patients had greater than 25% of the left ventricle at risk; all had anterior ST depression. The group with anterior ST depression also showed a significantly greater lateral extent of their acute perfusion defects—49 degrees from the midinferior wall compared with 23 degrees in patients without anterior ST depression. The septal border of the perfusion defect was similar in the 2 groups, approximately −45 degrees. There were no measurable anterior perfusion defects in either group.

Conclusions.—In patients with inferior-wall AMI, anterior ST depression provides a simple and easily obtained indicator of myocardium at risk. Patients without anterior ST depression may receive less potential benefit from thrombolytic therapy. There is significant overlap, however, between patients with and without anterior ST depression.

▶ This study indicates that "the presence of anterior ST-segment depression during acute inferior wall infarction is associated with greater myocardium at risk and a more lateral extent of the acute perfusion defect. There was no evidence in any patient of an [separate] anterior perfusion abnormality" during technetium sestamibi imaging "in association with anterior ST depression." Moreover, the prevalence of left anterior descending coronary artery stenosis in the group with anterior ST-segment depression was the same as in the group without anterior ST-segment depression. Thus, the absence of anterior ST-segment depression may identify a subset of low-risk patients with inferior-wall AMI who may have less potential benefit from thrombolytic therapy or primary coronary angioplasty.—R.A. O'Rourke, M.D.

Prognostic Value of Ambulatory ST Segment Monitoring Compared With Exercise Testing at 1–3 Months After Acute Myocardial Infarction

Currie P, Ashby D, Saltissi S (Royal Liverpool Univ, England; Univ of Liverpool, England)

Eur Heart J 15:54–60, 1994   119-95-37–2

Introduction.—Several studies have found significant increases in cardiac events and rate of mortality in patients with myocardial infarction in whom ischemic ST-segment depression develops while they are on ambulatory monitoring before hospital discharge. The predictive value of ST-segment monitoring has not been established, however. The prognostic value of ambulatory ST-segment monitoring was compared with that of exercise treadmill testing in patients with myocardial infarction.

Patients and Methods.—One hundred thirty-three men and 44 women (mean age, 58 years) were included. Thirty-five had received thrombolytic therapy, and 38 had had a previous myocardial infarction. Ambulatory monitoring was performed a mean of 38 days after myocardial infarction. All but 7 patients also underwent exercise treadmill testing. Patients were followed for at least 1 year for major cardiac events, including myocardial infarction, cardiac death, and coronary revascularization.

Results.—Fifty-six patients (32%) had transient ST depression on ambulatory monitoring. In 94% of cases, these episodes were asymptomatic. The mean follow-up from ambulatory monitoring was 374 days. There were 28 major cardiac events, including 7 deaths, 9 nonfatal reinfarctions, 7 coronary artery bypass procedures, and 5 instances of coronary angioplasty. The presence of ST depression on ambulatory monitoring did not predict fatal or nonfatal cardiac events. The severity of ST depression, however, was predictive of outcome after adjusting for clinical variables and coronary prognostic indices. The ST deviation on exercise testing was significantly associated with increased cardiac events during follow-up. The ST depression on ambulatory monitoring did not identify any additional events in patients with a positive exercise test. Once variables from exercise testing were considered, no factor available from ambulatory monitoring was predictive of outcome.

Conclusions.—The finding of ST-segment depression on ambulatory monitoring 1–3 months after myocardial infarction is inferior in predictive value to the results of exercise treadmill testing. Any value of ambulatory monitoring is limited to patients who have marked ST depression. However, ambulatory monitoring may be an acceptable alternative to treadmill testing in patients who cannot perform an exercise test.

▶ This study in the late recovery phase after acute myocardial infarction is consistent with studies in other patient groups comparing ambulatory ECG monitoring for ST-segment depression with exercise ECG testing for risk-stratifying patients with coronary artery disease. ST-segment depression on ambulatory ECG monitoring was very common and did not predict increased fatal or nonfatal cardiac events. By contrast, ST depression during exercise testing was associated with increased cardiac events. Also, the addition of ambulatory ECG monitoring to exercise ECG testing did not improve the prediction of cardiac events. Although ambulatory ECG monitoring may be useful in certain patients unable to perform an exercise test, the positive predictive value for cardiac events is low, and the use of myocardial perfusion imaging or echocardiographic wall-motion assessment during pharmacologic stress (adenosine, dipyridamole, or dobutamine) yields much better specificity.—R.A. O'Rourke, M.D.

Troponin T and Myoglobin at Admission: Value of Early Diagnosis of Acute Myocardial Infarction

Bakker AJ, Koelemay MJW, Gorgels JPMC, van Vlies B, Smits R, Tijssen JGP, Haagen FDM (Medisch Centrum Leeuwarden, Amsterdam; Academisch Medisch Centrum, Amsterdam)
Eur Heart J 15:45–53, 1994   119-95-37-3

Introduction.—Immunologic estimation of cardiospecific troponin T, a polypeptide subunit of the myofibrillar regulatory troponin complex, has been proposed as a reliable marker of myocardial damage. Troponin T is released into the serum at the same time as the MB isoenzyme of creatine kinase (CK-MB) but remains elevated for as long as several weeks after acute myocardial infarction (AMI), whereas CK-MB is increased for only a few days.

Methods.—The predictive power of troponin T and myoglobin estimates was compared with that of CK, CK-MB activity, and the ECG in 290 consecutive patients suspected of having AMI. All patients were admitted within 12 hours of the onset of chest pain. Catalytic activity of CK-MB was measured by immunoinhibition and by the serum level of

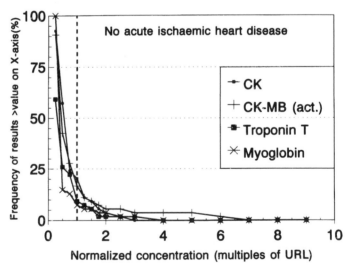

Fig 37–2.—Frequency (y-axis) of results greater than the normalized concentration on *x*-axis for the various biochemical markers at admission in patients with no acute ischemic heart disease. *URL*, upper reference limit; CK, for male 130 units/L, for female 90 units/L; *CK-MB activity* = 15 units/L; *troponin T* = .1 µg; myoglobin = 57.9 µg/L. (Courtesy of Bakker AJ, Koelemay MJW, Gorgels JPMC, et al: *Eur Heart J* 15:45–53, 1994.)

cardiac troponin T using an enzyme-linked immunosorbent assay. In addition, serum myoglobin was estimated by a turbidimetric method.

Findings.—For all anylates, fewer than 95% of the results obtained at the time of admission were within the reference range (Fig 37–2). For patients admitted 4–12 hours after the onset of chest pain, the likelihood ratio for ischemic ECG changes was 2.85. In those seen within 4 hours of the onset, an abnormal or normal myoglobin level was the measure most predictive of AMI. Troponin T had the highest sensitivity of all the markers (64%), but its specificity was only 74%; it was often elevated in patients with unstable angina. Logistic regression analysis indicated that the ECG and myoglobin concentration were the best predictors of AMI in patients seen within 4 hours of the onset of chest pain, and the ECG, CK-MB activity, and serum myoglobin were best in those seen at 4–12 hours.

Implications.—Troponin T is a sensitive indicator of myocardial damage and, along with the serum myoglobin, produces fewer false positive results than the CK and CK-MB in patients without acute ischemic heart disease. Patients seen at a very early stage are best evaluated by a myoglobin estimate and ECG. The troponin T level appears to be a marker of minor myocardial damage in patients with unstable angina.

▶ The patient's history of chest pain and the ECG have been the primary methods for screening for myocardial infarction or ischemia. In patients with suspected myocardial infarction, however, the ECG is diagnostic only in the minority. In addition, the presence of new, nonspecific ECG changes in patients with chest pain has a predictive value of less than 50% for myocardial infarction.

The established enzymatic criteria for myocardial infarction, namely serial quantitative analysis of plasma CK-MB every 4–6 hours, are regarded as the most specific, sensitive, and cost-effective means of diagnosing myocardial injury. However, experience to date with the most reliable quantitative assays have shown the plasma levels of CK-MB can reliably exclude infarction *only* after a minimum of 6–8 hours since the onset of chest pain. To this interval must be added the time required for the assay to be performed.

As the authors note, "in recent years, several different approaches have been developed to overcome the disadvantages in measuring total CK and CK-MB activity." The measurement of serum myoglobin, although less specific, has been used for the early diagnosis and monitoring of AMI. More recently, the serum level of the cardiospecific regulatory protein troponin T has been reported to be a sensitive and specific marker for myocardial damage, the troponin T in the serum increasing simultaneously with CK-MB.

In this study, the diagnostic *sensitivity* of troponin T was considerably better than that of myoglobin, total CK, and CK-MB activity in patients with a diagnosis of acute myocardial ischemia. However, the concentration of troponin T was also often elevated, unlike the concentrations of myoglobin, total CK, and CK-MB in patients with unstable angina pectoris.

In another study of markers of AMI, Wu and associates (1) demonstrated that the sensitivity of cardiac troponin T serum levels for the diagnosis of acute infarction was improved at 0–3, 3–6, and 6–9 hours after the onset of symptoms than corresponding results for serum CK-MB. However, the specificity of the markers from 49 patients without AMI was 46% and 79% for troponin T and CK-MB, respectively.

In a separate study (2), a new, automated enzyme immunoassay was used to evaluate the clinical usefulness of serum troponin T levels in the laboratory diagnosis of AMI. Serum concentration of troponin T was compared with total CK activity, CK-MB myoglobin concentrations, and lactate dehydrogenase activity in 173 patients. A concentration of troponin T of .2 μg/L was determined to be the best discriminator for AMI. At this level, the sensitivity of troponin T was .98 at the ninth hour after chest pain; specificity was .88. Only myoglobin had a high sensitivity during the first 2 hours after onset of the symptoms. The total CK had a sensitivity of greater than .97 from 8 to 38 hours, but troponin T had a consistently high sensitivity for a longer duration of between 8 and 126 hours after the onset of chest pain.

Recently, there has been considerable interest in several preliminary reports concerning the sensitivity of CK-MB and CK-MM subforms for detecting myocardial infarction during the first 6 hours after the onset of symptoms (3–5). In a report by Puleo and associates (3), the sensitivity of the CK-MB subforms for detecting myocardial infarction in the first 6 hours after the onset of symptoms was 95.7%, as compared with only 48% for the conventional CK-MB assay. Specificity was 93.9% among patients hospitalized without myocardial infarction and 96.2% among those sent home. The assay of CK-MB subforms reliably detected myocardial infarction within the first 6 hours after the onset of symptoms, and its use could reduce admission to the coronary unit by as much as 50% to 70%. The usefulness of early diagnosis of AMI by measuring plasma CK subforms resulted in more effective triage in the emergency department and the early administration of thrombolytic therapy to appropriate patients, as well as the earlier detection of coronary reocclusion and reinfarction (5).—R.A. O'Rourke, M.D.

References

1. Wu AHB, Valdes R, Apple FS, Gornet T, Stone MA, Mayfield-Stokes S, Ingersoll-Stroubos AM, Wiler B: Cardiac troponin-T immunoassay for diagnosis of acute myocardial infarction. *Clin Chem* 40:900–907, 1994.
2. Burlina A, Zaninotto M, Secchiero S, Rubin D, Accorsi F: Troponin T as a marker of ischemic myocardial injury. *Clin Biochem* 27:113–121, 1994.
3. Puleo PR, Meyer D, Wathen C, Tawa CB, Wheeler S, Hamburg RJ, Ali N, Obermueller SD, Triana JF, Zimmerman JL, Perryman MB, Roberts R: Use of a rapid assay of subforms of creatine kinase MB to diagnose or rule out acute myocardial infarction. *N Engl J Med* 331:561–566, 1994.
4. Hossein-Nia M, Kallis P, Brown PA, Chester MR, Kaski JC, Murday AJ, Treasure T, Holt DW: Creatine kinase MB isoforms: Sensitive markers of ischemic myocardial damage. *Clin Chem* 40:1265–1271, 1994.
5. Roberts R, Kleinman NS: Earlier diagnosis and treatment of acute myocardial infarction necessitates the need for a "new Diagnostic Mind-set." *Circulation* 89:872–881, 1994.

Diagnosis of Perioperative Myocardial Infarction With Measurement of Cardiac Troponin I
Adams JE III, Sicard GA, Allen BT, Bridwell KH, Lenke LG, Dávila-Román VG, Bodor GS, Ladenson JH, Jaffe AS (Washington Univ, St Louis, Mo; Vanderbilt Univ, Nashville, Tenn)
N Engl J Med 330:670–674, 1994   119-95-37-4

Introduction.—Among patients undergoing noncardiac surgical procedures, perioperative myocardial infarction is a common problem that can be difficult to diagnose. Detection of myocardial infarction in these patients would be facilitated by a serum marker more specific than MB creatine kinase for cardiac injury but just as sensitive. Serum cardiac troponin I was evaluated for this purpose.

Methods.—Ninety-six patients undergoing vascular surgery and 12 undergoing spinal surgery were included. Before surgery, each patient underwent measurement of MB creatine kinase, total creatine kinase, and cardiac troponin I. Electrocardiograms and 2-dimensional echocardiograms were also obtained. After surgery, blood samples were evaluated every 6 hours, and ECGs were evaluated daily. A second echocardiogram was obtained 3 days after surgery. The echocardiographic finding of a new abnormality in segmental wall motion was considered to indicate a perioperative infarction.

Results.—According to these criteria, perioperative myocardial infarction was diagnosed in 8 patients. Cardiac troponin I was elevated in all 8, and MB creatine kinase was elevated in 6. Of the remaining 100 patients, none of whom had evidence of perioperative myocardial infarc-

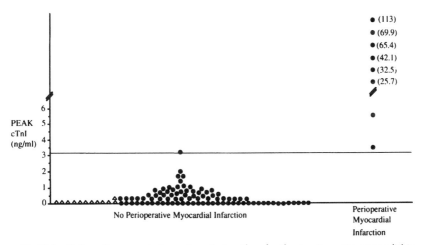

Fig 37–3.—Peak cardiac troponin I mass in patients with and without perioperative myocardial infarction. The upper reference limit for cardiac troponin I mass is 3.1 ng per mL. The *triangles* denote patients undergoing spinal surgery, and the *circles* indicate those undergoing vascular surgery. (Courtesy of Adams JE III, Sicard GA, Allen BT, et al: *N Engl J Med* 330:670–674, 1994.)

tion, 19 had elevated MB creatine kinase values, and 1 had a slight elevation in cardiac troponin I (Fig 37–3). Specificities were 99% for cardiac troponin I vs. 81% for MB creatine kinase.

Conclusions.—Cardiac troponin I is a sensitive and specific serum marker for perioperative myocardial infarction. Its greater specificity avoids the high false positive diagnosis rate observed with MB creatine kinase, and it should be simpler and more cost-effective than routine echocardiography.

▶ As the authors state, "Cardiac troponin I is a regulatory protein with a high specificity for cardiac injury. [Because] it is not found in skeletal muscle during neonatal development, or during adulthood, even after acute or chronic skeletal muscle injury," elevations in plasma concentrations do not occur unless acute myocardial necrosis is present. This study in a relatively small number of patients suggests that the measurement of cardiac troponin I can distinguish between patients with perioperative elevations of MB creatine kinase because of skeletal muscle injury and those with increased values because of myocardial injury.—R.A. O'Rourke, M.D.

Rapid Diagnosis of Coronary Reperfusion by Measurement of Myoglobin Level Every 15 Min in Acute Myocardial Infarction

Miyata M, Abe S, Arima S, Nomoto K, Kawataki M, Ueno M, Yamashita T, Hamasaki S, Toda H, Tahara M, Atsuchi Y, Nakao S, Tanaka H (Kagoshima Univ, Japan; Minami Kyushu Chuo Natl Hosp, Kagoshima, Japan; Kagoshima Municipal Hosp, Japan; et al)
J Am Coll Cardiol 23:1009–1015, 1994   119-95-37–5

Background.—Intravenous thrombolytic therapy has important benefits in the treatment of acute myocardial infarction. When thrombolysis is used, some rapid and noninvasive assessment of coronary reperfusion is needed to allow initiation of further treatment. Myoglobin, which is released early from infarcted, necrotic myocardium, may be the best available biochemical marker for rapid detection of reperfusion. The value of plasma myoglobin measurement in the assessment of coronary reperfusion was examined.

Methods.—Sixty-three patients with acute myocardial infarction were studied. All had total occlusion of the infarct-related artery, as confirmed by coronary angiography. Forty-five patients were reperfused and 18 were not. Both groups underwent measurement of myoglobin, creatinine kinase (CK), and CK-MB fraction isoenzyme (CK-MB) every 15 minutes. A 10-minute turbidimetric latex agglutination assay was used to measure myoglobin. In addition, coronary angiography was performed every 5–8 minutes to evaluate the condition of the infarct-related artery.

Results.—During the 1-hour monitoring period, all 3 biochemical markers increased at a significantly greater rate after treatment and

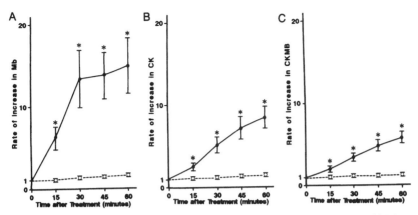

Fig 37-4.—Plots showing the time course curves of the rate of increase in myoglobin (*Mb*) (**A**), CK (**B**), and CK-MB (**C**) from the start of treatment to 60 minutes. The rates of increase in Mb, CK, and CK-MB in the reperfused group (*filled circles*) were significantly higher than those in the nonperfused group (*open circles*) at 15, 30, 45, and 60 minutes after treatment. **P* < .01 vs. the nonreperfused group. Values shown are mean value ± SE. (Courtesy of Miyata M, Abe S, Arima S, et al: *J Am Coll Cardiol* 23:1009–1015, 1994.)

reperfusion in the reperfused group than in the nonreperfused group. The reperfused patients had a significantly higher rate of myoglobin increase than the corresponding rates of CK and CK-MB increase at 15, 30, and 45 minutes after reperfusion (Fig 37-4). At a reperfusion cutoff level of 2 or greater for myoglobin, 1.8 or greater for CK, and 1.5 or greater for CK-MB, myoglobin had a predictive accuracy of 95% at 15 minutes after reperfusion, compared with 68% for CK and 73% for CK-MB.

Conclusions.—In patients with acute myocardial infarction, measuring plasma myoglobin every 15 minutes allows rapid and accurate detection of coronary reperfusion. This method allows earlier detection of coronary reperfusion without coronary angiography, compared with previously reported methods. Blinded, prospective studies are needed to confirm the discriminatory power of myoglobin for clinical use.

▶ When thrombolytic agents are administered intravenously to patients with acute myocardial infarction who do not undergo emergent coronary arteriography, it often is important to determine rapidly, accurately, and noninvasively whether coronary reperfusion has occurred so that further therapy interventions can be initiated in those who are at high risk. Several "methods for evaluating the results of reperfusion therapy utilize the washout phenomenon accompanying reperfusion of such biochemical markers" as CK, CK-MB isoenzyme, myoglobin, and CK-MM and CK-MB subforms.

In this study, the authors measured myoglobin levels every 15 minutes and could detect a rapid increase after reperfusion. Using the optimal cutoff levels for myoglobin, CK, and CK-MB within 60 minutes after reperfusion, the sensitivity and predictive accuracy for the measurement of myoglobin were significantly higher than those for CK and CK-MB at 15 minutes after reperfusion. However, as the authors state, "the evaluation of coronary perfusion by measuring myoglobin levels without coronary angiography has several problems." The first problem is the lack of specificity of myoglobin for cardiac muscle. "Second, myoglobin levels are difficult to interpret in the presence of renal failure because myoglobin is normally cleared rapidly by the kidney." Third, "in patients with spontaneous reperfusion before hospital admission, plasma myoglobin [often] will not increase in response to reperfusion therapy because it may have been previously washed out." Fourth, reocclusion often occurs after initially successful thrombolytic therapy. "In this study, the presence or absence of reperfusion within the 1st 90 minutes was examined, and patients with reocclusion occurring more >90 min after reperfusion were not investigated." Finally, "the influence of collateral [coronary] arteries on the rate of increase in serum myoglobin remains unresolved. . . ."

In a related study, Abe and associates (1) measured serum cardiac troponin T concentration and plasma CK-MB activities every 15 minutes in patients with acute myocardial infarction and attempted reperfusion therapy. The change in troponin T and the change in CK-MB levels in the reperfused groups were significantly higher than those in the nonreperfused groups 60 minutes after treatment was initiated. The sensitivity, specificity, and predictive accuracy of Δtroponin T greater than .5 ng/mL as well as ΔCK-MB 25 mU/mL were 100%, 100%, and 100% in patients with successful coronary angioplasty and 92%, 100%, and 96% in patients with successful thrombolytic therapy, respectively. Therefore, coronary reperfusion could be detected accurately 1 hour after the initiation of treatment using increases in cardiac troponin T as well as CK-MB levels in patients undergoing successful coronary angioplasty or successful thrombolytic therapy.

In another study, Jaffe and associates (2) studied the conjoint use of CK-MM and MB isoforms (subforms) in detecting coronary recanalization with thrombolytic therapy. Their preliminary data in 33 patients suggest that reperfusion criteria based on rates of change in the percentage of $CK-MB_2$ are more sensitive than those based on the percentage of $CK-MM_3$. However, criteria based on the percentage of $CK-MM_3$ were more likely to identify patients in need of an intervention to maintain coronary artery patency. More information concerning the usefulness of CK subforms in determining the status of the infarct-related coronary artery is being obtained in multicenter clinical trials involving thrombolytic therapy and primary coronary angioplasty.—R.A. O'Rourke, M.D.

References

1. Abe S, Arima S, Yamashita T, Miyata M, Okino H, Toda H, Nomoto K, Ueno M, Tahara M, Kiyonaga K, Nakao S, Tanaka H: Early assessment of reperfusion therapy using cardiac troponin T. *J Am Coll Cardiol* 23:1382–1389, 1994.
2. Jaffe AS, Eisenberg PR, Abendschein DR: Conjoint use of MM and MB creatine kinase isoforms in detection of coronary recanalization. *Am Heart J* 127:1461–1466, 1994.

Combination Antithrombotic Therapy in Unstable Rest Angina and Non–Q-Wave Infarction in Nonprior Aspirin Users: Primary End Points Analysis From the ATACS Trial

Cohen M, Adams PC, Parry G, Xiong J, Chamberlain D, Wieczorek I, Fox KAA, Chesebro JH, Strain J, Keller C, Kelly A, Lancaster G, Ali J, Kronmal R, Fuster V, Antithrombotic Therapy in Acute Coronary Syndromes Re (Hahnemann Univ Hosp, Philadelphia; Royal Victoria Infirmary, Newcastle Upon Tyne, England; Royal Sussex County Hosp, Brighton, England; et al)

Circulation 89:81–88, 1994   119-95-37–6

Background.—There is evidence that acute coronary syndromes, including unstable angina and non–Q-wave myocardial infarction, are triggered by the presence of platelet-rich thrombus over a ruptured plaque. Aggressive antithrombotic treatment encompassing both platelet inhibition and anticoagulation might be more beneficial than either measure by itself. Data from a prospective, randomized, open-label, multicenter trial were reviewed to compare combined treatment with aspirin and anticoagulation with aspirin alone, both added to conventional antianginal treatment.

Method.—Two hundred fourteen adult patients who had unstable rest angina or non–Q-wave infarction and had not used aspirin regularly were studied. The patients were randomized to receive either aspirin alone in a daily dose of 162.5 mg or aspirin in the same dose combined with a loading dose of heparin, 100 units/kg, given as an IV bolus. Subsequent heparin infusion was adjusted to maintain the activated partial thromboplastin time at twice the control level for 3–4 days. Warfarin was begun on day 2 or 3, and heparin was withdrawn when the prothrombin time was 1.3–1.5 times control. Standard antianginal treatment included metoprolol, isosorbide dinitrate, and, for high-risk patients, nifedipine. Diltiazem was used if β-blocker treatment was contraindicated. The 2 treatment groups were similar at baseline, except that more aspirin-only patients had hypertension.

Results.—After 12 weeks, 28% of patients assigned to receive aspirin alone and 19% of those receiving combined antithrombotic treatment had had a primary event (recurrent angina, myocardial infarction, or death from any cause). Post hoc analysis indicated that 27% of patients given aspirin alone and 10% of those given combination treatment had primary events. The difference was significant after adjusting for a history of hypertension and the diastolic pressure at entry to the study. Slightly more patients given aspirin alone underwent revascularization. Major bleeding occurred in 3% of patients receiving combined treatment but in none of those receiving aspirin alone.

Implication.—Aggressive antithrombotic treatment with aspirin plus anticoagulation is appropriate for patients with unstable rest angina or non–Q-wave myocardial infarction who have not been using aspirin.

▶ As Cohen et al. state, "The relative risk reduction in [myocardial] infarction or death occurring within the first 5 days in patients on combination [antithrombotic] therapy versus aspirin alone" for unstable *rest* angina was similar to that reported in 2 previous trials. The influence of combination therapy on the subset of patients with non–Q-wave infarctions was similar but less convincing, with a trend in favor of combination therapy. Because *routine* myocardial revascularization with either coronary angioplasty or urgent bypass graft surgery has not been shown to reduce acute mortality or improve long-term survival compared with aggressive medical therapy in such patients, the combination antithrombotic regimen added to antianginal drugs has become the standard, *early-phase* medical management for unstable rest angina. I agree that a more effective antithrombotic therapy must be identified for prior aspirin users and for patients with non–Q-wave infarction.

In a seemingly conflicting report, Holdright and associates (1) compared the effects of heparin and aspirin vs. aspirin alone on transient myocardial ischemia and on inhospital prognosis in patients with unstable angina at rest or with exertion. Two hundred eighty-five consecutive patients with "unstable angina" were randomized to receive either IV heparin plus oral aspirin (150 mg/day) or aspirin alone. There were no significant differences between the 2 treatment arms in the number of patients with transient myocardial ischemia (ECG ST-segment monitoring); the incidence of inhospital myocardial infarction or death was significantly greater in patients with transient myocardial ischemia. In contrast to the study by Cohen et al., the findings of Holdright and colleagues suggest that combination therapy with heparin andaspirin has noadvantages as compared with aspirinalone. Combination antithrombotictherapy did not alter the presence of transient myocardial ischemia onthe inhospital prognosis as compared with aspirin in patients with a clinical diagnosis of "unstable angina," many of whom did *not* have angina at rest in contrast to patients in the Antithrombotic Therapy in Acute Coronary Syndromes Research Group trial. Differences in patient population, inclusion criteria, end-point definitions, and study protocols obviously often result in findings that appear to be contradictory.—R.A. O'Rourke, M.D.

Reference

1. Holdright D, Patel D, Cunningham D, Thomas R, Hubbard W, Hendry G, Sutton G, Fox K: Comparison of the effect of heparin and aspirin versus aspirin alone on transient myocardial ischemia and in-hospital prognosis in patients with unstable angina. *J Am Coll Cardiol* 24:39–45, 1994.

Effects of Tissue Plasminogen Activator and a Comparison of Early Invasive and Conservative Strategies in Unstable Angina and Non–Q-

Wave Myocardial Infarction: Results of the TIMI IIIB Trial
Braunwald E, for the TIMI IIIB Investigators (Harvard Med School, Boston)
Circulation 89:1545–1556, 1994   119-95-37–7

Objective.—Coronary thrombosis is a major factor in the pathogenesis of unstable angina and non–Q-wave myocardial infarction (NQMI). The effects of thrombolytic therapy are not clear, however, and the role of early coronary arteriography followed by revascularization in these disorders has not been established. The results of the Thrombolysis in Myocardial Ischemia (TIMI IIIB) trial, designed to determine the effects of thrombolytic therapy and an early invasive strategy on the clinical outcome of unstable angina and NQMI, were reported.

Incidence of Death, Myocardial Infarction Death or Myocardial Infarction, and Stroke Within 42 Days

	TPA	Placebo	P†
All patients			
Death	2.3	2.0	.67
MI	7.4	4.9	.04
Q wave, %	43	39	NS
Before hospital discharge, %	87	83	NS
Death or MI	8.8	6.2	.05
Stroke	1.6	0.8	.14
Patients with evolving non–Q-wave MI			
Death	3.4	4.9	.41
MI	5.6	5.4	.92
Death or MI	8.1	8.6	.85
Stroke	1.7	0.8	.38
Patients with unstable angina			
Death	1.8	0.6	.07
MI	8.3	4.6	.01
Death or MI	9.1	5.0	.01
Stroke	1.6	0.8	.23

Abbreviations: TPA, tissue plasminogen activator; *MI,* myocardial infarction (fatal or nonfatal).
Note: Based on Kaplan–Meier estimation.
† Calculated from the log-rank statistic.
(Courtesy of Braunwald E, for the TIMI IIIB Investigators: *Circulation* 89:1545-1556, 1994.)

Methods.—A total of 1,473 patients with unstable angina or NQMI were included. All were seen within 24 hours of the onset of ischemic chest pain at rest. The patients were randomized to receive initial therapy with either tissue plasminogen activator (tPA) or placebo. They were further randomized to either an early invasive strategy—consisting of early coronary arteriography followed by revascularization, if possible—or an early conservative strategy—consisting of coronary arteriography followed by revascularization if the initial medical therapy failed. Both groups were placed on bed rest and given anti-ischemic medications, aspirin, and heparin.

Results.—At 6 weeks, approximately 55% of both the tPA- and placebo-treated patients had died, had a myocardial infarction, or did not respond to initial therapy. Seven percent of tPA-treated patients had fatal or nonfatal myocardial infarction after randomization, compared with 4.9% of the placebo-treated patients (table). Four patients in the tPA group had intracranial hemorrhages, compared with none in the control group. There was also no significant difference in the main outcomes of the early strategy groups. At 6 weeks, 18.1% of the conservative group and 16.2% of the invasive group had died, had myocardial infarction, or had an unsatisfactory symptom-limited exercise test. However, the average length of stay, incidence of rehospitalization, and days of rehospitalization were all significantly lower in the patients treated by the early invasive strategy.

Conclusions.—With treatment, low 6-week rates of mortality and myocardial infarction or reinfarction can be achieved in patients with unstable angina or NQMI. Results are similar whether an early conservative or an early invasive strategy is used. However, the invasive approach may reduce hospital days, rehospitalization, and need for antianginal drugs. Thus, attempting thrombolysis may not be helpful and may even be harmful.

▶ Considering the lack of clinical benefit, the higher incidence of myocardial infarction, and the .55% incidence of intracranial hemorrhage, thrombolytic therapy with tPA should not be used routinely in patients with unstable angina or NQMI.

In the TIMI IIIB trial, "the most serious end points of death and nonfatal myocardial infarction as well as the prespecified composite primary end point . . . occurred with similar frequencies in patients assigned to the 2 strategies. While more postdischarge rehospitalizations and anti-ischemic medications were required in patients randomized to the early conservative strategy, fewer cardiac catheterizations and PTcA were performed compared with" patients randomized to the early invasive strategy. Although the early invasive strategy provided more rapid relief of angina than the early conservative strategy, the anginal status by 6 weeks was similar, as was the incidence of death or myocardial infarction.

It should be emphasized that the TIMI IIIB investigators compared 2 *management strategies:* routine early coronary arteriography followed by revascularization in patients with suitable lesions and a more conservative approach in which coronary arteriography and revascularization were performed if intensive medical management failed. Thus, the results of early invasive and conservative strategies for patients with unstable angina or NQMI are similar to the findings previously reported in several clinical trials concerning patients with Q-wave myocardial infarction who received thrombolytic therapy.—R.A. O'Rourke, M.D.

Halving of Mortality at 1 Year by Domiciliary Thrombolysis in the Grampian Region Early Anistreplase Trial (GREAT)
Rawles J, for the GREAT Group (Univ of Aberdeen, Scotland)
J Am Coll Cardiol 23:1–5, 1994   119-95-37–8

Objective.—In patients with acute myocardial infarction, thrombolytic therapy appears to be more effective the earlier it is given. Although this conclusion is based on a great deal of theoretic, experimental, and clinical evidence, its clinical importance remains unclear. Whether thrombolytic therapy could be administered at home, how much time could be saved in comparison to hospital administration, and whether earlier thrombolytic therapy resulted in decreased mortality were determined.

Methods.—Three hundred eleven patients with suspected acute myocardial infarction who were seen within 4 hours of onset of symptoms were included. The participating general medical practices were located 16-62 miles from the study hospital; the practitioners were given paired ampules of anistreplase, 30 units, and matching placebo, which were randomly labeled for home or hospital injection. The hospital injection

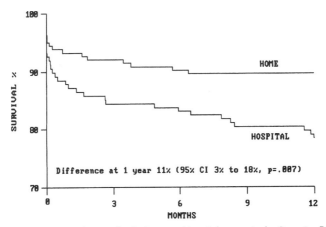

Fig 37–5.—One-year survival curves for the home and hospital groups in the Grampian Region Early Anistreplase Trial. *Abbreviation: CI*, confidence interval. (Courtesy of Rawles J, for the GREAT Group: *J Am Coll Cardiol* 23:1–5, 1994.)

was sent to the hospital along with the patient. The patients were followed for 1 year.

Results.—One hundred sixty-three patients received anistreplase at home, and 148 received it in the hospital. The anistreplase injections were given at home a median of 101 minutes after onset of symptoms and in the hospital at a median of 240 minutes. In-home thrombolysis injection saved a median of 130 minutes. At 1 year of follow-up, 10% of the patients receiving anistreplase at home had died, compared with 22% of those receiving anistreplase in the hospital. This amounted to a relative mortality rate reduction of 52%, with a 95% confidence interval of 14% to 89% (Fig 37–5).

Conclusions.—In-home administration of thrombolytic therapy by general practitioners is feasible and saves significant time compared with in-hospital administration (more than 2 hours in this study). Routine prehospital thrombolysis would likely yield similar time savings. Prehospital administration of thrombolytic drugs appears to reduce the 1-year mortality rate from acute myocardial infarction by half. Earliest-possible thrombolytic therapy may have greater clinical benefits than previously recognized.

▶ The investigators in the GREAT group are "the first to report a significant reduction in mortality rate with prehospital as compared with hospital administration of thrombolytic therapy." Anistreplase was used because it is given in an IV bolus injection rather than by slow IV infusion. The authors note that, "compared with hospital administration, domiciliary thrombolysis resulted in a time saving of > 2 h."

In 5 other randomized studies of prehospital thrombolysis, there was considerable overlap in the times of prehospital and inhospital injections. Many of the patients in *both* the hospital groups and the prehospital groups received thrombolytic therapy during the first 2 hours after the onset of symptoms, a time when thrombolysis is most efficacious.

Rawles et al. relate that, in the Myocardial Infarction Triage Intervention (MITI) Project (1), "the time difference between prehospital and in-hospital thrombolysis was only 33 min, and nearly all patients received therapy within 3 h of symptom onset. There was no significant difference in left ventricular ejection fraction or myocardial infarct size between the two groups."—R.A. O'Rourke, M.D.

Reference

1. Weaver WD, Cerqueira M, Hallstrom AP, et al: For the MITI Project Group. The myocardial infarction, triage intervention trial of prehospital versus hospital initiated thrombolytic therapy. JAMA 270:1211–1216, 1993.

Immediate Coronary Angioplasty Versus Intravenous Streptokinase in Acute Myocardial Infarction: Left Ventricular Ejection Fraction,

Hospital Mortality and Reinfarction

de Boer MJ, Hoorntje JCA, Ottervanger JP, Reiffers S, Suryapranata H, Zijlstra F (Hosp de Weezenlanden, Zwolle, The Netherlands)
J Am Coll Cardiol 23:1004–1008, 1994   119-95-37–9

Background.—Both IV thrombolysis and immediate percutaneous transluminal coronary angioplasty are frequently used in patients with acute myocardial infarction, but they have only recently been compared in randomized trials. Angioplasty has resulted more often in a patent infarct vessel and less marked residual stenosis, but it is not clear whether this translates into clinical benefit.

Patients and Methods.—Three hundred one patients, aged 75 years and younger, with acute myocardial infarction were randomly assigned to have immediate coronary angioplasty or to receive IV streptokinase (1.5 million units in 1 hour). More than 80% of patients in each group were men.

Results.—The hospital mortality rate was 7% in the thrombolysis group and 2% in the angioplasty group. The respective rates of recurrent myocardial infarction were 10% and 1%. Significantly more patients treated with streptokinase either died or had a nonfatal reinfarction (15% vs. 3%). The mean left ventricular ejection fraction was 50% in angioplasty patients and 44% in those given thrombolytic treatment.

Conclusion.—Immediate coronary angioplasty without first giving a thrombolytic agent promotes better ventricular function in patients with acute myocardial infarction and lowers both the hospital mortality rate and the risk of reinfarction compared with IV thrombolysis.

▶ Three reports comparing immediate coronary angioplasty with thrombolytic therapy for acute myocardial infarction were reviewed last year (1). de Boer and associates extended their previous trial to determine whether the better coronary artery patency and less recurrent myocardial ischemia with angioplasty, as compared with thrombolysis, would result in a more satisfactory clinical outcome. The results indicate that immediate angioplasty (when feasible) without the previous administration of a thrombolytic agent is associated with better left ventricular systolic function and a lower inhospital incidence of recurrent myocardial infarction and death as compared with treatment with IV streptokinase.—R.A. O'Rourke, M.D.

Reference

1. 1994 YEAR BOOK OF MEDICINE, p 324.

A Pilot, Early Angiographic Patency Study Using a Direct Thrombin Inhibitor As Adjunctive Therapy to Streptokinase in Acute Myocardial Infarction

Lidón R-M, Théroux P, Lespérance J, Adelman B, Bonan R, Duval D, Lévesque J (Montreal Heart Inst)

Circulation 89:1567–1572, 1994   119-95-37–10

Introduction.—Many patients with acute myocardial infarction experience reocclusion after successful reperfusion, an event associated with poorer left ventricular function and a worse prognosis. The potential benefits of using Hirulog as an adjunctive therapy to streptokinase were evaluated. Hirulog, a direct thrombin inhibitor, has been shown in experimental studies to be superior to heparin and antiplatelet therapy in enhancing patency.

Patients and Methods.—Forty-five patients were identified within 6 hours of the onset of chest pain. A 12-lead ECG was obtained, and the

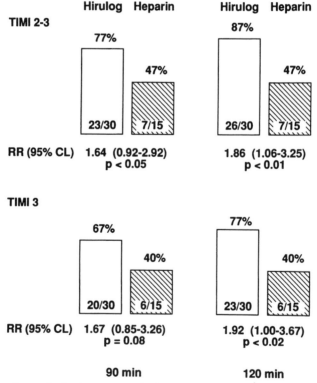

Fig 37–6.—Bar graphs showing TIMI 2 and 3 flow and TIMI 3 flow observed 90 and 120 minutes after the initiation of streptokinase and of Hirulog or heparin. *Abbreviation:* RR, relative risk of success with 95% confidence limits (CL). (Courtesy of Lidón R-M, Théroux P, Lespérance J, et al: *Circulation* 89:1567–1572, 1994.)

indication for thrombolysis was immediately established. Inclusion criteria included ST-segment elevation of at least 1 mm in 2 contiguous ECG leads. Randomization was double blind to Hirulog or heparin on a 2:1 ratio. Patients were given the study drugs immediately before or simultaneously with streptokinase. All had previously received aspirin, 325 mg orally. The infusions of Hirulog and heparin were discontinued before the second angiogram. The major end points of the study were restoration of Thrombolysis in Myocardial Infarction (TIMI) grade 2 or 3 flow at 90 and 120 minutes after the start of streptokinase and absence of reocclusion at late angiogram obtained 3–7 days later.

Results.—The 30 patients in the Hirulog group and the 15 in the heparin group were similar in baseline characteristics, except that the Hirulog patients were less frequently smokers and were more likely to have experienced a previous infarction. Coronary angiography documented a TIMI 2 or 3 flow after 90 minutes in 77% of patients in the Hirulog group and in 47% of patients in the heparin group; at 120 minutes, this outcome was achieved by 87% and 47% of patients, respectively. Hirulog had a similar advantage when TIMI 3 flow was recorded (Fig 37–6). The only patient with reocclusion at late angiogram was in the heparin group. Chest pain was relieved sooner, and serious bleeding events were less common with Hirulog than with heparin.

Conclusions.—In this pilot study, Hirulog was clearly superior to heparin when used as an adjunctive therapy to streptokinase. The early patency rate was significantly improved with administration of Hirulog, and severe bleeding complications occurred less frequently than with heparin.

▶ As the authors note, "this study suggests that Hirulog, one of the new direct thrombin inhibitors, can potentiate the thrombolytic efficacy of streptokinase, resulting in an enhanced rate of early patency of the infarct-related coronary artery." The initial infusion rate of Hirulog was .5 mg/kg/hour, and heparin was given at 1,000 units/hr. After 12 hours, the infusion rate of Hirulog was reduced to .1 mg/kg/hour, whereas the rate of heparin infusion was titrated to maintain an activated partial thromboplastin time 2–2.5 times control.

In the TIMI 5 trial (1), a pilot trial of hirudin vs. heparin given with front-loaded tissue-type plasminogen activator and aspirin was initiated in 246 patients with acute myocardial infarction. The antithrombin agent hirudin appeared to offer several advantages over heparin. Hirudin improved the combination of early and sustained TIMI grade 3 flow, as well as coronary artery patency at 18–36 hours, and resulted in a more stable clinical course; the inhospital death and reinfarction rates were lowered.

In 3 subsequent reports (2–4), surprisingly high rates of intracranial hemorrhage were associated with the administration of 2 plasminogen activators (streptokinase and tissue-type plasminogen activator) and 2 intravenously administered anticoagulants (heparin and hirudin). Subsequent trials using hirudin and heparin as adjunctive therapy have been designed with a lower hirudin bolus and infusion rate and a lower rate of heparin infusion. Infusion of both antithrombins are being titrated to a target activated partial thromboplastin time of 55–85 seconds.—R.A. O'Rourke, M.D.

References

1. Cannon CP, McCabe CH, Henry TD, for the TIMI 5 Investigators: A pilot trial of recombinant desulfatohirudin compared with heparin in conjunction with tissue-type plasminogen activator and aspirin for acute myocardial infarction: Results of the thrombolysis in myocardial infarction (TIMI) 5 trial. *J Am Coll Cardiol* 23:993–1003, 1994.
2. Antman EM, for the TIMI 9A Investigators: Hirudin in acute myocardial infarction: Safety report from the Thrombolysis and Thrombin Inhibition in Myocardial Infarction (TIMI) 9A trial. *Circulation* 90:1624–1630, 1994.
3. The Global Use of Strategies to Open Occluded Coronary Arteries (GUSTO) IIa Investigators: Randomized trial of intravenous heparin versus recombinant hirudin for acute coronary syndromes. *Circulation* 90:1631–1637, 1994.
4. Neuhaus K-L, von Essen R, Tebbe U, Jessel A, Heinrichs H, Mäurer W, Döring W, Harmjanz D, Kötter V, Kalhammer E, Simon H, Horacek T: Safety observations from the pilot phase of the randomized r-hirudin for improvement of thrombolysis (HIT-III) study. *Circulation* 90:1638–1642, 1994.

Clinical Importance of Thrombocytopenia Occurring in the Hospital Phase After Administration of Thrombolytic Therapy for Acute Myocardial Infarction

Harrington RA, for the Thrombolysis and Angioplasty in Myocardial Infarction Study Group (Duke Univ Med Ctr, Durham, NC)

J Am Coll Cardiol 23:891–898, 1994   119-95-37–11

Introduction.—Thrombolytic measures have reduced the mortality rate associated with acute myocardial infarction, but bleeding remains a major problem and may be associated with thrombocytopenia.

Method.—The frequency and sequelae of thrombocytopenia were examined in 1,001 patients with myocardial infarction who received recombinant tissue–type plasminogen activator, urokinase, or combined thrombolytic treatment in varying doses. All patients also received heparin, aspirin, and a calcium channel blocker.

Findings.—Thrombocytopenia, defined as a nadir platelet count of less than 100,000/μL or a 50% or greater reduction from baseline, developed in 16.4% of patients. The risk was similar for the various thrombolytic regimens. The occurrence of thrombocytopenia correlated with a lower initial ejection fraction and with triple-vessel coronary artery disease. Thrombocytopenia was associated with more frequent bleeding, a more complicated hospital course, and higher hospital mortality even after adjusting for a number of important prognostic variables. Patients whose lowest platelet count was less than 100,000/μL had a hospital mortality rate of 21.9%.

Conclusions.—Thrombocytopenia is frequent in patients given thrombolytic treatment for acute myocardial infarction. Its occurrence is strongly associated with excessive bleeding and increased mortality. The platelet count should be monitored on a daily basis.

▶ The common occurrence of thrombocytopenia after thrombolytic therapy may result from several causes, including heparin-induced thrombocytopenia, the use of intra-aortic balloon counterpulsation, the mechanical trauma and local consumption of platelets associated with cardiopulmonary bypass, and the possible antiplatelet effects of the thrombolytic agents and the fibrinolytic state they produce.

In a randomized, double-blind, placebo-controlled trial, the Anticoagulants in the Secondary Prevention of Events in Coronary Thrombosis (ASPECT) research group (1) assessed the effect of long-term oral anticoagulant therapy on mortality in 3,404 hospital survivors of myocardial infarction. Anticoagulant treatment, as compared with placebo treatment, significantly reduced the incidence of recurrent myocardial infarction (hazard ratio, .47) and of cerebrovascular events (hazard ratio, .6). However, major bleeding complications were observed in 73 patients who received anticoagulation, as compared with 19 who received placebo, during the mean follow-up of 37 months. Because this trial did not include patients treated with aspirin, no efficacy estimates for the comparison of anticoagulant and aspirin treatment can be derived from these data.

In several large, ongoing clinical trials, low-dose aspirin, low-dose warfarin, and various combinations of anticoagulant and antiplatelet therapy are being compared for the secondary prevention of acute coronary syndromes and for the prevention of embolic stroke.—R.A. O'Rourke, M.D.

Reference

1. Anticoagulants in the Secondary Prevention of Events in Coronary Thrombosis (ASPECT) Research Group: Effect of long-term oral anticoagulant treatment of mortality and cardiovascular morbidity after myocardial infarction. *Lancet* 343:499–503, 1994.

Acute Intervention With Captopril During Thrombolysis in Patients With First Anterior Myocardial Infarction: Results From the Captoprii and Thrombolysis Study (CATS)
Kingma JH, For The CATS Investigators (St. Antonius Hosp, Nieuwegein, The Netherlands)
Eur Heart J 15:898–907, 1994   119-95-37–12

Hypothesis.—Experimental work suggests that concomitant administration of captopril should enhance the effects of thrombolysis during acute myocardial infarction. In addition, ongoing treatment should preserve left ventricular function in the chronic phase of infarction.

Study Design.—The effects of captopril were examined in a double-blind, placebo-controlled trial. Two hundred ninety-eight patients with a first anterior myocardial infarction who received IV streptokinase within 6 hours of the onset of symptoms were enrolled. The patients were randomly assigned to receive either 6.25 mg of captopril or placebo starting at the time of streptokinase infusion. The dose was titrated to 25 mg 3 times daily and continued for 3 months, as long as the systolic blood pressure remained at 95 mm Hg or higher.

Results.—Hypotension occurred only slightly more frequently in the captopril group during titration. At 3 months, the rate was 26.8% in the captopril group and 18.1% in the placebo group. Left ventricular end-diastolic and end-systolic volumes tended to be lower in the captopril group at all intervals. Ventricular arrhythmias were less frequent in the actively treated patients. Their levels of norepinephrine and angiotensin-converting enzyme activity were significantly lower than in the placebo group, as was the peak creatine kinase. The mortality rate was low in both groups, but heart failure was 34% less frequent in the patients who received captopril.

Conclusion.—Captopril therapy at the time of thrombolysis was associated with less frequent heart failure in these patients with a first myocardial infarct, and the drug was well tolerated.

▶ The long-term use of the angiotensin-converting enzyme inhibitor captopril in patients with asymptomatic left ventricular dysfunction after myocardial infarction reduces mortality, the incidence of heart failure, and the rate of reinfarction. However, treatment with IV enalapril within 24 hours of the onset of symptoms of myocardial infarction and subsequent oral therapy did not modify the 6-month rate of survival. A modest, but significant favorable effect on mortality by captopril and lisinopril, respectively, has been observed when treatment is started within the first 24 hours after myocardial infarction.

In this randomized, double-blind, placebo-controlled trial, 298 patients with a first *anterior* myocardial infarction who were eligible for thrombolytic therapy were treated with 6.25 mg of captopril or placebo started immediately after streptokinase infusion with captropril then titrated to 25 mg 3 times a day. After the first dose, hypotension was reported in 18 patients receiving placebo and 31 patients receiving captopril. Left ventricular volumes were significantly increased in both groups at 3 months but were somewhat smaller in the captopril-treated group. The incidence of accelerated idioventricular rhythm and nonsustained ventricular tachycardia was lower in patients receiving captopril than in those receiving placebo. This incidence was paralleled by transiently lower norepinephrine levels during thrombolysis. Also, enzymatic-determined infarct size was smaller in the captopril group. A 34% lower incidence of heart failure occurred during 3 months of follow-up in the captopril group. Thus, the initiation of early captopril therapy should be seriously considered for patients with anterior myocardial infarctions who are receiving thrombolytic therapy when hypotension is absent.—R.A. O'Rourke, M.D.

GISSI-3: Effects of Lisinopril and Transdermal Glyceryl Trinitrate Singly and Together on 6-Week Mortality and Ventricular Function After Acute Myocardial Infarction

Gruppo Italiano per lo Studio della Sopravvivenza nell'Infarto Miocardico (GISSI-3 Coordinating Centre, Milan, Italy)
Lancet 343:1115–1122, 1994   119-95-37–13

Introduction.—Deteriorating left ventricular function is the strongest predictor of mortality after acute myocardial infarction. The effects on mortality and ventricular function of lisinopril, an angiotensin-converting enzyme (ACE) inhibitor, were compared with the effects of transdermal glyceryl trinitrate (GTN) in a large, controlled, multicenter open trial.

Methods.—A total of 19,394 patients with chest pain and ECG findings consistent with acute myocardial infarction were randomly assigned to 1 of 4 treatment groups. The groups received either lisinopril alone, transdermal GTN alone, combined lisinopril and transdermal GTN, or neither therapy for 6 weeks. Patients were also treated with thrombolysis, IV β-blockers, and aspirin when appropriate. Left ventricular function was assessed at 6 weeks.

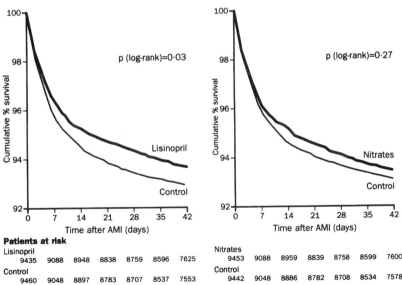

Fig 37–7.—Six-week survival in lisinopril, nitrates, and respective control groups. (Courtesy of Gruppo Italiano per lo Studio della Sopravvivenza nell'Infarto Miocardico: *Lancet* 343:1115–1122, 1994.)

Results.—Mortality risk was reduced by 11% in the patients treated with lisinopril compared with the control group, whereas mortality risk was slightly but not significantly reduced in patients treated with GTN (Fig 37-7). Lisinopril also reduced the number of patients with a severely diminished left ventricular ejection fraction. In the group treated with both lisinopril and GTN, the fewest patients experienced severe left ventricular deterioration. The limiting adverse reactions were hypotension and renal function impairment, which occurred more frequently with lisinopril therapy.

Discussion.—There was a significant reduction in mortality and in left ventricular dysfunction with lisinopril treatment. The lisinopril protocol was also safe; the hypotension episodes did not produce clinically relevant cardiac events. The lack of significant effect with transdermal GTN alone, but significant effect of combined lisinopril and GTN therapy, suggests that there may be a cumulative, synergistic benefit.

▶ This GISSI-3 protocol was specifically designed not only to test the drug effects of the ACE inhibitor lisinopril and transdermal GTN, but also to assess the benefit-risk ratio of the combination of these drugs in the whole population of patients with acute myocardial infarction and in elderly patients and women who are at higher risk of cardiac mortality.

Lisinopril, started within 24 hours of the onset of symptoms, produced a significant reduction in the overall mortality and the combined outcome measurement of mortality and severe left ventricular dysfunction. The systematic administration of transdermal GTN did not show any independent effect on the same outcome parameters. The combined administration of lisinopril and GTN also produced significant reductions in overall mortality and the combined end point. The favorable effect on the combined end point with lisinopril alone or together with GTN definitely was present in the predefined high-risk populations (elderly patients and women). Vasodilator therapy with an ACE inhibitor alone appears applicable and beneficial for most patients with a depressed left ventricular systolic function.—R.A. O'Rourke, M.D.

Long-Term Outcome After Intravenous Magnesium Sulphate in Suspected Acute Myocardial Infarction: The Second Leicester Intravenous Magnesium Intervention Trial (LIMIT-2)
Woods KL, Fletcher S (Univ of Leicester, England)
Lancet 343:816–819, 1994   119-95-37–14

Background.—The second Leicester Intravenous Magnesium Intervention Trial (LIMIT-2) was intended to determine whether doubling the serum magnesium level during acute myocardial infarction would lessen the mortality rate. Early analysis showed that the mortality rate at 28 days was reduced by 24% in patients who received magnesium and that left ventricular failure in the coronary care unit was reduced 25%. The long-term results are now available.

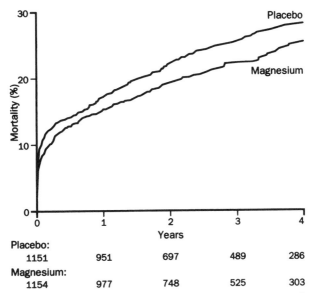

Fig 37–8.—Mortality from all causes in the trial groups. The number of patients at risk in each group at the beginning of each year are shown. (Courtesy of Woods KL, Fletcher S: *Lancet* 343:816–819, 1994.)

Trial Design.—A total of 2,316 patients suspected of having acute myocardial infarction were randomly assigned in a double-blind manner to receive either an IV load of 8 mmol of magnesium sulfate, followed by a 24-hour infusion of 65 mmol, or a loading dose and infusion of saline. The median time of randomization was 3 hours after the onset of symptoms.

Results.—Deaths resulting from all causes were reduced 16% in the magnesium group (Fig 37–8). The difference in long-term survival was entirely attributable to reduced mortality from ischemic heart disease, which was 21% lower in the magnesium-treated group. There was no indication that patients who were hypotensive initially were unequally allocated to the active-treatment and placebo groups.

Conclusion.—Intravenously administered magnesium sulfate improves long-term survival when given at an early stage of acute myocardial infarction.

▶ "In LIMIT-2, magnesium given for the first 24 h after admission reduced the incidence of left ventricular failure by 25% with a corresponding reduction in mortality rate from ischaemic heart disease during a mean follow-up of 2.7 years."

A loading dose of magnesium was given before any thrombolytic therapy; in those patients not given thrombolytic therapy, magnesium was infused early enough to increase the serum magnesium level for the time when spontaneous reperfusion is most likely to occur.

Woods and Fletcher also report that, in the ISIS-4 study (1), "intravenous magnesium sulphate had no effect on mortality. The dose of magnesium was almost identical to that in LIMIT-2 but with open control. However, the time from onset of symptoms to randomisation was substantially longer" (median, 8 hours). "The protocol specified that thrombolytic therapy should be given first and the lytic phase completed before trial randomisation." Therefore, the likelihood of reperfusion, either induced or spontaneous, occurring during magnesium treatment was less. It is uncertain "whether the antiplatelet and coronary vasodilator actions of magnesium salts make any contribution to myocardial protection in acute myocardial infarction."

The results of LIMIT-2 indicate that early IV magnesium sulfate may be a useful addition to standard therapy. Its role needs further definition as to when and for whom.—R.A. O'Rourke, M.D.

Reference

1. ISIS Collaborative Group: ISIS-4: Randomised study of intravenous magnesium in over 50 000 patients with suspected acute myocardial infarction *Circulation* 4:1559, 1993.

38 Chronic Coronary Heart Disease

Practice Guidelines and Reminders to Reduce Duration of Hospital Stay for Patients With Chest Pain: An Interventional Trial
Weingarten SR, Riedinger MS, Conner L, Lee TH, Hoffman I, Johnson B, Ellrodt AG (Cedars-Sinai Med Ctr, Los Angeles; Brigham and Women's Hosp, Boston)
Ann Intern Med 120:257–263, 1994   119-95-38–1

Introduction.—Practice guidelines have been developed to reduce the inappropriate use of coronary care units, but the efficacy and acceptability of these guidelines have not been thoroughly studied. Although guidelines and decision aids are now frequently used for patients admitted to coronary care and intermediate care units, few have actually been tested in clinical practice.

Study Plan.—At a large teaching community hospital, a guideline was evaluated prospectively in 375 patients admitted with chest pain to coronary care and intermediate care units. On an alternate-month basis for 1 year, the physicians treating these patients, whose risk of complications was considered to be low, received personalized written and verbal reminders concerning a recommended 2-day hospital stay. All patients were initially evaluated by utilization review coordinators. Research nurse reviewers retrospectively determined the correct risk classification according to information available in the medical record.

Results.—Compliance with the guideline increased by at least 50% and by as much as 69% when concurrent reminders were provided. The hospital stay decreased from a mean of 3.5 to a mean of 2.6 days. The intervention was associated with a total cost reduction averaging $1,397 per patient. There was no significant difference in the rates of complications between patients admitted to the hospital during control and intervention periods. There were also no significant differences in health status, patient satisfaction, or complications recorded 1 month after discharge.

Conclusions.—Concurrent feedback of practice guideline recommendations can significantly alter physician behavior and patient care. Practice guidelines have the potential to reduce health care costs for low-risk patients with chest pain without increasing the risk of complications.

▶ There is considerable interest and motivation for decreasing the duration of hospitalization of patients admitted because of chest pain that may represent an acute or chronic coronary artery syndrome. Several abstracts in the previous chapter concern the earlier diagnosis or exclusion of acute myocardial infarction using techniques that detect evidence of myocardial necrosis.

Patients admitted with chest pain who were considered to be at *low risk* and in whom the diagnosis of acute myocardial infarction was *excluded* did well with the application of a practice guideline recommending a 2-day hospital stay. The concurrent reminders to the physician reduced hospital costs in this low-risk subset of patients without an apparent increase in morbidity and mortality resulting from shorter-term hospitalization. The reduced hospital stay was not offset by increased outpatient diagnostic testing. Importantly, when direct feedback of guideline recommendations was withdrawn, physician practice reverted to that observed before initiation of the reminder intervention. Thus, a reduced hospital stay for low-risk patients with chest pain can be a reality when physician "motivation" is appropriate.—R.A. O'Rourke, M.D.

Echocardiographic Correlates of Survival in Patients With Chest Pain
Fleischmann KE, Goldman L, Robiolio PA, Lee RT, Johnson PA, Cook EF, Lee TH (Harvard Med School, Boston)
J Am Coll Cardiol 23:1390–1396, 1994   119-95-38-2

Background.—One reason the prognostic usefulness of echocardiographic data in patients with acute chest pain remains unclear is the qual-

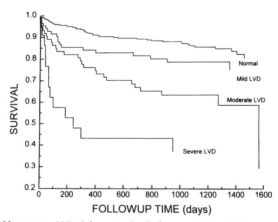

Fig 38–1.—*Abbreviation:* LVD, left ventricular dysfunction. Kaplan–Meier survival curves for patients stratified by left ventricular function. (Courtesy of Fleischmann KE, Goldman L, Robiolio PA, et al: *J Am Coll Cardiol* 23:1390–1396, 1994.)

itative nature of routine echocardiographic readings. Qualitative measurements have not been integrated into risk stratification algorithms, which tend to use quantitative assessments. Echocardiographic predictors of survival were identified in patients with chest pain.

Methods.—Five hundred thirteen patients underwent transthoracic 2-dimensional and Doppler echocardiography within 1 month of emergency department visits for acute chest pain. Clinical and ECG data were recorded at the time of initial evaluation; echocardiographic data were subsequently obtained from official hospital reports. Follow-up survival data were obtained from medical records or the Massachusetts Bureau of Vital Statistics.

Results.—Twenty percent of patients had died a mean of 28.5 months after the index visit; in 57% of these patients, the primary cause of death was cardiovascular. In univariate analysis, several echocardiographic variables correlated significantly with overall mortality: structural abnormalities of the mitral and aortic valves, aortic regurgitation, mitral regurgitation, left ventricular enlargement, moderate or severe depression of global left ventricular function, and regional wall motion abnormalities. The incidence of mortality increased steadily with severity of abnormal global left ventricular function and mitral regurgitation (Fig 38-1). Mortality rate ratios were highest for severe left ventricular enlargement, severe left ventricular dysfunction, and 3+ or 4+ mitral regurgitation.

Conclusion.—Qualitative echocardiographic data of left ventricular dysfunction and mitral regurgitation are independent correlates with prognosis in patients with acute chest pain, including those without myocardial infarction. Additional data are needed to determine whether these findings can be generalized.

▶ These data are consistent with "findings from previous reports that have established global left ventricular systolic function as an potent prognostic factor for patients after acute myocardial infarction." It also has been previously shown that moderate-to-severe mitral regurgitation caused by acute myocardial infarction is an independent predictor of mortality (1).

This retrospective analysis in patients seen in an emergency department with chest pain is a basis for prospective studies using 2-dimensional and Doppler echocardiographic data to determine whether the incremental benefit of transthoracic echocardiography for risk stratification is cost-effective.

In another study related to patients with chest pain, Gaspoz and associates (2) determined the safety and cost of a new, short-stay unit for low-risk patients. Patients were admitted to 2 beds with telemetry monitoring within a 10-bed holding unit adjacent to the emergency department. Guidelines for admission were a probability of acute myocardial infarction of 10% or less, an anticipated stay of fewer than 48 hours, and the absence of clinical indicators of myocardial ischemia, arrhythmias, or depressed left ventricular systolic function.

The rate of recurrent myocardial infarction or cardiac deaths during 6 months after the initial presentation of the 592 patients admitted to the coronary observation unit was similar to that of the 924 comparison patients before and after adjustments for clinical factors influencing the triage strategy and initial diagnosis. Their median total costs at 6 months were significantly lower than for comparison patients admitted to the wards, to stepdown or intermediate care units, or to the coronary care units.

These results suggest that the coronary observation unit is a safe and cost-saving option to other triage strategies for patients with a low risk of acute myocardial infarction admitted from the emergency department.—R.A. O'Rourke, M.D.

References

1. 1993 YEAR BOOK OF MEDICINE, p 355.
2. Gaspoz J-M, Lee TH, Weinstein MC, Cook EF, Goldman P, Komaroff AL, Goldman L: Cost-effectiveness of a new short-stay unit to "rule out" acute myocardial infarction in low risk patients. *J Am Coll Cardiol* 24:1249–1259, 1994.

Morning Increase in Ambulatory Ischemia in Patients With Stable Coronary Artery Disease: Importance of Physical Activity and Increased Cardiac Demand
Parker JD, Testa MA, Jimenez AH, Tofler GH, Muller JE, Parker JO, Stone PH (Harvard Med School, Boston; Harvard School of Public Health, Boston; Queen's Univ, Kingston, Ont, Canada)
Circulation 89:604–614, 1994   119-95-38-3

Introduction.—Acute cardiac ischemic events tend to occur in the first hours after awakening in the morning, and reversible episodes of myocardial ischemia exhibit a similar pattern. A better understanding of how ambulatory ischemia develops may help determine appropriate interventions.

Study Plan.—A double-blind, randomized, placebo-controlled trial was carried out at 2 clinical centers to determine whether the concentration of ambulatory ischemia in the morning results from physical activity or whether it reflects a basic endogenous circadian phenomenon, such as altered coronary vasomotor tone. Initially, patients received either nadolol in a maximum dose of 120 mg/day or a placebo for 5–7 days. The mean dose was 100 mg/day. The patients then were admitted for ambulatory ECG monitoring for 2 days: 1 day of regular activities, and 1 during which the usual morning activities were deferred.

Results.—In the 19 patients evaluated, nadolol reduced the systolic blood pressure and heart rate in the hospital phase. Most ECG manifestations of cardiac ischemia were significantly reduced by nadolol compared with placebo use. In placebo recipients, ischemic episodes were most numerous between 8 AM and noon on the day of regular activity but occurred 3–4 hours later when activity was deferred. Treatment with nadalol abolished the peak of ischemic episodes at the time activity began in the morning. No circadian variation in ischemic episodes was evident during treatment with nadolol. In patients given nadolol, the increase in heart rate before ischemic episodes occurring in the late afternoon or at night was significantly less than in those occurring at other times.

Implications.—The peak in myocardial ischemia noted in the morning hours is related to physical activity rather than any endogenous phenomenon. β-Blockade is associated with ischemic episodes that do not follow an increase in heart rate, events that may result in part from episodic coronary vasoconstriction. Combined treatment with a β-blocker and either an organic nitrate or a calcium channel antagonist may effectively prevent these episodes.

▶ The data from this study indicate that "the morning increase in ambulatory myocardial ischemia [that occurs in patients with chronic stable coronary artery disease] is closely related to the morning increase in physical activity and not to an endogenous phenomenon occurring at that time of the day." A long acting β-blocker reduced the frequency of ischemic episodes occurring in the morning and early afternoon, but only those episodes associated with an increase in heart rate. These results are consistent with observations by others that the use of β-adrenergic blockers reduces the likelihood of myocardial infarction and sudden death occurring during the morning hours. Because both an increase in myocardial oxygen demand and episodic coronary vasoconstriction may be responsible for episodes of myocardial ischemia, the "combination of a β-adrenergic blocking agent with either an organic nitrate or a calcium antagonist ["double" or "triple" therapy] may be particularly valuable because both of these latter agents have been reported to be effective in the management of ischemic events not mediated by increases in heart rate."

The primary objective of the Asymptomatic Cardiac Ischemia Pilot (ACIP) study (1) was to compare the 12-week efficacy of 3 treatment strategies for suppressing myocardial ischemia and to assess the feasibility of a prognosis trial in patients with asymptomatic cardiac ischemia. In this multicenter trial, patients were randomly assigned to 1 of the 3 strategies: First, angina-guided medical therapy; second, angina-guided plus ambulatory ECG ischemia-guided medical therapy; and finally, either percutaneous transluminal coronary angioplasty or coronary bypass surgery (revascularization strategy). The results of ACIP presented at the November 1994 American Heart Association Scientific Sessions suggest the probability of a more favorable prognosis in patients receiving revascularization therapy for recurrent episodes of asymptomatic cardiac ischemia.—R.A. O'Rourke, M.D.

Reference

1. Pepine CJ, and associates for the ACIP Investigators: The asymptomatic cardiac ischemia pilot (ACIP) study: Design of a randomized clinical trial, baseline data

and implications for a long-term outcome trial. *J Am Coll Cardiol* 24:1–10, 1994.

Coronary Vasodilator Reserve, Pain Perception, and Sex in Patients With Syndrome X

Rosen SD, Uren NG, Kaski J-C, Tousoulis D, Davies GJ, Camici PG (Hammersmith Hosp, London)
Circulation 90:50–60, 1994   119-95-38–4

Background.—Because of the anginal quality of the chest pain and the ST-segment changes on the stress ECG, an ischemic cause for syndrome X has been suspected. The function of the coronary microcirculation and its relationship to pain perception were investigated.

Methods.—Myocardial blood flow (MBF) was measured at rest and after IV dipyridamole administration using positron emission tomography with $H_2^{15}O$, and coronary vasodilator reserve was calculated as $MBF_{dipyridamole}/MBF_{rest}$. Changes in ECG and chest pain after dipyridamole administration in patients with syndrome X were compared with those in patients with coronary artery disease (CAD).

Findings.—Resting and postdipyridamole MBFs were homogeneous throughout the left ventricle in patients with syndrome X and in controls. In the respective groups, MBF was 1.05 vs. 1 mL/min^{-1}/g^{-1} at rest and 2.73 vs. 3 mL/min^{-1}/g^{-1} after dipyridamole. Coronary vasodilator reserves were 2.66 and 3.06 in patients and controls, respectively, and, after correction of resting MBF for rate-pressure product, were 2.35 and 2.34. Women with syndrome X had greater resting MBFs than men, 1.18 vs. .88 mL/min^{-1}/g^{-1}, respectively. The occurrence of chest pain after dipyridamole administration was as frequent in patients with syndrome X as in those with CAD.

Conclusions.—There were no differences between patients with syndrome X and controls in MBF at rest or after dipyridamole, respectively, even though patients with syndrome X have chest pain to the same extent as patients with CAD after dipyridamole. These findings cast more doubt on the proposition that ischemia is the basis of chest pain in syndrome X, at least in most patients.

▶ There continues to be considerable controversy regarding the incidence of patients with *classic angina pectoris* who have normal coronary arteriograms and no evidence of inducible coronary vasospasm or the implications. In this study, a well-defined group of patients with syndrome X were matched with true normal controls. The results indicate that global and regional myocardial blood flow and coronary vascular reserve are comparable in patients with syndrome X and normal controls. Among patients with syndrome X, there was no relationship between myocardial blood flow, chest pain, and ECG changes during stress. However, an abnormal perception of chest pain could be demonstrated in many patients with syndrome X and may be related to activation and interactions of the central and sympathetic nervous systems.

In a randomized, double-blind, placebo-controlled study, Cannon and associates (1) showed that imipramine, but not clonidine, improved the symptoms of patients with chest pain and normal coronary arteriograms, probably through a visceral analgesic effect. The reduction in sensitivity to cardiac pain among patients who received imipramine was unrelated to a change in esophageal mortality or to the psychiatric profile. Because the symptomatic benefit of imipramine was independent of the results of cardiac, esophageal, or psychiatric testing before treatment, this drug may have wide applicability in the management of chest pain in patients with normal coronary arteriograms who continue to have symptoms despite reassurance that their prognosis is good.—R.A. O'Rourke, M.D.

Reference

1. Cannon RO, Quyyumi AA, Mincemoyer R, Stine AM, Gracely RH, Smith WB, Geraci MF, Black BC, Uhde TW, Waclawiw MA, Maher K, Benjamin SB: Imipramine in patients with chest pain despite normal coronary angiograms. N *Engl J Med* 330:1411–1417, 1994.

Lack of Pharmacologic Tolerance and Rebound Angina Pectoris During Twice-Daily Therapy With Isosorbide-5-Mononitrate
Thadani U, Maranda CR, Amsterdam E, Spaccavento L, Friedman RG, Chernoff R, Zellner S, Gorwit J, Hinderaker PH (Univ of Oklahoma, Health Sciences Ctr, Oklahoma City; McGill Univ, Montreal; Univ of California, Sacramento; et al)
Ann Intern Med 120:353–359, 1994   119-95-38–5

Introduction.—Several methods have been attempted to reduce nitrate tolerance and extend antianginal effects. Isosorbide-5-mononitrate (IS-5-MN) at 20 mg exerts a prolonged effect and produces tolerance but remains inadequate therapy on a dosing schedule at 8 AM and 8 PM. Exercise performance, side effects, and anginal attacks with an alternative dosing schedule were evaluated in a double-blind, placebo-controlled, randomized study.

Methods.—All antianginal drugs, except β-blockers, were discontinued. After 1 week of single-blind placebo, 116 patients were randomized to 20 mg of IS-5-MN at 8 AM and 3 PM or placebo for 2 weeks. Evaluations included symptom-limited exercise tests and review of angina diaries.

Findings.—Patients taking IS-5-MN walked significantly longer at 2, 5, and 7 hours after the morning dose and at 2 and 5 hours after the afternoon dose (Fig 38-2). Neither anginal attacks nor nitroglycerin consumption was increased in the IS-5-MN group. Nineteen patients (32%)

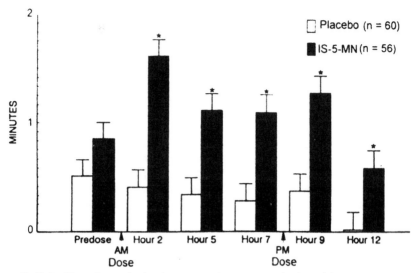

Fig 38–2.—Change in exercise duration among patients receiving placebo and those receiving isosorbide-5-mononitrate (IS-5-MN) therapy. Mean changes in total exercise duration from respective pretherapy baseline values after 8 AM and 3 PM doses of IS-5-MN and placebo. Total exercise duration increased significantly (P < .01) with IS-5-MN compared with placebo at 2, 5, and 7 hours after the 8 AM dose and at 2 and 5 hours after the 3 PM dose (hours 9 and 12 after the 8 AM dose). Exercise time before the 8 AM dose did change significantly. Mean values ± SE are shown by the *vertical bars.* *P < .01. (Courtesy of Thadani U, Maranda CR, Amsterdam E, et al: *Ann Intern Med* 120:353–359, 1994.)

taking IS-5-MN and 9 (15%) taking placebo complained of headaches, but only 2 of these patients discontinued therapy.

Conclusions.—Pharmacologic tolerance to nitrates is avoidable with 20 mg of IS-5-MN given once in the morning and again 7 hours later. Such a regimen is both safe and effective with or without concurrent β-blockers. Alternate dosing schedules of other long-acting oral nitrates are needed to evaluate whether tolerance can be minimized. Additional study is required to determine the effects of concomitant IS-5-MN and calcium channel blockers.

▶ As the authors note, "tolerance defined as a decrease in magnitude and duration of effects despite constant or increased dose . . . is a serious concern during long-term nitrate therapy." Isosorbide-5-mononitrate is the major active metabolite of isosorbide dinitrate, is nearly 100% bioavailable after oral administration, and has prolonged antianginal effects.

In this study, IS-5-MN, administered 20 mg twice daily given 7 hours apart, "was well tolerated and improved exercise performance for 7 hours after the morning dose and for 5 hours after the afternoon dose without evidence of development of pharmacologic tolerance. No rebound increase in anginal attacks was found."

Thadani et al. conclude with the following: "Many patients in our study did not have angina during daily activities even though all had angina during treadmill exercise. Thus, whether patients who have frequent episodes of angina during daily activity will have a rebound increase in frequency during periods of low plasma nitrate levels at night cannot be ascertained from these results." Also, in specific patients, additional therapy with β-blockers or calcium antagonists may be necessary for prevention of anginal episodes.

In another study concerning nitrate therapy for myocardial ischemia, Mahmarian and associates (1) demonstrated that transdermal nitroglycerin patch therapy reduces the extent of exercise-induced myocardial ischemia. Their double-blind, placebo-controlled trial used quantitative thallium-201 tomography to define ischemic myocardial perfusion defects. Short-term, intermittent nitroglycerin patch therapy significantly reduced myocardial ischemia, particularly in patients with large ischemic perfusion defects.

Several studies have used exercise thallium-201 perfusion scintigraphy to temporally assess the reduction or elimination of ischemia after successful coronary angioplasty. Importantly, the study by Mahmarian et al. convincingly demonstrates that scintigraphic evidence of myocardial ischemia can also be markedly reduced by antianginal drug therapy.—R.A. O'Rourke, M.D.

Reference

1. Mahmarian JJ, Fenimore NL, Marks GF, Francis MJ, Morales-Ballejo H, Verani MS, Pratt CM: Transdermal nitroglycerin patch therapy reduces the extent of exercise-induced myocardial ischemia: Results of a double-blind, placebo-controlled trial using quantitative thallium-201 tomography. *J Am Coll Cardiol* 24:25–32, 1994.

Effects of Coronary Angioplasty, Coronary Bypass Surgery, and Medical Therapy on Employment in Patients With Coronary Artery Disease: A Prospective Comparison Study

Mark DB, Lam LC, Lee KL, Jones RH, Pryor DB, Stack RS, Williams RB, Clapp-Channing NE, Califf RM, Hlatky MA (Duke Univ, Durham, NC; Stanford Univ, Calif)

Ann Intern Med 120:111–117, 1994   119-95-38-6

Background.—Coronary bypass surgery and coronary angioplasty have been shown to relieve angina and improve exercise tolerance compared with medical therapy. The high economic cost of these procedures could be partially offset by improved return-to-work rates. Studies from the 1970s failed to show an effect of bypass surgery on return-to-work rates, but bypass surgery was done more effectively in the 1980s with less morbidity and mortality. Return-to-work rates were compared in patients treated with bypass surgery, coronary angioplasty, and medical therapy between 1986 and 1990.

Methods.—All 1,252 patients were younger than 65 years and employed and had been referred for diagnostic cardiac catheterization. Quality-of-life and job status information was gathered immediately before catheterization and again 1 year later. Questions regarding func-

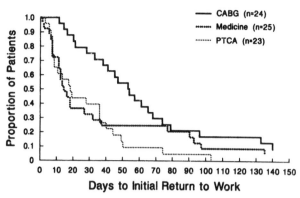

Fig 38–3.—Kaplan-Meier plot of time to initial return to work by treatment group for 72 patients. The x-axis shows days from diagnostic cardiac catheterization until return to work. The y-axis shows the proportion of patients returning to work at each time interval. The .5 point indicates the median value; the area under each curve indicates the mean value for that group: angioplasty, 27 days; bypass surgery, 67 days; and medicine, 45 days. *Abbreviations:* CABG, coronary artery bypass graft; PTCA, percutaneous transluminal coronary angioplasty. (Courtesy of Mark DB, Lam LC, Lee KL, et al: *Ann Intern Med* 120:111–117, 1994.)

tional, psychological, general health, and socioeconomic status were included.

Results.—At 1 year, 84% of patients who had angioplasty were still working, compared with 79% of patients who had bypass surgery and 76% of patients who received medical therapy. Approximately 87% of those who returned to work went back to the same job and the same hours as before treatment. Evaluation of a random subset revealed that patients who had angioplasty returned to work earlier than those who had bypass surgery (Fig 38–3).

Discussion.—These results were obtained from recently treated patients. There was no significant difference in employment rates after 1 year for patients who had coronary angioplasty, coronary bypass surgery, or medical therapy. However, the same positive outcome was assigned to patients whether they returned to work after 1 week or 6 months of recuperation. The participants were part of a lower-risk subset of the coronary artery disease population.

▶ In this group of patients at relatively low risk, "neither angioplasty nor bypass surgery as an initial treatment strategy had any long-term advantage compared with medical therapy in maintaining employment status up to 1 year for patients with coronary artery disease. However, among patients who do return to work, angioplasty is associated with a significantly shorter recuperation period than is bypass surgery and with lower indirect costs due to decreased productivity in the months after the procedure than either bypass surgery or medicine."

In the first large-scale, prospective observational treatment comparison of coronary angioplasty, bypass graft surgery, and medicine, Mark and associates (1) confirmed the previously reported survival advantages for coronary artery bypass graft surgery instead of medical therapy for 3-vessel disease and severe 2-vessel disease, particularly with a severe stenosis involving the proximal left anterior descending coronary artery. The data indicate that for patients with less severe coronary disease, the primary treatment choices are either medicine or coronary angioplasty. An analysis of the data from 9,263 patients with symptomatic coronary artery disease referred for cardiac catheterization between 1984 and 1990 indicates that treatment decisions are based not only on probability of survival differences, but also on relief of symptoms, quality-of-life outcomes, and patient preferences.—R.A. O'Rourke, M.D.

Reference

1. Mark DB, Nelson CL, Califf RM, Harrell FE, Lee KL, Jones RH, et al: Continuing evolution of therapy for coronary artery disease: Initial results from the era of coronary angioplasty. *Circulation* 89:2015–2025, 1994.

39 Coronary Angioplasty, Atherectomy, and Stents

A Randomized Study of Coronary Angioplasty Compared With Bypass Surgery in Patients With Symptomatic Multivessel Coronary Disease
Hamm CW, for the German Angioplasty Bypass Surgery Investigation (Univ Hosp Eppendorf, Hamburg, Germany; et al)
N Engl J Med 331:1037–1043, 1994   119-95-39–1

Introduction.—Coronary artery bypass grafting (CABG) has become standard therapy for symptomatic patients with multivessel coronary artery disease. Percutaneous transluminal coronary angioplasty (PTCA), which is standard therapy for symptomatic patients with single-vessel disease, has also been extended to selected patients with multivessel disease. The 2 alternatives were compared in a randomized study of patients with multivessel disease who required complete revascularization.

Methods.—Of 8,981 patients with multivessel coronary artery disease at 8 centers screened for inclusion in the German Angioplasty Bypass Surgery Investigation, 359 were randomly selected to undergo CABG or PTCA. All patients needed complete revascularization of at least 2 major vessels supplying different regions of the myocardium, and all procedures were judged clinically necessary and technically feasible. The pa-

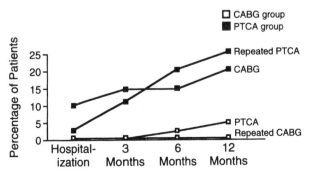

Fig 39–1.—Rate of further interventions (CABG or PTCA) in the 2 treatment groups during initial hospitalization and 3, 6, and 12 months later. (Courtesy of Hamm CW, for the German Angioplasty Bypass Surgery Investigation: N Engl J Med 331:1037–1043, 1994.)

tients received the routine surgical or angioplastic care at their hospital; decisions made during the procedures and throughout follow-up were left to the discretion of the treating physicians. The outcomes of the 2 groups were compared 1 year after the procedures.

Results.—The CABG group underwent grafting of an average of 2.2 vessels, and the PTCA group had dilation of an average of 1.9 vessels. Median hospitalization was 19 days with CABG vs. 5 days with PTCA. The procedure was associated with Q-wave myocardial infarction in 8% of the CABG group vs. 2% of the PTCA group. There was no significant difference in in-hospital mortality: 2.5% with CABG and 1% with PTCA. Discharge assessments showed freedom from angina in 93% of the CABG group vs. 82% of the PTCA group.

In the year after the procedure, 44% of the PTCA group required further interventions: a second PTCA in 23%, CABG in 18%, and both in 3%. By contrast, only 6% of the CABG group required a second procedure: a second CABG in 1% and PTCA in 5% (Fig 39–1). One-year follow-up assessments showed freedom from angina in 74% of the CABG group and 71% of the PTCA group. Both groups had comparable improvements in exercise capacity, although significantly more patients in the CABG group did not require antianginal medications: 22% vs. 12%.

Conclusions.—For properly selected patients with symptomatic multivessel coronary artery disease, CABG and PTCA yield approximately equal improvements in angina after 1 year of follow-up. However, patients undergoing PTCA are more likely to require further interventions and antianginal medications to achieve the same outcome as those undergoing CABG. On the other hand, patients undergoing CABG are more likely to have an acute myocardial infarction during the procedure. The findings will be useful in clinical decision-making; the results will be assessed again at 5 and 10 years after treatment.

▶ This report discusses the results of 1 of 6 randomized trials comparing coronary angioplasty to coronary artery bypass surgery for multivessel disease that either have been completed or are in various stages of patient follow-up.

In the Emory Angioplasty Versus Surgery Trial (EAST) (1), follow-up clinical information was collected every 6 months, and coronary arteriography and thallium stress perfusion imaging were performed at 1 and 3 years after randomization to angioplasty or bypass surgery. The primary end point was a composite of death, a Q-wave myocardial infarction, and a large ischemic defect identified on thallium imaging at 3 years. The primary end point occurred in 27.3% of the surgery group and 28.8% of the angioplasty (PTCA) group and was no different. Death occurred in 6.2% of the surgery group and 7.1% of the PTCA group. At 3 years, the proportions of patients in the surgical group (CABG) who required repeat bypass surgery (1%) or angioplasty (13%) were significantly lower than the proportions in the PTCA group (22% and 41%, respectively; $P < .001$). Angina was more frequent in the angioplasty group than in the CABG group.

The reports of these prospective randomized comparisons of angioplasty and bypass grafting in patients with multivessel coronary artery disease have been consistent. In patients who are good candidates for either procedure, angioplasty and surgery had similar rates of procedure-related mortality (1% to 2.5%). Patients who underwent bypass grafting were more likely to have procedure-related Q-wave myocardial infarctions (8% to 10%, as compared with 2% to 3% for angioplasty). Not surprisingly, surgically-treated patients were hospitalized for a longer time. Subsequently, those who underwent bypass grafting had less angina, required less antianginal medications, and were much less likely to require another revascularization procedure.

Although some patients with multivessel coronary artery disease are excellent candidates for angioplasty, bypass surgery will continue to be the preferred revascularization procedure for large numbers of them (2). Many patients with multivessel disease are not optimal candidates for angioplasty, and only 4% to 10% of those screened in the multicenter trials were enrolled in the randomized study. Many of the potential study group had 1 or more occluded coronary arteries, and some had sufficient narrowing of the left main coronary artery to preclude safe angioplasty. Also, the favorable results of surgery on survival in patients with multivessel coronary disease who have stenosis of the proximal left anterior descending (LAD) coronary artery and in those with 3-vessel coronary artery disease and left ventricular systolic dysfunction are well documented.

For patients with single-vessel or multivessel disease (not involving the proximal LAD) and normal left ventricular systolic function, the selection of medical therapy, angioplasty, or bypass graft surgery should be based on specific circumstances. When nonmedical therapy is selected, the choice of angioplasty or bypass surgery should be made recognizing that surgery is associated with a greater initial morbidity but results in more effective relief of angina and in far less repeated procedures during the next 2 or 3 years. Coronary angioplasty is associated with a lower initial morbidity rate but a greater likelihood of recurrent angina, need for antianginal medications, and subsequent revascularization procedures.

In another important clinical, single-center, randomized study, Goy and associates (3) comparatively examined coronary angioplasty and left internal mammary artery (LIMA) coronary bypass surgery in patients with isolated proximal LAD coronary artery stenosis, preserved left ventricular systolic function, and documented myocardial ischemia. Sixty-eight patients were assigned to angioplasty and 66 to LIMA graft surgery. The incidence of in hospital complications was 2% for the surgical approach and 3% for angioplasty; clinical and functional status improved similarly in both groups. However, patients in the PTCA group took more antianginal drugs. At the median follow-up of 2.5 years, 86% of the LIMA-treated group and 43% of the PTCA-treated patients were free from adverse cardiac events. The difference was a result of re-stenosis often requiring subsequent surgical or percutaneous revascularization in the angioplasty group. Rates of cardiac death and myocardial infarction did not differ between the 2 groups.—R.A. O'Rourke, M.D.

References

1. King SB, Lembo NJ, Weintraub WS, Kosinski AS, Barnhart HX, Kutner MH, Alazraki NP, Guyton RA, Zhao X-Q, for the Emory Angioplasty Versus Surgery Trial (EAST): A randomized trial comparing coronary angioplasty with coronary bypass surgery. N Engl J Med 331:1044–1050, 1994.
2. Hillis LD, Rutherford JD: Coronary angioplasty compared with bypass grafting. N Engl J Med 331:1086–1087, 1994.
3. Goy JJ, Eeckhout E, Burnand B, Vogt P, Stauffer J-C, Hurni M, Stumpe F, Ruchat P, Sadeghi H, Kappenberger L: Coronary angioplasty versus left internal mammary artery grafting for isolated proximal left anterior descending artery stenosis. Lancet 343:1449–1453, 1994.

Similar Results of Percutaneous Transluminal Coronary Angioplasty for Women and Men With Postmyocardial Infarction Ischemia

Welty FK, Mittleman MA, Healy RW, Muller JE, Shubrooks Jr SJ (Harvard Med School, Boston)

J Am Coll Cardiol 23:35–39, 1994   119-95-39–2

Purpose.—Women undergo revascularization procedures less often than men, perhaps because of expectations of worse outcomes and less symptomatic improvement. None of the outcome studies of coronary angioplasty for postmyocardial infarction ischemia has included enough women to evaluate them as a separate group. Gender differences in the outcome of coronary angioplasty performed for postmyocardial infarction ischemia were identified.

Methods.—The analysis included 505 consecutive patients undergoing coronary angioplasty within an 8½-year period for recurrent myocardial ischemia after acute myocardial infarction. There were 341 men and 164 women, mean ages 57 and 63 years, respectively. Both groups were followed for a mean of 34 months. They were compared for morbidity and mortality rates during and after the procedure.

Results.—The 2 groups were no different in extent of coronary artery disease, number of vessels treated, or completeness of vascularization. Success rates of the procedure were 91% in men and 89% in women. The need for coronary artery bypass surgery was 4% vs. 3%, and mortality rates at coronary angioplasty were less than 1% in both groups. Similarly, follow-up showed no differences in the need for bypass, repeat angioplasty, reinfarction, or death (Fig 39–2). The combined end point of all 4 events was equal in both sexes—27%. Fifty-four percent of the women had recurrent angina, compared with 43% of the men, despite the fact that they were similar in extent of coronary artery disease and frequency of incomplete revascularization.

Conclusions.—Procedural morbidity and mortality and long-term outcome are very similar for men and women undergoing coronary angioplasty for postinfarction ischemia. The only significant difference is that women are more likely to have recurrent ischemia develop, with a rela-

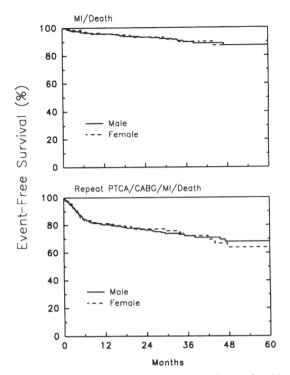

Fig 39–2.—The 5-year Kaplan–Meier actuarial event-free survival curves for 139 women and 301 men after successful percutaneous transluminal coronary angioplasty (*PTCA*) for postmyocardial infarction ischemia. Freedom from myocardial infarction (*MI*) and death (**upper panel**), and freedom from repeat angioplasty, coronary artery bypass grafting (*CABG*), MI, and death (**lower panel**). Men are indicated by *solid lines*, women by *dashed lines*. (Courtesy of Welty FK, Mittleman MA, Healy RW, et al: *J Am Coll Cardiol* 23:35–39, 1994.)

tive risk of 1.7. Concerns about the safety of coronary angioplasty in women should not restrict its use for female patients with myocardial infarction complicated by ischemia.

▶ These long-term follow-up results indicate that women with postinfarct myocardial ischemia treated with coronary angioplasty have similar unadjusted rates for repeat angioplasty, coronary bypass surgery, reinfarction, and death as do men even though the women were an average of 6 years older. The increased incidence of recurrent postprocedure angina for women as compared with men has also been observed after coronary artery bypass graft surgery.

In another study concerning coronary angioplasty (1), the frequency of silent ischemia was determined by stress thallium scintigraphy in 490 patients examined 6 months after successful coronary angioplasty. Of 112 patients with positive scintigraphic findings 6 months after angioplasty, 67 (60%) had no angina during exercise testing. The symptomatic patients and those with silent ischemia had similar degrees of re-stenosis. Ischemia, whether silent or symptomatic, correlated with an increased risk of recurrent ischemic events but *not* with death. The results of this study are of interest when considering whether "routine" thallium scintigraphy is indicated as a cost-effective method for assessing patients after coronary angioplasty performed for relief of symptoms who do not have recurrent symptoms but who may have silent re-stenosis. Identification of subsets of asymptomatic, postangioplasty patients who may be at higher risk for future cardiac events may be feasible. For example, patients with unstable ST-T-waves on the resting ECG or an abnormal ECG response to exercise are likely in this category.

Other recent articles of interest concerning coronary angioplasty and restenosis include a study by Golino and associates (2) demonstrating that serotonin is released into the coronary circulation during angioplasty and may contribute to the occurrence of vasoconstriction distal to the dilated site. This vasoconstriction could be attenuated by ketanserin, a serotonin$_2$ receptor antagonist. Also, the EPIC investigators (3) have demonstrated that the ischemic complications of coronary angioplasty and atherectomy are reduced using a monoclonal antibody directed against the platelet IIb/IIIa glycoprotein receptor; however, the risk of bleeding is increased (3).—R.A. O'Rourke, M.D.

References

1. Pfisterer M, Rickenbacher P, Kiowski W, Muller-Brand J, Burkart F: Silent ischemia after percutaneous transluminal coronary angioplasty: Incidence and prognostic significance. *J Am Coll Cardiol* 22:1446–1454, 1993.
2. Golino P, Piscione F, Benedict CR, Anderson HV, Cappelli-Bigazzi M, Indolfi C, Condorelli M, Chiariello M, Willerson JT: Local effect of serotonin released during coronary angioplasty. *N Engl J Med* 330:523–528, 1994.
3. Califf RM, for the EPIC Investigators: Use of a monoclonal antibody directed against the platelet glycoprotein IIb/IIIa receptor in high-risk coronary angioplasty. *N Engl J Med* 330:956–961, 1994.

Percutaneous Excimer Laser Coronary Angioplasty: Results in the First Consecutive 3,000 Patients
Litvack F, for the ELCA Investigators (Univ of California, Los Angeles)
J Am Coll Cardiol 23:323–329, 1994   119-95-39-3

Background.—Preliminary reports of excimer laser coronary angioplasty suggest that it is an effective and relatively safe procedure, even in patients with lesions not ideal for balloon angioplasty. The procedure uses a pulsed, 308-nm ultraviolet laser transmitted by optical fibers to reduce coronary stenoses. The results of the first 3,000 patients treated in an excimer laser coronary angioplasty registry were reported.

Methods.—The patients were treated at 33 centers within a 4-year period. All were enrolled in a prospective, nonrandomized fashion. A total of 3,592 lesions were treated; 75% of the patients were men, and 68% were in the Canadian Cardiovascular Society functional class III or IV.

The procedures were performed with 1.3 to 2.4-mm diameter catheters and with energy densities of as much as 70 mJ/mm². A standard angioplasty technique and conventional guide catheters were used. Criteria for procedural success were a final stenosis of 50% or less, without inhospital Q-wave myocardial infarction, coronary artery bypass surgery, or death.

Results.—The success rate was 90% and was consistent across the experience. The length and complexity of the treated lesions had no significant effect on success or complication rates. Inhospital bypass surgery was performed in 4% of patients, 2% had Q-wave myocardial infarction, and .5% died. The procedure was complicated by coronary artery perforation in 1% of lesions, although the rate of this complication decreased to .3% in the latter 1,000 procedures. Thirteen percent of lesions were associated with angiographic dissection, 3% with transient occlusion, and 3% with sustained occlusion. Most procedures were performed in American College of Cardiology–American Heart Association type B2 and C lesions; there were no significant differences in short-term outcome between these 2 types.

Conclusions.—Percutaneous excimer laser coronary angioplasty is a safe procedure with good short-term results. The results are good even in patients with complex lesions that are not amenable to percutaneous transluminal coronary angioplasty, such as aorto-ostial lesions, long lesions, total occlusions that are crossable with a wire, diffuse disease, and vein grafts. As experience with the laser procedure increases, mainly complex lesions are selected and the incidence of perforation declines. Excimer laser angioplasty may increase the opportunities for intervention in selected patients with complex coronary artery disease.

▶ Relatively high success rates with laser coronary angioplasty were seen in the patient study data for aorto-ostial vein grafts and totally occluded lesions (1). "Perforation, perhaps the most feared potential complication of laser angioplasty, occurred in only .4% of the last 1,000 patients compared with 1.6% of the first 2,000." Angiographic follow-up was available at 6 months in only 50% of the 2,184 patients who had completed follow-up. The data are difficult to interpret in relation to previous angioplasty experiences because of potential bias not to perform recatheterization in patients without recurrent symptoms, the relatively high rate of prior coronary angioplasty, and the preponderance of long, complex lesions and vein grafts. All are factors associated with high re-stenosis rates.—R.A. O'Rourke, M.D.

Reference

1. 1994 Year Book of Medicine, p 376.

Clinical and Angiographic Results of Transluminal Extraction Coronary Atherectomy in Saphenous Vein Bypass Grafts

Safian RD, Grines CL, May MA, Lichtenberg A, Juran N, Schreiber TL, Pavlides G, Meany TB, Savas V, O'Neill WW (William Beaumont Hosp, Royal Oak, Mich)

Circulation 89:302–312, 1994   119-95-39–4

Introduction.—Transluminal extraction coronary (TEC) atherectomy is a novel approach to removing clot and atheromatous material that may prove useful in patients who have stenosed saphenous vein bypass grafts. Conventional angioplasty may have limited use in this setting because of the risk of distal embolization, failure to reestablish flow, or high rate of restenosis.

Objective and Methods.—A total of 158 saphenous vein graft lesions in 146 consecutive patients were treated by TEC atherectomy. About half the patients had unstable angina, and 8% had angina develop within a month of myocardial infarction. Angioplasty or other measures had been tried in 22% of lesions. Patients were pretreated with aspirin and given heparin during and after the procedure, as well as intracoronary urokinase if a visible thrombus or a diffusely diseased or totally occluded graft was present.

Operative Results.—The atherectomy instrument was successfully advanced through 91% of the lesions. The minimum luminal diameter increased from .9 to 1.5 mm after atherectomy and to 2.3 mm after percutaneous transluminal coronary angioplasty (PTCA). The mean stenosis diameter decreased from 75% to 58% after atherectomy, and to 36% after PTCA. A reduction of 20% or more was achieved in 39% of lesions. A smooth luminal contour was achieved in 32% of lesions after atherectomy and in half the lesions at the time of the final angiography. Distal embolization occurred in 12% of lesions and no-reflow in 9%. One lesion abruptly closed and remained closed. The hospital mortality rate was 2%. Ten patients (7%) required hemodynamic support.

Clinical Outcome.—Of 118 patients followed up for a mean of 6 months after discharge from the hospital, 63% had improvement in anginal symptoms and 16% were worse. Angiography gave evidence of restenosis (stenosis exceeding 50%) in 69% of the 105 evaluable lesions. Thirty total occlusions were found, but only 19 patients required late revascularization and none had late infarction.

Conclusions.—Transluminal extraction coronary atherectomy is of limited use in patients with stenosed vein bypass grafts. Re-stenosis and late occlusion are frequent sequelae. Nevertheless, the procedure may be considered in patients having old, diffusely degenerated vein grafts if a second coronary bypass surgery is not feasible.

▶ A major problem for physicians caring for patients with coronary artery disease is the increasing number who have been successfully treated with vein bypass graft surgery but who are seen with recurrent symptoms 8 to 15 years after the initial myocardial revascularization procedure because of "graft atherosclerosis." Alternative successful methods of myocardial revascularization rather than repeat coronary artery bypass surgery are needed for many of these patients. Because of the disappointing acute and long-term results of coronary angioplasty, several new technologies are being considered as alternative strategies for revascularization of patients with stenoses in saphenous vein bypass grafts. Several current randomized studies are assessing the merits of stent placement or directional atherectomy as compared with balloon angioplasty for treating bypass graft disease.

Atherectomy with TEC appeared to offer many theoretical advantages over other percutaneous devices for treatment of stenotic vein grafts. However, as the authors note, the use of TEC atherectomy is limited in such cases because of the "small size of the device and the suboptimal angiographic results, often requiring adjunctive balloon angioplasty. Although the incidence of serious clinical complications is similar to that of other percutaneous interventions in vein grafts, there is a high incidence of restenosis and late vessel occlusion." Other interventional techniques such as directional atherectomy, high-speed mechanical rotational atherectomy, stent placement, or their combinations will likely produce lesser complications and better results in patients with stenoses of saphenous vein bypass grafts.—R.A. O'Rourke, M.D.

A Randomized Comparison of Coronary-Stent Placement and Balloon Angioplasty in the Treatment of Coronary Artery Disease
Fischman DL, for the Stent Restenosis Study Investigators (Jefferson Med College, Philadelphia)
N Engl J Med 331:496–501, 1994   119-95-39–5

Objective.—Because preliminary evidence suggests that a stent may reduce the risk of re-stenosis after coronary balloon angioplasty, stent placement was compared with standard balloon angioplasty in patients with symptomatic coronary artery disease in a prospective, randomized study.

Methods.—From 20 participating centers, 410 patients with symptoms of ischemic heart disease and new coronary lesions were randomized to undergo standard balloon angioplasty or elective placement of a Palmaz-Schatz stent. All patients had at least 70% stenosis and a lesion extending for 15 mm or less in a vessel 3 mm or more in diameter.

Results.—Clinical success was achieved in 96% of patients given a stent and in 90% of those who had angioplasty. Seven stented patients and 3 in the angioplasty group had abrupt closure of the treated vessel after leaving the catheterization laboratory. Major events (death, myocardial infarction, bypass surgery, repeat angioplasty) occurred within 2 weeks of treatment in 6% of the stented group and 8% of those with angioplasty. Bleeding and vascular complications occurred in 7% and 4%

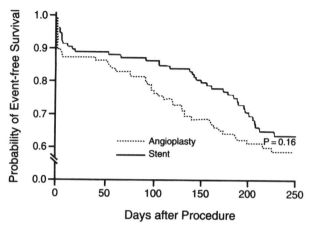

Fig 39–3.—Kaplan-Meier survival curves for major cardiac events (death, myocardial infarction, coronary artery bypass surgery, and repeated angioplasty). (Courtesy of Fischman DL, for the Stent Restenosis Study Investigators: N Engl J Med 331:496–501, 1994.)

of the groups, respectively. Stented patients were hospitalized twice as long as angioplasty patients. Angiography confirmed a larger immediate gain in luminal diameter in the stented group, and a larger net gain was confirmed at follow-up. On long-term follow-up, the number of deaths and infarcts was comparable in the 2 groups, but fewer stented patients had revascularization of the target lesion. Event-free survival was 80.5% in the stented group and 76% in the angioplasty group (Fig 39–3). More stented patients remained free of angina.

Conclusions.—In selected patients, elective placement of a coronary stent is clinically more effective than balloon angioplasty. Major cardiac events are not more frequent after stent placement, and the need for later revascularization is reduced.

▶ In this trial, stent placement was compared with balloon angioplasty for the treatment of new focal coronary stenoses in larger vessels. The re-stenosis rate was reduced significantly from 42.1% in the angioplasty group to 31.6% in the stent group, but the probability of an increase in survival at 250 days after the procedure was *no different*.

The authors' Discussion section included the following:

Several limitations of stent placement need to be emphasized. Stent thrombosis occurred in 3.4 percent of patients who underwent stent placement as an elective procedure and in 21.4 percent of those in whom stent placement was used as a bailout technique. These thrombotic events occurred 2 to 14 days after placement of the stent, with six instances of thrombosis after discharge, and invariably resulted in major clinical complications. Furthermore, the intense anticoagulation, antiplatelet regimen associated with stent placement resulted in nearly twice the number of hemorrhagic and peripheral vascular complications associated with angioplasty, as well as a prolonged hospital stay.

Although the frequency with which follow-up angiography was performed was relatively high in both groups, there was a higher rate of angiographic follow-up in the stent group (92 percent vs. 83 percent, P = 0.008). This difference, which may bias the rate of restenosis in favor of stent placement, is a limitation of the study.

In a previous multicenter report by Savage and Associates (1), a remarkably low thrombotic occlusion rate of 5% was noted in 300 consecutive patients undergoing coronary artery stent placement with a 1-year mortality rate of less than 1%. The re-stenosis rate of 14% for previously untreated lesions and of 39% when the stent was placed in patients with previous angioplasty was similar to previous reports. Re-stenosis has a low mortality rate provided that appropriate clinical management is used, including coronary artery bypass surgery or repeat angioplasty. Interestingly, many patients who had re-stenosis because of clinical stability did not require repeat angioplasty or bypass surgery.

Shömig et al. (2) quantitatively assessed the angiographic lumen changes in 164 patients after emergency coronary artery stenting and in the group of 31 patients who required repeat angioplasty within the stent. The angiographic results of emergency coronary artery stenting compared favorably with those of conventional angioplasty. In-stent balloon redilation in patients with re-stenosis was associated with excellent short-term results, and the re-stenosis rate was not different from that reported for nonstented vessels.—R.A. O'Rourke, M.D.

References

1. Savage MP, Fischman DL, Schatz RA, et al., for the Palmaz-Schatz Stent Study Group: Long-term angiographic and clinical outcome after implantation of a balloon-expandable stent in the native coronary circulation. *J Am Coll Cardiol* 24:1207–1212, 1994.
2. Schömig A, Kastrati A, Dietz R, Rauch B, Neumann F-J, Katus HH, Busch U: Emergency coronary stenting for dissection during percutaneous transluminal coronary angioplasty: Angiographic follow-up after stenting and after repeat angioplasty of the stented segment. *J Am Coll Cardiol* 23:1053–1060, 1994.

40 Valvular Heart Disease

Percutaneous Transatrial Mitral Commissurotomy: Immediate and Intermediate Results
Arora R, Kalra GS, Murty GSR, Trehan V, Jolly N, Mohan JC, Sethi KK, Nigam M, Khalilullah M (G B Pant Hosp, New Delhi, India)
J Am Coll Cardiol 23:1327–1332, 1994   119-95-40-1

Background.—Percutaneous transatrial mitral commissurotomy has become an effective nonoperative treatment alternative for patients with symptomatic mitral stenosis. Immediate outcomes have been shown to be comparable to those achieved with closed and open mitral valvotomy. The immediate and follow-up results of percutaneous transatrial mitral commissurotomy in a large series of patients with rheumatic mitral stenosis were analyzed.

Patients and Methods.—Six hundred patients underwent percutaneous transatrial mitral commissurotomy by the double-balloon or flow-guided Inoue balloon technique. The patients were 446 females and 154 males, aged 8 to 60 years. Four percent of the patients had atrial fibrillation. Ten percent had mitral regurgitation of grade 2 or less, and 2% had densely calcific valve. Every 3 months, all patients were clinically and echocardiographically assessed.

Findings.—The procedure was successful in 98% of the patients. Optimal commissurotomy was attained in 93.6%, with an increase in mitral valve area from .75 to 2.2 cm² and a reduction in transmitral end-diastolic gradient from 27.3 to 3.8 mm Hg. In 34.6% of the patients, mitral regurgitation developed or increased. One percent of the patients with mitral regurgitation needed mitral valve replacement. Cardiac tamponade developed in 1.3%. Six patients (1%) died. During a mean follow-up of 37 months, re-stenosis occurred in 1.7%.

Conclusions.—Percutaneous transatrial mitral commissurotomy is a safe and effective procedure in patients with rheumatic mitral stenosis. The intermediate outcomes of the technique in this patient population are gratifying.

▶ In this study of 600 patients, "optimal" mitral valve balloon commissurotomy was achieved in 94% of patients who had a mean follow-up period of 37 ± 8 months. The hemodynamic improvement obtained in these patients is comparable to the results reported previously. The procedure was successful in all pregnant patients with no adverse effects to the fetus. A comparative analysis of 2 large patient groups with nearly equal numbers revealed that both the double-balloon and Inoue balloon techniques are equally effective. An atrial septal defect was found in 92% of 50 patients who had transesophageal echocardiography immediately after percutaneous transatrial mitral commissurotomy. However, at 6 months, it persisted in only 4%; the mean closure time was 4.6 ± 2.2 weeks. During the 3 years of average follow-up, echocardiographic re-stenosis was observed in only 10 (2%) of patients.—R.A. O'Rourke, M.D.

Percutaneous Balloon Valvuloplasty Compared With Open Surgical Commissurotomy for Mitral Stenosis

Reyes VP, Raju BS, Wynne J, Stephenson LW, Raju R, Fromm BS, Rajagopal P, Mehta P, Singh S, Rao P, Satyanarayana PV, Turi ZG (Wayne State Univ, Detroit; Nizam's Inst of Med Sciences and MediCiti, Hyderabad, India)

N Engl J Med 331:961–967, 1994   119-95-40-2

Background.—Percutaneous balloon mitral valvuloplasty may provide an adequate alternative to open surgical commissurotomy in the treatment of rheumatic mitral valve stenosis. The outcomes of both methods of treatment were compared in a randomized, prospective study.

Methods.—Sixty patients with severe mitral stenosis were randomly assigned to either balloon valvuloplasty or open surgical commissurotomy. All patients underwent cardiac catheterization before the procedure, and again to determine the mitral valve area at 1 week, 6 months, and 3 years after treatment.

Results.—Thirty patients were assigned to each treatment group, and all were available for follow-up. Hemodynamic variables at baseline, 1 week, 6 months, and 3 years after treatment are shown in Figure 40–1. An initial improvement was seen in mitral valve areas in both groups from a mean of .9 cm² to 2.1 cm² in the balloon-valvuloplasty group, and from .9 cm² to 2 cm² in the open surgery group. Although overall improvement was maintained in both groups during 3 years, mitral valve areas were greater in the patients who underwent balloon-valvuloplasty at the end of the follow-up than in the surgery group (2.4 cm² vs. 1.8 cm², respectively). Three patients in the balloon-valvuloplasty group and 4 in the surgery group had re-stenosis. Within the balloon-valvuloplasty group, 1 patient died of an apparent stroke after 2.5 years and 4 had residual atrial septal defects. Two patients in the balloon-valvuloplasty group and 1 in the surgery group were considered to have severe mitral regurgitation. A total of 72% of the patients who underwent balloon valvuloplasty and 57% of the surgery group were considered free of cardiovascular symptoms at 3 years.

Conclusion.—For patients with severe mitral stenosis, both balloon valvuloplasty and open surgical commissurotomy resulted in sustained improvement during a 3-year period. However, in this patient group, balloon valvuloplasty appeared superior to surgery in providing a larger mitral valve area and less mitral regurgitation, as well as improved mitral

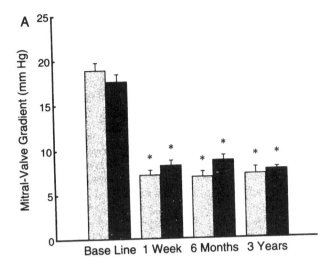

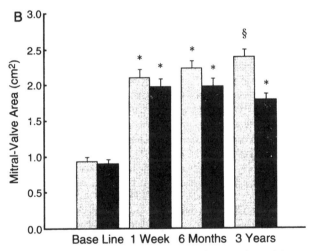

Fig 40–1.—Hemodynamic variables at baseline and 1 week, 6 months, and 3 years after balloon mitral valvuloplasty or open surgical commissurotomy. The *asterisk* indicates $P < .001$ for the comparison with the baseline value. The *section mark* in (**B**) indicates $P < .001$ for the comparison with the surgery group. The *bars* indicate the standard errors. (Courtesy of Reyes VP, Raju BS, Wynne J, et al: N Engl J Med 331:961–967, 1994.)

valve gradient, pulmonary artery wedge pressure, pulmonary artery pressure, and hemodynamic measurements during exercise. Such results suggest that balloon valvuloplasty provides a successful, less invasive, and more cost-effective treatment than open surgical commissurotomy, and it should be considered for patients with uncomplicated mitral valve stenosis.

▶ This study, like the previous one (Abstract 119-95-40–1), supports the use of mitral valve balloon commissurotomy as the treatment of choice for many patients with mitral stenosis who have favorable mitral valve anatomy. The theoretical advantage that controlled surgical separation of fused commissures under direct vision would lead to a larger mitral valve area and less mitral regurgitation was not substantiated. However, open surgical commissurotomy will continue to be used preferentially for patients with severe subvalvular disease, calcification, or thrombus who are considered to be candidates for repair procedures rather than for mitral valve replacement.—R.A. O'Rourke, M.D.

Significant Tricuspid Regurgitation is a Marker for Adverse Outcome in Patients Undergoing Percutaneous Balloon Mitral Valvuloplasty

Sagie A, Schwammenthal E, Newell JB, Harrell L, Joziatis TB, Weyman AE, Levine RA, Palacios IF (Harvard Med School, Boston; Tel Aviv Univ, Israel; Westfalicshe Wilhelms-Universitat, Munster, Germany)
J Am Coll Cardiol 24:696–702, 1994   119-95-40–3

Background.—Percutaneous mitral balloon valvuloplasty has recently become an accepted alternative to surgery in patients with mitral stenosis. With the new technique, however, residual tricuspid regurgitation may persist after the procedure, especially when the lesion has contributed to irreversible right heart dilation or is of organic origin. The association between the presence of tricuspid regurgitation before mitral valvuloplasty and immediate and long-term adverse outcomes in patients

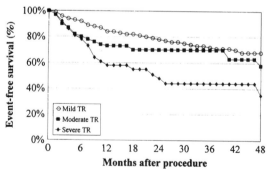

Fig 40–2.—Kaplan-Meier estimates of event-free survival rate after balloon mitral valvuloplasty among 318 patients with mild, moderate, or severe tricuspid regurgitation (TR). Events were defined as mitral valve surgery, repeat balloon valvuloplasty, New York Heart Association functional class III or IV, and death before mitral valve surgery. (Courtesy of Sagie A, Schwammenthal E, Newell JB, et al: *J Am Coll Cardiol* 24:696–702, 1994.)

with different degrees of tricuspid regurgitation who had balloon mitral valvuloplasty was investigated.

Methods.—Three hundred eighteen consecutive patients undergoing the procedure within a 5-year period were included in the analysis. The mean patient age was 54 years. All had had color Doppler echocardiographic studies before balloon mitral valvuloplasty. Sixty-nine percent had no or mild tricuspid regurgitation; 19%, moderate regurgitation; and 12%, severe regurgitation. The patients were followed up for 6 to 62 months.

Findings.—Although initial success rates did not differ among the 3 groups with varying degrees of tricuspid regurgitation, patients with more severe regurgitation had less optimal results, reflected by a smaller absolute increase in the mitral valve area. The estimated 4-year event-free survival rate was reduced in the group with severe tricuspid regurgitation (Fig 40-2). At 4 years, the event-free survival rates in the groups with mild, moderate, and severe tricuspid regurgitation were 68%, 58%, and 35%, respectively. Survival rates at 4 years were 94% for mild, 90% for moderate, and 69% for severe tricuspid regurgitation. Tricuspid regurgitation independently predicted late outcome.

Conclusions.—Patients with severe tricuspid regurgitation treated with percutaneous balloon mitral valvuloplasty have advanced mitral valve and pulmonary vascular disease, suboptimal immediate results, and poor late outcomes, with a 4-year major event-free probability of only 35%. Associated severe tricuspid regurgitation should be corrected during mitral valve surgery. Careful follow-up with echocardiography is indicated for patients with severe tricuspid regurgitation undergoing percutaneous balloon mitral valve commissurotomy. Patients with persistent tricuspid regurgitation at follow-up should be considered for possible tricuspid valve surgery.

▶ The clinical recognition of the presence, etiology, and severity of tricuspid regurgitation associated with mitral stenosis has assumed increased importance because of its effects on the outcome of mitral valve surgery. Lesser degrees of tricuspid regurgitation are likely to diminish after the mitral valve lesion is corrected. However, more severe tricuspid regurgitation may persist and lead to progressive right ventricular dysfunction.

This study defines the impact of significant tricuspid regurgitation on late outcome in patients undergoing balloon mitral valve commissurotomy. Patients with severe tricuspid regurgitation undergoing balloon mitral valvulotomy also had a poor outcome at late follow-up, which is consistent with the observations made in patients who have undergone mitral valve surgery for mitral stenosis.—R.A. O'Rourke, M.D.

Mitral Valve Replacement Versus Mitral Valve Repair: A Doppler and Quantitative Stress Echocardiographic Study

Tischler MD, Cooper KA, Rowen M, LeWinter MM (Med Ctr Hosp of Vermont, Burlington; Univ of Vermont, Burlington)
Circulation 89:132–137, 1994   119-95-40-4

Introduction.—Patients with pure chronic mitral regurgitation who undergo mitral valve replacement (MVR) generally have a significantly reduced left ventricular ejection fraction when measured at rest after surgery. In contrast, this reduction during rest is not seen in patients who undergo mitral valve repair (MV repair). Left ventricular performance during exercise after MV repair and MVR was compared.

Methods.—Two groups of 10 patients with pure chronic mitral regurgitation who underwent either MVR or standard MV repair were matched for age, sex, preoperative left ventricular ejection fraction, and time since surgery. Left ventricular function was monitored at rest and during upright bicycle exercise with continuous Doppler and 2-dimensional echocardiography and blood pressure measurements.

Results.—The patients in both groups exercised for comparable lengths of time. Patients in the MV repair group had significantly higher left ventricular stroke volume, higher ejection fraction (Fig 40–3), and lower end-systolic wall stress than those in the MVR group during both rest and exercise. More of the patients in the MV repair group maintained an ellipsoidal left ventricular chamber, whereas patients in the MVR group tended to have a more spherical chamber develop during exercise. Both at rest and during exercise, patients in the MVR group had a higher mean transmitral diastolic gradient.

Discussion.—The reduced ejection fraction seen in the MVR group was partially the result of increased end-systolic circumferential wall

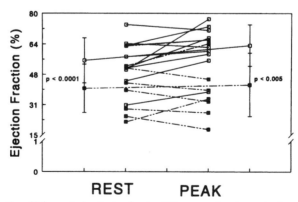

Fig 40–3.—Plot of left ventricular ejection fraction (%) at rest and peak exercise in patients with MV repair (*connected open squares*) and MVR (*connected solid squares*). (Courtesy of Tischler MD, Cooper KA, Rowen M, et al: *Circulation* 89:132–137, 1994.)

stress. Chordal preservation has been implicated in moderating wall stress. In patients in the MV repair group with a preserved chordal apparatus, improved rest and exercise left ventricular ejection fractions were related to decreased end-systolic wall stress and maintaining an ellipsoidal-chamber structure.

▶ Mitral valve repair and, as the authors state, "more recently, MVR with chordal preservation have been shown to preserve left ventricular ejection performance at rest in patients with chronic mitral regurgitation." In this study, the differences in left ventricular ejection fraction and wall stress with MV repair as compared with replacement, became more marked at peak exercise, which is not surprising considering the high degree of correlation between rest and peak values. These data confirm prior studies performed at rest comparing MVR with and without chordal preservation. They indicate that the functional advantages at rest are maintained and even potentiated during exercise. Thus, chordal preservation results in improved left ventricular ejection fraction and stroke volume. This is due, in part, to reduced end-systolic wall stress and the maintenance of a more elliptical-chamber geometry, the latter improving left ventricular filling.

In another study, Chua and associates (1) reviewed the results of MV repair for mitral regurgitation in 323 consecutive patients, 97 of whom had preoperative atrial fibrillation. Neither the operative mortality nor the 5-year survival differed significantly for patients with preoperative atrial fibrillation as compared with sinus rhythm. The 2 groups have a similar prevalence of late thromboembolic events. At late follow-up, 80% of patients with long-standing atrial fibrillation at surgery continued to have atrial fibrillation, whereas none of the patients with recent-onset atrial fibrillation at surgery had atrial fibrillation at late postoperative follow-up. Thus, a case can be made for the early repair of *severe* mitral regurgitation once atrial fibrillation ensues, even in asymptomatic patients with a normal left ventricular ejection fraction.—R.A. O'Rourke, M.D.

Reference

1. Chua YL, Schaff HV, Orszulak TA, Morris JJ: Outcome of mitral valve repair in patients with preoperative atrial fibrillation: Should the Maze procedure be combined with mitral valvuloplasty? *J Thorac Cardiovasc Surg* 107:408–415, 1994.

Echocardiographic Prediction of Survival After Surgical Correction of Organic Mitral Regurgitation
Enriquez-Sarano M, Tajik AJ, Schaff HV, Orszulak TA, Bailey KR, Frye RL (Mayo Clinic and Mayo Found, Rochester, Minn)
Circulation 90:830–837, 1994   119-95-40–5

Predicted 5-Year Survival of Operative Survivors

	Ejection Fraction		
Variable	≥60%	50%-60%	<50%
No risk factor	93 (1.44)*	90 (2.13)	83 (3.57)
Class III-IV, no CAD	87 (2.81)	81 (4.13)	70 (6.86)
Class I-II and CAD	87 (2.86)	81 (4.20)	70 (6.96)
Class III-IV and CAD	75 (5.52)	66 (8.06)	49 (13.19)

Abbreviation: CAD, coronary artery disease.
* Numbers indicate, in patients surviving the operative period, probability of 5-year survival as a percentage and yearly mortality (*in parentheses*).
(Courtesy of Enriquez-Sarano M, Tajik AJ, Schaff HV, et al: *Circulation* 90:830–837, 1994.)

Background.—In patients who have successful surgical repair of mitral regurgitation, left ventricular dysfunction is a common cause of death. The role of preoperative echocardiographic left ventricular variables in predicting postoperative survival and their clinical implications are not clear.

Methods.—Four hundred nine patients undergoing surgery between 1980 and 1989 for pure, isolated, organic mitral regurgitation were studied. All had had a preoperative echocardiogram within 6 months of surgery.

Findings.—The overall 5-year survival was 75%, 58% for 10-year survival, and 44% for 12-year survival. The operative mortality improved from 10.7% between 1980 and 1984 to 3.7% between 1985 and 1989. In a multivariate analysis, age, date of operation, and functional class predicted operative mortality, whereas left ventricular function did not. In the last 4 years studied, the operative mortality was 12.3% in patients 75 years of age or older and only 1.1% in patients younger than 75 years of age. In a multivariate analysis, the best predictor of late survival in operative survivors was echocardiographic ejection fraction (EF) (table), followed by age, creatinine level, systolic blood pressure, and presence of coronary artery disease. The 10-year survival was 32% for patients with EFs of less than 50%, 53% in those with EFs of 50% to 60%, and 72% for those with EFs of 60% or more. Compared with EFs of 60% or more, the hazard ratio for patients with EFs below 50% was 2.79 and for those with EFs of 50% to 60%, 1.81. The best predictor of late survival was echocardiographic EF, even when combined with left ventricular angiographic variables. Among patients with EFs of 60% or greater, survival at 10 years was better in patients with class I or II disease than in those with class III or IV disease, those rates being 82% and 59%, respectively. In combined multivariate analyses, the preoperative predictors of operative and late mortality continued to be significant, independent of the type of surgical correction done.

Conclusions.—In patients with organic mitral regurgitation, operative mortality has been substantially reduced, to a low 1.1% in those younger than 75 years of age. Age and symptoms but not left ventricular function predict operative mortality. The strongest predictor of late survival is left ventricular EF measured by echocardiography. Surgery should be considered early, even in the absence of severe symptoms, in patients with severe mitral regurgitation before left ventricular dysfunction occurs.

▶ As the authors note, age, symptoms, and left ventricular EF should be the 3 primary variables considered when recommending surgical correction for patients with moderate-to-severe mitral regurgitation. The presence or absence of significant coronary artery disease is also important. Both a progressive decline in the operative mortality and technical advances using valve repair have increased the popularity of earlier mitral valve surgery.

Patients who are in functional classes III and IV should continue to be evaluated for immediate surgery. Even though the operative mortality has decreased in patients age 75 years or older, it is still significant and surgery is indicated on the basis of the symptoms. In patients younger than age 75 years, the current operative mortality is extremely low and surgery is often considered for patients with no or minimal symptoms (class I or II). In patients with a left ventricular EF of less than 50%, the late mortality is higher, but surgery is not contraindicated and usually improves symptoms.—R.A. O'Rourke, M.D.

Thromboembolic and Bleeding Complications in Patients With Mechanical Heart Valve Prostheses
Cannegieter SC, Rosendaal FR, Briët E (Univ Hosp Leiden, The Netherlands)
Circulation 89:635–641, 1994   119-95-40–6

Introduction.—Valve thrombosis may lead to systemic embolism in patients with mechanical heart valve prostheses; treatment is with oral anticoagulant drugs. Reliable estimates of the risks and benefits of this therapy are needed to provide rational answers to a number of important clinical questions, including the optimal intensity of anticoagulation for different patient groups and the risks of temporarily interrupting anticoagulation. To obtain more precise estimates of the risks and benefits of anticoagulant therapy in patients with mechanical heart valves, a meta-analytic study was performed.

Methods.—The analysis included 46 studies on the incidence of thromboembolic and/or bleeding complications in patients with mechanical heart valve prostheses. The inclusion criteria were defined to select only comparable studies of acceptable quality. The studies, published between 1970 and 1992, included 13,088 patients who were studied for a total of 53,467 patient-years. Univariate and multivariate analyses were performed to estimate the influence of antithrombotic therapy, valve position, and valve type.

Results.—Without antithrombotic therapy, the incidence of major embolism was 4 per 100 patient-years. This risk declined to 2.2 per 100 patient-years with antiplatelet therapy and to 1 per 100 patient-years with warfarin therapy. The prosthesis type and site had important effects on the risk of embolic complications. The risk was almost doubled with prostheses in the mitral position vs. the aortic position. The risk was lower with tilting disk valves and bileaflet valves than with caged-ball valves. Among warfarin-treated patients, the incidence of major bleeding was 1.4 per 100 patient-years. The addition of antiplatelet therapy increased this risk significantly without any further decrease in the risk of thromboembolism.

Conclusions.—In patients with mechanical heart valves, warfarin treatment appears to reduce the yearly incidence of major embolism from about 4% to 1%. This benefit counterbalances the risk of major bleeding associated with warfarin therapy, which is 1.4% yearly. The risk of embolism is significantly affected by the type and size of the prosthesis, which in turn affect the optimal intensity of anticoagulation therapy.

▶ Thromboembolism and anticoagulant-related bleeding are still the most frequently encountered complications of mechanical heart valve prostheses. As the authors note, "Without anticoagulation, the risk of major embolism is about 4 per 100 patient-years. Aspirin reduces the risk of major embolism by about 40% compared with no treatment but is only about half as effective as cumarin therapy. Dipyridamole does *not* [emphasis mine] appear to have any effect on the prevention of thromboembolism either alone or when given in combination with aspirin." The risk of major bleeding resulting from warfarin therapy is less than 1.4% per year, so the benefit-risk ratio in these patients is acceptable. For patients receiving warfarin therapy, the incidence of major embolism is almost twice as high with prosthetic valves in the mitral position as compared with those in the aortic position. Both tilting disk valves and bileaflet valves have a lesser incidence of major embolism than do the caged ball valves.

Hayashi and associates (1) studied the efficacy of combined warfarin and antiplatelet therapy after St. Jude valve replacement for mitral valve disease. A total of 125 patients were assigned to receive treatment with warfarin alone, whereas the remaining 70 received warfarin together with antiplatelet agents that included dipyridamole in 14 patients and ticlopidine in 56 patients. If the maximum platelet aggregation rate by collagen was not reduced, 10–40 mg of aspirin was added to the daily regimen (29 patients). At 10 years, patients in the warfarin plus antiplatelet group had an actuarial survival rate of 98.3% compared with 90.3% of patients given warfarin only. Actuarial stroke-free and complication-free rates at 10 years were 95.3 and 89.4%, respectively, for patients receiving combined treatment vs. 84.3% and 67.9% in those receiving warfarin. Only hemorrhagic complications were not noted in patients given warfarin and antiplatelet drugs.

In this study, a higher survival rate, lower incidence of cerebrovascular strokes, and better quality of life with fewer postoperative complications were obtained with the combination of warfarin and antiplatelet therapy after St. Jude valve replacement for mitral valve disease. These data indicate the possible advantages of combined warfarin plus antiplatelet antithrombotic treatment after mechanical valve replacement.—R.A. O'Rourke, M.D.

Reference

1. Hayashi J-I, Nakazawa S, Oguma F, Miyamura H, Eguchi S: Combined warfarin and antiplatelet therapy after St Jude medical valve replacement for mitral valve disease. *J Am Coll Cardiol* 23:672–677, 1994.

Vasodilator Therapy in Chronic Asymptomatic Aortic Regurgitation: Enalapril Versus Hydralazine Therapy

Lin M, Chiang H-T, Lin S-L, Chang M-S, Chiang BN, Kuo H-W, Cheitlin MD (Veterans Gen Hosp–Kaohsiung, Taiwan, Republic of China; Natl Yang-Ming Med College, Taiwan, Republic of China; Inst of Public Health, Taichung, Taiwan, Republic of China; et al)
J Am Coll Cardiol 24:1046–1053, 1994   119-95-40–7

Background.—The conventional treatment of patients with chronic aortic regurgitation has been to prevent decompensation of the left ventricle for as long as possible. The ability of pharmacologic treatment to prevent or delay myocardial dysfunction is still unclear. The long-term effects of enalapril vs. hydralazine therapy on left ventricular volume, mass, and function, as well as on the renin-angiotensin system in chronic asymptomatic aortic regurgitation were investigated.

Methods.—Seventy-six patients with chronic asymptomatic aortic regurgitation were enrolled in the study and were randomized to receive either enalapril or hydralazine. Echocardiographic evaluations, treadmill exercise tests, and neurohumoral assays were carried out at 6 and 12 months after initiation of treatment.

Results.—Seventy patients completed the 12-month follow-up. No significant changes in heart rate and ECG pattern of left ventricular hypertrophy were seen in the hydralazine group. However, highly significant changes in systolic blood pressure occurred, along with mild changes in diastolic blood pressure. The enalapril-treated patients had a slight slowing down of heart rate and a significant reduction in systolic blood pressure compared with baseline values. Both groups had improved exercise duration and decreased pulse pressure. Only enalapril therapy achieved significant inhibition of the renin-angiotensin system. The left ventricular mean wall stress was significantly reduced in both groups, although the hydralazine-treated patients did not have much change in the left ventricular mass index. In contrast, the enalapril group had both a significant reduction in the left ventricular mass index and the left ventricular end-diastolic volume index. A statistically significant reduction in the left ventricular end-diastolic volume index was observed between the 2 groups

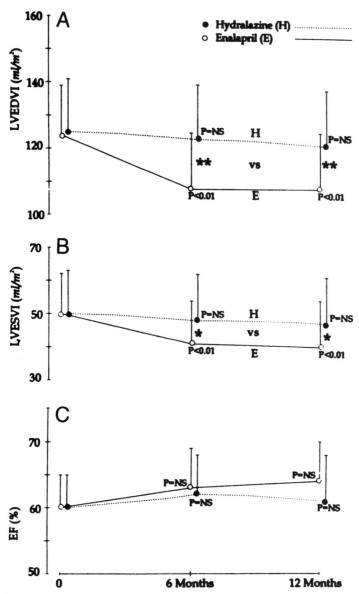

Fig 40–4.—Changes in left ventricular end-diastolic (*LVEDVI*) and end-systolic (*LVESVI*) volume indices and ejection fraction (*EF*) over time for the 2 study groups. Left ventricular end-diastolic (**A**) and end-systolic (**B**) volume indices did not change significantly in the hydralazine-treated group but decreased significantly in the enalapril-treated group. Ejection fraction (**C**) increased slightly in both the enalapril- and hydralazine-treated groups (P = NS). *P < .05. **P < .01. (Courtesy of Lin M, Chiang H-T, Lin S-L, et al: *J Am Coll Cardiol* 24:1046–1053, 1994.)

after 6 and 12 months of follow-up (Fig 40–4). Enalapril was associated with greater changes in the left ventricular end-diastolic volume index than hydralazine showing a multiple r^2 analysis value of 72%.

Conclusion.—Both hydralazine and enalapril treatment resulted in a decreased left ventricular mean wall stress. However, enalapril achieved significant sustained left ventricular volume and mass regression over a long-term follow-up. Enalapril also successfully inhibited the renin-angiotensin system, whereas hydralazine did not. Early unloading therapy with enalapril has advantages over pure arteriolar vasodilators (e.g., hydralazine).

▶ On the basis of this study, an angiotensin-converting enzyme inhibitor seems to have advantages for left ventricular afterload reduction in elderly patients with aortic regurgitation as compared with the arterial dilator, hydralazine. It must be emphasized that this trial included asymptomatic patients with chronic mild-to-severe (less than one third of patients) aortic regurgitation as quantitated by Doppler echocardiography only. Many of the patients apparently had systemic hypertension. Enalapril therapy had variable effects on left ventricular dimensions, hypertrophy, volume, and function. Only enalapril significantly suppressed the renin-angiotensin system as shown by the increase in plasma renin activity and the decrease in the plasma aldosterone concentration. On the basis of clinical and experimental observations, the beneficial effect of enalapril is likely caused by balanced vasodilatory activity and renin-angiotensin system inhibition.

Whether chronic vasodilator therapy favorably affects the natural history of asymptomatic *severe* aortic regurgitation remains to be convincingly demonstrated. The long-term effect of vasodilator therapy in patients with severe aortic regurgitation and a very low left ventricular ejection fraction (less than 20%) also needs further delineation. In both situations, a nonsurgical management approach is often selected.—R.A. O'Rourke, M.D.

41 Cardiomyopathy/Heart Failure

The Relation of Alcoholic Myopathy to Cardiomyopathy
Fernandez-Sola J, Estruch R, Grau JM, Pare JC, Rubin E, Urbano-Marquez A
(Univ of Barcelona; Jefferson Med College, Philadelphia)
Ann Intern Med 120:529–536, 1994   119-95-41–1

Background.—Excessive drinking is a common cause of congestive cardiomyopathy. Whereas nutritional deficiency once was thought to play a key role in its development, at present, a direct toxic effect of alcohol on the myocardium is implicated. Dose-related effects have been observed in both cardiac and skeletal muscle.

Study Population.—A cross-sectional study was planned to examine the relationship between skeletal muscle disease and degenerative changes in cardiac muscle in patients with chronic alcoholism. Twenty-four patients with chronic alcoholism and dilated cardiomyopathy, 24 alcoholics with normal cardiac function, 12 patients with dilated cardiomyopathy attributed to coronary disease, and 12 with idiopathic cardiomyopathy were studied, along with 24 normal individuals and 5 young men who had died suddenly of traumatic causes.

Methods.—Deltoid muscle strength was clinically assessed, and cardiac status was determined by radionuclide angiography and echocardiography. Deltoid muscle biopsy samples were obtained from the patients who were alcoholics and normal individuals and endomyocardial biopsy specimens of the left ventricle from the alcoholics with cardiomyopathy.

Findings.—Muscle strength was diminished in alcoholic patients with cardiomyopathy compared with that of alcoholic patients whose cardiac function was normal and that of nonalcoholics with cardiomyopathy. More than 80% of the alcoholic patients with cardiomyopathy had myopathic changes in skeletal muscle, compared with only 1 of the alcoholic patients having normal cardiac function. Interstitial fibrosis, myocytic hypertrophy, and myocytolysis were consistently observed in cardiac biopsy samples. The severity of these changes correlated with reduced skeletal muscle strength.

Implication.—The finding that cardiac dysfunction is related to clinical myopathy in alcoholic patients with dilated cardiomyopathy suggests that skeletal muscle weakness may be a marker of myocardial damage in this setting.

▶ Interestingly, histologic changes characteristic of skeletal myopathy were found in biopsy specimens of 20 of the 24 patients with alcoholic cardiomyopathy as compared with only 1 of the 24 patients with chronic alcoholism who had a normal left ventricular ejection fraction.

In patients with congestive heart failure, the reported poor correlation between exercise performance and measured cardiac function raises the possibility that impaired skeletal muscle function may limit exercise performance. Consistent with these reports, patients with nonalcoholic dilated cardiomyopathy and heart failure had less skeletal muscle strength than did a control group. However, *alcoholic* patients with dilated cardiomyopathy were still substantially weaker. Although the pathogenesis of muscle damaged mediated by ethanol remains to be clarified, the correlation between cardiac and skeletal muscle damage suggests that ethanol exerts similar toxic effects on both types of striated muscle. However, not all patients who consume excessive amounts of alcohol have either cardiomyopathy or skeletal myopathy develop, and other environmental and genetic factors may also play a role.

Another study (1) provided a clinical pathologic review of 673 consecutive patients with dilated cardiomyopathy. The most common causes of dilated cardiomyopathy were idiopathic origin (47%), idiopathic myocarditis (12%), and "coronary artery disease" (11%). Other identifiable causes of dilated cardiomyopathy were present in 31% of the total cases. The cause was attributed to alcohol abuse in 3.4% of cases.

In an echocardiographic study of acute global left ventricular dysfunction in HIV infection, De Castro and associates (2) prospectively studied 136 HIV-positive patients with serial echocardiograms. During a mean follow-up of 415 days, 7 patients, all in the AIDS subgroup, had clinical and echocardiographic findings of acute global left ventricular dysfunction develop; of these, 6 (85%) died of congestive heart failure. The mean survival time from the onset of symptoms was 41 days. Necropsy findings in 5 patients revealed acute lymphocytic myocarditis in 3, cryptococcal myocarditis in 1, and interstitial edema and fibrosis in 1. In only 1 patient was left ventricular dysfunction reversible with treatment.

In another study (3), the histologic and immunopathologic results of 37 endomyocardial biopsy samples were determined in patients infected with HIV-1 who were evaluated for unexplained left ventricular systolic dysfunction. All patients had moderate-to-severe global left ventricular hypokinesia on 2-dimensional echocardiography. Four patients had myocarditis secondary to known etiologies. Of the remaining 33 samples, 17 demonstrated histologic evidence of idiopathic active or borderline myocarditis. Importantly, immunohistologic findings showed induced expression of major histocompatibility class I antigen on myocytes and the infiltration of CD8+ T lymphocytes. These results suggest that cardiotropic virus infection and myocarditis may be important in the pathogenesis of symptomatic HIV-associated cardiomyopathy.—R.A. O'Rourke, M.D.

References

1. Kasper EK, Agema WRP, Hutchins GM, Deckers JW, Hare JM, Baughman KL: The causes of dilated cardiomyopathy: A clinicopathologic review of 673 consecutive patients. *J Am Coll Cardiol* 23:586–590, 1994.

2. DeCastro S, d'Amati G, Gallo P, Cartoni D, Santopadre P, Vullo V, Cirelli A, Migliau G: Frequency of development of acute global left ventricular dysfunction in human immunodeficiency virus infection. *J Am Coll Cardiol* 24:1018–1024, 1994.

3. Herskowitz A, Wu T-C, Willoughby SB, Vlahov D, Ansari AA, Beschorner WE, Baughman KL: Myocarditis and cardiotropic viral infection associated with severe left ventricular dysfunction in late-stage infection with human immunodeficiency virus. *J Am Coll Cardiol* 24:1025–1032, 1994.

Exercise Capacity and Systolic and Diastolic Ventricular Function After Recovery From Acute Dilated Cardiomyopathy

Semigran MJ, Thaik CM, Fifer MA, Boucher CA, Palacios IF, William G (Massachusetts Gen Hosp, Boston; Harvard Med School, Boston)
J Am Coll Cardiol 24:462–470, 1994   119-95-41–2

Objective.—Because persistent structural abnormalities of the ventricle could restrict exercise capacity or ventricular function in patients recovering from acute dilated cardiomyopathy, function was examined in 18 such patients who were seen within 6 months of the onset and who subsequently had a normal resting left ventricular ejection fraction (LVEF).

Methods.—The patients were studied a mean of nearly 5 months after the onset of ventricular dysfunction, when symptoms of heart failure had resolved. A transvenous right ventricular biopsy was performed in 13 patients. Three patients with myocarditis received immunosuppressive treatment for 6 months. Cardiac scintigraphy with indium-111–labeled monoclonal antimyosin and radionuclide angiography were performed, along with exercise testing and radionuclide studies of left ventricular diastolic function.

Results.—The 13 patients with biopsy specimen findings of myocyte necrosis recovered more rapidly than the others. Recovered patients had lower values of oxygen consumption both at peak exercise and at anaerobic threshold than did controls, and their end-systolic and end-diastolic left ventricular volumes at rest and on exercise were greater. Stroke volumes were comparable in the patients and controls. The patients had lower left ventricular filling at rest and slower normalized early peak filling rates normalized for end-diastolic volume. During an average follow-up of approximately 3 years, 2 patients had recurrent symptoms of heart failure and a decline in LVEF.

Conclusion.—Patients who have recovered from acute dilated cardiomyopathy may have a normal resting LVEF, but they have persisting abnormalities in aerobic exercise capacity and left ventricular systolic and diastolic function.

▶ Even though patients with dilated cardiomyopathy typically have a mortality rate of 7% to 10% per year resulting from progressive heart failure or arrhythmias, individual patients vary in both their clinical course and the severity of residual ventricular dysfunction. All the post–acute dilated cardiomyopathy patients had a normal LVEF at rest and were in functional class I at exercise testing. These data indicate that the prognosis of patients who recover from an episode of dilated cardiomyopathy is often favorable despite persistent abnormalities in left ventricular systolic and diastolic function.

Although the clinically measured resting LVEF was within normal limits in these patients, it remained lower than that of age- and gender-matched controls, despite the concurrent treatment with vasodilator therapy. In the cardiomyopathy patient group, the diastolic function at rest was abnormal, and the peak left ventricular filling rate, which was normalized for either end-diastolic volume or stroke volume, was depressed.—R.A. O'Rourke, M.D.

Improved Exercise Hemodynamic Status in Dilated Cardiomyopathy After Beta-Adrenergic Blockade Treatment

Andersson B, Hamm C, Persson S, Wikström G, Sinagra G, Hjalmarson Å, Waagstein F (Göteborg Univ, Sweden; Univ of Hamburg, Germany; Univ of Lund, Sweden; et al)
J Am Coll Cardiol 23:1397–1404, 1994   119-95-41–3

Purpose.—In patients with congestive heart failure, treatment with β-adrenergic blocking drugs may have beneficial effects on exercise hemodynamic studies. However, there have been no large, randomized studies of this. As part of the Metoprolol in Dilated Cardiomyopathy Trial, the potential benefits of β-adrenergic blockade on exercise hemodynamics and myocardial metabolism were examined.

Methods.—The double-blind, placebo-controlled trial included 41 patients with idiopathic dilated cardiomyopathy; all had an ejection fraction of less than .4. Hemodynamic status was studied at rest and during supine submaximal exercise before and after 6 months of treatment with placebo or metoprolol; the mean final dose was 130 mg. In addition, 19 patients were studied for myocardial metabolism.

Results.—The exercise cardiac index improved significantly in the metoprolol group, from 4.3 to 5.4 L/min/m², compared with 4.8 to 4.7 L/min/m² in the placebo group. With metoprolol, the stroke work index improved from 35 to 58 g/m/m², exercise systolic arterial pressure from 155 to 165 mm Hg, and exercise oxygen consumption index from 406 to 507 mL/min/m²; none of these variables improved significantly in the placebo group. The duration of exercise increased by 63 seconds in the metoprolol group, whereas it decreased by 24 seconds in the placebo group. The metoprolol group also had an increase in the net myocardial lactate extraction, suggesting that they had less myocardial ischemia. Although peripheral norepinephrine levels tended to decrease at rest and during exercise, the myocardial net spillover was unchanged.

Conclusions.—In patients with dilated cardiomyopathy, β-adrenergic blockade with metoprolol can improve hemodynamic status at rest and especially during exercise. These benefits are accompanied by improved or stable myocardial metabolic findings. The effects of β-blockers in protecting against sympathetic overstimulation are consistent with the internal unloading rather than increased inotropic stimulation.

▶ Many ongoing studies are assessing the usefulness of β-adrenergic blockade in the treatment of patients with dilated cardiomyopathy. The clinical benefit of β-blockers in the treatment of certain patients with dilated cardiomyopathy is well documented. However, methods of defining those patients who are likely to do better with β-adrenergic blockade remain to be elucidated.

In this study, the patient group receiving metoprolol treatment responded favorably, as compared with placebo-treated patients. Metoprolol patients had improved hemodynamic status, increased myocardial lactate extraction, higher ejection fractions, and lower arterial norepinephrine levels.

In a 6-month, double-blind, placebo-controlled, randomized trial (1), the impact of metoprolol therapy was examined in 50 patients with heart failure, known coronary artery disease, and an ejection fraction of .4 or less. The use of the β-blocker was associated with a significant reduction in the number of hospital admissions, overall improved functional class, increased ejection fraction, and greater increment in exercise duration. The cautious use of titrated doses of metoprolol appeared to be safe and beneficial when added to standard heart failure therapy in patients with dilated cardiomyopathy associated with coronary artery disease. The study group was too small to show any difference in mortality resulting from metoprolol therapy.

In the Cardiac Insufficiency Bisoprolol Study (CIBIS) (2), progressively increasing doses of the β-blocker given to 641 patients with chronic failure of various etiologies and a left ventricular ejection fraction of less than 40% improved the clinical functional status. Subgroup analysis suggested that the benefit from β-blockade therapy was greater for those with "nonischemic" cardiomyopathy. However, an improvement in survival due to β-blocker therapy again was not demonstrated.

In a clinical trial designed to explain the mechanism for the benefit of β-blockers in certain patients with congestive heart failure, Maisel (3) found that patients with dilated cardiomyopathy who were treated with metoprolol had enhanced cell-mediated immunity and improved T-cell function; these improvements appeared to correlate with an improvement in left ventricular ejection fraction.

In a multicenter clinical trial (4), a dose-effect response to bucindolol, a nonselective β-blocker with a mild vasodilator action, was evaluated in 141 patients with class II or III heart failure caused by either idiopathic dilated cardiomyopathy or "ischemic" dilated cardiomyopathy. After 12 weeks of treatment, patients given the highest dose of bucindolol had an improvement of 7.8 ejection fraction units as measured by radionuclide ventriculography as compared with 1.8 units for those receiving placebo. Although all doses of bucindolol typically lowered the systolic blood pressure during exercise, no changes in the New York Heart Association functional class or quality of life were noted. Results of this study suggest that in patients with depressed left ventricular systolic function, β-blockade with bucindolol produces a dose-related improvement in the left ventricular ejection fraction. The long-term clinical salutory effects of this approach are being evaluated in an appropriately designed multicenter clinical trial.

In another randomized study (4) of 40 patients with idiopathic dilated cardiomyopathy, carvedilol, a new β-blocker with associated vasodilator effects, produced a short-term reduction in both the heart rate and pulmonary wedge pressures. Long-term administration increased the resting and peak exercise cardiac stroke volume, and stroke work indices and further reduced right heart pressures. Long-term carvedilol therapy also improved the resting left ventricular ejection fraction, submaximal exercise capacity, quality of life, and functional clinical class.—R.A. O'Rourke, M.D.

References

1. Fisher ML, Gottlieb SB, Plotnick GD, Greenberg NL, Patten RD, Bennett SK, Hamilton BP: Beneficial effects of metoprolol in heart failure associated with coronary artery disease: A randomized trial. *J Am Coll Cardiol* 23:943–950, 1994.
2. CIBIS Investigators and Committees: A randomized trial of beta-blockade in heart failure: The cardiac insufficiency bisoprolol study (CIBIS). *Circulation* 90:1765–1773, 1994.
3. Maisel AS: Beneficial effects of metoprolol treatment in congestive heart failure: Reversal of sympathetic-induced alterations of immunologic function. *Circulation* 90:1774–1780, 1994.
4. Bristow MR, for the Bucindolol Investigators: Dose-response of chronic beta-blocker treatment in heart failure from either idiopathic dilated or ischemic cardiomyopathy. *Circulation* 89:1632–1641, 1994.
5. Metra M, Nardi M, Giubbini R, Dei Cas L: Effects of short- and long-term carvedilol administration at rest and exercise hemodynamic variables, exercise capacity and clinical conditions in patients with idiopathic dilated cardiomyopathy. *J Am Coll Cardiol* 24:1678–1687, 1994.

Randomised Trial of Low-Dose Amiodarone in Severe Congestive Heart Failure

Doval HC, for Grupo Estudio de la Sobrevida en la Insuficiencia Cardiaca en Argentina (GESICA) (GESICA, Capital Federal, Argentina)
Lancet 344:493–498, 1994   119-95-41–4

Purpose.—Many patients with severe congestive heart failure die suddenly, and many of these deaths are attributed to ventricular arrhythmias. However, there is no evidence that prophylactic administration of

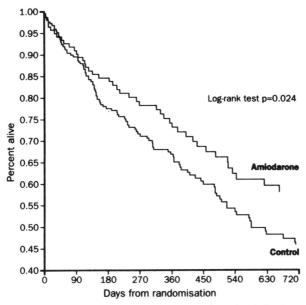

Fig 41–1.—Total mortality in 24-month period. (Courtesy of Doval HC, for Grupo Estudio de la Sobrevida en la Insuficiencia Cardiaca en Argentina: *Lancet* 344:493–498, 1994.)

antiarrhythmic drugs improves survival. The antiarrhythmic drug amiodarone is useful in patients with symptomatic complex arrhythmias, especially those in whom other agents have failed. The effects of low-dose amiodarone on mortality in patients with severe chronic heart failure were assessed in a prospective, multicenter trial.

Methods.—The study included 516 patients who were receiving optimal standard treatment for advanced chronic heart failure. None had symptoms of ventricular arrhythmias. After stratification for the presence of nonsustained ventricular tachycardia, the patients were randomly assigned to receive either amiodarone, 300 mg/day, or standard treatment only. The patients were followed for as many as 24 months.

Results.—On intention-to-treat analysis, 33.5% of the amiodarone-treated group died vs. 41% of the control group, for a risk reduction of 28% (Fig 41–1). The risk of sudden death was reduced by 27% and that of progressive heart failure by 23%. Amiodarone was also associated with a 31% reduction in risk of dying or being admitted to the hospital for worsening heart failure. This finding was present in all patient subgroups and was independent of the presence of nonsustained ventricular tachycardia. Six percent of patients experienced side effects from amiodarone.

Conclusions.—In patients with severe heart failure, low-dose amiodarone treatment can effectively and reliably reduce mortality and hospital admission. The benefits of the drug are independent of the presence of complex ventricular arrhythmias. Separate studies will be needed to determine amiodarone efficacy in patients with less severe heart failure or less impairment of left ventricular systolic function.

▶ In comparison to the usual current treatment for heart failure, the addition of low-dose amiodarone reduced the mortality and hospital admissions for congestive heart failure and improved the functional class of survivors. The reduced mortality and hospital admission in patients with severe heart failure appeared to be independent of the presence of complex ventricular arrhythmias.

Although the low dose of amiodarone used was associated with a low incidence of side effects (6%), the *routine* use of low-dose amiodarone in patients with severe heart failure cannot be recommended at this time.—R.A. O'Rourke, M.D.

Effect of Acute Magnesium Administration on the Frequency of Ventricular Arrhythmia in Patients With Heart Failure

Sueta CA, Clarke SW, Dunlap SH, Jensen L, Blauwet MB, Koch G, Patterson JH, Adams Jr KF (Univ of North Carolina, Chapel Hill)
Circulation 89:660–666, 1994   119-95-41–5

Introduction.—Ventricular arrhythmia and sudden death are common in patients with congestive heart failure. Currently used antiarrhythmic drugs have only limited efficacy in this situation and may lead to proarrhythmia and hemodynamic deterioration. Although parenteral magnesium has potential therapeutic benefits, there have been few studies of its antiarrhythmic effect in patients with heart failure. A prospective, randomized, double-blind, placebo-controlled, crossover study was performed to determine whether acute augmentation of serum magnesium concentration could reduce the frequency and severity of ventricular arrhythmia in patients with symptomatic heart failure.

Methods.—Thirty patients with symptomatic heart failure were studied; their mean left ventricular ejection fraction was 23%, and all were in New York Heart Association class II or III. None had symptomatic ventricular arrhythmia, and none were taking antiarrhythmic drugs, calcium channel antagonists, or β-blockers. The patients were randomized to receive 5% dextrose in water (D5W) or magnesium chloride in D5W, given as a .3-mEq/kg bolus over 10 minutes, followed by a maintenance infusion of .08 mEq/kg/hr for 24 hours. Magnesium analysis and ambulatory ECG recordings were performed in both groups.

Results.—In the magnesium chloride group, the mean magnesium concentration was 3.6 mg/dL 30 minutes after the bolus and 4.2 mg/dL at 24 hours. The serum potassium concentration was not significantly affected by magnesium administration. On "blinded" analysis, the magnesium chloride group showed significant reductions in total ventricular

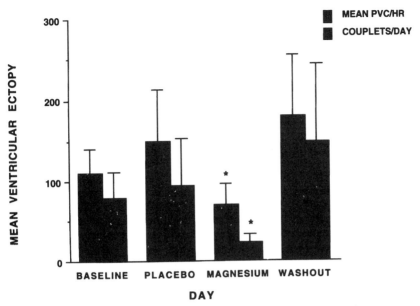

Fig 41–2.—Bar graph shows frequency (mean ± SEM) of total premature ventricular contractions per hour (PVC/HR) (*solid bar*) and couplets per day (*hatched bar*) on baseline (*n* = 29), placebo (*n* = 30), magnesium (*n* = 30), and washout (*n* = 16) days. An *asterisk* indicates a statistically significant difference (P < .01) between magnesium and placebo, baseline, or washout days. (Courtesy of Sueta CA, Clarke SW, Dunlap SH, et al: *Circulation* 89:660–666, 1994.)

ectopy per hour, 70 vs. 149 in the placebo group; couplets per day, 23 vs. 94; and episodes per day of ventricular tachycardia, .8 vs. 2.6 (Fig 41-2).

Conclusions.—In patients with symptomatic congestive heart failure, IV magnesium chloride can reduce the frequency of ventricular arrhythmia. Magnesium administration is well tolerated, with no adverse effects on blood pressure or heart rate. Further studies in a larger group of patients are needed to determine the dose-response relationship and the effect of long-term oral magnesium therapy on ventricular arrhythmias.

▶ This article reports findings of the first randomized, placebo-controlled trial to study the antiarrhythmic effect of acute parenteral magnesium administration on ventricular arrhythmias in patients with symptomatic heart failure. The use of IV magnesium for acute infarction patients is discussed in Chapter 2. Magnesium infusion significantly reduced ventricular ectopy by 53%, couplets by 76%, and episodes of ventricular tachycardia by 53% in the heart failure patients. However, only 30 patients were studied, and, thus, the impact of the parenteral administration of magnesium on symptomatic ventricular arrhythmias or on the incidence of sudden death in patients with congestive heart failure could not be assessed. Also, it is unknown whether similar beneficial effects on arrhythmia frequency would occur during chronic oral administration of magnesium.

In a study by Moser et al. (1), deaths among 566 consecutive patients followed up after the treatment for advanced heart failure were prospectively categorized as sudden death, death due to heart failure, or noncardiac death. Sudden death occurred 2.5 times more frequently between 6 AM and noon than in the 3 other 6-hour time intervals. The morning peak occurred both in patients with coronary artery disease and in those with nonischemic causes of heart failure. Despite a variety of potential mechanisms for sudden death and underlying causes of heart disease in patients with heart failure, the 24-hour distribution of sudden death in these patients is similar to that observed in other patient groups. Morning surges in sympathetic nervous system activity may promote a variety of mechanisms for sudden death, including ischemic- and non–ischemic-related arrhythmias.

Serial quantitative coronary arteriography is often used to assess progression of coronary artery disease, but it is a relatively insensitive technique for the detection of coronary artery disease in *cardiac transplant* recipients. Recently, Pinto and associates (2) used intracoronary ultrasound (ICUS) to assess the progression of intimal proliferation in cardiac transplant recipients. Serial intracoronary ultrasound often demonstrated progression of intimal thickening at specific sites in cardiac transplant patients. Progression of intimal proliferation often occurs in the presence or absence of initially increased intimal thickening or of angiographic disease at the time of the initial studies. The ICUS technique provides an alternative method for the early detection of intimal thickening of coronary arteries in the transplanted hearts, an important consideration for patients at high risk for having "painless" severe coronary atherosclerosis develop during follow-up.—R.A. O'Rourke, M.D.

References

1. Moser DK, Stevenson WG, Woo MA, Stevenson LW: Timing of sudden death in patients with heart failure. *J Am Coll Cardiol* 24:963–967, 1994.
2. Pinto FJ, Chenzbraun A, Botas J, Valantine HA, Goar FG, Alderman EL, Oesterle SN, Schroeder JS, Popp RL: Feasibility of serial intracoronary ultrasound imaging for assessment of progression of intimal proliferation in cardiac transplant recipients. *Circulation* 90:2348–2355, 1994.

42 Noninvasive Testing

Prognostic Value of Thallium-201 Single-Photon Emission Computed Tomographic Myocardial Perfusion Imaging According to Extent of Myocardial Defect: Study in 1,926 Patients With Follow-Up at 33 Months
Machecourt J, Longère P, Fagret D, Vanzetto G, Wolf JE, Polidori C, Comet M, Denis B (Centre Hospitalier Universitaire, Grenoble, France)
J Am Coll Cardiol 23:1096–1106, 1994   119-95-42-1

Background.—Thallium single-photon emission CT (SPECT) allows better assessment of the extent of myocardial perfusion defect than planar scintigraphy. However, no studies of large patient populations have been done to determine its prognostic value.

Methods.—From 1987 to 1989, 3,193 patients were studied. Patients with unstable angina, myocardial infarction during the previous month,

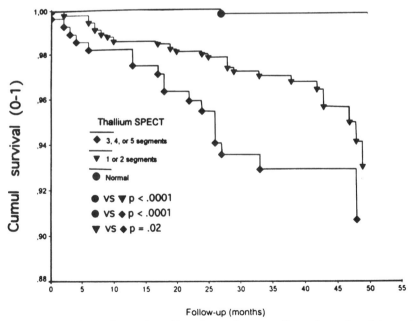

Fig 42–1.—Cardiovascular cumulative (*Cumul*) survival rate according to the number of abnormal segments on initial thallium SPECT imaging. (Courtesy of Machecourt J, Longère P, Fagret D, et al: *J Am Coll Cardiol* 23:1096–1106, 1994.)

or earlier revascularization were excluded, leaving 1,926 patients in the final group. The mean follow-up after stress thallium SPECT imaging was 33 months. Left ventricle thallium SPECT imaging was divided into 6 segments.

Findings.—After normal thallium SPECT imaging in 715 patients, the annual total and cardiovascular death rates were .42% and .10% per year, respectively. These rates were significantly greater after abnormal thallium SPECT imaging. The number of abnormal segments was significantly related to cardiovascular mortality during follow-up or the occurrence of nonfatal events. The best SPECT variable for long-term prognosis was the extent of the defect on the initial scan. Compared with clinical variables such as gender, previous myocardial infarction, and exercise ECG, thallium SPECT imaging provided additive prognostic information (Fig 42–1).

Conclusions.—Normal thallium SPECT imaging indicates a low risk in patients with stable angina. The extent of myocardial defect is an important prognostic predictive factor.

▶ In this large group of patients who were selected and assessed because of suspected angina or stable myocardial ischemia, the presence and extent of the myocardial perfusion abnormality on initial thallium SPECT imaging performed with exercise or dipyridamole stress were the most predictive indices of prognosis. As the authors write, "The results indicate that a patient with normal stress thallium-201 tomography has a coronary risk that is comparable to one chosen at random from the general population." This is not surprising, considering that no evidence of prior infarction or stress-induced ischemia could be demonstrated by a relatively sensitive technique. Thus, as the authors note, it seems possible to avoid the risk and additional cost of coronary arteriography in such patients, except in specific circumstances such as angina that do not respond to medical therapy. In patients with abnormal thallium SPECT imaging, the more widespread the initial perfusion defect is, the worse the cardiovascular prognosis. An individual patient has a particularly high risk when 3 or more abnormal SPECT segments are observed.—R.A. O'Rourke, M.D.

Dipyridamole–Thallium Scintigraphy and Gated Radionuclide Angiography to Assess Cardiac Risk Before Abdominal Aortic Surgery
Baron J-F, Mundler O, Bertrand M, Vicaut E, Barré E, Godet G, Samama CM, Coriat P, Kieffer E, Viars P (Hôpital Pitié-Salpétrière, Paris; Hôpital Lariboisière, Paris; Hôpital Fernand Widal, Paris)
N Engl J Med 330:663–669, 1994   119-95-42–2

Objective.—A significant proportion of patients with atherosclerosis of the abdominal aorta also have coronary artery disease. This situation has led to the use of preoperative cardiac risk assessment in patients scheduled for abdominal aortic surgery. The usefulness of dipyridamole-thallium single-photon emission CT (SPECT) to assess myocardial perfusion and radionuclide angiography to measure left ventricular ejection fraction was investigated as preoperative cardiac risk evaluation.

Methods.—A total of 457 consecutive patients were undergoing elective abdominal aortic surgery. All patients received both SPECT and radionuclide angiography in prospective fashion before surgery. Subsequently, all had inclusion graft procedures involving the abdominal aorta. Multivariate analyses were used to predict the adverse cardiac outcomes of mortality and major cardiac morbidity.

Results.—At least 1 postoperative complication developed in 19% of patients. Sixty-one had prolonged myocardial ischemia, 22 had myocardial infarction, 20 had congestive heart failure, and 2 had severe ventricular tachyarrhythmia. There were 20 postoperative deaths, half from cardiac causes. The SPECT myocardial perfusion data did not accurately predict adverse cardiac outcomes. The best predictors were solid clinical evidence of coronary artery disease, odds ratio (OR) 2.6, and age older than 65 years, OR 2.3. Left ventricular failure was the only adverse outcome predicted by data on left ejection fraction. The only variable that predicted death was age older than 65 years, OR 26.4.

Conclusions.—Dipyridamole-thallium SPECT and radionuclide angiography do not predict adverse cardiac outcomes in patients undergoing elective abdominal aortic surgery. Thus, routine preoperative use of these procedures does not appear to be justified. The most important predictors are definite clinical evidence of coronary artery disease and advanced age.

▶ As Baron et al. note, "Many studies have identified preoperative clinical markers that correlate with adverse postoperative cardiac outcomes." The most frequently reported markers are advanced age, history of myocardial infarction, angina pectoris, abnormal baseline ECG, hypertension, diabetes mellitus, congestive heart failure, and cardiac arrhythmias. Several clinical scoring systems have been identified with multivariate discriminant analysis.

As noted in the Discussion section of the article, "The principal finding of this study is that definite clinical evidence of coronary artery disease and [older] age are the two most important variables correlated with adverse cardiac outcomes in patients undergoing abdominal aortic surgery." Preoperative dipyridamole–thallium SPECT imaging and radionuclide ventriculography did provide additive information in certain patients before surgery, but the tests, in general, were not predictive of adverse cardiac outcomes in a large number of patients undergoing abdominal aortic surgery. I agree with the authors that, on the basis of these data, the considerable expense of "routine" preoperative assessment with dipyridamole–thallium scintigraphy and radionuclide ventriculography would seem unwarranted and often will not change the management strategies in patients either at *very high* risk or *very low* risk.

In a related, retrospective study of only 53 patients, Takase and associates (1) compared the prognostic value of clinical risk indexes, resting echocardiography, and dipyridamole stress thallium-201 myocardial imaging for perioperative cardiac events in patients undergoing major nonvascular surgery. A combination of the 2 noninvasive techniques predicted acute ischemic events (thallium myocardial perfusion imaging) and left ventricular decompensation (echocardiography) during or immediately after surgery. Clinical risk factor assessment did not predict cardiac events in this patient population but provided a framework for deciding whether to perform noninvasive testing.

Although the results of various studies comparing clinical prognostic indices and the results of noninvasive testing for risk stratification of patients prior to vascular and nonvascular surgery differ, an integrated approach with noninvasive testing applied to obtain more information on patients thought to be at intermediate risk on clinical grounds seems to be logical.

In a study of 936 patients *several months* after recovery from an acute coronary event, Krone and associates (2) performed treadmill testing with planar thallium-201 scintigraphy to determine the risk of a coronary event in patients who were followed for an average of 23 months. Although thallium-201 scintigraphy and exercise testing variables identified patients at risk for subsequent cardiac events, the poor predictive value of these tests in these patients with stable coronary artery disease severely limited their usefulness. It should be pointed out that more than 21% of the possible candidates for the study underwent bypass surgery during or soon after hospital admission and were not enrolled in the risk stratification performed several months after recovery from the acute coronary event. Also, many patients underwent myocardial revascularization based on the result of the stress thallium scintigraphy, the variable that was being assessed for prognostic significance.

In another study, Grover-McKay and associates (3) compared thallium-201 SPECT scintigraphy with IV dipyridamole and with arm exercise. The 2 forms of stress were comparable for detecting the presence or absence of significant coronary artery disease when care was taken not to oversubtract background radioactivity on thallium images obtained after arm exercise. The pathophysiology of exercise and vasodilator imaging is somewhat different. Many laboratories include a short period of arm crank or hand-grip exercise after dipyridamole IV injection as part of the dipyridamole stress test and claim that the sensitivity and specificity of the scintigraphy are somewhat increased by the combined stress.—R.A. O'Rourke, M.D.

References

1. Takase B, Younis LT, Byers SL, Shaw LJ, Labovitz AJ, Chaitman BR, Miller DD: Comparative prognostic value of clinical risk indexes, resting two-dimensional echocardiography, and dipyridamole stress thallium-201 myocardial imaging for perioperative cardiac events in major nonvascular surgery patients. *Am Heart J* 126:1099–1106, 1993.
2. Krone RJ, Gregory JJ, Freedland KE, Kleiger RE, Wackers FJ, Bodenheimer MM, Benhorin J, Schwartz RG, Parker JO, Van Voorhees L, Moss AJ: Limited

usefulness of exercise testing and thallium scintigraphy in evaluation of ambulatory patients several months after recovery from an acute coronary event: Implications for management of stable coronary heart disease. *J Am Coll Cardiol* 24:1274–1281, 1994.

3. Grover-McKay M, Milne N, Atwood JE, Lyons KP: Comparison of thallium-201 single-photon emission computed tomographic scintigraphy with intravenous dipyridamole and arm exercise. *Am Heart J* 127:1516–1520, 1994.

Dobutamine Stress Echocardiography: Sensitivity, Specificity, and Predictive Value for Future Cardiac Events

Afridi I, Quiñones MA, Zoghbi WA, Cheirif JB (Baylor College of Medicine, Houston; VA Hosp, Houston)
Am Heart J 127:1510–1515, 1994   119-95-42–3

Background.—Echocardiographic imaging during or immediately after exercise testing in patients with coronary artery disease (CAD) increases the test's sensitivity and specificity. In patients who are unable to exercise because of peripheral vascular disease, obstructive lung disease, or neurologic or musculoskeletal disorders, dobutamine stress echocardiography (DE) has been used as an alternative to test for ischemic heart dis-

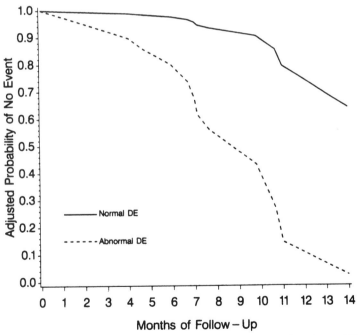

Fig 42–2.—Probability of not having a cardiac event in patients with normal vs. abnormal DE test. Probability was adjusted for age, preexisting CAD, ischemic ECG changes during DE, and baseline left ventricular ejection fraction. (Courtesy of Afridi I, Quiñones MA, Zoghbi WA, et al: *Am Heart J* 127:1510–1515, 1994.)

ease. The value of DE in predicting future cardiac events in patients with known or suspected CAD was studied retrospectively.

Methods.—Seventy-seven patients undergoing DE were included in the analysis. An echocardiogram was done at baseline, followed by imaging during IV dobutamine infusion initiated at 10 μg/kg/min with incremental increases of 10 μg/kg/min every 3 minutes. The maximum dose given was 40 μg/kg/min. Dobutamine stress echocardiography was done for preoperative cardiac assessment in 30 patients, chest pain in 23, assessment of ischemia in 18, and suspected re-stenosis in 6. Results were classified on the basis of wall-motion response as normal, fixed abnormal, or ischemic. The patients were followed up for an average of 10 months.

Findings.—Fourteen patients had cardiac events during that time. Seven had congestive heart failure and 6 had myocardial infarction. The last patient died of cardiac causes. Normal wall-motion response, recorded in 40 patients, was associated with a 5% incidence of cardiac events, compared with a 50% incidence in patients with an ischemic response. Twenty-six percent of the patients with fixed abnormal wall motion had cardiac events (Fig 42-2). Dobutamine echocardiography had an overall sensitivity of 85% for predicting future cardiac events. The test identified CAD with a sensitivity of 71% in 45 patients undergoing coronary angiography within 2 months of DE.

Conclusions.—Dobutamine stress echocardiography appears to be a safe, well-tolerated test in general, with a high sensitivity and specificity for detecting CAD. In patients with known or suspected CAD, the wall-motion response during DE may be used for risk stratification. The maximal heart rate achieved during the test may affect its predictive value.

▶ This study, like several other reports, indicates that DE with the assessment of regional wall motion during progressive IV infusion of dobutamine has a sensitivity and specificity for predicting cardiac events similar to other noninvasive techniques currently used in patients unable to exercise to the point of induced myocardial ischemia.

Dobutamine echocardiography is also being used for the assessment of myocardial viability with the finding of a low-dose (2.5–7.5 μg/kg/min) improvement in regional left ventricular contractility followed by a higher-dose (20–40 μg/kg/min) depression of function in the same region being a marker of depressed myocardium distal to coronary artery stenoses that likely will improve functionally after myocardial revascularization. Several clinical studies are in progress comparing various myocardial perfusion imaging protocols using thallium, low- and high-dose DE wall-motion responses, and metabolic and myocardial perfusion imaging with positron emission tomography in patients in whom the postprocedure response of hypokinetic and akinetic ventricular wall motion to coronary angioplasty or bypass graft surgery is uncertain. Such studies are particularly relevant to potential coronary bypass surgical patients with severe CAD and a very low (less than 20%) ejection fraction.—R.A. O'Rourke, M.D.

Assessment of Viable Myocardium by Dobutamine Transesophageal Echocardiography and Comparison With Fluorine-18 Fluorodeoxyglucose Positron Emission Tomography

Baer FM, Voth E, Deutsch HJ, Schneider CA, Schicha H, Sechtem U (Universität zu Köln, Cologne, Germany)
J Am Coll Cardiol 24:343–353, 1994   119-95-42–4

Background.—In patients with chronic myocardial infarction and impaired left ventricular function, it is important to distinguish between left ventricular dysfunction attributable to irreversible myocardial damage resulting in fibrotic scar formation and akinetic but viable myocardium. Past studies have indicated that postischemic myocardial dysfunction can be transiently reversed by moderate inotropic stimulation. Moreover, this response may be measured by echocardiographic detection of wall motion or wall thickening. Whether low-dose dobutamine transesophageal echocardiography can detect residual viable myocardium in patients with chronic myocardial infarction was investigated.

Methods.—Forty patients with angiographically documented coronary artery disease and regional akinesia or dyskinesia by left ventriculography were studied. All the patients underwent rest and dobutamine transesophageal echocardiography (dobutamine 5, 10, and 20 μg/kg of body weight per minute) and fluorine 18-fluorodeoxyglucose positron emission tomography (PET) at rest. Three representative short-axis positron emission tomograms and a transverse 4-chamber view were used for wall motion and fluorine-18 fluorodeoxyglucose–uptake analysis in corresponding myocardial regions. An asynergic segment was considered viable by transesophageal echocardiography if dobutamine-induced systolic wall motion could be seen. The PET segments were considered viable if the mean segmental fluorine-18 fluorodeoxyglucose uptake was greater than 50% of the maximal uptake.

Results.—Viable myocardium in at least 1 segment of a basally akinetic region was found by dobutamine transesophageal echocardiography in 53% of the patients. Infarct-related viability by fluorine-18 fluorodeoxyglucose uptake was observed in 63% of the patients. These results yielded a diagnostic agreement between both techniques in 90% of the study population. In 235 basally akinetic or dyskinetic segments, data on myocardial viability were concordant by the 2 techniques in 210 (89%) segments. The positive and negative predictive accuracy of dobutamine transesophageal echocardiography for viability estimated by fluorine-18 fluorodeoxyglucose uptake was 81% and 97%, respectively. This uptake was significantly different for segments remaining akinetic during dobutamine infusion and segments with a dobutamine-induced contraction reserve.

Conclusion.—Low-dose dobutamine transesophageal echocardiography is a safe, effective, inexpensive, and widely available method of providing high-quality images for identifying residual myocardial viability in patients with chronic myocardial infarction.

▶ The quest continues for a widely available and accurate noninvasive technique for determining the presence of viable myocardium in patients with major regional wall-motion abnormalities and depressed left ventricular systolic function who are candidates for myocardial revascularization. Although PET is an accurate method for determining zones of metabolic-perfusion mismatch in areas that are likely to improve their contractility after revascularization, it is not widely available. Other imaging techniques are more readily available but may be less sensitive and specific in determining the presence of viable myocardium.

In this study, the results of dobutamine transesophageal echocardiography was compared with those using metabolic imaging with PET in 40 patients with arteriographically documented coronary artery disease and regional akinesis or dyskinesis by left ventriculography. Even though the positive and negative predictive accuracy of dobutamine transesophageal echo for determining viability can be estimated by comparing the results with PET, the true test of any technique for assessing viability is the comparison of affected myocardial segments before and after myocardial revascularization.

On the same subject, Dilsizian and associates (1) assessed myocardial viability in patients with chronic coronary artery disease by comparing technetium sestamibi imaging and thallium reinjection imaging with metabolic imaging using fluorodeoxyglucose PET imaging (1). Their data indicated that same-day rest then stress sestamibi imaging will incorrectly identify at least one third of myocardial regions as both irreversibly impaired and not viable compared with both thallium redistribution-reinjection imaging and PET. However, the identification of reversible and viable myocardium was greatly enhanced with technetium sestamibi if an additional redistribution image was acquired after the rest sestamibi injection. Thus, the usefulness of imaging with sestamibi for determining the presence or absence of myocardial viability remains to be demonstrated.—R.A. O'Rourke, M.D.

Reference

1. Dilsizian V, Arrighi JA, Diodati JG, Quyyumi AA, Alavi K, Bacharach SL, Marin-Neto JA, Katsiyiannis PT, Bonow RO: Myocardial viability in patients with chronic coronary artery disease: Comparison of 99mTc-sestamibi with thallium reinjection and [18F]fluorodeoxyglucose. *Circulation* 89:578–587, 1994.

Diagnostic Role of Doppler Echocardiography in Constrictive Pericarditis

Oh JK, Hatle LK, Seward JB, Danielson GK, Schaff HV, Reeder GS, Tajik AJ
(Mayo Clinic and Mayo Found, Rochester, Minn)
J Am Coll Cardiol 23:154–162, 1994   119-95-42–5

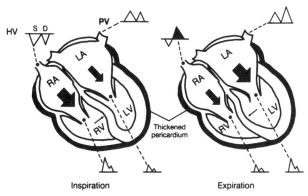

Inspiration   Expiration

Fig 42–3.—Schematic of respiratory variation in transvalvular and central venous flow velocities in constrictive pericarditis. With inspiration, the driving pressure gradient from pulmonary capillaries to left cardiac chambers decreases, resulting in decreased mitral inflow and diastolic pulmonary venous (PV) flow velocity. The decreased left ventricular filling results in ventricular septal shift to the left (*small arrow*), allowing augmented flow to the right-sided chambers shown as increased tricuspid inflow and diastolic hepatic venous (HV) flow velocity because the cardiac volume is relatively fixed as a result of the thickened shell of pericardium. The opposite changes occur during expiration. *Abbreviations: D,* diastole; *LA,* left atrium; *LV,* left ventricle; *RA,* right atrium; *RV,* right ventricle; *S,* systole. (Courtesy of Oh JK, Hatle LK, Seward JB, et al: *J Am Coll Cardiol* 23:154–162, 1994.)

Introduction.—Patients with constrictive pericarditis have been reported to have a typical Doppler pattern consisting of respiratory variation in ventricular filling and central venous flow velocities (Fig 42–3). However, these studies included only small numbers of patients with known constrictive pericarditis. The diagnostic value of Doppler echocardiography was evaluated in patients with suspected constrictive pericarditis.

Methods.—Twenty-eight patients—21 men and 7 women (mean age, 55 years)—had suspected constrictive pericarditis and underwent comprehensive 2-dimensional and Doppler echocardiography, followed by exploratory thoracotomy with or without pericardiectomy. The Doppler flow velocity data were assessed without knowledge of the clinical and surgical findings. Postoperative Doppler studies were performed in 21 patients.

Results.—The operative diagnosis was constrictive pericarditis in 25 patients; 2 patients had normal pericardium and 1 had pericardial restriction. Preoperative Doppler echocardiography made the correct diagnosis in 22 of the patients with constriction and showed restriction in the other 3. Restriction was correctly diagnosed by Doppler in the 1 patient with this diagnosis; in the 2 patients with normal pericardium, Doppler showed constriction in 1 case and normal findings in the other. Among patients with confirmed constriction, postoperative Doppler showed normal findings in 14 of 19 and pericardial restriction in the rest. Symptoms resolved in all but 2 of the patients with normalized Doppler findings, whereas all 5 patients with restrictive pericarditis on postoperative Doppler remained symptomatic.

Conclusions.—In patients with suspected constrictive pericarditis, Doppler echocardiography with simultaneous respiratory recording is a highly sensitive diagnostic technique. Doppler studies may also predict the functional response to pericardiectomy. Once the Doppler diagnosis of constriction has been made, cardiac catheterization appears to offer no further diagnostic information.

▶ Dr. Hatle previously described characteristic Doppler patterns of constrictive pericarditis based on respiratory variation in transvalvular and central venous flow velocity profiles (1).

Because echocardiography is commonly obtained in patients with dyspnea, peripheral edema, jugular venous distention, or abnormal cardiac auscultation, it may provide the first diagnostic clue for constrictive pericarditis, as it did in 29% of the authors' patients.

Pericardial exploration and pericardiectomy may be recommended for certain patients on the basis of characteristic clinical symptoms and signs of constriction accompanied by typical 2-dimensional and Doppler findings. In patients with typical Doppler velocity patterns of constriction but other unusual or complex clinical features, CT or MRI may be necessary to demonstrate thickened pericardium before surgical management is selected.

In another study using Doppler echocardiography, Pai and associates (1) concluded that the peak-to-peak and onset-to-onset A-wave transmit times from the mitral valve to the left ventricular outflow tract are easily obtained Doppler parameters that reflect left ventricular late diastolic stiffness as determined by high-fidelity left ventricular pressure tracings and angiographic volume assessments in patients with coronary artery disease.

Additional reports concerning noninvasive testing include a description of the usefulness of transthoracic echocardiography for documenting the improvement in right ventricular function and septal wall motion that occurs after successful single-lung transplantation for patients with end-stage pulmonary disease (2) and the better sensitivity of exercise echocardiography as compared with either transesophageal atrial pacing or dipyridamole echocardiography for diagnosing coronary artery disease in patients (3).—R.A. O'Rourke, M.D.

References

1. Pai RG, Suzuki M, Heywood JT, Ferry DR, Shah PM: Mitral A velocity wave transit time to the outflow tract as a measure of left ventricular diastolic stiffness: Hemodynamic correlations in patients with coronary artery disease. *Circulation* 89:553–557, 1994.
2. Scuderi LJ, Bailey SR, Calhoon JH, Trinkle JK, Cronin TA, Zabalgoitia M: Echocardiographic assessment of right and left ventricular function after single-lung transplantation. *Am Heart J* 127:636–642, 1994.
3. Marangelli V, Iliceto S, Piccinni G, De Martino G, Sorgente L, Rizzon P: Detection of coronary artery disease by digital stress echocardiography: Comparison of exercise, transesophageal atrial pacing and dipyridamole echocardiography. *J Am Coll Cardiol* 24:117–124, 1994.

43 Arrhythmias

Prevalence of Atrial Fibrillation in Elderly Subjects (the Cardiovascular Health Study)
Furberg CD, for the CHS Collaborative Research Group (Bowman Gray School of Medicine, Winston-Salem, NC)
Am J Cardiol 74:236–241, 1994   119-95-43–1

Background.—Atrial fibrillation (AF), a common arrhythmia among the elderly, can cause embolic stroke. In most reports of the prevalence and correlates of AF, the study participants were selected and hospital-based. The Cardiovascular Health Study baseline data were used to describe the prevalence of AF, to compare prevalence among individuals with and without clinical and subclinical cardiovascular disease, and to identify the correlates of AF in a sample from an elderly population.

Methods and Findings.—The Cardiovascular Health Study, a population-based, longitudinal study of risk factors for coronary artery disease and stroke, included 5,201 men and women aged 65 years and older. At baseline, AF was diagnosed in 4.8% of the women and 6.2% of the men. Prevalence was strongly associated with advanced age in women. The prevalence of AF was 9.1% in individuals with clinical cardiovascular disease, 4.6% in those with evidence of subclinical but not clinical cardiovascular disease, and 1.6% in those with neither clinical nor subclinical disease. Factors independently associated with the prevalence of AF included a history of congestive heart failure, valvular heart disease and stroke, echocardiographic evidence of enlarged left atrial dimension, abnormal mitral or aortic valve function, treated systemic hypertension, and older age.

Conclusions.—The prevalence of AF in men and women with clinical cardiovascular disease was 9.1%, which is similar to what was obtained previously. In addition, AF was associated with subclinical disease, especially subclinical atrial/valvular disease. In the absence of clinical or subclinical cardiovascular disease, AF was very uncommon.

▶ The incidence of atrial fibrillation is increasing both because the population is aging and because more patients are surviving the acute phase of a cardiac illness that formerly would have been fatal. An important objective is to terminate atrial fibrillation and prevent subsequent episodes. When this is not possible, the ventricular rate should be controlled and thromboembolic complications prevented.

Multiple factors including the age of the patient, the duration of the arrhythmia, the left atrial size, and the type and severity of associated cardiac or noncardiac disease affect the success rate of antiarrhythmic drug therapy in reverting atrial fibrillation to sinus rhythm, which varies in between 35% and 75% of patients. It has not been determined which drug is most effective, because alternative antiarrhythmic drugs have rarely been compared in the same patient. The electroshock reversion of atrial fibrillation has a higher success rate than pharmacologic reversion. However, approximately 50% of patients have recurrences of atrial fibrillation within 6 months.—R.A. O'Rourke, M.D.

Warfarin Versus Aspirin for Prevention of Thromboembolism in Atrial Fibrillation: Stroke Prevention in Atrial Fibrillation II Study

McBride R, for the Stroke Prevention in Atrial Fibrillation Investigators (Statistics and Epidemiology Research Corp, Seattle)
Lancet 343:687–691, 1994

119-95-43–2

Introduction.—Although warfarin is an established preventive treatment for stroke in patients with atrial fibrillation, its value relative to as-

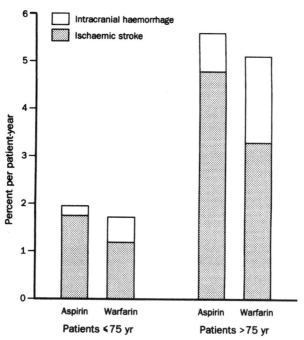

Fig 43–1.—Combined rate of ischemic stroke and intracranial hemorrhage according to antithrombotic therapy and age group. (Courtesy of McBride R, for the Stroke Prevention in Atrial Fibrillation Investigators: *Lancet* 343:687–691, 1994.)

pirin has not been defined. The Stroke Prevention in Atrial Fibrillation II (SPAF-II) study compared the effectiveness of these 2 treatments.

Study Design.—Warfarin and aspirin were compared for the prevention of stroke and embolism in 2 parallel, randomized trials involving 715 patients younger than the age of 75 years and 385 patients older than 75 years (Fig 43–1).

Results.—In the younger group of patients, warfarin decreased the absolute rate of primary events by .7% per year, so that the primary event rate was 1.3% per year. The rate with aspirin was 1.9% per year. The rate of primary events in low-risk younger patients assigned to aspirin was .5% per year. Among the older patients, warfarin decreased the rate of primary events by 1.2% per year, so that the rate was 3.6%. With aspirin in this group, the event rate was 4.8% per year.

Conclusion.—The SPAF-II study was designed to compare the reduction in ischemic stroke by warfarin compared with aspirin in patients with atrial fibrillation. Only a modest benefit of warfarin over aspirin was achieved. Patients younger than 75 years of age with few risk factors are at low risk for thromboembolism when treated with aspirin. Younger patients with risk factors may require warfarin. In older patients, the rate of stroke was high regardless of which agent was used, and the search for better preventive modalities for this group continues.

▶ As the authors note, "This study, designed to evaluate the magnitude of reduction in ischaemic stroke by warfarin over aspirin in patients with atrial fibrillation, revealed only a modest benefit in patients of any age." Although the results of this study are in accord with the substantial risk reduction rate by warfarin over aspirin reported by others, patients in the younger age group in the SPAF II cohort had a low risk of stroke when taking aspirin and, as a result, "would not benefit enough to justify the risk, expense, and inconvenience of lifelong anticoagulation." The impressive relative risk "reduction by warfarin over aspirin becomes negligible in terms of the absolute decrease in the rate of stroke in this age group."

In older patients taking warfarin, the high rate of bleeding occurred at similar dosing intensity and despite careful management of anticoagulation. As the investigators write in their Discussion section:

Previous trials of anticoagulation in patients with atrial fibrillation that reported lower rates of major haemorrhage in the elderly (> 75 years) involved fewer hypertensive patients, shorter periods of anticoagulant exposure, and lower intensities of anticoagulation. Since the prevalence of atrial fibrillation increases with advancing age, most strokes occur in the over 75 age group. For these patients the rate of stroke, if both ischaemic and hemorrhagic types are considered, was substantial in those assigned to either aspirin or warfarin in the doses used.

Rigid, generalized recommendations for antithrombotic prophylaxis are not justified, because patients with atrial fibrillation at high risk and low risk can be identified by age and other clinical features. Several multicenter studies comparing the efficacy of lower-dose warfarin therapy in combination with aspirin as compared with warfarin therapy alone or aspirin therapy alone are currently in progress.

In another study concerning the incidence of thromboemboli in patients with nonvalvular atrial fibrillation, Mügge and associates (1) demonstrated that patients with nonrheumatic atrial fibrillation are a heterogenous group with respect to left atrial appendage function as assessed by transesophageal echocardiography function. One subgroup of patients had "low-flow profile" left atrial appendage filling and emptying patterns by Doppler echocardiography that are similar to those seen in patients with rheumatic atrial fibrillation. Eighty percent of the patients within this low-flow profile subgroup as compared with only 5% of the "high-flow profile" subgroup had the spontaneous left atrial echo contrast phenomenon—an indicator of increased risk for thrombus formation and thromboembolic complications.—R.A. O'Rourke, M.D.

Reference

1. Mügge A, Kühn H, Nikutta P, Grote J, Lopez AG, Daniel WG: Assessment of left atrial appendage function by biplane transesophageal echocardiography in patients with nonrheumatic atrial fibrillation: Identification of a subgroup of patients at increased embolic risk. *J Am Coll Cardiol* 23:599–607, 1994.

Comparative Effects of the Combination of Digoxin and *d1*-Sotalol Therapy Versus Digoxin Monotherapy for Control of Ventricular Response in Chronic Atrial Fibrillation
Brodsky M, for the *d1*-Sotalol Atrial Fibrillation Study Group (Univ of California, Irvine)
Am Heart J 127:572–577, 1994   119-95-43–3

Background.—Patients with chronic atrial fibrillation who had insufficient control of rapid ventricular response with digoxin therapy alone were studied. The efficacy and safety of *d1*-sotalol in controlling the ventricular response in atrial fibrillation at rest and during exercise were evaluated.

Methods.—To be eligible for the multicenter, randomized, double-blind, parallel, placebo-controlled study, patients needed to have a resting heart rate greater than 80 beats/min. After 6 minutes of exercise, the heart rate needed to be greater than 120 beats/min and to have increased 50 beats/min or more. During a 2-week, single-blind, placebo period, the patients received digoxin treatment. Digoxin treatment was continued, and the patients were randomly selected to receive *d1*-sotalol, 80 mg/day, in divided doses; *d1*-sotalol, 160 mg/day, in divided doses; or placebo for 4 weeks. Exercise treadmill testing and ambulatory ECG recordings were done during screening and after 4 weeks of double-blind therapy.

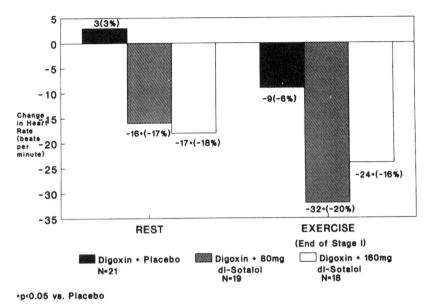

Fig 43–2.—Change in mean ventricular rate during rest and exercise. (Courtesy of Brodsky M, for the *d1*-Sotalol Atrial Fibrillation Study Group: *Am Heart J* 127:572–577, 1994.)

Results.—Sixty patients entered the study. Compared with treatment with digoxin and placebo, treatment with digoxin and either dose of *d1*-sotalol resulted in a significant reduction in the ventricular response rate at rest and in response to exercise (Fig 43–2). The 2 doses of *d1*-sotalol did not significantly differ in their effects on heart rate at rest or during exercise. There were no significant differences observed among treatment groups in the presence or absence of symptoms or in improvement or worsening of symptoms.

Conclusion.—Compared with digoxin therapy alone, the addition of *d1*-sotalol at a dose of either 80 or 160 mg/day significantly reduced the rapid ventricular response of chronic atrial fibrillation at rest and during exercise.

▶ The ventricular rate in patients with atrial fibrillation can usually be controlled pharmacologically. Digitalis slows the ventricular rate in patients at rest but does not prevent inappropriate acceleration of the ventricular rate during exercise. This can be controlled by the addition of calcium antagonists such as verapamil and diltiazem to digitalis or by β-adrenergic blocking drugs. Clonidine has also been shown to improve the control of the ventricular rate during activity. However, these drugs have negative inotropic properties that limit their use in patients with preexisting impairment of left ventricular function. In such patients, these drugs should be administered under close supervision starting with very low doses. This study shows that *d1*-sotalol, a class III antiarrhythmic agent with β-adrenergic–blocking properties (class II) can be safely used as an effective adjunct to digoxin for control of ventricular response in chronic atrial fibrillation.

The relative efficacy of IV digitalis, β-blockers, and calcium antagonists in the initial control of heart rate or reversion to sinus rhythm in patients presenting with atrial fibrillation is being assessed in several ongoing clinical trials.—R.A. O'Rourke, M.D.

Radiofrequency Catheter Modification of Atrioventricular Conduction to Control the Ventricular Rate During Atrial Fibrillation

Williamson BD, Man KC, Daoud E, Niebauer M, Strickberger SA, Morady F (Univ of Michigan, Ann Arbor)
N Engl J Med 331:910–917, 1994   119-95-43–4

Introduction.—Patients with atrial fibrillation and ventricular rates refractory to drug therapy are often candidates for ablation of the atrioventricular junction and insertion of a permanent pacemaker. A radiofrequency catheter technique was used in 19 consecutive patients with atrial fibrillation and uncontrolled ventricular rates to modify atrioventricular conduction.

Methods.—Isoproterenol was infused at 4 μg/minute. Two catheters were positioned at the His bundle and in the right ventricle. A third catheter, positioned on the posterior thorax, delivered radiofrequency energy during atrial fibrillation at 12 to 38 W for as long as 60 seconds. Application of energy was immediately discontinued when the RR interval lengthened or the ventricular rate noticeably slowed. Patients were monitored for at least 48 hours. Exercise stress tests and Holter monitoring were done at 2 days and 3 months.

Results.—Atrioventricular conduction was successfully modified in 14 of 19 patients (74%). Inadvertent atrioventricular block occurred in 4 patients (21%), requiring permanent pacemaker insertion, and ablation of the atrioventricular junction was done in 1 patient (5%). Significant decreases in the mean ventricular rates were noted at 2 days and 3 months in the minimal rates, while at rest, and after walking. The mean maximal ventricular rate did increase by 25% from 2 days to 3 months but was still approximately 25% lower than baseline. Improvement was significant as measured by the overall Canadian Cardiovascular Society functional class and according to symptom relief. At 5 months, 1 patient who had been successfully treated died suddenly, possibly because of underlying heart disease.

Conclusion.—The risk for inadvertent atrioventricular block when radiofrequency energy is used is about 20%. The procedure may be an alternative for patients who are symptomatic enough for ablation of the atrioventricular junction and permanent pacemaker implantation.

▶ The inability to control the ventricular rate with drugs in certain patients with atrial fibrillation and in patients' intolerance of the drugs have stimulated a search for other methods to reach that goal. An important step has been the electrical ablation of the bundle of His. The interruption of conduction through the bundle of His requires implantation of a permanent pacemaker to guarantee an adequate ventricular rate. This is currently facilitated by the availability of pacemakers that adapt their rate to the physiologic needs of the body.

In this study, another method of reducing the ventricular rate during atrial fibrillation using radiofrequency energy to modify atrioventricular nodal conduction was presented.

The results indicate that atrioventricular conduction can be slowed by radiofrequency ablation and that clinical improvement is achieved. However, it is difficult to estimate the practical value of this approach. It seems appropriate to wait for perspective studies in which this modification procedure is compared with His-bundle ablation and physiologic ventricular pacing. The optimal treatment for such patients with chronic atrial fibrillation will be determined by several factors including morbidity, mortality, quality of life, and cost (1).—R.A. O'Rourke, M.D.

Reference

1. Wellens HJJ: Atrial fibrillation: The last big hurdle in treating supraventricular tachycardia. N Engl J Med 331:944–945, 1994.

Use of the Signal-Averaged Electrocardiogram for Predicting Inducible Ventricular Tachycardia in Patients With Unexplained Syncope: Relation to Clinical Variables in a Multivariate Analysis

Steinberg JS, Prystowsky E, Freedman RA, Moreno F, Katz R, Kron J, Regan A, Sciacca RR (College of Physicians and Surgeons of Columbia Univ, New York; Northside Cardiology, Indianapolis, Ind; Univ of Utah, Salt Lake City; et al)

J Am Coll Cardiol 23:99–106, 1994   119-95-43–5

Purpose.—Inducible ventricular tachycardia, as well as other important diagnostic findings, may be detected on electrophysiologic study of patients with unexplained syncope. Inducible ventricular tachycardia is predictable from the signal-averaged ECG; however, the value of this prediction has never been examined in a large patient sample. Predictors of electrically induced ventricular tachycardia were examined in a sample of 189 patients with unexplained syncope, including an assessment of the value of the signal-averaged ECG in varying patient subsets.

Methods.—The patients were evaluated at 6 hospitals with signal-averaged ECG and electrophysiologic studies. Signal-averaged ECG recordings were analyzed at a central laboratory and were not used in deciding whether to perform the electrophysiologic studies. The value of these

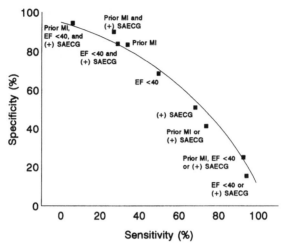

Fig 43–3.—Receiver operator curve for single and combination clinical variables. *Abbreviations: EF* <40, ejection fraction <.40; *MI*, myocardial infarction; (+) *SAECG*, positive result on signal-averaged ECG. (Courtesy of Steinberg JS, Prystowsky E, Freedman RA, et al: *J Am Coll Cardiol* 23:99–106, 1994.)

recordings was examined in patient subsets with differing pretest probabilities of ventricular tachycardia.

Results.—Twenty-eight patients (15%) had inducible ventricular tachycardia. On univariate analysis, significant predictors of this result were a history of myocardial infarction, reduced left ventricular ejection fraction, and abnormal signal-averaged ECG results. The latter was the most sensitive (70%) but had low specificity (55%). Independent predictors on multivariate analysis were an abnormal signal-averaged ECG and a history of myocardial infarction. Patients with both of these factors had a 17-fold increase in risk for ventricular tachycardia. When there was no history of myocardial infarction, no other test was useful in indicating risk of inducible ventricular tachycardia.

Conclusions.—Signal-averaged ECG is the most sensitive noninvasive test for predicting inducible sustained ventricular tachycardia on electrophysiologic study in patients with unexplained syncope. However, the results are false positive in many patients. A history of myocardial infarction plus signal-averaged ECG is the most efficient screening process to predict electrically induced ventricular tachycardia (Fig 43–3). The findings of this multicenter, prospective study will aid the clinician in selecting the type and sequence of diagnostic testing for patients with unexplained syncope.

▶ Of the 3 noninvasive tests available, the signal-averaged ECG was superior to determination of the left ventricular ejection fraction and ambulatory ECG monitoring for ventricular ectopic activity in predicting the likelihood of ventricular arrhythmia on electrophysiologic testing. As noted in the article, "The only historical variable used in the multivariate model that contributed predicted value was a history of previous myocardial infarction." Also, "In the absence of a previous myocardial infarction (low risk group), ventricular tachycardia risk prediction was very difficult, even with the addition of the signal-averaged ECG and other noninvasive data."

As in other studies, the presence of a positive signal-averaged ECG in patients with recent infarction and a left ventricular ejection fraction of less than 40% indicates a high likelihood of inducible ventricular tachycardia.—R.A. O'Rourke, M.D.

Electrical Alternans and Vulnerability to Ventricular Arrhythmias
Rosenbaum DS, Jackson LE, Smith JM, Garan H, Ruskin JN, Cohen RJ (Massachusetts Gen Hosp, Boston; Harvard Univ, Cambridge, Mass)
N Engl J Med 330:235–241, 1994   119-95-43–6

Introduction.—Electrical alternans (ECG beat-to-beat alternating amplitude) has recently been linked with sudden cardiac death. However, the prognostic significance of electrical alternans has not been systematically evaluated. It was hypothesized that a pattern of repolarization alternans predicts vulnerability to arrhythmias.

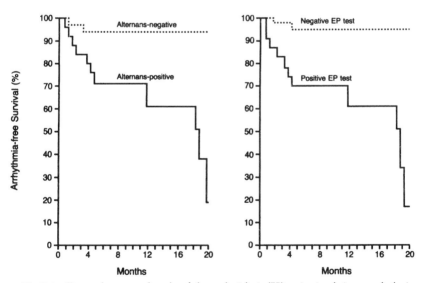

Fig 43–4.—T-wave alternans and results of electrophysiologic (*EP*) testing in relation to arrhythmia-free survival among 66 patients. **Left,** arrhythmia-free survival according to Kaplan–Meier life-table analysis is compared in patients with T-wave alternans (alternans ratio > 3.0) and without it (ratio ≤ 3.0). Note that the presence of T-wave alternans is a strong predictor of reduced arrhythmia-free survival. **Right,** arrhythmia-free survival among patients with positive EP tests is compared with that among patients in whom ventricular arrhythmias were not induced on EP testing (negative EP test). The predictive value of EP testing and T-wave alternans is essentially the same in these plots. (Courtesy of Rosenbaum DS, Jackson LE, Smith JM, et al: *N Engl J Med* 330:235–241, 1994.)

Methods.—Eighty-three patients referred for electrophysiologic testing were prospectively analyzed. A technique was developed to detect alternans not otherwise visible on the ECG. The relationships between alternans patterns and arrhythmia-free survival, and between electrical alternans and electrophysiologic testing were calculated.

Results.—Electrical alternans could be visually detected on only 2 of 36 baseline ECGs in which there was a significant alternans on the frequency spectrum. Alternans occurred most frequently in the T wave, followed by the ST segment, and seldom in the QRS complex. These patterns were consistent during varied stimulation rates. The ST-segment and T-wave alternans were independent significant predictors of inducible ventricular arrhythmia; QRS alternans did not predict arrhythmia. Also, T-wave alternans significantly predicted reductions in arrhythmia-free survival; its predictive value was equal to that of electrophysiologic testing (Fig 43–4).

Discussion.—The hypothesized relationship between repolarization alternans and vulnerability to arrhythmia is supported. These patterns can be detected noninvasively and can identify candidates for invasive electrophysiologic testing. The pathophysiologic mechanisms involved in electrical alternans require further study.

▶ The authors used a signal-processing technique to measure electrical alternans at the microvolt level. Subtle alternation of the ST segment or T wave was an independent marker of vulnerability to inducible ventricular arrhythmias and clinical arrhythmic events.

Rosenbaum et al. note that "unlike signal averaging, electrical alternans is a measure of beat-to-beat changes in amplitude and not absolute amplitude." It is also applicable to patients with bundle-branch block, whereas signal averaging usually is not. Also, "In this study, electrical alternans was detected in patients with bundle-branch block and bore the same relation to the results of electrophysiologic study and arrhythmia-free survival in those patients as in patients without bundle-branch block." The quantitative relationship between repolarization alternans and vulnerability to arrhythmias that was described here could be used to determine which patients are most likely to benefit from an invasive electrophysiologic testing.—R.A. O'Rourke, M.D.

Clinical Outcome of Patients With Malignant Ventricular Tachyarrhythmias and a Multiprogrammable Implantable Cardioverter-Defibrillator Implanted With or Without Thoracotomy: An International Multicenter Study
Saksena S, for the PCD Investigator Group (Passaic, NJ)
J Am Coll Cardiol 23:1521–1530, 1994   119-95-43–7

Introduction.—Implantable cardioverter-defibrillator systems have been almost exclusively implanted using epicardial lead systems requiring

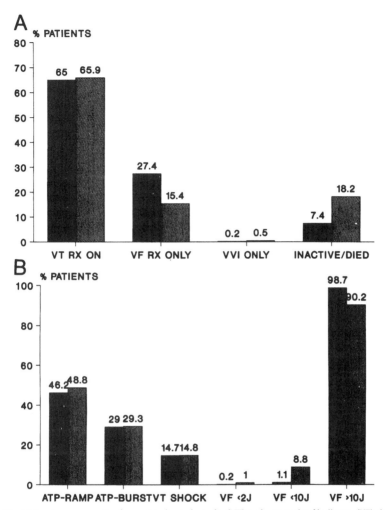

Fig 43–5.—A, programming for ventricular tachycardia (VT) and ventricular fibrillation (VF) therapies (RX) as defined by the device or demand ventricular pacing in the study population at follow-up. Ventricular tachycardia therapy is independently programmed in addition to VF therapy in the VT RX ON group. Ventricular fibrillation therapy is used alone in the VF RX ONLY group. Neither was used, but demand ventricular pacing was active, in the VVI ONLY group. INACTIVE includes patients with active antitachycardia therapies. **B,** initial electrical therapy for VT or VF stratified by lead system for study population. ATP indicates antitachycardia pacing for VT. (Courtesy of Saksena S, for the PCD Investigator Group: *J Am Coll Cardiol* 23:1521–1530, 1994.)

thoracotomy. This implantation approach carries a significant perioperative risk. Newer developments include endocardial lead systems that do not require thoracotomy and third-generation implantable cardioverter-defibrillators with bradycardia or antitachycardia pacing. The impact of these developments on safety and clinical outcome were studied in a prospective, international, multicenter, clinical trial.

Methods.—Patients who had sustained drug-refractory ventricular tachycardia after sudden cardiac arrest or ventricular fibrillation and were at risk for recurrent cardiac arrest or ventricular fibrillation underwent implantation or a third-generation cardioverter-defibrillator using either epicardial leads (616 patients), requiring thoracotomy or sternotomy, or endocardial leads (605 patients), inserted from the cephalic or subclavian vein. Patient outcome was evaluated 1 month and every 3 months after implantation for 3 years.

Results.—The perioperative mortality rate was 3.6% with direct epicardial implantation, 4.2% with generator implantation and the epicardial lead system, and .8% with the endocardial lead system, with direct or generator implantation. Ventricular tachycardia and ventricular fibrillation therapy were independently programmed and activated in equal proportions of the patients in each group, but ventricular fibrillation therapy alone was more common with endocardial implantation, and more patients with epicardial implantation were classified as inactive because of the higher mortality rate (Fig 43–5). With epicardial implantation, the 2-year survival rate free of sudden-death was 97.3%, and the 2-year total survival rate was 81.9%. With endocardial implantation, the 2-year survival rate free of sudden death was 99.8%, and the total survival was 87.6%. Spontaneous arrhythmia events occurred in 51.8% and 42% of the patients with epicardial and endocardial implantation, respectively.

Discussion.—The lesser mortality risk with implantation and the greater patient survival associated with endocardial lead systems recommends this as the front-line implantation technique.

▶ Implantable cardioverter-defibrillator systems are being recommended as the potential therapeutic solution to the large and increasing health care problem of sudden unexpected cardiac death. The PCD Investigator Group estimates that 20,000 implantations are performed annually at a cost of over 1 billion dollars.

The conclusion of this multicenter study is that the efficacy and safety of multiprogrammable hybrid pacemaker-cardioverter-defibrillator devices used in conjunction with either epicardial or endocardial leads are established. I agree that the endocardial lead systems should be the first-line implantation technique used because of the lower implantation mortality risk. Also, "Endocardial leads, by reducing patient risk for device implantation mortality, can significantly contribute to patient survival." This article states a limitation of this approach: "the inability to implant endocardial leads in 11.8% of patients for long-term use is a current limitation."

In another study, Wood and associates (1) describe the outcome of 66,276 spontaneous ventricular tachyarrhythmia detections recorded in a group of 393 patients after implantation of the Telectronics Guardian ATP 4210 implantable cardioverter-defibrillator. This device incorporates datalogging capabilities. A total of 74.4% of the episodes terminated spontaneously without any delivered therapy, 22.1% terminated after antitachycardia pacing, and 1.7% terminated after shock therapy. Antitachycardia pacing was activated without formal testing in 47% of all patients receiving this therapy and was successful in 96% of all episodes requiring this therapy. Acceleration of tachycardia to shock therapy occurred in 1.3% of all episodes and in 30.5% of patients receiving antitachycardia pacing. These data indicate that most ventricular tachyarrhythmia detections by the noncommitted implantable cardioverter-defibrillator resolve spontaneously, whereas most receiving therapy can be treated with antitachycardia pacing.—R.A. O'Rourke, M.D.

Reference

1. Wood MA, Stambler BS, Damiano RJ, Greenway P, Ellenbogen KA, Guardian ATP 4210 Multicenter Investigators Group: Lessons learned from data logging in a multicenter clinical trial using a late-generation implantable cardioverter-defibrillator. *J Am Coll Cardiol* 24:1692–1699, 1994.

44 Other Topics

Progression of Aortic Dilatation and the Benefit of Long-Term β-Adrenergic Blockade in Marfan's Syndrome
Shores J, Berger KR, Murphy EA, Pyeritz RE (Johns Hopkins Univ, Baltimore, Md)
N Engl J Med 330:1335–1341, 1994   119-95-44–1

Background.—Progressive enlargement of the aortic root is the most serious clinical feature of Marfan syndrome. In untreated patients, the associated aortic dissection and regurgitation shorten life expectancy by as much as one third. β-Adrenergic blockade might have the effect of protecting the aortic root by reducing the impulse (rate of pressure change) of left ventricular ejection and the heart rate.

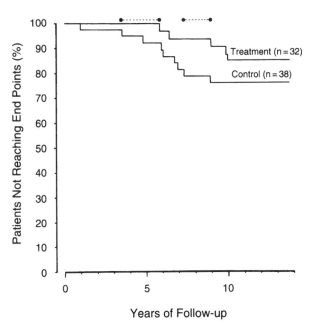

Years of Follow-up

Fig 44–1.—Kaplan–Meier survival analysis based on the clinical end points in the study (death, congestive heart failure, or aortic regurgitation, aortic dissection, or cardiovascular surgery). The *dashed lines* at the top indicate the periods when the 90% confidence limits for the difference between the curves did not include zero. The curves diverge the most in the middle years but do not intersect at any point. (Courtesy of Shores J, Berger KR, Murphy EA, et al: *N Engl J Med* 330:1335–1341, 1994.)

Study Plan.—A randomized, open-label study of propranolol was undertaken in adult and adolescent patients with classic Marfan syndrome. Thirty-two patients were given propranolol in an initial dose of 10 mg 4 times daily, and the dose was increased until the heart rate remained less than 100 beats per minute during exercise or the systolic time interval, corrected for heart rate, increased 30%. The 38 other patients of similar age and cardiovascular characteristics were untreated. The patients were followed clinically for about 10 years on average and had the dimensions of the aortic root monitored by M-mode echocardiography.

Results.—The mean dose of propranolol was 212 mg/day, and the mean serum drug level on optimal dosing was 135 ng/mL. The rate of dilatation of the aortic root was significantly less in propranolol-treated patients than in the controls (Fig 44–1). Nine control patients and only 3 who actually took their prescribed drug reached a clinical end point: death, congestive heart failure, aortic regurgitation, aortic dissection, or cardiovascular surgery. Two of the control patients died. Only 1 patient required dose reduction, because of third-degree atrioventricular block.

Discussion.—β-Adrenergic blockade effectively slows the development of aortic root dilatation in some patients with Marfan syndrome. It may be advantageous to use a β_1-selecive agent such as atenolol, which has a longer therapeutic half-life and fewer side effects than propranolol.

▶ Two types of benefits were evident in this important study of patients with Marfan syndrome and mild-to-moderate dilatation of the aortic root who received long-term β-adrenergic blockade with propranolol. The "rates of increase in aortic root size were lower in the treated patients as a group and in most of them individually" than the progression of aortic dilatation in the untreated patients. Second, fewer patients in the treatment group achieved 1 or more of the 5 predetermined end points for withdrawal from the study.

Propranolol was initiated in the Marfan patients because of its negative inotropic and chronotropic effects. However, the lesser aortic dilatation in the patients treated with β-blockers could be due to other mechanisms such as the effect of the drug on collagen. A prospective investigation of the effect of long-term oral β-adrenergic blockade on the elastic properties of the aorta in patients with Marfan syndrome should provide important mechanistic information.

These results support the use of daily β-blocker therapy in doses that reduce the heart rate response to exercise in most patients with Marfan syndrome and mild-to-moderate aortic root dilatation.—R.A. O'Rourke, M.D.

Normalization of Cardiac Structure and Function After Regression of Cardiac Hypertrophy
Habib GB, Mann DL, Zoghbi WA (Veterans Affairs Med Ctr, Houston; Methodist Hosp, Houston; Baylor College of Med, Houston)
Am Heart J 128:333–343, 1994   119-95-44–2

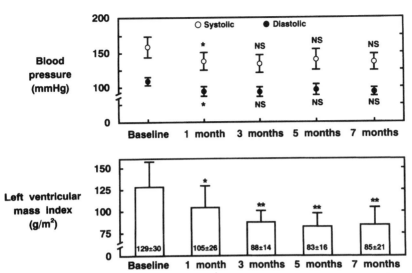

Fig 44–2.—Top, effect of antihypertensive treatment on blood pressure. Analysis of variance showed significant overall decrease in systolic and diastolic blood pressure during treatment (P < .001) at 1 month compared with control, with no further significant change after 1 month (NS, P > .05 compared with values at 1 month). **Bottom,** effect of treatment on left ventricular mass index. Analysis of variance showed significant overall decrease in left ventricular mass index during treatment (P < .01). Post hoc analysis showed significant decrease in left ventricular mass index (*P < .05) at 1 month and further significant decrease in left ventricular mass index at 3, 5, and 7 months compared with values obtained at 1 month (**P < .001). There was no significant change in left ventricular mass index after 3 months of treatment. (Courtesy of Habib GB, Mann DL, Zoghbi WA: *Am Heart J* 128:333-343, 1994.)

Background.—Left ventricular hypertrophy has been found to regress after pharmacologic treatment of patients who are hypertensive. However, the impact of regression of left ventricular hypertrophy on systolic function and on left and right ventricular diastolic function is still controversial.

Methods.—Twenty-seven patients who were hypertensive patients (mean age, 43 years) were assessed for left ventricular mass, systolic function, and left and right ventricular diastolic function. Echocardiographic and Doppler studies were done before and 1, 3, 5, and 7 months after treatment. At the same time, left ventricular mass and ventricular function were assessed in 27 age-matched normotensive controls.

Findings.—Antihypertensive treatment with long-acting nifedipine significantly reduced diastolic blood pressure by 15 mm Hg at 1 month and throughout the study (Fig 44-2). Hemodynamic unloading was associated with a decline in the left ventricular mass index from 129 g/m² at baseline to 105 g/m² after 1 month and 88 g/m² at 3 months of treatment. The final value remained the same over the next 4 months. After 3 months of treatment, the hypertensive and control groups had similar left ventricular mass indices. Systolic function was unaffected throughout treatment and did not differ from that in the control group. However, patients with a shortening fraction that was initially depressed had a higher increase in shortening fraction during therapy than those with an initially normal shortening fraction and improvement in the relationship between the shortening fraction and end-systolic wall stress during therapy. In the first 3 months of therapy, ventricular filling dynamics improved, then remained the same. Ventricular filling dynamics in the hypertensive and control groups were comparable.

Conclusions.—Pharmacologic unloading of the left ventricle in patients with mild-to-moderate hypertension normalizes the left ventricular mass index as well as left and right ventricular filling dynamics. Thus, left ventricular mass index normalization is not only possible but accompanied by a normalization of left and right ventricular filling dynamics. In addition, a substantial regression of left ventricular hypertrophy can be safely attained with no apparent deterioration in left ventricular systolic performance.

▶ As anticipated, this study substantiates other reports showing that antihypertensive treatment reduces the left ventricular mass index in patients with mild-to-moderate hypertension. It demonstrated that antihypertensive treatment with a calcium antagonist results in normalization of left ventricular mass, left and right ventricular filling dynamics, and, often, in left ventricular systolic function. "In patients with an initially depressed left ventricular shortening fraction, there was a significant improvement in systolic function during treatment, as evidenced by an increase in shortening fraction . . . and in the relationship between shortening fraction and end-systolic stress." This did not occur in hypertensive patients with an initially normal shortening fraction.—R.A. O'Rourke, M.D.

Call Mosby Document Express at **1 (800) 55-MOSBY** to obtain copies of the original source documents of articles featured or referenced in the YEAR BOOK series.

PART FIVE

THE DIGESTIVE SYSTEM

NORTON J. GREENBERGER, M.D.

Introduction

The 53 articles selected for the Gastroenterology section of the 1995 YEAR BOOK OF MEDICINE were chosen from more than 2,500 articles reviewed. This year, as in years past, I have tried to achieve a balance between articles dealing with the basic mechanisms of diseases and those providing important and useful clinical information. I would like to comment on some of the key articles selected.

The chapter on the esophagus includes articles on the treatment of gastroesophageal reflux disease. This is a disorder that affects over 60 million Americans. Seven percent of the United States population experiences symptoms of gastroesophageal reflux daily. The studies indicate that omeprazole is a very effective drug in effecting long-term remissions and is also cost-effective. Barrett's esophagus is a disorder that affects approximately 750,000 Americans and is a significant risk factor for development of adenocarcinoma of the esophagus. The incidence of adenocarcinoma of the esophagus has increased dramatically during the past 10-20 years and, accordingly, surveillance strategies for monitoring patients with Barrett's esophagus have become necessary.

The chapter on the stomach highlights the critical role of *Helicobacter pylori* and duodenal ulcer disease. I am still grappling with the concept that the vast majority of patients with duodenal ulcer disease, in essence, have an infectious process. Recent data indicate that in patients with duodenal ulcer disease and *H. pylori*, eradication of *H. pylori* will lower the recurrence rate of duodenal ulcer to approximately 2% per year. The National Institutes of Health held a consensus conference on *H. pylori*, and these recommendations are discussed in detail. In essence, patients with peptic ulcer disease and *H. pylori* should receive a minimum of 2 drugs for 2 weeks. This is a rapidly evolving area and the recommendations are changing every 6 months. Other articles deal with exciting advances in physiologic regulation of satiety and implications for obese patients.

The section on the small bowel contains a classic article on the pathophysiology of potassium absorption secretion. Other selections include articles dealing with interesting side effects of omeprazole (bacterial overgrowth in small bowel) and details of the massive outbreak of cryptosporidiosis that resulted in over 400,000 cases in Milwaukee, Wisconsin. A provocative article links enteric infection with *Ancylostoma caninum* and eosinophilic enteritis. The interesting question of food intolerance is discussed in an authoritative article as well.

The selections in the chapter on the colon contain 2 articles on ulcerative colitis, one of which is a landmark study detailing a 25-year experience with over 1,000 patients. The vexing problem of colorectal cancer, with special attention to occult blood testing and flexible sigmoidoscopy, is also discussed. Loss of chromosome 18q carries with it a poor prognosis in patients with colorectal cancer, and this is discussed in detail. The efficacy of antidepressant medications in the treatment of patients with irritable bowel syndrome is also worth reading.

Recurrent themes characterize the section on the liver, in which 2 articles deal with hepatitis B and 3 articles deal with hepatitis C. Treatment recommendations for patients with chronic hepatitis C have also changed, and this is discussed in detail. Treatment of portal hypertension and bleeding varices is also reviewed with special reference to the relative effectiveness of sclerotherapy and transjugular intrahepatic portal system shunts. Other articles include screening for hemochromatosis, ursodiol treatment of primary biliary cirrhosis, an extensive review of Budd–Chiari syndrome, and outcome indicators in alcoholic hepatitis.

A seminal article on the effects of dietary cholesterol on cholesterol and bile acid homeostasis in patients with gallstone disease is also presented. The section on the pancreas contains a much-needed article detailing the correlation of pancreatic morphology and exocrine functional impairment in patients with chronic pancreatitis. That study indicates that if the endoscopic retrograde pancreatogram (ERCP) is abnormal, there is a strong likelihood that there will be exocrine functional impairment. Diagnosis and management of pancreatitis with end-stage renal disease offers some new insights. Risk factors for pancreatic cancer are also discussed in 2 articles.

Finally, I have chosen to include selected citations of important editorial opinions concerning many of these articles.

Norton J. Greenberger, M.D.

45 Esophagus

Omeprazole v Ranitidine for Prevention of Relapse in Reflux Oesophagitis: A Controlled Double Blind Trial of Their Efficacy and Safety
Dent J, Yeomans ND, Mackinnon M, Reed W, Narielvala FM, Hetzel DJ, Solcia E, Shearman DJC (Royal Adelaide Hosp, Australia; Western Hosp, Footscray, Australia; Flinders Med Ctr, Bedford-Park, Australia; et al)
Gut 35:590–598, 1994   119-95-45–1

Background.—In a previous study of omeprazole in severe reflux esophagitis, it was discovered that, although healing rates were unprecedentedly high, relapse occurred quite frequently after treatment was withdrawn. Omeprazole's efficacy in the suppression of acid secretion increases in the first 3–5 days of repeat treatment because of increased bioavailability. A weekend dosing regimen with omeprazole was compared with a daily dosing schedule with omeprazole or ranitidine as maintenance therapy for reflux esophagitis.

Methods.—The study included 159 patients who had achieved endoscopic healing of reflux esophagitis with omeprazole treatment (20 mg every morning for 4–8 weeks). All patients had erosive reflux esophagitis

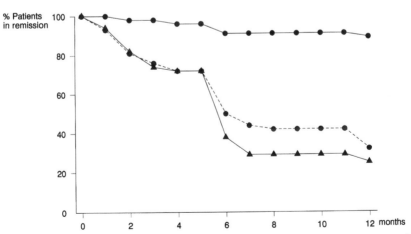

Fig 45–1.—Percentage of patients remaining in remission while receiving 1 of the regimens, over 12 months. *Solid line*, 20 mg of omeprazole every morning; *dashed line*, 20 mg on weekends; *triangles*, 150 mg of ranitidine twice daily. (Courtesy of Dent J, Yeomans ND, Mackinnon M, et al: *Gut* 35:590–598, 1994.)

of at least grade 2 severity at baseline. The second phase of the study was a 12-month, randomized, double-blind trial of maintenance therapy with either daily omeprazole, 20 mg every morning; weekend omeprazole, 20 mg on 3 consecutive days per week; or daily ranitidine, 150 mg twice daily. Endoscopy with gastric biopsy was performed at 6 and 12 months or if symptomatic recurrence developed. Serum gastrin was monitored as well.

Results.—The proportion of patients in remission at 12 months, as estimated by the actuarial life-table method, was 89% with daily omeprazole vs. 32% with weekend omeprazole and 25% with daily ranitidine (Fig 45-1). Almost all of the patients who remained relapse free with the latter 2 regimens initially had milder disease. During the healing phase, median gastrin concentrations increased slightly but remained within the range of normal. There was no change in gastrin concentrations during the maintenance phase of treatment. There were no unusual pathologic findings nor any adverse effects of drug treatment.

Conclusion.—For patients with reflux esophagitis who respond favorably to acute treatment with daily omeprazole, maintenance treatment with daily omeprazole is safe and effective in the prevention of relapse and its associated symptoms. Maintenance therapy with weekend omeprazole or daily ranitidine is ineffective. The amount of acid suppression is significantly related to successful maintenance of healing and symptom control.

▶ This carefully done comprehensive study confirms that omeprazole is the most effective agent currently available for prevention of relapse in reflux esophagitis. Several findings in this investigation merit further emphasis:
- The relapse rate in patients with endoscopically verified grade 2 or greater esophagitis is high if such patients are not on a maintenance regimen after initial healing with omeprazole.
- After initial healing of esophagitis with omeprazole, switching to standard doses of an H₂-blocker such as ranitidine results in a high relapse rate, which in this study approximated 70%.
- Weekend therapy with 3 days of omeprazole was even less effective than daily ranitidine.

Abstract 119-95-45-2 demonstrates the effectiveness of long-term (i.e., 5 years) maintenance therapy with omeprazole. Further, the safety issue concerning extended use of omeprazole is also discussed.—N.J. Greenberger, M.D.

Long-Term Treatment With Omeprazole for Refractory Reflux Esophagitis: Efficacy and Safety
Klinkenberg-Knol EC, Festen HPM, Jansen JBMJ, Lamers CBHW, Nelis F, Snel P, Lückers A, Dekkers CPM, Havu N, Meuwissen SGM (Free Univ Hosp, Amsterdam; Groot Ziekengasthuis, 's Hertogenbosch, The Netherlands; State

Univ, Leiden, The Netherlands; et al)
Ann Intern Med 121:161–167, 1994

119-95-45–2

Background.—Omeprazole is approved for the long-term treatment of reflux esophagitis in some European countries. In the United States, its use is approved only for short-term therapy. The results of omeprazole treatment for up to 64 months were reported.

Methods.—Ninety-one patients with gastroesophageal reflux resistant to H$_2$-receptor antagonist treatment were studied. In all patients, the disease was subsequently responsive to 40 mg of omeprazole daily. Open maintenance treatment consisted of omeprazole daily at a dose of 20 mg in 86 patients and 40 mg in 5. The mean follow-up was 48 months, with a range of 36 to 64 months.

Findings.—Forty-seven percent of the patients taking 20 mg of omeprazole daily had esophagitis recurrence. All of these patients rehealed after the dose was doubled. Eighteen percent of 40 patients had a second relapse after a mean follow-up of 24 months. These relapses were

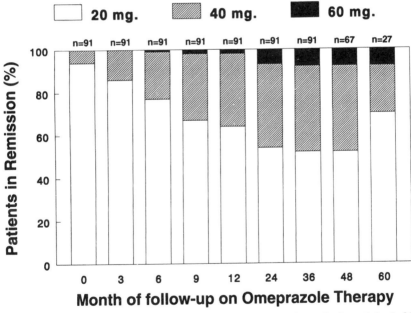

Fig 45–2.—Cumulative remission rates with dose adjustments required to maintain remission in 91 patients with reflux esophagitis during maintenance treatment with omeprazole. Cumulative remission rate in 91 patients after 36 months: 100% confidence interval (CI) 96% to 100%; in 67 patients after 48 months: (100% CI, 95% to 100%); and in 27 patients after 60 months: (100% CI, 87% to 100%). The 5 patients receiving 40 mg of omeprazole at 0 months of follow-up were not healed after the acute treatment period of 12 weeks and continued to receive this dose. The other patients receiving 40 mg of omeprazole represent a first relapse, whereas the patients receiving 60 mg of omeprazole represent a second relapse. (Courtesy of Klinkenberg-Knol EC, Festen HPM, Jansen JBMJ, et al: *Ann Intern Med* 121:161–167, 1994.)

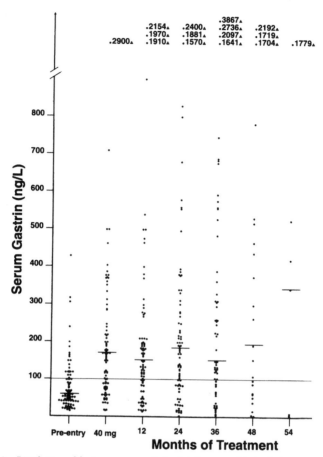

Fig 45–3.—Distribution of fasting serum gastrin levels (all measured individual values) during maintenance treatment with omeprazole. *Horizontal line* indicates normal values (less than 100 ng/L). 40 mg = acute treatment period. (Courtesy of Klinkenberg-Knol EC, Festen HPM, Jansen JBMJ, et al: *Ann Intern Med* 121:161–167, 1994.)

treated successfully with another 20-mg dose increment for a mean of 36 months (Fig 45–2). The median gastrin levels rose initially from 60 ng/L before the study to 162 ng/L with therapy, reaching a plateau during maintenance. Eleven percent of the patients had very high gastrin levels. The incidence of micronodular hyperplasia rose from 2.5% at the first biopsy to 20% at the final one. There was a corresponding progression of gastritis to subatrophic or atrophic gastritis from less than 1% to 25%, which was more marked in patients with very high serum gastrin concentrations (Fig 45–3).

Conclusion.—In this series of patients with gastroesophageal reflux resistant to treatment with H₂-receptor antagonists, omeprazole maintenance treatment was effective for at least 5 years. Treatment was associated with a persistent elevation in serum gastrin concentrations and in micronodular argyrophil cell hyperplasia and subatrophic or atrophic gastritis.

▶ This study provides valuable information on long-term therapy of reflux esophagitis with omeprazole. Note that approximately 30% of 91 patients required treatment with 40 mg of omeprazole daily. Median gastrin levels increased from 60 to 162 ng/mL with therapy, which is not surprising because omeprazole is a more potent inhibitor of gastric acid secretion than H_2-blockers, even when the latter are given in higher than conventional dosages. Ten of 91 (11%) patients developed marked hypergastrinemia with serum gastrin levels greater than 500 ng/mL. This compares with earlier reports documenting similar hypergastrinemia in 2 of 31 (6.5%) and 4 of 74 (5.4%) patients receiving long-term omeprazole cited by Klinkenberg-Knol. As Freston (1) points out in the editorial accompanying this article, the study by Klinkenberg-Knol et al. confirms previous reports of long-term studies that found hyperplasia of enterochromaffin-like cells *but no evidence* of dysplasia, carcinoid tumors, or other neoplastic changes.

For monitoring patients on long-term omeprazole, Freston (1) recommends measuring serum gastrin levels after 1 year of continuous therapy. If gastrin levels greater than 500 ng/L are recorded, it could reflect development of chronic atrophic gastritis and diminished acid secretion, and under these circumstances patients might not require omeprazole. Klinkenberg-Knol et al. point out that some of their patients with hypergastrinemia had food retention at endoscopy, suggesting delayed gastric emptying and antral distention, thus raising the interesting question of possible use of prokinetic drugs such as cisapride.

Finally, I call attention to a study by Kuster et al. (2), who have provided an interesting analysis of predictive factors for long-term outcome of 107 patients with gastroesophageal reflux disease (GERD) who were followed for 6 years. Long-term treatment need was defined as major if daily H_2-blockers or surgery was required. Three factors were independent predictors of major therapeutic needs: First, a decreased lower esophageal sphincter pressure; second, radiologic evidence of reflux; and finally, erosive esophagitis. The initial clinical scores reflecting severity of symptoms did not correlate with the clinical course or outcome.—N.J. Greenberger, M.D.

References

1. Freston JW: Omeprazole, hypergastrinemia and gastric carcinoid tumors. *Ann Intern Med* 121:232–233, 1994.
2. Kuster E, Pos E, Toledo-Pimentel V, et al: Predictive factors of the long-term outcome in gastroesophageal reflux disease: Six year follow-up of 107 patients. *Gut* 35:8–14, 1994.

Omeprazole Versus H₂-Receptor Antagonists in Treating Patients With Peptic Stricture and Esophagitis

Marks RD, Richter JE, Rizzo J, Koehler RE, Spenney JG, Mills TP, Champion G (Univ of Alabama, Birmingham; Yale Univ, New Haven, Conn)

Gastroenterology 106:907–915, 1994   119-95-45-3

Introduction.—Most patients with peptic stricture have coexistent reflux esophagitis. Nevertheless, the primary therapy for these patients with dysphagia is dilatation of the peptic stricture. It was hypothesized that healing the esophagitis may be an equally important treatment approach in relieving dysphagia. The efficacy of omeprazole and H₂-receptor antagonists (H₂RA) in healing esophagitis was compared and the impact of this healing on relieving dysphagia was assessed.

Methods.—A total of 34 dysphagic patients with both peptic stricture and esophagitis were assigned to 2 groups: those with moderate, grade 2 esophagitis or those with severe, grade 3 or 4 esophagitis. The patients in each group were then randomly assigned to receive either omeprazole or H₂RA. All the patients underwent serial dilatation at baseline and thereafter only when dysphagia occurred at least once a week or when requested by the patient. Esophagitis healing was assessed by upper gastrointestinal endoscopy at 3 and 6 months of treatment.

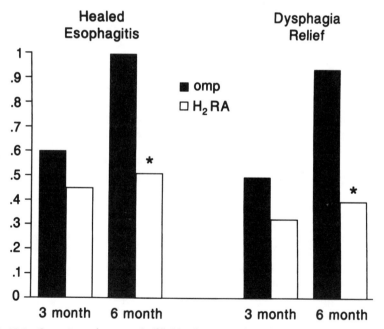

Fig 45–4.—Comparison of omeprazole (*filled bars*) vs. H₂RA (*open bars*). By 6 months, patients treated with omeprazole had significantly higher esophagitis healing rates and dysphagia relief rates (dysphagia scale) than patients treated with H₂RA. *Asterisk* indicates $P < 0.01$. (Courtesy of Marks RD, Richter JE, Rizzo J, et al: *Gastroenterology* 106:907–915, 1994.)

Results.—Patients with healed esophagitis had significantly more relief of dysphagia at 3 months (61%) and 6 months (88%) than did patients whose esophagitis was not healed (20% and 0%, respectively). Dilatation was required in all unhealed patients but in only 44% of the healed patients. Significantly more patients taking omeprazole than those taking H_2RA were healed at 3 months (61% vs. 47%) and at 6 months (100% vs. 53%). Similar differences were found in the numbers of patients experiencing relief of dysphagia (Fig 45-4). The therapeutic benefit of omeprazole was particularly strong among patients with more severe esophagitis. Fewer patients treated with omeprazole required dilatation, and those who did require dilatation needed fewer sessions. There was a lower cost burden for healing esophagitis using omeprazole than H_2RA.

Discussion.—These findings indicate than dysphagia relief is associated with healing esophagitis in patients with peptic stricture. Omeprazole was superior to H_2RA in healing esophagitis, relieving dysphagia, and decreasing the need for stricture dilatation and was more cost-effective.

▶ This study found that medical healing of coexistent esophagitis in patients with peptic stricture decreased dysphagia and, in addition, decreased the need for stricture dilatation over a 6-month period. Further, omeprazole was superior to H_2-blockers in relieving dysphagia and decreasing dilatation requirement, presumably because it was more effective in healing coexistent esophagitis.—N.J. Greenberger, M.D.

A Guide for Surveillance of Patients With Barrett's Esophagus
Provenzale D, Kemp JA, Arora S, Wong JB (Tufts Univ, Boston)
Am J Gastroenterol 89:670–680, 1994   119-95-45–4

Background.—Barrett's esophagus, or columnar metaplasia of the distal esophagus caused by chronic gastroesophageal reflux, is found in up to 20% of patients undergoing endoscopy for gastroesophageal reflux. These patients have an increased risk of esophageal adenocarcinoma—30 to 125 times higher than the general population. It has been recommended that patients with confirmed Barrett's esophagus should have periodic endoscopic surveillance with biopsy. However, there has been little research into whether the morbidity of endoscopy and the cost of such surveillance—nearly $350 million yearly, based on an estimated 700,000 affected patients—are justified. Decision analysis methods were used to examine the effectiveness and cost-effectiveness of endoscopic surveillance in patients with Barrett's esophagus.

Methods.—A Markov model was used to examine the effects of 12 different strategies in a computer cohort simulation of 10,000 men with Barrett's esophagus. The strategies ranged from no surveillance with esophagectomy performed only if cancer was detected to yearly surveillance with esophagectomy performed for high-grade dysplasia. Parame-

Results of Procedures for 10,000 Patients

Strategy	Cumulative Incidence of Cancer (%)	Remaining Life Expectancy*	Quality-Adjusted Life Expectancy	No. of Endoscopies	No. of Endoscopic Complications	Surgeries
No surveillance:						
A: Esophagectomy for cancer	27.48	20.63	20.47	48,100	63	2,300
B: Esophagectomy for high grade dysplasia	24.23	20.93	20.64	34,600	45	2,600
Endoscopic surveillance—esophagectomy for cancer						
C_5: Surveillance every 5 yr	18.11	21.62	21.04	200,900	260	3,000
C_4: Surveillance every 4 yr	17.34	21.72	21.08	223,200	290	3,100
C_3: Surveillance every 3 yr	16.59	21.82	21.12	253,500	330	3,200
C_2: Surveillance every 2 yr	15.92	21.92	21.15	296,200	390	3,300
C_1: Surveillance every 1 yr	15.37	22.01	21.15	360,000	470	3,500
Endoscopic surveillance—esophagectomy for high grade dysplasia‡						
D_5: Surveillance every 5 yr	7.33	22.65	21.60	149,600	200	4,000
D_4: Surveillance every 4 yr	6.00	22.78	21.64	167,800	220	4,200
D_3: Surveillance every 3 yr	4.73	22.90	21.67	192,800	250	4,400
D_2: Surveillance every 2 yr	3.67	23.01	21.67	228,700	300	4,600
D_1: Surveillance every 1 yr	2.96	23.06	21.59	283,400	370	4,800

* Average remaining life expectancy for a healthy 55-year-old man is 24.5 years.

‡ Strategies with esophagectomy for high-grade dysplasia result in fewer endoscopic complications and surgeries than those with esophagectomy for cancer. Over time, more patients in the former strategies undergo esophagectomy, and therefore, these patients do not undergo further endoscopies or have further endoscopic complications, resulting in fewer procedures and complications overall in these strategies.

(Courtesy of Provenzale D, Kemp JA, Arora S, et al: Am J Gastroenterol 89:670–680, 1994.)

ters for the analysis were taken from published reports, if available, or from experts in the field.

Results.—Aggressive surveillance significantly reduced the incidence of cancer and increased life expectancy and quality-adjusted life expectancy. On average, patients had to undergo 4–10 times more endoscopies than patients with no surveillance to realize this benefit. Endoscopic complications were similarly increased, and the lifetime number of surgeries was doubled. Despite the marked reduction in cancer, life expectancy gains were modest; this was because of the low overall risk of cancer, surgical risk, and morbidity related to endoscopy and esophagectomy (table).

From the standpoint of life expectancy, yearly surveillance with surgery for high-grade dysplasia was the optimal method. However, after adjustment for morbidity and quality of life, surveillance every 2 or 3 years was preferred. Performing endoscopy every 5 years yielded a smaller increase in life expectancy but an incremental cost-effectiveness ratio similar to that of common medical practices.

Conclusion.—In deciding on the optimal surveillance strategy for patients with Barrett's esophagus, the most important factors are the cumulative incidence of cancer and the quality of life after esophagectomy. At a cancer incidence of 1%, surveillance every 4 years will maximize quality-adjusted survival for patients who accept quality-of-life adjustments. If the cancer incidence is 2%, surveillance every 2 years is optimal; if cancer risk is higher than 2%, yearly surveillance is optimal.

▶ I would like to restate the authors' analysis, which suggests that:

- Annual endoscopic surveillance yields the greatest life expectancy but is associated with a lower quality-adjusted life expectancy.
- Endoscopy every 2–3 years yields the greatest quality-adjusted life expectancy but is expensive.

Two recent studies have implicated a mutation of the tumor suppressor gene *p53* in the progression of Barrett's epithelium to invasive esophageal carcinoma (1). While it is well established that adenocarcinoma in Barrett's esophagus is often preceded by mucosal dysplasia, understanding of this dysplasia/carcinoma sequence remains incompletely defined. Harmack et al. (2) studied the participation of *p53* mutations in 30 patients with Barrett's esophagus and adenocarcinoma. Sixteen (53%) of the tumors overexpressed *p53*, 10 of which had adjacent dysplastic Barrett's mucosa; in all 10 patients this dysplastic mucosa also overexpressed *p53*. This occurred predominantly in areas of high-grade vs. low-grade dysplasia. Importantly, none of the dysplastic mucosa adjacent to 11 tumors lacking *p53* overexpression showed detectable values of *p53*.

Casson et al. (1) studied 20 patients with Barrett's esophagus, 10 of whom had an associated adenocarcinoma. *p53* gene mutations were detected in 7 of 10 patients with primary esophageal adenocarcinoma and in 6 patients with associated Barrett's epithelium, 3 of whom had high-grade dysplasia. Of

10 patients with Barrett's epithelium alone, 6 had *p53* mutations with mild or no dysplasia histologically.

Further prospective studies of p53 mutations in patients with Barrett's esophagus may facilitate identification of the patients at highest risk for developing malignancy.—N.J. Greenberger, M.D.

References

1. Casson AG, Manoloupolos B, Traster H: Clinical implications of p53 gene mutation in the progression of Barrett's epithelium to invasive esophageal cancer. *Am J Surg* 167:52–57, 1994.
2. Harmack RH, Shephert NA, Moorghen H, et al: Adenocarcinoma rising in Barrett's esophagus: Evidence for the participation of p53 dysfunction in the dysplasia/carcinoma sequence. *Gut* 35:764–768, 1994.

46 Stomach and Duodenum

Empirical H₂-Blocker Therapy or Prompt Endoscopy in Management of Dyspepsia

Bytzer P, Hansen JM, Schaffalitzky de Muckadell OB (Odense Univ, Denmark)

Lancet 343:811–816, 1994   119-95-46–1

Background.—The recommended treatment for patients with dyspepsia is H₂-blocking agents on an empirical basis followed by endoscopy if the symptoms are unresponsive or recurrent. The impact on diagnosis,

TABLE 1.—Clinical and Demographic Characteristics of Patients Assigned Prompt Endoscopy or Empirical H₂-Blocker Treatment

	Group 1 (n = 208)	Group 2 (n = 206)
Demographic details		
Age (yr)*	44·9 (17·0)	43·6 (16·0)
M/F	87/121	89/117
History		
History of dyspepsia (yr)*	8·9 (12·6)	7·6 (11·2)
Length of present episode (mo)*	4·1 (6·1)	5·0 (8·6)
Sick-leave days preceding month†	0 (0–2)	0 (0–3)
Percentage of patients:		
Smoker	58	52
Previous H₂-blocker therapy	16	20
Family history of ulcer	31	31
Epigastric pain	86	92
Heartburn	63	71
Night pain	48	57
Vomiting	32	33
Overall assessment of dyspepsia (%):		
No/minimal influence‡	1	4
Minor influence‡	43	38
Moderate influence‡	48	46
Debilitating symptoms	8	12
Quality of life§	10·0 (10·2)	10·0 (9·9)

* Mean standard deviation.
† Median interquartile range.
‡ Effect on lifestyle.
§ Percent of total possible dysfunction.
(Courtesy of Bytzer P, Hansen JM, Schaffalitzky de Muckadell OB: *Lancet* 343:811-816, 1994.)

TABLE 2.—Outcome After 1 Year for Per-Protocol Patients

	Group 1 (n = 187)	Group 2 (n = 186)
Overall assessment of dyspepsia (%)		
No symptoms	40	41
Symptoms improved	33	32
Symptoms unchanged	21	23
Symptoms worse	6	4
% of patients with:		
Epigastric pain	43	49
Heartburn	39	42
Vomiting	10	10
Quality of life*	5.3 (8.5)	4.8 (6.9)
Satisfaction with medical care (%)		
Very satisfied	46	18
Satisfied	48	35
Dissatisfied	6	44
Very dissatisfied	0	3

* Percent total possible dysfunction.
(Courtesy Bytzer P, Hansen JM, Schaffalitzky de Muckadell OB: *Lancet* 343: 811–816, 1994.)

dyspeptic symptoms, quality of life, patient satisfaction, and health care costs associated with empirical H_2-blocker treatment were compared with those of prompt endoscopy before drug treatment.

Methods.—The patients included in the study were those who would normally receive empirical therapy from the general practitioner (Table 1). Four hundred fourteen patients were randomized. Group 1 patients received prompt endoscopy, and group 2 patients received empirical therapy with ranitidine, 150 mg twice a day for 4 weeks. Three hundred seventy-three completed the 1-year follow-up.

Findings.—Thirty-three percent of the patients in group 1 had a lesion, identified on endoscopy, that could explain dyspeptic symptoms (Table 2). Peptic ulcer was the most common lesion. Sixty-six percent of the patients in group 2 had endoscopy during the study period. Group 2 patients undergoing endoscopy reported significantly fewer days without symptoms per week than patients who did not have endoscopy. Fifty-seven more endoscopies were performed in group 1 than in group 2. The empirical treatment strategy was costlier, primarily because of the greater number of sick-leave days and the cost of ulcer drug use.

Conclusion.—Prompt endoscopy is a cost-effective approach in patients with dyspeptic symptoms severe enough to warrant the current strategy of empirical H_2-blocker therapy. Prompt endoscopy is recommended only for patients with dyspepsia of unknown cause.

▶ It has been traditional to manage patients with recent onset of dyspepsia by empirically prescribing H_2-blockers if a patient did not have "alert" or "alarm" features. If "alert" findings such as a history of weight loss, nausea, emesis, early satiety, family history of duodenal ulcer disease, abnormal physical findings, hemoccult-positive stools, or anemia were present, then endoscopy was clearly indicated. This approach was endorsed by the American College of Physicians (1) and is widely practiced today.

The controlled trial by Bytzer et al. questions the efficacy of this policy. Bytzer found that the empirical treatment strategy was associated with higher costs (mostly related to drug costs and sick-leave days) and lower patient satisfaction than the strategy of prompt endoscopy before treatment. Talley (2) has succinctly summarized the advantages of early investigation. Therapy can be targeted to peptic ulcer disease and eradication of *Helicobacter pylori*, NSAID-induced lesions, gastroesophageal reflux disease, non-ulcer dyspepsia, and gastric cancer. With regard to cost-effectiveness, it should also be noted that in several countries, the cost of 2 months of H_2-blocker therapy exceeds the cost of esophagogastroduodenoscopy.—N.J. Greenberger, M.D.

References

1. Health and Public Policy Committee: The American College of Physicians. *Ann Intern Med* 102:265–269, 1985.
2. Talley NJ: Commentary. ACP Journal Club. *Ann Intern Med* 121 (suppl 2):31, 1994.

Helicobacter Pylori Infection and the Risk for Duodenal and Gastric Ulceration

Nomura A, Stemmermann GN, Chyou P-H, Perez-Perez GI, Blaser MJ (Kuakini Med Ctr, Honolulu, Hawaii; Univ of Cincinnati, Ohio; Vanderbilt Univ, Nashville, Tenn)
Ann Intern Med 120:977–981, 1994   119-95-46-2

Background.—It seems likely that infection by *Helicobacter pylori* increases the risk of duodenal and gastric ulcer disease. Infection has been found in up to 100% of duodenal ulcer and 86% of gastric ulcer patients, and its eradication correlates with significantly fewer recurrences of duodenal ulceration. These findings may, however, merely reflect the frequent association of antral gastritis that is caused by the same organism.

Study Plan.—A case-control study was planned, using as a population base 5,443 Japanese-American men living in Hawaii who were examined and had a phlebotomy in the period 1967–1970. After a hospital surveillance period longer than 20 years, 150 patients with gastric ulcers and 65 with duodenal ulcers were identified. Stored sera from these patients and from age-matched control subjects were examined for IgG antibody against *H. pylori* using an enzyme-linked immunosorbent assay.

Findings. —A significant titer of specific antibody was found in 93% of patients with gastric ulcers and 78% of the matched control subjects, for an odds ratio of 3.2. Antibody was found in 92% of case patients with duodenal ulcers and 78% of controls, for an odds ratio of 4. When comparing patients with the highest antibody titers with those who were antibody-negative, an odds ratio of 6.8 was found. The association remained significant for both types of ulcer disease, even when diagnosed 10 years or longer after serum sampling.

Discussion. —Preexisting infection by *H. pylori* increases the risk of ulcer disease. It is estimated that 44% of the total risk of hospitalization with gastric or duodenal ulcers can be ascribed to previous *H. pylori* infection. Duodenal ulcer disease may reflect a synergy between infection by *H. pylori* and the presence of gastric metaplasia in the duodenum.

▶ This paper by Nomura et al. is important for 2 reasons. First, they demonstrate that both duodenal and gastric ulcers are causally related to this infection. Secondly, they document a correlation between the level of antibody response to the bacterium and the likelihood of an ulcer developing. Some additional important questions are raised.

The primary questions are: *When and how is* H. pylori *infection acquired?* Webb et al. (1) related the prevalence of infection with *H. pylori* in 47 adults aged 18–65 years to their living conditions in childhood, in order to identify risk factors for infection. Seroprevalence of *H. pylori* increased with age (29% at less than 30 years to 63% at 55–65 years). After appropriate adjustments, subjects from large families whose childhood homes were crowded or who regularly shared a bed in childhood were significantly more likely to be seropositive. The authors conclude that close person-to-person contact in childhood is an important determinant of seropositivity for *H. pylori* in adulthood. Further support for familial clustering of *H. pylori* infections derives from the work of Malaty et al. (2) These investigations showed that for infected patients with gastritis, 68% of their spouses also had the infection, whereas for normal control index cases, *H. pylori* infection was present in the spouse only 9% of the time. The report by Cullen et al. (3) suggests that *H. pylori* infection is predominantly acquired at a younger age. Of 86 subjects who were seronegative in 1969, only 6 (7%) were seropositive in 1990, suggesting that *H. pylori* infection is infrequently acquired during adult life.

Once a person is infected with H. pylori, *what determines whether an individual will develop a duodenal ulcer?* The answer may lie in strain differences in the organism. Crabtree et al. (4) demonstrated that strains of *H. pylori* that elaborate a 120-kDa protein have pathogenic characteristics that are associated with active gastritis and peptic ulceration. Crabtree suggests that patients in whom peptic ulceration does not develop may be infected with 120-KDa negative strain of *H. pylori*. Another possibility is that the genetic makeup of the host may determine which infection with *H. pylori* results in peptic ulceration.—N.J. Greenberger, M.D.

References

1. Webb PM, Knight T, Greaves S, et al: Relation between infection with *H. pylori* and living condition in childhood: Evidence for person to person transmission in early life. *B M J* 308:750–753, 1994.
2. Malaty HM, Graham DY, Klein PD, et al: Transmission of *Helicobacter pylori* infection: Studies in families of healthy individuals. *Scand J Gastroenterol* 26:927–932, 1991.
3. Cullen DJE, Cullen BJ, Christiansen KJ, et al: When is *Helicobacter pylori* infection acquired? *Gut* 34:1681–1682, 1993.
4. Crabtree JE, Taylor VD, Wyatt I, et al: Mucosal IgA recognition of *Helicobacter pylori* 120 kDa protein, peptic ulceration and gastric pathology. *Lancet* 338:332–335, 1991.

Duodenal Ulcer Treated With *Helicobacter pylori* Eradication: Seven-Year Follow-Up

Forbes GM, Glaser ME, Cullen DJE, Warren JR, Christiansen KJ, Marshall BJ, Collins BJ (Royal Perth Hosp, Western Australia, Australia; Univ of Virginia, Charlottesville)
Lancet 343:258–260, 1994   119-95-46-3

Introduction.—The reduction of recurrence of duodenal ulcer resulting from *Helicobacter pylori* eradication treatment (HET) is well documented, but most of the follow-up has been for ≤ 2 years. The long-term effect of HET was examined in a cohort of patients who participated in the first controlled trial of HET.

Methods.—Sixty-three of the original 100 patients from the trial conducted from 1985 to 1986 were available and agreeable to follow-up. Records of care rendered for complaints consistent with duodenal ulcer were reviewed. Patients were interviewed and upper gastrointestinal en-

Incidence of Duodenal Ulcer Relapse Compared With *H. pylori* Status at Time of Relapse

H pylori status	Current DU relapse	Proven DU relapse	Clinical DU relapse
H p+	5 (n=25)	9 (n=26)	11 (n=26)
H p–	1 (n=38)	3 (n=37)	8 (n=37)
p	<0.05	<0.01	<0.1

Abbreviations: H p+ and –, *H. pylori* positive and negative; DU, duodenal ulcer.
One patient currently H p– had proven DU relapse accompanied by persistence of *H. pylori* 4–8 years after the initial study; hence, he was H p+ in the proven and clinical groups for statistical analysis. *n* is the number with specified *H. pylori* status.
(Courtesy of Forbes GM, Glaser ME, Cullen DJE, et al: *Lancet* 343:258–260, 1994.)

doscopy and 3 gastric antral biopsies were done by a blinded gastroen-terologist. Relapse of duodenal ulcer was classified as current-active at endoscopy; proven-demonstrated by endoscopy or barium meal since the original study and before this study; or clinical-patient reports of symptoms identical to those that led to the original diagnosis of duode-nal ulcer whether confirmed by examination or not.

Results. The mean period from the original study to the present study was 6.5 years. At completion of the original study, 28 patients were *H. pylori*–positive and 35 were negative. At the new examination, 5 of the positive patients tested negative because of interim HET. Of the 35 pa-tients known to be negative from the prior study, 32 remained negative, and 1 more had a relapse and was *H. pylori*–positive but underwent ad-ditional HET and became negative again. The other 2 were found to be positive at this examination (table). At follow-up endoscopy for the new study, 20% of currently *H. pylori*–positive patients were found to have active duodenal ulcers compared with 3% of the negative group. Proven relapse had occurred in significantly more *H. pylori*–positive than *H. pylori*–negative patients (35% vs. 8%). Clinical relapse was noted by 42% of positive and 22% of negative patients. During the interim years, 3 pa-tients received H_2-receptor antagonists, 6 received further HET, and 3 who reported clinical duodenal ulcer relapse had been receiving nonste-roidal anti-inflammatory drugs.

Discussion.—Other studies have shown, in small numbers of patients undergoing serial endoscopy, that reinfection is uncommon for up to 4 years after HET. These data reveal an annual reinfection rate of 1.2%. As found in shorter term studies, no spontaneous loss of *H. pylori* was identified. Of the 37 patients from the original study who could not be reevaluated, 21 tested negative—similarly proportionate to the group that was studied. The reports of duodenal ulcer relapse may be underes-timated because of silent duodenal ulcer disease. In spite of these criti-cisms, HET is an alternative that may reduce costs and be used more fre-quently as HET regimens are refined.

▶ This study clearly demonstrates that the recurrence of duodenal ulcer-ation after eradication of *H. pylori* is markedly reduced, and freedom from relapse extends to at least 7 years after treatment. In 27 duodenal ulcer stud-ies involving 1,881 patients, the annual relapse rate was 58% (571/988) in *H. pylori*–positive patients compared to 2.6% (23/893) in *H. pylori*–negative patients (1). Furthermore, most ulcers in the latter category occurred in pa-tients taking NSAIDs.

Tytgat (1) also cited various factors that have been studied in relation to *H. pylori* eradication. Compliance is an obvious factor. The antibiotic efficacy is also reduced in smokers vs. nonsmokers. Acquired resistance to metronida-zole may be significantly associated with smoking.

Tytgat (1) has also summarized the efficacy of various treatment regimens in several studies comprising over 2,000 patients. The key findings are as follows:

Regimen	*H. pylori* eradication rate
Bismuth–tetracycline–metronidazole	95%
Amoxicillin–omeprazole	70% to 85%
Amoxicillin–omeprazole–metronidazole	90%

The simplest effective regimen in terms of patient compliance is the combination of omeprazole, 20 mg b.i.d., and amoxicillin, 1 g b.i.d. If patients do not clear their *H. pylori* infections with this regimen, the standard bismuth–metronidazole–tetracycline regimen can be tried. Alternative regimens include omeprazole plus clarithromycin with or without metronidazole.

To summarize briefly, over 90% of patients with duodenal ulcer disease have *H. pylori* infection, and eradication of the infection will reduce the relapse rate to approximately 2% per year.—N.J. Greenberger, M.D.

Reference

1. Tytgat GNJ: Review article: Treatments that impact favourably upon the eradication of *Helicobacter pylori* and ulcer recurrence. *Adv Pharmacol Ther* 8:359–368, 1994.

Duodenal Ulcer Healing by Eradication of *Helicobacter pylori* Without Anti-Acid Treatment: Randomised Controlled Trial
Hosking SW, Ling TKW, Chung SCS, Yung MY, Cheng AFB, Sung JJY, Li AKC (Chinese Univ, Hong Kong, Shatin)
Lancet 343:508–510, 1994   119-95-46–4

Background.—In patients with duodenal ulcers who are treated with H_2-blockers, healing occurs faster if *Helicobacter pylori* is eradicated concurrently. This raises the question of whether eradication of *H. pylori* alone—without suppression of acid secretion—is sufficient to allow ulcer healing.

Endoscopic and Biopsy Results at Completion of Trial		
	Omeprazole, bismuth, tetracycline, and metronidazole	**Bismuth, tetracycline, and metronidazole**
Duodenal ulcer		
Healed	63	60
Unhealed (*H pylori* positive)	4 (0)	5 (1)
H pylori		
Eradicated	66	61
Not eradicated	1	4

(Courtesy of Hosking SW, Ling TKW, Chung SCS, et al: *Lancet* 343:508–510, 1994.)

Methods.—The subjects were 153 patients with *H. pylori* infection and duodenal ulcers. One group received 1 week of treatment 4 times a day with bismuth subcitrate, 120 mg; tetracycline, 500 mg; and metronidazole, 400 mg. The other group received omeprazole, 20 mg/day for 4 weeks, in addition to 1 week of treatment with the 3-drug regimen. At baseline and 4 weeks after treatment, the patients underwent endoscopy and antral biopsy.

Results.—One hundred thirty-two patients were evaluable. Ninety-two percent of those receiving just the 3-drug regimen had healing of their duodenal ulcers, as did 95% of those receiving omeprazole as well. Eradication of *H. pylori* was achieved in 94% of those receiving only the 3-drug regimen and in 98% of those receiving omeprazole as well (table). The omeprazole group obtained more effective symptom alleviation during the first week of treatment.

Conclusion.—For most patients with duodenal ulcers, 1 week of treatment with bismuth, tetracycline, and metronidazole can effectively eradicate *H. pylori* and heal the ulcer. Although concurrent omeprazole can lead to more rapid reduction of ulcer pain, it has no effect on ulcer healing. As long as *H. pylori* is eradicated, duodenal ulcers associated with this organism will heal without acid suppression.

▶ A similar study was carried out by Logan et al. (1). Forty-five patients with duodenal ulcers and *H. pylori* infection were treated for 7 days with a triple-drug regimen consisting of tripotassium dicitrate bismuthate (120 mg q.i.d.), amoxicillin (500 mg q.i.d.), and metronidazole, 400 mg 5 times/day on days 5–7. At the second endoscopy done at a median interval of 20 days from the start of treatment, 33 of 44 (75%) duodenal ulcers had healed. Ten of the remaining 11 duodenal ulcers were smaller, and those 10 healed within the next 2 weeks with no further treatment.

Both this study, as well as the study by Hoskins in which eradication of *H. pylori* without antiacid treatment resulted in healing of duodenal ulcers, provide further support for a causal role of *H. pylori* in the pathogenesis of duodenal ulcer. However, treatment of duodenal ulcer with antibiotics alone is not recommended for several reasons, most notably because the eradication of *H. pylori* with such a regimen is only 60% to 65%. The failure to eradicate *H. pylori* is associated with an increased likelihood of duodenal ulcer relapse. Current recommendations call for treatment with both antisecretory and antimicrobial agents in either a 2-drug or 3-drug regimen.—N.J. Greenberger, M.D.

Reference

1. Logan RPH, Grummett PA, Misrenica JJ, et al: One week's anti-*Helicobacter pylori* treatment for duodenal ulcer. *Gut* 38:15–18, 1994.

Helicobacter pylori in **Peptic Ulcer Disease**
Hall WH, for the NIH Consensus Development Panel on *Helicobacter pylori* in Peptic Ulcer Disease (National Insts of Health, Bethesda, Md)
JAMA 272:65–69, 1994   119-95-46–5

Background.—Peptic ulcer disease affects as much as 10% of the United States population and results in much human suffering and high economic cost. Despite the use of therapeutic agents, peptic ulcer disease has a high rate of recurrence, even after complete healing. Specialists were brought together from gastroenterology, surgery, infectious diseases, epidemiology, and pathology to address questions that included the following: (1) What is the causal relationship of *Helicobacter pylori* to upper gastrointestinal disease? (2) How is *H. pylori* infection diagnosed and eradicated? and (3) Are patients with peptic ulcer disease benefited by eradicating *H. pylori* infection?

Discussion.—There is a well-established causal relationship between *H. pylori* and chronic superficial gastritis. The strongest evidence for the pathogenic role of *H. pylori* in peptic ulcer disease is the decrease in recurrence of ulcers after the infection is eradicated. There is no convincing evidence of an association of *H. pylori* infection with nonulcerative dyspepsia. In patients with nonulcerative dyspepsia, the incidence of *H. pylori* is no higher than in the general population.

Of invasive diagnostic tests, the sensitivity and specificity of histologic demonstration of *H. pylori* by Giemsa or Warthin-Starry stains and urease testing are greater than 90%. Noninvasive tests also have excellent sensitivity and specificity (greater than 95%), and include serologic tests for IgG antibodies to *H. pylori* antigens and breath tests of urease activity which use urea labeled with carbon 14 or carbon 13. In patients who have recently taken antibiotics, bismuth compounds, or omeprazole, all the tests may be falsely negative, except for the serologic assays. There is no accurate method of monitoring the eradication of *H. pylori* that is also readily available, inexpensive, and noninvasive. Therapy consisting of bismuth subsalicylate, tetracycline, and metronidazole can result in eradication rates of about 90%. If the combination of omeprazole and amoxicillin is given, omeprazole should be given at least twice per day, and both drugs should be started at the same time because immediate pretreatment with omeprazole lowers the efficacy of the combination of the 2 drugs. Regimens with 2 or 3 drugs should last 2 weeks.

In patients with peptic ulcers, the principal benefit of eradicating *H. pylori* infection is a substantial reduction in the risk of ulcer recurrence. More definitive data are needed to evaluate whether eradicating *H. pylori* prevents future problems in patients with peptic ulcer and a history of bleeding or other complications.

Conclusion.—Treatment with antimicrobial agents and antisecretory drugs is required for patients with peptic ulcer with *H. pylori* infection.

The value of treatment of patients with nonulcerative dyspepsia and *H. pylori* infection has not been determined.

▶ The primary recommendations from the National Institutes of Health consensus conference on *H. pylori* and peptic ulcer disease can be summarized as follows:

- Ulcer patients with *H. pylori* infection require treatment with antimicrobial agents in addition to antisecretory drugs, whether on first presentation or with recurrence. Either 2-drug or 3-drug regimens should be followed for 2 weeks. Multiple agents have been studied in various combinations. Omeprazole plus amoxicillin or bismuth, metronidazole and tetracycline or omeprazole plus ranitidine are 2 frequently used regimens.

- The value of treatment of patients with nonulcer dyspepsia remains to be determined. One problem here relates to different types of dyspepsia, i.e., gastroesophageal reflux type dyspepsia, dysmotility type dyspepsia, and nonulcer dyspepsia. More detailed studies on the effect of eradicating *H. pylori* in the latter group of patients are clearly needed.

- Prophylactic antimicrobial therapy is not indicated in asymptomatic *H. pylori*–infected patients. Approximately 80% to 90% of such patients will not have evidence of peptic ulceration.—N.J. Greenberger, M.D.

Helicobacter pylori Infection and Gastric Lymphoma

Parsonnet J, Hansen S, Rodriguez L, Gelb AB, Warnke RA, Jellum E, Orentreich N, Vogelman JH, Friedman GD (Stanford Univ, Calif; Cancer Registry of Norway, Oslo; Norwegian Cancer Society, Oslo; et al)
N Engl J Med 330:1267–1271, 1994   119-95-46–6

Background.—Circumstantial evidence suggests that *Helicobacter pylori* infection may increase the risk of gastric non-Hodgkin's lymphoma. A nested case-control study was done to further explore this possibility.

Methods.—Two large cohorts of a total of 230,593 participants were included. Thirty-three patients with gastric non-Hodgkin's lymphoma were matched with 4 controls each on the basis of cohort, age, sex, and date of serum collection. In addition, 31 patients with nongastric non-Hodgkin's lymphoma from 1 of the cohorts, each of whom had been previously matched to 2 control subjects, were assessed for comparison. Serum samples from all persons were assessed for *H. pylori* IgG using an enzyme-linked immunosorbent assay.

Findings.—By a median of 14 years after serum collection, 33 cases of gastric non-Hodgkin's lymphoma had occurred. Patients with gastric lymphoma were significantly more likely than matched control subjects to have signs of previous *H. pylori* infection. Findings in the 2 cohorts were similar. In the group with nongastric lymphoma, a median of 6 years elapsed between serum collection and development of disease.

Odds Ratios and 95% Confidence Intervals for the Association of *H. pylori* Infection with Gastric Non-Hodgkin's Lymphoma and Nongastric Non-Hodgkin's Lymphoma

TYPE OF LYMPHOMA	NO. OF PATIENTS	*H. PYLORI* INFECTION*		MATCHED ODDS RATIO	95% CONFIDENCE INTERVAL
		PATIENTS	CONTROLS		
		% infected			
Gastric	33	85	55	6.3	2.0–19.9
Nongastric	31	65	59	1.2	0.5–3.0

* Infection status was determined by serum enzyme-linked immunosorbent assay.
(Courtesy of Parsonnet J, Hansen S, Rodriguez L, et al: N Engl J Med 330:1267-1271, 1994.)

Nongastric non-Hodgkin's lymphoma was unassociated with previous *H. pylori* infection (table).

Conclusion.—Non-Hodgkin's lymphoma of the stomach but not other sites is associated with previous infection with *H. pylori*. Although a causative role for this infection is possible, it has yet to be proven.

▶ Mucosa-associated lymphoid transformation (MALT) lymphomas are B-cell lymphomas that arise from lymphoid aggregates in the lamina propria. A recent study (1) provides evidence that *H. pylori* is an important pathogenetic factor in this subgroup of gastric lymphomas. In the report by Wotherspoon, et al. (1), MALT lymphomas regressed completely in 5 of 6 patients in response to eradication of the *H. pylori* infection. This report by Parsonnet and colleagues indicates that non-Hodgkin's lymphoma affecting the stomach, but not other sites, is associated with previous *H. pylori* infection. However, Parsonnet et al. are more circumspect in ascribing a causative role for *H. pylori*. Nonetheless, it seems reasonable as a first step in treatment to eradicate *H. pylori* in patients with MALT gastric lymphomas and concurrent *H. pylori* infection.—N.J. Greenberger, M.D.

Reference

1. Wotherspoon AC, Doglioni C, Diss TC, et al: Regression of primary low-grade B-cell gastric lymphoma of mucosa-associated lymphoid tissue after eradication of *Helicobacter pylori*. Lancet 342:575–577, 1993.

A Controlled Study of Ranitidine for the Prevention of Recurrent Hemorrhage From Duodenal Ulcer

Jensen DM, Cheng S, Kovacs TOG, Randall G, Jensen ME, Reedy T, Frankl H, Machicado G, Smith J, Silpa M, Van Deventer G (Univ of California, Los Angeles; Kaiser Permanente, Los Angeles; Valley Med Ctr, Van Nuys, Calif; et al)

N Engl J Med 330:382–386, 1994   119-95-46-7

Introduction.—Despite the fact that bleeding is the most common complication of duodenal ulcer, few controlled trials of maintenance treatment have been conducted in patients with documented hemorrhage. There are, in fact, no randomized, controlled, double-blind studies documenting a significant reduction in complications as a result of medical treatment. Nevertheless, several uncontrolled studies do indicate that maintenance treatment can lower the risk of recurrent bleeding.

Study Design.—A double-blind, placebo-controlled study of maintenance ranitidine therapy was carried out in 65 adults having endoscopically confirmed bleeding from a duodenal ulcer. All had been hospitalized because of upper gastrointestinal bleeding and had either a 5% drop in hematocrit or had been transfused. Most patients were entered in the study about 3 months after the index bleeding episode. The patients were randomized to receive either 150 mg of ranitidine or placebo at

Outcome According to Treatment Group

Outcome	Placebo Group (N = 33)	Ranitidine Group (N = 32)
	no. of patients (%)	
Recurrence of bleeding ulcer	12 (36)	3 (9)*
Recurrence without bleeding	11 (33)	6 (19)
Symptomatic	7 (21)	4 (12)
Asymptomatic†	4 (12)	2 (6)
Other treatment failure	0	2 (6)‡
Dropped out	9 (27)	6 (19)
Medical reason	1 (3)§	2 (6)¶
Adverse event	0	1 (3)‖
Noncompliance or refusal	7 (21)	3 (9)
Moved	1 (3)	0

* $P < 0.05$ for the comparison with the placebo group.

† Determined on endoscopy performed at exit from the study.

‡ One patient was withdrawn after 3 symptomatic recurrences without bleeding, and 1 was withdrawn because a symptomatic ulcer had not healed after 8 weeks of treatment.

§ One patient was withdrawn when endoscopy for a symptomatic ulcer revealed a nonbleeding visible vessel.

¶ One patient was withdrawn after a spider bite followed by a cerebrovascular accident, and 1 patient was withdrawn after a myocardial infarction.

‖ One patient was withdrawn because of moderate thrombocytopenia that developed in the first month of coded treatment.

(Courtesy of Jensen DM, Cheng S, Kovacs TOG, et al: N Engl J Med 330:382–386, 1994.)

night and were followed for up to 3 years. Endoscopy was repeated at the end of the study or when symptoms persisted and did not respond to antacids.

Results.—During a mean follow-up of 61 weeks, 3 of 32 ranitidine-treated patients and 12 of 33 placebo recipients had recurrent bleeding. Half of the recurrent episodes were unaccompanied by symptoms (table). One patient who received ranitidine withdrew because of asymptomatic thrombocytopenia which developed in the first month of treatment.

Implications.—Patients with duodenal ulcers who have bled in the past are at risk of recurrent bleeding when not receiving maintenance treatment. If these patients were treated, a substantial reduction in hospital costs could be expected.

▶ This study demonstrates that long-term maintenance therapy with ranitidine is safe and reduces the risk of recurrent bleeding in patients initially seen with an endoscopically documented hemorrhage from a duodenal ulcer. However, some important information is not available in this study. It would be of considerable interest to know the *H. pylori* status of all the patients in both the placebo and ranitidine treatment groups. It is tempting to speculate that ulcer recurrence both with and without bleeding recurred in *H. pylori*–positive patients. That this seems likely derives from a recent presentation (1) in which Tytgat reviewed 4 recent studies relating *H. pylori* status to recurrent bleeding from duodenal ulcer with reference to the role of H₂ receptor blockers given alone or in conjunction with a regimen to eradicate *H. pylori.* Long-term treatment after ranitidine alone resulted in a 50% reduction in recurrent bleeding from a duodenal ulcer, findings not dissimilar to those reported by Jensen et al. However, no patients in whom *H. pylori* was eradicated had recurrent ulceration with bleeding. However, it should be noted that the duration of follow-up in an indeterminate number of these patients did not approach 3 years. Pending a longer follow-up and the full-length publication of the data, it does seem appropriate to determine *H. pylori* status in patients with bleeding duodenal ulcer and attempt to eradicate *H. pylori* in the approximately 75% of such patients with bleeding ulcers who will be *H. pylori*–positive. It may well be possible to avoid the expense of long-term H₂ blocker therapy in this subset of patients.—N.J. Greenberger, M.D.

Reference

1. Tytgat G: State of the art lecture. *Helicobacter pylori:* How to treat. Third United European Gastroenterology Week, Oslo, June 28, 1994.

Risk Factors for Gastrointestinal Bleeding in Critically Ill Patients

Cook DJ, for the Canadian Critical Care Trials Group (McMaster Univ, Hamilton, Ont, Canada)
N Engl J Med 330:377–381, 1994   119-95-46-8

Objective.—Because measures used to prevent stress ulceration are expensive and may themselves have adverse effects, the frequency of significant gastrointestinal bleeding in critically ill patients was studied prospectively.

Study Population.—The study included consecutive patients older than 16 years of age who, in a 1-year period, were admitted to 4 university-affiliated medical–surgical ICUs. Patients with evidence of upper gastrointestinal bleeding were excluded. Physicians were asked to withhold measures intended to prevent stress ulceration except in head-injured or burn injury patients, organ transplant recipients, and those given a diagnosis of peptic ulcer or gastritis in the past 6 weeks.

Observations.—Of the 2,252 eligible patients, 674 received prophylaxis against stress ulceration. Their Acute Physiology and Chronic Health Evaluation scores were comparable with those of the other patients, although their mortality rate was higher (16.8% vs. 6.7%). The 100 overt bleeding episodes included 33 clinically significant episodes, defined as overt bleeding with either hemodynamic compromise or a need for transfusion. On multiple regression analysis, the only independent risk factors for clinically important bleeding were prolonged respiratory failure necessitating mechanical ventilation and coagulopathy. Only 2 affected patients lacked both risk factors. Bleeding occurred in 3.4% of the patients given prophylaxis and in .6% of the others.

Implication.—Because clinically important gastrointestinal bleeding develops in relatively few critically ill patients, prophylaxis against stress ulceration may be withheld unless coagulopathy is present or the patient requires mechanical ventilation.

▶ Accumulating data indicate that the incidence of clinically important stress-related gastrointestinal bleeding (GIB) is lower than previously believed. The above article documents that clinically significant GIB occurred in only .1% of patients without respiratory failure or coagulopathy compared with a 3.7% incidence figure if 1 or both of these risk factors was present.

A recent report by Ben-Menacham et al. corroborates these findings. Of 300 medical ICU admissions, 100 were randomized to a control group, 100 to a group receiving sucralfate, and 100 to a group receiving IV cimetidine, the latter to maintain an intragastric pH of $\geq$ 4. Clinically important GIB was defined as endoscopically verified, stress-related gastritis plus any 1 of 3 additional criteria: first, persistent hematemesis that did not clear with 1.5-L saline lavage; second, a 3-point decrease in hematocrit accompanied by red blood or guaiac-positive "coffee grounds" material that cleared with lavage; and finally, any unexplained 6-point decrease in hematocrit during a 48-hour period. The incidences of clinically important stress-related GIB were 6%, 5%, and 5% in the control, sucralfate, and cimetidine groups, respectively. Ben-Menacham and colleagues conclude that neither cimetidine nor sucralfate prophylaxis affected the already low incidence of stress-related hemorrhage in the ICU.—N.J. Greenberger, M.D.

Reference

1. Ben-Menacham T, et al: Prophylaxis for stress-related gastric hemorrhage in the medical intensive care unit. *Ann Intern Med* 121:568–575, 1994.

Risks of Bleeding Peptic Ulcer Associated With Individual Non-Steroidal Anti-Inflammatory Drugs
Langman MJS, Weil J, Wainwright P, Lawson DH, Rawlins MD, Logan RFA, Murphy M, Vessey MP, Collin-Jones DG (Univ of Birmingham, England; Glasgow Royal Infirmary, Scotland; Univ of Newcastle upon Tyne, England; et al)
Lancet 343:1075–1078, 1994   119-95-46-9

Introduction.—Nonsteroidal anti-inflammatory drug (NSAID) therapy has been linked to an increased risk of peptic ulcer complications. However, controversy exists regarding the relative toxicity of individual NSAIDs. A large, multicenter, case-control study was performed to assess the associations between NSAID use and other risk factors for peptic ulcer bleeding in a geriatric population.

Methods.—Questionnaires detailing all previous drug intake, smoking habits, alcohol consumption, and a history of gastrointestinal disease

	Cases	Hospital controls	Community controls	Odds ratio (95% CI)*
		Risks of Ulcer Complications Associated With NSAID Use During Previous 3 Months		
Azapropazone	22	2	2	31·5 (10·3–96·9)
Diclofenac	71	30	31	4·2 (2·6–6·8)
Ibuprofen	88	61	75	2·0 (1·4–2·8)
Indomethacin	57	16	14	11·3 (6·3–20·3)
Ketoprofen	31	2	4	23·7 (7·6–74·2)
Naproxen	90	23	21	9·1 (5·5–15·1)
Piroxicam	57	13	11	13·7 (7·1–26·3)
Any non-aspirin NSAID	411	169	182	4·5 (3·6–5·6)
Not on NSAID or aspirin†	457	807	657	1·0

* All odds ratios from unconditional logistic regression model with terms for aspirin use, smoking, alcohol, previous peptic ulcer, and history of dyspepsia. For azapropazone, to obtain convergence, aspirin use was not included.
† Reference category.
(Courtesy of Langman MJS, Weil J, Wainwright P, et al: *Lancet* 343:1075–1078, 1994.)

were completed by 1,144 patients, aged 60 years and older, admitted for gastric or duodenal bleeding and by age- and sex-matched controls, including 1,126 inpatients admitted for nonrelated complaints and 989 community controls.

Results.—Current smoking and drinking were slightly more likely among peptic ulcer patients than among controls. Peptic ulcer patients were also more likely than controls to have active rheumatoid arthritis and to have taken nonaspirin NSAIDs during the 3 months preceding the interview. The risk of peptic ulcer bleeding was increased with the use of all nonaspirin NSAIDs. The risk was lowest with ibuprofen and diclofenac; intermediate for indomethacin, naproxen, and piroxicam; and highest with azapropazone and ketoprofen (table). The risk patterns were consistent regardless of the duration of use, but the risk was substantially greater for patients who had started taking a nonaspirin NSAID within 1 month of the interview than for earlier use, and this risk increased in a dose-dependent manner.

Discussion.—Use of the various NSAIDs carried different, but consistent, risks of peptic ulcer bleeding, which were independent of other risk factors. Therefore, NSAIDs should not be routinely administered. They should be given only to patients who do not improve with non-NSAID analgesics, and then the least toxic NSAIDs should be given at the lowest effective doses.

▶ A similar study by Garcia-Rodriguez and Jick (1) supports the findings reported by Langman and colleagues. Garcia-Rodriguez and Jick evaluated a study sample comprising 1,457 cases of upper gastrointestinal bleeding (UGIB) and 10,000 control subjects identified from computerized records. The adjusted estimate of relative risk of UGIB associated with current NSAID use was 4.7. The single most important predictor of UGIB was a previous upper gastrointestinal bleed. For all NSAIDs, the risk was greater for high doses than for low doses. Although the estimate of risk associated with individual NSAIDs varied widely, *users of azapropazone and piroxicam* had the highest risk of UGIB among the NSAIDs studied. These findings are in accord with the data provided by Langman et al.—N.J. Greenberger, M.D.

Reference

1. Garcia-Rodriguez LA, Jick H: Risk of upper gastrointestinal bleeding and perforation associated with individual non-steroidal anti-inflammatory drugs. *Lancet* 343:769–772, 1994.

Satiety Effects of Cholecystokinin in Humans
Lieverse RJ, Jansen JBMJ, Masclee AAM, Lamers CBHW (Univ of Leiden, The Netherlands; Univ of Nijmegen, The Netherlands)
Gastroenterology 106:1451–1454, 1994   119-95-46–10

Background.—Cholecystokinin may increase satiety in several species, including human beings. Other biological actions of cholecystokinin are stimulation of pancreatic exocrine enzyme secretion, inhibition of gastric emptying, and stimulation of intestinal peristalsis. The satiety effects of an infusion of cholecystokinin-33 in doses leading to physiologic plasma cholecystokinin levels in lean and obese subjects were examined.

Methods.—Cholecystokinin-33 (1 Ivy Dog Unit/kg ideal wt per hour) was infused IV into 32 healthy men and women; 14 were obese, 18 were lean. Infusions were given randomly in a double-blind fashion for 1 hour. Desire to eat, feelings of hunger, fullness, and prospective feeding intentions were measured at 15-minute intervals.

Results.—The subjects receiving the infusion of cholecystokinin reported significant decreases in desire to eat, feelings of hunger, and prospective feeding intentions. The increase in feelings of fullness was nearly significant. There were no clear differences between obese and lean subjects, except for a more marked decrease in fullness and an increase in prospective feeding intentions during saline infusion in lean subjects.

Discussion.—Infusion of cholecystokinin-33 leading to physiologic plasma levels significantly increases satiety in human beings. However, there are still several problems with using cholecystokinin to treat obesity.

▶ This important study has shown that it is possible to induce satiety in humans with physiologic doses of cholecystokinin, leading to plasma levels comparable to those obtained after a meal. The additional interesting observation was the finding of a more marked *decrease* in satiety over time during saline infusion in lean compared with obese subjects.

Other physiologic signals that influence food intake are discussed in the following article (Abstract 119-95-46–11).—N.J. Greenberger, M.D.

Effect of Intravenous Human Gastrin-Releasing Peptide on Food Intake in Humans
Gutzwiller J-P, Drewe J, Hildebrand P, Rossi L, Lauper JZ, Beglinger C (Univ Hosp, Basel, Switzerland)
Gastroenterology 106:1168–1173, 1994   119-95-46–11

Background.—A number of peptides normally secreted from the gastrointestinal tract during eating suppress food intake if given before meals. Some of these peptides, notably the bombesin-like peptides, may act as regulatory signals to end food ingestion. One of them, gastrin-releasing peptide (GRP), has close structural homology to bombesin and has proven to be a strong stimulator of gastric acid secretion, exocrine pancreatic secretion, and gallbladder contraction in human beings.

Study Plan.—A randomized, double-blind study was carried out in 20 healthy young men to delineate the effects of infused synthetic human GRP on food intake. Either saline or GRP in a dose of 10, 40, or 160 pmol/kg per hour was infused for 1 hour before presentation of a standard meal. The subjects scored their feelings of hunger and fullness every 15 minutes.

Results.—Infusion of GRP reduced caloric intake in a dose-dependent manner. The 19% reduction in food intake was not statistically significant. None of the subjects described abdominal discomfort or other adverse reactions. They felt less hungry and more full after the 2 higher doses of GRP. All doses of GRP led to an early feeling of fullness in the pre-meal period. In a separate study of 8 subjects, infusion of loxiglumide, a specific cholecystokinin octapeptide receptor antagonist, did not influence the total energy intake from food or the amounts of food or fluid consumed.

Conclusion.—These findings support a role for GRP/bombesin-like peptides as endogenous signals that help regulate food intake. The intake-reducing effect of GRP-like peptides is probably independent of endogenous cholecystokinin.

▶ In a landmark paper, Zhang et al. (1) recently reported the isolation of a gene (the *ob* gene) through elaborate cloning methods, and this gene appears to be an important regulator of body fat and body weight. The investigation demonstrates that the mouse and human genes are nearly identical. The gene appears to be switched on solely or largely in fat tissue, resulting in generation of a hormone that triggers responses in the hypothalamus, considered a major controller of appetite. In the mouse model studied by Zhang et al., a mutant version of the gene would either fail to make the hormone altogether or would produce too little of it.—N.J. Greenberger, M.D.

Reference

1. Zhang Y, Proenca R, Maffei M, et al. Positional cloning of the mouse *obese* gene and its human homologue. *Nature* 372:425–531, 1994.

47 Small Bowel

Pathophysiology of Potassium Absorption and Secretion by the Human Intestine
Agarwal R, Afzalpurkar R, Fordtran JS (Baylor Univ, Dallas)
Gastroenterology 107:548–571, 1994   119-95-47–1

Background.—The renal transport of potassium has been extensively analyzed; however, little attention has been given to its intestinal absorption. Studies of the human intestine in vivo were reviewed, and the role of intestinal absorption in potassium homeostasis under normal conditions and when physiology is deranged by disease were clarified.

Results.—Total body exchangeable potassium averages 46 mEq/kg in men and 39 mEq/kg in women, yet only 1.5% to 2.5% of total body potassium is found in the extracellular fluid. The average diet provides about 90 mEq/day of potassium, of which 90% is absorbed. Rich dietary

---

TABLE 1.—Mechanisms of Increased Fecal K$^+$ Excretion
in Diarrhea

Major effects
  K$^+$ obligation by poorly absorbed anion ingested by mouth (e.g.,
    sulfate, phosphate)
  K$^+$ obligation by organic anions derived from bacterial
    metabolism of unabsorbed carbohydrates
  K$^+$ obligation by unabsorbed or actively secreted chloride
  Increased K$^+$ secretion caused by secondary hyperaldosteronism
Minor Effect
  Washout secondary to increased fecal water output
Some possible mechanisms that have apparently not been
    investigated in humans
  Malabsorption of K$^+$ caused by small bowel disease
  Obligation of K$^+$ by unabsorbed fatty acids in patients with
    steatorrhea
  Ingestion of K$^+$ salts administered to prevent K$^+$ depletion
  Increased active K$^+$ secretion or decreased active K$^+$ absorption
  Increased passive K$^+$ secretion in response to abnormally high
    electrical gradients or change in intestinal permeability
  Induction of K$^+$ channels by polypeptides or toxins

(Courtesy of Agarwal R, Afzalpurkar R, Fordtran JS: *Gastroenterology* 107:548–571, 1994.)

TABLE 2.—Speculation on Factors That May Promote the Development of Hypokalemia in Individuals With Diarrhea

1. High fecal K^+ output as seen mainly in secretory diarrhea and augmented by secondary hyperaldosteronism
2. Low dietary K^+ intake
3. Failure of kidneys to conserve K^+ normally (<10 mEq/day)
   A. Secondary hyperaldosteronism combined with a factor that causes Na^+ delivery to the distal tubules. The secondary hyperaldosteronism is caused by volume contraction due to high fecal Na^+ and water losses. The factors that cause Na^+ delivery to the distal tubule (in spite of volume contraction) include short-term oral or intravenous salt loads (not enough to replete volume status and thereby reverse hyperaldosteronism), metabolic alkalosis, or the excretion of other poorly absorbed anions such as ketoanions and D-Lactate
   B. Polydipsia,* resulting in water diuresis, which increases urinary K^+ excretion
   C. Magnesium depletion[129,130]
4. Shift of K^+ from ECF to ICF
   A. B_2 agonists (e.g., epinephrine) released in response to volume contraction
   B. Metabolic alkalosis
   C. ? aldosterone

---

* Severe polydipsia and polyuria may occur in patients with chronic diarrhea. Polydipsia apparently does not contribute to the diarrhea but by increasing urinary flow rate may contribute to urinary K+ losses.
(Courtesy of Agarwal R, Afzalpurkar R, Fordtran JS: *Gastroenterology* 107:548-571, 1994.)

sources include potatoes, beans, bananas, oranges, cantaloupes, black strap molasses, beef, and turkey. When dietary potassium is zero, obligatory renal potassium loss averages 6.3 mEq/day. Normal fecal potassium excretion averages around 10 mEq/day when a normal diet is consumed. However, in cases of deficiency, fecal potassium decreases to about 3.5 mEq/day. Most intestinal absorption of potassium occurs in the small intestine (the contribution of the colon is minimal). Hyperaldosteronism brings an increase in fecal potassium excretion by about 3 mEq/day in patients with otherwise normal intestinal tracts. Oral cation exchange resin can also increase fecal potassium excretion to 40 mEq/day. Diarrhea does not appear to disturb the absorption of potassium per se; however, fecal potassium losses are increased in patients with diarrhea by unabsorbed anions (which obligate potassium) and by electrochemical gradients secondary to active chloride secretion (Table 1). In patients with diarrhea, total body potassium can be reduced by both loss of muscle mass as the result of malnutrition and by reduced net absorption of potassium; however, only the latter causes hypokalemia (Table 2). Studies emphasize the importance of dietary potassium intake, renal potassium excretion, and fecal potassium losses in determining whether hypokalemia will develop.

▶ I selected this review article for inclusion in the 1995 YEAR BOOK OF MEDICINE because it is the best single article on potassium absorption and secretion by the human intestine in health and disease. Two of the big tables are included in the abstract, but they give only a hint of the wealth of information in the paper. The reader would be well served by reading the article in its entirety.—N.J. Greenberger, M.D.

Duodenal Bacterial Overgrowth During Treatment in Outpatients With Omeprazole
Fried M, Siegrist H, Frei R, Froehlich F, Duroux P, Thorens J, Blum A, Bille J, Gonvers JJ, Gyr K (Univ Hosp, Lausanne, Switzerland; Univ Hosp, Basel, Switzerland)
Gut 35:23–26, 1994   119-95-47-2

Introduction.—Omeprazole is a potent inhibitor of gastric acid secretion. Little information is available, however, on the gastric and duodenal bacterial flora during treatment with omeprazole, and it is not known whether small bacterial overgrowth occurs during therapy. A controlled, prospective study examined the bacterial content of duodenal juice of patients with peptic ulcer disease after treatment with omeprazole.

Patients and Methods.—Nine patients were treated with 20 mg and 16 patients with 40 mg of omeprazole for a mean of 5.7 weeks. The entire daily dose was taken with breakfast. All patients underwent endoscopy 1 day after the end of treatment. Fifteen patients with suspected peptic ulcer disease and referred for endoscopy served as controls.

Results.—Bacterial overgrowth in the duodenum was detected in 14 patients treated with omeprazole. The frequency of bacterial overgrowth was not influenced by dose size. No significant bacterial overgrowth was observed in untreated controls. The most commonly identified types of bacteria were hemolytic and nonhemolytic streptococci. Although most bacteria belonged to species colonizing the oral cavity and pharynx, fecal type bacteria were found in 7 of 14 patients and anaerobic bacteria in 3 of 14 patients. The number of bacteria in duodenal juice was distinctly higher in omeprazole-treated patients than in controls. These findings may prove to have clinical significance, particularly during long-term use of omeprazole by high-risk groups.

▶ Despite lack of Food and Drug Administration approval, many patients with difficult-to-manage gastroesophageal reflux disease remain on extended treatment with omeprazole. In view of the findings of Fried et al., it seems likely that a small but significant number of patients will develop clinically significant bacterial overgrowth. Accordingly, development of unexplained weight loss, diarrhea, and anemia in a patient given long-term omeprazole treatment should prompt an evaluation for abnormal bacterial proliferation in the proximal small bowel.

Another consequence of the potent long-lasting inhibition of gastric secretions induced by omeprazole is impaired absorption of cyanocobalamine (vitamin B_{12}) (1). Marcuard et al. demonstrated that at the end of a 2-month treatment period, vitamin B_{12} absorption decreased from 3.2% to 0.9% in participants receiving 20 mg of omeprazole daily. In patients taking 40 mg of omeprazole daily, vitamin B_{12} absorption decreased from 3.4% to 0.9%. Because normal individuals have a finite supply of vitamin B_{12} (approximately 2,000 μg, equivalent to a 4- to 5-year supply if utilized at the rate of 1 μg/day), it would seem prudent to monitor serum cyanocobalamine levels in patients on long-term therapy with omeprazole and, especially, after 3 years.—N.J. Greenberger, M.D.

Reference

1. Marcuard SP, Albernaz L, Khazane F: Omeprazle therapy causes malabsorption of cyanocobalamine (vitamin B_{12}). *Ann Intern Med* 120:211–215, 1994.

A Massive Outbreak in Milwaukee of Cryptosporidium Infection Transmitted Through the Public Water Supply

Mac Kenzie WR, Hoxie NJ, Proctor ME, Gradus MS, Blair KA, Peterson DE, Kazmierczak JJ, Addiss DG, Fox KR, Rose JB, Davis JP (Bureau of Public Health, Madison, Wis; City of Milwaukee Bureau of Labs, Wis; City of Milwaukee Dept of Health, Wis; et al)
N Engl J Med 331:161–167, 1994   119-95-47-3

Background.—An outbreak of acute watery diarrhea took place in Milwaukee early in the spring of 1993. Observations of very turbid water at 1 of 2 local water treatment plants suggested that the water supply probably was the source of infection.

Epidemiologic Findings.—After a marked increase in turbidity was noted at Milwaukee's southern water treatment plant, *Cryptosporidium* oocysts were identified in water made from ice in that part of the city, and the plant was shut down. The rate of isolation of *Cryptosporidium* increased more than 100-fold, but rates for other enteric pathogens remained stable. *Cryptosporidium* was found in the stools of 8 of 11 individuals having gastrointestinal illness who were evaluated within 48 hours of the onset of illness.

Clinical Aspects.—*Cryptosporidium* infection was confirmed in the laboratory in 285 individuals, 46% of whom were hospitalized. Diarrhea was universal and was watery in more than 90% of infected patients (table). The diarrhea lasted a median of 9 days, and at its peak produced 12 stools a day. Three fourths of patients lost a median of 10 lb of body

Clinical Characteristics of Case Patients With Laboratory-Confirmed
Cryptosporidium Infection and Survey Respondents With Clinical Infection

CHARACTERISTIC	LABORATORY-CONFIRMED INFECTION (N = 285)		CLINICAL INFECTION* (N = 201)		P VALUE†
Symptoms — no. of patients or respondents (%)					
Diarrhea	285	(100)	201	(100)	NA
Watery diarrhea	265	(93)	201	(100)	NA
Abdominal cramps	238	(84)	168	(84)	0.9
Fatigue	247	(87)	145	(72)	<0.001
Loss of appetite	230	(81)	147	(73)	0.03
Nausea	199	(70)	119	(59)	0.01
Fever	162	(57)	72	(36)	<0.001
Chills	65	(64)‡	91	(45)	0.04
Sweats	55	(54)‡	83	(41)	0.04
Muscle or joint aches	152	(53)	100	(50)	0.6
Headache	53	(52)‡	122	(61)	0.2
Vomiting	136	(48)	37	(18)	<0.001
Cough	68	(24)	56	(28)	0.3
Sore throat	48	(17)	35	(17)	0.7
Mean duration of diarrhea — days	12		4.5		0.001§
Mean maximal no. of stools/day	19		7.7		0.001§
Mean maximal temperature — °C	38.3		38.1		0.09§
Mean duration of vomiting — days	2.9		2.0		0.07§
Mean maximal no. of vomiting episodes/day	3.9		2.6		0.36§

* The criterion for clinical infection was the reported presence of watery diarrhea.
† Unless otherwise noted, Yates' correction has been applied to P values. NA denotes not applicable.
‡ Data are from 101 case patients interviewed during phase 1 of the study.
§ By Kruskal-Wallis test. (Courtesy of Mac Kenzie WR, Hoxie NJ, Proctor ME, et al: N Engl J Med 331:161–167, 1994.)

weight. Immunocompromised patients, (17% of the total) had more diarrheal stools than the others and were more likely to be hospitalized.

Magnitude of the Outbreak.—A household survey indicated that 30% of 1,663 individuals surveyed had had diarrhea during the epidemic period. The rate was highest for those living near the water plant that had been implicated. It was estimated that, of the total population of 1,610,000 in greater Milwaukee, 419,000 individuals had watery diarrhea during the survey period, compared with an expected 16,000 cases.

Implications.—This outbreak was ascribed to *Cryptosporidium* oocysts that passed the filtration system of a water treatment plant. These plants should consider continuously monitoring treated water for turbidity. In addition, routine stool tests for *Cryptosporidium* might be performed in all those having watery diarrhea.

▶ *Cryptosporidium* has been recognized increasingly as a cause of gastrointestinal illness in both immunocompetent and immunodeficient individuals. In immunocompetent people, cryptosporidiosis is a self-limited illness, but in immunocompromised patients, *Cryptosporidium* infection can be unrelenting and extremely difficult to eradicate. Waterborne outbreaks of *Cryptosporidium* have been reported with contaminated well water, untreated surface water, and filtered public water supplies. The massive outbreak of watery diarrhea in Milwaukee is unprecedented in that over 400,000 people were estimated to have had watery diarrhea attributable to *Cryptosporidium*. As the authors point out in their discussion, intensive efforts and cooperation between the medical community and those who provide and regulate drinking water in the United States will be required to prevent future waterborne outbreaks by this emerging pathogen.—N.J. Greenberger, M.D.

Occult Enteric Infection by *Ancylostoma caninum*: A Previously Unrecognized Zoonosis

Croese J, Loukas A, Opdebeeck J, Prociv P (Townsville Gen Hosp, Queensland, Australia; Univ of Queensland, Australia)
Gastroenterology 106:3–12, 1994   119-95-47–4

Introduction.—An extraordinarily high prevalence of eosinophilic enteritis and of abdominal pain associated with peripheral blood eosinophilia occurred in northern Queensland, Australia. The infection in 1 patient was found to originate from a single hookworm, and because a higher porportion of the patients were dog owners than the general population of the area, a dog hookworm was posited as the cause. Sera from these and other patients were tested for the presence of *Ancylostoma caninum*.

Methods.—Sera from 7 groups of patients were tested for the presence of *A. caninum* with an enzyme-linked immunosorbent assay (ELISA) and Western blot (WB). Three groups of patients had the infections found in the test population: eosinophilic enteritis and abdominal pain with and without blood eosinophilia. The 4 control groups were composed of patients with other gastrointestinal diseases, other patients with hookworm, and 2 groups with anonymous serum samples, 1 from the area where the infected patients lived and 1 from an area where *A. caninum* is not endemic. Eighteen of the patients with the target infections provided serum samples at least 6 months later for convalescent ELISA evaluation. Symptoms and demographic, clinical, and outcome data were reviewed.

Results.—The ELISA was positive for the presence of *A. caninum* in 71% of the patients with eosinophilic enteritis, in 67% of the patients

Clinical, Demographic, and Serologic Results, by Patient Group

	A1 (n = 42) Eosinophilic enteritis	A2 (n = 105) Pain and blood eosinophilia	A3 (n = 84) Obscure pain	B (n = 40) Other diseases	C (n = 4) Hookworm infection
Age (yr)					
Mean	38	37	38	46	46
Range	13–72	11–80	13–71	15–79	31–61
Males (%)	26 (62)	58 (55)	31 (37)	24 (60)	1 (25)
Atopy					
No. sampled (%)[a]	39 (93)	92 (88)	74 (88)	30 (75)	4 (100)
No. atopic (%)[b]	2 (5)	11 (12)	8 (11)	2 (7)	0 (0)
Dog ownership					
No. sampled (%)[a]	35 (83)	75 (71)	66 (79)	23 (58)	4 (100)
No. of owners (%)[b]	28 (80)	59 (79)	52 (79)	14 (61)	4 (100)
Pain classification					
No. with acute pain (%)[a]	13 (31)	20 (19)	6 (7)		0
No. with recurrent pain (%)[a]	19 (45)	38 (36)	42 (50)		3 (75)
No. with chronic pain (%)[a]	9 (21)	47 (45)	34 (40)		1 (25)
No. with diarrhea (%)[a]	2 (5)	12 (11)	0		0
Radiology					
No. sampled (%)[a]	25 (60)	8 (8)	1 (1)		1 (25)
No. with diagnostic changes (%)	25 (100)	0	0		1 (100)
Colonoscopy					
No. sampled (%)[a]	15 (36)	35 (33)	40 (48)		3 (75)
No. with ulceration (%)[b]	4 (27)	3 (9)	1 (3)		3 (100)
No. who underwent biopsy (%)[c]	10 (67)	18 (51)	0		3 (100)
No. with diagnostic histology (%)	8 (80)	0	0		3 (100)

(continued)

Table (*continued*)

Laparotomy					
No. sampled (%)[a]	23 (55)	7 (7)	4 (5)		1 (25)
No. with positive gross findings (%)[b]	22 (96)	0	0		1 (100)
No. who underwent biopsy (%)[c]	12 (52)	2 (29)	0		1 (100)
No. with diagnostic histology (%)[b]	11 (92)	0	0		1 (100)
Histology					
No. sampled (%)[a]	22 (52)	18 (17)	8 (10)		4 (100)
No. who underwent diagnostic histology (%)[b]	18 (82)	0	0		4 (100)
Treatment					
No. treated (%)[a]	17 (40)	47 (45)	9 (11)		3 (75)
No. with positive outcome (%)[b]	14 (82)	46 (98)	8 (89)		3 (100)
ELISA					
No. sampled (%)[a]	21 (50)	64 (61)	79 (94)	40 (100)	3 (75)
No. positive (%)[b]	15 (71)	43 (67)	24 (30)	3 (8)	1 (33)
Western Blot					
No. sampled (%)[a]	3 (7)	14 (13)	2 (2)	40 (100)	3 (75)
No. positive (%)[b]	3 (100)	14 (100)	2 (100)	4 (10)	3 (100)

[a]Number and percentage of the total group sampled.
[b]Number and percentage of the sample classified positive.
[c]Number and percentage of the sample who underwent biopsy.
[d]Number and percentage of biopsies diagnosed as eosinophilic enteritis.
(Courtesy of Croese J, Loukas A, Opdebeeck J, et al: *Gastroenterology* 106:3-12, 1994.)

with abdominal pain associated with blood eosinophilia, and 30% of those without blood eosinophilia. Among the control groups, a positive ELISA was found in 8% of the patients with other gastrointestinal diseases and in 1 of the 4 patients with a feeding single hookworm. All sera in the study population that were tested with WB analysis had positive results, as did all 3 sera from those with hookworm infection, whereas only 4 of 40 controls had positive WB results (table). A positive ELISA after 6 months was more common among patients with recurrent pain.

Discussion.—The presence of A. *caninum* was verified in the sera of patients with abdominal pain, blood eosinophilia, and eosinophilic enteritis. However, neither sexual maturation nor successful colonization of A. *caninum* was seen in any patients, indicating that the infection in human beings will always resolve spontaneously.

▶ This provocative study indicates that in Australia, occult human A. *caninum* infections are common and are characterized by eosinophilic enteritis and obscure abdominal pain with or without blood eosinophilia. Importantly, the diagnosis can be confirmed by serology. The findings suggest that a subset of patients with eosinophilic enteritis may have had the disease process initiated by an occult infection with A. *caninum*. Accordingly, it seems reasonable to determine whether patients with eosinophilic enteritis have pets and, if so, to test the patient for serum antibodies for A. *caninum*. It will be interesting to determine whether there is a significant reservoir of infected domestic pets in other countries such as the United States and the United Kingdom.—N.J. Greenberger, M.D.

A Population Study of Food Intolerance
Young E, Stoneham MD, Petruckevitch A, Barton J, Rona R (Amersham Hosp, England; Guy's and St Thomas's Hosp, London)
Lancet 343:1127–1130, 1994   119-95-47–5

Objective.—Immunologic food intolerance has only recently been described. There is no simple specific in vitro or in vivo test for food intolerance, making investigation of this problem difficult; dietary exclusion and repeated, controlled challenge is the best way to establish that a food intolerance is present. The prevalence of reactions to foods was examined in a British population study.

Methods.—Two random samples of 7,500 households were identified: 1 from households in a single United Kingdom Health Authority area and another from households nationwide. Individuals from the former sample who reported food intolerance in a questionnaire were invited to take part in an interview. If the reported food intolerance was relevant to food testing, the patient was invited to take part in a double-blind, placebo-controlled food-challenge study (Fig 47–1). Eight foods commonly perceived to cause reactions in the United Kingdom were se-

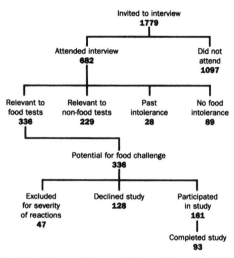

Fig 47–1.—Flow chart of participants. (Courtesy of Young E. Stoneham MD, Petruckevitch A. et al: *Lancet* 343:1127–1130, 1994.)

lected for study: cow's milk, eggs, wheat, soya, citrus fruit, fish or shell-fish, nuts, and chocolate.

Results.—About 20% of respondents in both samples complained of food intolerance. The most commonly implicated foods were chocolate, additives, citrus fruit, fish and shellfish, and cow's milk. Patients reporting atopic symptoms were more likely to report food reactions than those without such symptoms. Ninety-three patients completed the

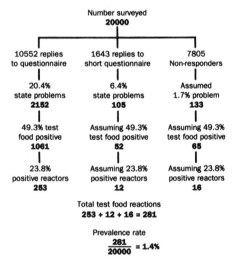

Fig 47–2.—Method used to calculate prevalence. (Courtesy of Young E, Stoneham MD, Petruckevitch A, et al: *Lancet* 343:1127–1130, 1994.)

food-challenge study; 19% of these patients had a positive reaction. Depending on the definition of a reaction, the estimated prevalence of reactions in the population to the 8 foods tested ranged from 1.4% to 1.8% (Fig 47–2). Women were more likely than men to report food intolerance and to have a positive reaction on food challenge.

Conclusion.—Although up to one fifth of the British population reports food intolerance, controlled challenge testing suggests that the actual prevalence is between 1% and 2%. Intolerance to food in the population appears to be more common than intolerance to food additives, as assessed in a previous study. Objective assessment of food allergy requires double-blind, placebo-controlled food challenge studies.

▶ This article brings into sharp focus the distinction between perceived and actual food intolerance. The irritable bowel syndrome is one disorder for which it is important to take a detailed dietary history. The classic study by Nanda et al. (1) demonstrated that identification of food intolerance and adherence to a restricted diet resulted in either improvement or amelioration of irritable bowel symptoms in approximately half of the patients.

On a related matter, for an excellent update on advances in clinical nutrition, see the article by Fleming and Jeejeebhog (2).—N.J. Greenberger, M.D.

References

1. Nanda R, James R, Smith H, et al: Food intolerance and the irritable bowel syndrome. *Gut* 30:1099–1104, 1989.
2. Fleming CR, Jeejeebhog KN: Advances in clinical nutrition. *Gastroenterology* 106:1365–1373, 1994.

Serological Screening of Coeliac Disease: Choosing the Optimal Procedure According to Various Prevalence Values
Corrao G, Corazza GR, Andreani ML, Torchio P, Valentini RA, Galatola G, Quaglino D, Gasbarrini G, di Orio F (Univ of Milan, Italy; Univ of L'Aquila, Italy; Univ of Bologna, Italy; et al)
Gut 35:771–775, 1994   119-95-47–6

Background.—Celiac disease is characterized by villous atrophy of the small intestine induced by the ingestion of gluten that contains gliadins and prolamins. The diagnosis of celiac disease is often missed because the classic symptoms of weight loss and diarrhea are not frequently present. This disease can be definitively diagnosed by finding specific histologic hallmarks on jejunal or duodenal biopsy specimens. The diagnostic performance of class A and G antigliadin antibodies, of class A antiendomysium antibodies, and of various combinations of tests was assessed.

Methods.—A serum sample was collected from 93 consecutive outpatients having suspected malabsorption. Celiac disease was diagnosed in 44 patients according to duodenal histologic findings. Antibodies were measured with a microenzyme-linked immunosorbent assay and an indirect immunofluorescence technique.

Results.—Class G antigliadin antibodies had the worst predictive ability, and class A antigliadin and class A antiendomysium antibodies had the best. For class A antigliadin antibodies, the positive predictive value corrected for the disease prevalence expected for patients with relatives with celiac disease decreased to 30%; for the general population, the predictive value decreased to less than 2%. For antiendomysium antibodies, this value remained at 100% both for patients with relatives with celiac disease and for the general population. In a 2-step approach, class A antigliadin antibodies were measured in all patients, and a confirmation test of either antiendomysium antibodies or duodenal biopsy was used only for patients who tested positive for antigliadin antibodies; the positive predictive value was always 100%, regardless of which confirmation test was used.

Discussion.—In screening for asymptomatic celiac disease, antigliadin antibodies are useful if antiendomysium antibodies are also used as a confirmation test. Antiendomysium antibodies are a reasonable, valid alternative to the more invasive duodenal biopsy. However, duodenal biopsy is recommended for patients with suspected celiac disease.

▶ It is not generally appreciated that subclinical celiac sprue is common, especially in certain populations. Only a third of adults with this condition give a history of celiac disease in childhood. Accordingly, there has been considerable interest in cost-effective screening for subclinical celiac sprue. Catassi et al. (1) have reported their observations in 3,351 schoolchildren 11–15 years old who were screened for subclinical celiac sprue by serum assays of IgG and IgA antigliadin antibody (AGA) and IgA antiendomysial antibody (AEA). Seventy-one (2%) were recalled because of AGA positivity; 18 of these satisfied second level criteria and underwent intestinal biopsy. Celiac sprue was diagnosed in 11 subjects, most of whom had no serious symptoms. Thus, the prevalence of subclinical celiac sprue in this study group was 3.28 per 1,000.

Challacombe (2) has written a thoughtful editorial that accompanies the paper by Catassi. He raises the following issues:

• Current screening tests such as serum assays for AGA, AEA, and antireticulin antibody (ARA) are expensive and time-consuming, and positive results need to be verified by small-bowel biopsy.

• Population screening may be more feasible as tests become more reliable and cheaper.

• The indications for treatment of *asymptomatic* patients with celiac sprue need to be more clearly defined, as some adolescents with the disease do not adhere to a gluten-free diet and yet have no symptoms.

However, there is a clear indication for treating *symptomatic* celiac sprue with a gluten-free diet.—N.J. Greenberger, M.D.

References

1. Catassi C, Rätsch IM, Fabiani E: Coeliac disease in the year 2000: Exploring the iceberg. *Lancet* 343:200–203, 1994.
2. Challacombe D: When is a coeliac. *Lancet* 343:188, 1994.

48 Colon

Course of Ulcerative Colitis: Analysis of Changes in Disease Activity Over Years

Langholz E, Munkholm P, Davidsen M, Binder V (Univ of Copenhagen)
Gastroenterology 107:3–11, 1994   119-95-48–1

Background.—Although patients with ulcerative colitis have good outcomes in terms of mortality and cancer occurrence, the chronicity of the disease with intermittent flare-ups or continuous activity remains troublesome. No good estimates of individual disease courses exist. An analysis of changes in disease activity over the years was presented.

Methods.—Follow-up data were obtained from 1,161 patients with ulcerative colitis. The patients were followed from diagnosis to as long as 25 years. Probabilities of remission and relapse during the course of the disease were estimated using actuarial analysis and Markov chain analysis.

Findings.—Disease activity distribution remained remarkably constant each year. About half the patients were in clinical remission. The 10-year colectomy rate was 24%. After 25 years of follow-up, the cumulative probability of a relapsing course was 90%. The disease course changed

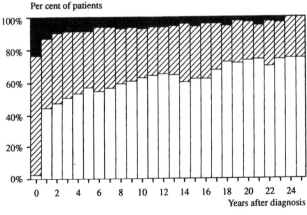

Fig 48–1.—Percentage of patients in remission (*white area*), with continuous disease activity within the year (*solid area*), and with intermittent disease activity within the year (*hatched area*) in all years after diagnosis. The calculation is based on all study patients in the actual year of observation except for patients undergoing colectomy. (Courtesy of Langholz E, Munkholm P, Davidsen M, et al: *Gastroenterology* 107:3–11, 1994.)

between remission and relapse with no significant predictors, except for disease activity in the foregoing years. Three to 7 years after diagnosis, one fourth of the patients were in remission. Eighteen percent had some disease activity every year, and 57% had intermittent relapses (Fig 48–1). Activity in the first 2 years after diagnosis was significantly associated with an increased probability of 5 consecutive years of disease activity. After 10 years, the probability of maintaining the ability to work was 92.8%.

Conclusion.—At any one time, about 50% of patients with ulcerative colitis will be in remission, although 90% have an intermittent course. Relapses are largely unpredictable. However, disease activity in foregoing years indicates continuing disease the following years with a probability of 70% to 80%.

▶ This comprehensive report of an unusually large series of 1,161 patients with ulcerative colitis provides a wealth of interesting information on the natural history of this disorder. The article should be read in its entirety as it provides the best current information on this disorder. I would like to call attention to the following salient observations:

- At any given time, approximately 50% of the patients were in clinical remission.
- The colectomy rate was 24% after 10 years and 30% after 15 years.
- Only 6 patients of 1,161 developed colorectal cancer during the observation period, and the calculated lifetime risk of developing colonic cancer while under treatment for ulcerative colitis was 3.5%.
- Although the relapse rate was 95% at 25 years and a majority had a relapse within 5 years of their first presentation, less than 1% had continuous disease activity.
- Patients whose ulcerative colitis was diagnosed in the latter years of the study seemed to have less relapse than those with earlier diagnoses. The reasons for this are not apparent.

N.J. Greenberger, M.D.

Cyclosporine in Severe Ulcerative Colitis Refractory to Steroid Therapy

Lichtiger S, Present DH, Kornbluth A, Gelernt I, Bauer J, Galler G, Michelassi F, Hanauer S (Mt Sinai School of Medicine, New York; Univ of Chicago)
N Engl J Med 330:1841–1845, 1994   119-95-48–2

Background.—Cyclosporine, which selectively inhibits immune responses mediated by T lymphocytes, has been found effective in patients with chronic corticosteroid-resistant Crohn's disease. In 1 uncontrolled trial, about 80% of patients with severe ulcerative colitis refractory to corticosteroid therapy responded to cyclosporine treatment. The effi-

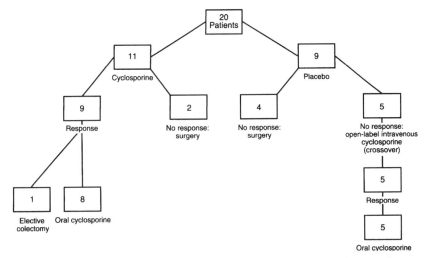

Fig 48–2.—Results of cyclosporine or placebo administration in 20 patients with severe ulcerative colitis. (Courtesy of Lichtiger S, Present DH, Kornbluth A, et al: *N Engl J Med* 330:1841-1845, 1994.)

cacy and safety of IV cyclosporine treatment in patients with severe ulcerative colitis were further explored.

Methods.—Twenty patients with severe ulcerative colitis were enrolled in the randomized, double-blind, controlled study. All had had no improvement after at least 7 days of IV corticosteroid treatment. Cyclosporine, 4 mg/kg of body weight per day, or placebo was administered. Response was defined as improvement in a numerical symptom score leading to hospital discharge and treatment with oral medications. Treatment failure resulted in colectomy. However, some patients given placebo had no response and no urgent need for surgery and were subsequently treated with cyclosporine.

Findings.—Responses occurred within a mean of 7 days of treatment initiation in 82% of the 11 patients given cyclosporine and in none of the 9 given placebo (Fig 48–2). The mean clinical activity score in patients given cyclosporine declined from 13 to 6. In the placebo group, this score declined from 14 to only 13. Adverse effects included paresthesias, occurring in 36% of patients in the cyclosporine group and in none of the placebo group, and hypertension, occurring in 36% of the cyclosporine group and 11% of the placebo group. There were no cases of nephrotoxicity or hepatotoxicity. One patient beginning cyclosporine had a grand mal seizure, and the drug was discontinued, averting further seizure activity.

Conclusion.—In these patients with severe corticosteroid-resistant ulcerative colitis, IV cyclosporine treatment was rapidly effective. Nearly 60% of the patients in an open trial maintained their clinical response to cyclosporine 6 months after discharge; many were later able to stop corticosteroid treatment and had endoscopic evidence of healing.

▶ Although the acute benefits of cyclosporine are apparent in severe corticosteroid-resistant ulcerative colitis (UC), the long-term benefits remain incompletely defined in this difficult to treat group of patients with severe and often refractory disease. In this regard, Baert and Hanauer (1) followed 12 patients with severe UC treated initially with IV cyclosporine. Twelve (of 18, or 66% who responded) were continued on oral cyclosporine at a dose of 8 mg/kg per day for a mean of 3 months, while azathioprine was added and corticosteroids were gradually tapered. Only 7 of the original 18 patients have remained in clinical remission. Life-table analysis of these data revealed a noncolectomy rate of 35.5% after 2.8 years.

Sandborn et al. (2) have assessed the efficacy and safety of cyclosporine enemas (350 mg/day for 4 weeks) in patients with mildly to moderately active left-sided ulcerative colitis. At 4 weeks, 8 of 20 patients (40%) who received cyclosporine had clinical improvement compared with 9 of 20 patients (45%) who received placebo. These findings indicate that cyclosporine enemas administered for 4 weeks are not efficacious in mildly to moderately active ulcerative colitis.

The efficacy of cyclosporine for treatment of Crohn's disease has also been evaluated. Feagan et al. (3) conducted a randomized, double-blind, placebo-controlled evaluation of the effect of 18 months of low-dose cyclosporine (2.5 mg/kg per day) treatment on the course of Crohn's disease in 305 patients. One hundred fifty-one patients received cyclosporine and 154 patients received a placebo in addition to their usual therapy. The main finding was that the addition of low-dose cyclosporine to conventional treatment of Crohn's disease did not improve symptoms or reduce requirements for other forms of therapy.—N.J. Greenberger, M.D.

References

1. Baert F, Hanauer S: Cyclosporine in severe steroid resistant ulcerative colitis. *Gastroenterology* 106:2190, 1994. (Abstract)
2. Sandborn WJH, Temaine WJ, Schroeder KN, et al: A placebo-controlled trial of cyclosporine enema for mildly to moderately active left-sided ulcerative colitis. *Gastroenterology* 106:1429–1435, 1994.
3. Feagan BG, McDonald IWD, Rochon J, et al: Low dose cyclosporine for the treatment of Crohn's disease. *N Engl J Med* 330:1846–1851, 1994.

A Swimming-Associated Outbreak of Hemorrhagic Colitis Caused by *Escherichia Coli* O157:H7 and *Shigella Sonnei*
Keene WE, McAnulty JM, Hoesly FC, Williams LP Jr, Hedberg K, Oxman GL, Barrett TJ, Pfaller MA, Fleming DW (Ctr for Disease Prevention and Epidemiology, Portland, Ore; Centers for Disease Control and Prevention, Atlanta,

Ga; Multnomah County Health Dept, Portland, Ore; et al)
N Engl J Med 331:579–584, 1994   119-95-48–3

Background.—A common cause of epidemic and sporadic disease, especially bloody diarrhea and hemolytic-uremic syndrome, is *Escherichia coli* O157:H7. Outbreaks have been traced to contaminated hamburger and other foods, drinking water, and person-to-person transmission. Simultaneous outbreaks of infection with *E. coli* O157:H7 and *Shigella sonnei* in the Portland, Oregon area were investigated.

Methods.—Cases were identified from routine surveillance reports. The activities of people with infections with *E. coli* O157:H7 and *S. sonnei* associated with use of a recreational park were compared with control groups. Environmental conditions at the park were evaluated and bacterial isolates were subtyped.

Results.—Park-related *E. coli* O157:H7 infections were identified in 21 people, all of them children. *S. sonnei* infections were identified in 38 people, most of them children. The infections did not result from food or beverage consumption, sewage leaks, or bathroom facilities. All case patients had been swimming, which was strongly associated with both types of infection. The case patients had spent more time in the lake and were more likely to have swallowed water than the control patients. Elevated numbers of enterococci, which were indicative of substantial fecal contamination, were detected in the swimming area, but not elsewhere in the lake.

Discussion.—The outbreak was caused by ingestion of lake water contaminated by fecal matter. This is supported by the elevated numbers of enterococci in the swimming area of the lake. Many of the bathers were toddlers who were not yet toilet trained. Small children should have alternatives for playing in water at parks.

▶ *Escherichia coli* O157:H7 is known to cause a hemorrhagic colitis and hemolytic uremic syndrome. Outbreaks are frequently traced to contaminated hamburger, but other foods such as unpasteurized apple cider and drinking water and person-to-person transmission have been reported. This report by Keene and associates calls attention to an outbreak traced to contaminated swimming water.

A recent letter (1) describes the largest reported milkborne outbreak of *E. coli* O157:H7 infection and the first to involve a heat-treated milk supply. Over 100 people were affected and over 90% of patients had consumed pasteurized milk in cartons or bottles from a local dairy. At least 7 cases were thought to be the result of secondary spread within households.—N.J. Greenberger, M.D.

Reference

1.   Upton P, Coia JE: Outbreak of *Escherichia coli* O157:H7 infection associated with pasteurized milk supply. *Lancet* 344:1015, 1994. (Letter to the Editor)

Aspirin Use and the Risk for Colorectal Cancer and Adenoma in Male Health Professionals

Giovannucci E, Rimm EB, Stampfer MJ, Colditz GA, Ascherio A, Willett WC
(Harvard Med School, Boston; Brigham and Women's Hosp, Boston; Harvard School of Public Health, Boston)
Ann Intern Med 121:241–246, 1994   119-95-48–4

Objective.—The evidence to date that nonsteroidal anti-inflammatory drugs reduce the risk of colorectal cancer, and possibly other gastrointestinal tumors, remains inconclusive. A prospective cohort study was planned to examine this purported association.

Methods.—A total of 47,900 male health professionals throughout the United States, 40–75 years of age, responded to a questionnaire mailed to them in 1986. Nearly 60% of those eligible were dentists and 20% were veterinarians. Optometrists, osteopaths, podiatrists, and pharmacists formed the rest of the cohort. Questionnaires concerning cancer and the use of aspirin were again sent in 1988 and 1990.

Findings.—Two hundred fifty-one new diagnoses of colorectal cancer were made during the study period. The regular use of aspirin at least twice a week was associated with a risk ratio for colorectal cancer of .68 (table). The relative risk of metastatic or fatal colorectal cancer was .51. These risk estimates were observed after controlling for age, history of polyps, previous endoscopy, parental history of colorectal cancer, smoking, body mass, level of physical activity, and the intake of red meat, alcohol, and vitamin E. Men who were regular users of aspirin in 1986 continued to have a lower risk of colorectal cancer when followed to 1992, regardless of subsequent aspirin use. Excluding those having endoscopy for fecal blood, men who used aspirin were at lower risk of having a colorectal adenoma diagnosed.

Conclusion.—Men who use aspirin regularly over the long term may be at substantially lower risk of colorectal cancer developing. Further

Relative Risk for Colorectal Cancer in Subsequent Time Periods by Aspirin Use in 1986

Aspirin Use in 1986	Follow-up		
	1986 to 1987	1988 to 1989	1990 to 1992
Total colorectal cancer			
Age-adjusted RR (95% CI)	0.78 (0.46 to 1.32)	0.72 (0.51 to 1.02)	0.67 (0.41 to 1.08)
Advanced colorectal cancer*			
Age-adjusted RR (95% CI)	0.50 (0.21 to 1.22)	0.50 (0.27 to 0.91)	0.43 (0.18 to 1.04)
Fatal colorectal cancer			
Age-adjusted RR (95% CI)	0.42 (0.15 to 1.18)	0.57 (0.24 to 1.37)	0.18 (0.03 to 1.00)

Abbreviations: RR, relative risks; CI, confidence interval.
*Patients with advanced cancers are those with metastases at diagnosis plus fatal cases.
(Courtesy of Giovannucci E, Rimm EB, Stampfer MJ, et al: *Ann Intern Med* 121:241–246, 1994.)

work is needed to determine the effective dose of aspirin and how long it must be used.

▶ These findings support the hypothesis that long-term use of aspirin may decrease substantially the incidence of colorectal cancer. The interesting finding of a particularly strong inverse association between aspirin use and metastatic cancer led the authors to suggest that aspirin-related bleeding could further decrease mortality by leading to earlier diagnosis and treatment of cancers.

The findings of Giovannucci et al. are in accord with an earlier report that also noted a reduced risk of fatal colon cancer in aspirin users (1).—N.J. Greenberger, M.D.

Reference

1. Thun MJ, Namboodiri MM, Heath CW Jr: Aspirin use and reduced risk of fatal colon cancer. N Engl J Med 325:1593–1596, 1991.

Fecal Occult Blood Screening for Colorectal Cancer: Is Mortality Reduced by Chance Selection for Screening Colonoscopy?
Lang CA, Ransohoff DF (Univ of Colorado, Denver; Univ of North Carolina; Chapel Hill)
JAMA 271:1011–1013, 1994   119-95-48–5

Purpose.—On fecal occult blood testing (FOBT) to screen for colorectal cancer, rehydration of slides has been found to increase positivity rates fourfold, from about 2% to 3% to about 8% to 16%. In 1 extensive experience, over 38% of patients screened annually underwent colonoscopy on the basis of FOBT results. With so many patients selected, it has

Results: Projected Cumulative Rate of Colonoscopy After 15 Years of Screening

FOBT Positivity Rate, %	Compliance With FOBT Screening, %	Compliance With Colonoscopy After a Positive FOBT, %	Cumulative Rate of Colonoscopy, %
2	80	80	10.1
5	80	80	23.2
8	80	80	34.4
10 (base case)	80	80	40.8
15	80	80	54.1
10	70	70	33.2
10	80	80	40.8
10	90	90	48.3
10	100	100	55.4

Note: Fifteen years of screening is interrupted for a 4-year period.
(Courtesy of Lang CA, Ransohoff DF: JAMA 271:1011–1013, 1994.)

been suggested that some of the mortality reductions achieved may be attributable to chance, with false positive FOBT results leading to "screening" colonoscopy. To assess the impact of such a mechanism on the benefits of FOBT screening, a simple mathematical model was constructed to define the contribution of chance when FOBT with slide rehydration is performed annually.

Methods.—The model, which incorporated published data, followed the clinical course of a hypothetical cohort of patients followed for up to 15 years in an FOBT screening program. Colonoscopy was performed only for patients with a positive FOBT. The base case compliance rate was 80% and the base case positivity rate was 10%.

Results.—The analysis suggested that one third to one half of the mortality reduction benefit was attributable to false positive FOBT results or chance (table). If 50 million older Americans were to be screened, FOBT without rehydration would have a 2% positivity rate and result in 1 million colonoscopies per year. With rehydration, a total of 5 million colonoscopies, at $750 per procedure, would be performed, at an additional annual cost of $3 billion. The costs would be even higher if they included colonoscopic surveillance for patients discovered to have adenomatous polyps.

Conclusion.—Annual FOBT screening with rehydration appears to be a haphazard method of selecting asymptomatic patients for colonoscopic examination. In terms of mortality reduction for effort expended, large-scale screening programs might do better to perform 1 or 2 screening colonoscopies rather than relying on yearly FOBT with rehydration. These issues must be considered carefully before screening FOBT with rehydration is recommended.

▶ The authors' analysis supports their conclusions that FOBT with rehydration reduces colon cancer mortality both by detecting bleeding cancers and adenomas and by leading to colonoscopic detection of nonbleeding neoplasms by the mechanism of chance.

The benefits of screening sigmoidoscopy have now been shown convincingly in case-control studies (1, 2). Accordingly, current recommendations call for a flexible sigmoidoscopic examination to be done on all individuals over age 50 years and every 5–10 years thereafter. The following article (Abstract 119-95-48–6) further demonstrates the efficacy offlexible sigmoidoscopy in that less than 1% of patients whose only lesions at sigmoidoscopy were small (< 1 cm), tubular adenomas had an advanced lesion proximally. This would appear to obviate the need for colonoscopy in such patients.

Selby (3) has questioned the need for FOBT screening after flexible sigmoidoscopy if the latter examination is normal or if only small tubular adenomas are found. He cautions that adding annual FOBT screening in this setting would more than double the costs of colorectal cancer screening, primarily by generating colonoscopies, most of which would be for false positive FOBTs. Finally, Selby points out that if flexible sigmoidoscopy is a screen for proximal disease, it needs to be determined whether FOBT adds any information on the proximal colon to that obtained by sigmoidoscopy. Further studies are needed to clarify this issue.—N.J. Greenberger, M.D.

References

1. Selby JV, Friedman GD, Quessenberry CP Jr, et al: A case control study of screening sigmoidoscopy and mortality from colorectal cancer. *N Engl J Med* 326:653–657, 1992.
2. Newcomb PA, Narfleet RG, Surawicz TS, et al: Screening sigmoidoscopy and colorectal cancer mortality. *J Natl Cancer Inst* 84:1572–1575, 1992.
3. Selby JV: Targeting colonoscopy. *Gastroenterology* 106:1702–1704, 1994.

Do Characteristics of Adenomas on Flexible Sigmoidoscopy Predict Advanced Lesions on Baseline Colonoscopy?

Zarchy TM, Ershoff D (Mullikin Med Ctr, Los Angeles; Univ of California, Los Angeles)
Gastroenterology 106:1501–1504, 1994　　　　　119-95-48–6

Introduction.—Current practice recommends colonoscopy for all patients with sigmoidoscopic evidence of benign neoplasms. Previous studies have shown that more lesions are found with colonoscopy than with sigmoidoscopy, but there have been no reports on the relative severity of the findings. A prospective study was undertaken to assess whether the adenomas found at flexible sigmoidoscopy predicted similar or more advanced lesions at colonoscopy.

Likelihood of Advance Lesion at Colonoscopy, Based on Polyp Characteristics at Sigmoidoscopy

Polyp characteristics	Advanced lesion colonoscopy (%)	Odds ratio
Number of polyps		
1	4.7	2.51
2+	11.1	
Size of largest polyp		
≤1 cm	4.2	2.65
>1 cm	10.3	
Histology of polyp(s)		
Tubular only	1.4 *	9.71
Villous/severe dysplasia	12.5	
Size and histology of polyp(s)		
Tubular and ≤1 cm	0.8 *	16.40
Villous and/or >1 cm	11.8	

*P < .01.
(Courtesy of Zarchy TM, Ershoff D: *Gastroenterology* 106:1501–1504, 1994.)

Methods.—Benign neoplasms were found at flexible sigmoidoscopy in 226 symptomatic and asymptomatic patients. They underwent follow-up colonoscopy within 1 year after sigmoidoscopy. The numbers and sizes of the polyps found at each examination were compared. All polyps were removed and analyzed histologically.

Results.—Most of the polyps found at sigmoidoscopy were smaller than 1 cm, and over half were only tubular adenomas. Sigmoidoscopy detected advanced lesions in 45% of the patients and polyps characterized histologically by villous or severe dysplasia in 39% of the patients. There were 24% more new neoplasms found with colonoscopy but no new cancer cases. Colonoscopy revealed advanced lesions not seen on sigmoidoscopy in only 6% of the patients. Sigmoidoscopic evidence of an advanced lesion or of polyps with villous or severe dysplasia significantly predicted colonoscopic findings of an advanced lesion (table). Conversely, there was a less than 1% likelihood of a colonoscopic finding of advanced lesions in patients without such findings at sigmoidoscopy. An advanced lesion was found in only 1 of 124 patients with a sigmoidoscopic finding of only small tubular adenoma.

Discussion.—These findings indicate that sigmoidoscopic findings regarding the size and histologic features of neoplasms predict subsequent colonoscopic findings. The routine recommendation of colonoscopy for all patients with any adenoma found at sigmoidoscopy should be reconsidered, particularly in patients with only small tubular adenoma.

▶ This paper demonstrates that small tubular adenomas, when discovered at sigmoidoscopy, are not markers for more severe or advanced lesions proximally. Advanced lesions were defined as neoplasms with villous or severe dysplasia histology and/or > 1 cm in diameter. The key observation was that less than 1% of patients whose only lesions at sigmoidoscopy were small tubular adenomas had an advanced lesion proximally. Grossman et al. (1) have reported similar findings documenting that 3% of persons with a single small tubular adenoma identified by rigid sigmoidoscopy and a negative family history of colorectal cancer had advanced lesions at colonoscopy. This slightly higher prevalence may be the result of performing rigid rather than 60-cm flexible sigmoidoscopic examinations. For an excellent brief review of this subject, see the editorial by Selby (2). As he points out, taken together, these studies indicate that a screening sigmoidoscopic program can be designed so that the colonoscopies generated are reduced in number and targeted to individuals who are most likely to benefit from them.—N.J. Greenberger, M.D.

References

1. Grossman S, Milos ML, Tekawa IS: Colonoscopic screening of persons with suspected risk factors for colon cancer: II. Past history of colorectal neoplasms. *Gastroenterology* 96:299–306, 1989.
2. Selby JV: Targeting colonoscopy. *Gastroenterology* 106:1702–1704, 1994.

Allelic Loss of Chromosome 18q and Prognosis in Colorectal Cancer

Jen J, Kim H, Piantadosi S, Liu Z-F, Levitt RC, Sistonen P, Kinzler KW, Vogelstein B, Hamilton SR (Johns Hopkins Univ, Baltimore, Md; Finnish Red Cross Blood Transfusion Service, Helsinki)

N Engl J Med 331:213–221, 1994   119-95-48–7

Background.—Determining prognosis and selecting patients with colorectal cancer for postoperative adjuvant treatment currently depend on pathologic and clinical staging. Chromosome 18q loss is a genetic event associated with tumor progression. The value of 18q allelic loss as a prognostic marker for colorectal cancer was studied.

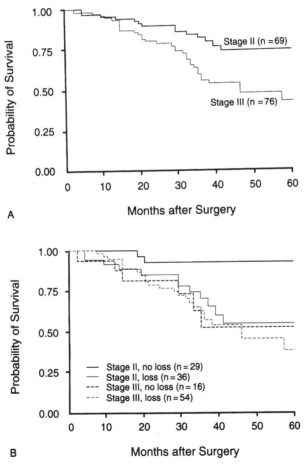

Fig 48–3.—Overall survival of patients with colorectal cancer, according to TNM stage alone (**A**) and both TNM stage and chromosome 18q allelic loss (**B**). (Courtesy of Jen J, Kim H, Piantadosi S, et al: *N Engl J Med* 331:213–221, 1994.)

Methods.—One hundred forty-five consecutively resected stage II or III colorectal carcinomas, formalin-fixed and paraffin-embedded, were studied. The status of chromosome 18q was examined with microsatellite markers and DNA from the tumors.

Findings.—Patients with stage II cancer and no evidence of allelic loss of chromosome 18q had a 5-year survival rate of 93%, compared with 54% of patients with stage II disease and allelic loss. Among patients with stage III disease, survival rates were 38% and 52% in those with and without allelic loss, respectively, In a univariate analysis, patients with chromosome 18q allelic loss had a 2.83 overall estimated hazard ratio for death. Chromosome 18q allelic loss remained a strong predictor after adjustments for tumor differentiation, vein invasion, and TNM stage (Fig 48-3).

Conclusion.—In patients with stage II colorectal cancer, the status of chromosome 18q has strong prognostic value. Patients with stage II disease and allelic loss have a prognosis similar to that of patients with stage III cancer, who may benefit from adjuvant treatment. Patients with stage II disease and no chromosome 18q allelic loss have a survival rate comparable to that of patients with stage I disease and may not need additional treatment.

▶ This study demonstrates that chromosome 18q allelic loss, is an important prognostic marker in patients with stage II colorectal cancer. The 5-year survival rate among patients with stage II disease and intact chromosome 18q was very good (93%), whereas in patients with chromosome 18q allelic loss, it was more comparable (54%) to the rate in patients with stage III disease (42%).

For an excellent brief review on this subject, see the editorial by Tempero and Anderson (1).—N.J. Greenberger, M.D.

Reference

1. Tempero M, Anderson J: Progress in colon cancer: Do molecular markers matter? *N Engl J Med* 331:267–268, 1994.

Benign Anal Lesions and the Risk of Anal Cancer
Frisch M, Olsen JH, Bautz A, Melbye M (Danish Epidemiology Science Ctr, Copenhagen; Danish Cancer Society, Copenhagen)
N Engl J Med 331:300–302, 1994   119-95-48-8

Introduction.—Inflammation from benign anal lesions, including hemorrhoids and anal fistulae, has long been considered to predispose to anal cancer. A recent review concluded that there was a causal association between benign anal disease and anal cancer. This association was reexamined in linkage of Danish national data on hospital discharge and cancer.

Relative Risk of Anal or Colorectal Cancer After Hospitalization for a Benign Anal Lesion, According to Sex and Age

INTERVAL FROM BENIGN LESION TO CANCER (YR)	CASES OF ANAL CANCER			CASES OF COLORECTAL CANCER		
	NO. OBSERVED	NO. EXPECTED	RR (95% CI)	NO. OBSERVED	NO. EXPECTED	RR (95% CI)
Men						
<1	3	0.29	10.4 (2.1–30.5)	63	27.14	2.3 (1.8–3.0)
1–4	4	1.01	4.0 (1.1–10.1)	109	95.16	1.1 (0.9–1.4)
5–13	2	0.89	2.3 (0.3–8.1)	85	86.06	1.0 (0.8–1.2)
Total (0–13)	9	2.19	4.1 (1.9–7.8)	257	208.37	1.2 (1.1–1.4)
Women						
<1	5	0.38	13.2 (4.2–30.7)	50	16.24	3.1 (2.3–4.1)
1–4	7	1.37	5.1 (2.0–10.5)	66	57.60	1.1 (0.9–1.5)
5–13	2	1.30	1.5 (0.2–5.6)	43	52.48	0.8 (0.6–1.1)
Total (0–13)	14	3.05	4.6 (2.5–7.7)	159	126.32	1.3 (1.1–1.5)
All subjects <60 yr†						
<1	4	0.30	13.3 (3.6–34.1)	32	11.03	2.9 (2.0–4.1)
1–4	5	1.24	4.0 (1.3–9.4)	63	48.99	1.3 (1.0–1.6)
5–13	3	1.42	2.1 (0.4–6.2)	66	65.36	1.0 (0.8–1.3)
All subjects ≥60 yr†						
<1	4	0.37	10.9 (2.9–27.9)	81	32.35	2.5 (2.0–3.1)
1–4	6	1.15	5.2 (1.9–11.4)	112	103.76	1.1 (0.9–1.3)
5–13	1	0.77	1.3 (0.0–7.3)	62	73.19	0.8 (0.6–1.1)
Total sample						
0–13	23	5.25	4.4 (2.8–6.6)	416	334.68	1.2 (1.1–1.4)

Abbreviations: RR, relative risk; CI, confidence interval.
Note: Benign anal lesions included fissures, fistulas, perianal or perirectal abscesses, and hemorrhoids.
†Age at the time of the first hospitalization for a benign anal lesion.
(Courtesy of Frisch M, Olsen JH, Bautz A, et al: *N Engl J Med* 331:300–302, 1994.)

Methods.—The analysis included 68,549 patients hospitalized with benign anal lesions between 1977 and 1989. The data on these patients were linked to the Danish Cancer Registry to identify all incident cases of epidermoid anal cancer. Eighty-nine percent of the sample were followed through the end of 1989 and 11% until death, for a median follow-up of over 6 years.

Results.—Twenty-three patients had epidermoid anal cancers and 416 had colorectal cancers. The relative risk of anal cancer, based on observed vs. expected cases, was 4.4 overall, 12 in the first year after hospitalization for benign anal lesions, 4.6 from 1 to 4 years, and 1.8 five or more years after hospitalization. The relative risk of colorectal cancer was 2.6 in the first year after hospitalization; this was the only period during which risk was significantly increased (table).

Conclusion.—A strong temporal association between the diagnosis of benign anal lesions and the diagnosis of anal cancer is apparent. However, the evidence does not support the theory that anal inflammation predisposes to epidermoid anal cancer. When presumably benign lesions are identified before anal cancer, they are probably the initial manifestations of an undetected cancer. A moderate increase in long-term risk of anal cancer, however, cannot be excluded.

▶ Recent studies (1, 2) from several countries have indicated that there have been significant increases in the incidence of epidermoid anal carcinoma. The increase has been more pronounced in women, urban dwellers, blacks, and never-married men (2). To illustrate, the incidence of anal cancer observed for white men in the San Francisco Bay area increased from 0.5/100,000 in 1973–1975 to 1.2/100,000 in 1988–1989. Further, these studies suggest that homosexual men are at special and increasing risk.

A study by Melbye et al. (2) established a strikingly increased relative risk of anal cancer among people with AIDS. Although the absolute risk of anal cancer in this group of homosexual men was about 1 per 1,000 cases, it bears emphasizing that anal dysplasia (including carcinoma in situ) may occur in up to 15% of severely immunosuppressed HIV-infected homosexual men without signs or symptoms of anal cancer. However, whether screening for anal dysplasia in such symptom-free individuals will be effective remains an open question.—N.J. Greenberger, M.D.

References

1. Melbye M, Rabin C, Frisch M, et al: Changing patterns of anal cancer incidence in the United States, 1940–1989. *Am J Epidemiol* 139:772–780, 1994.
2. Melbye M, Cote TR, Kessler L, et al: High incidence of anal cancer among AIDS patients. *Lancet* 343:636–639, 1994.

Improving Adjuvant Therapy for Rectal Cancer by Combining Protracted-Infusion Fluorouracil With Radiation Therapy After Curative Surgery
O'Connell MJ, Martenson JA, Wieand HS, Krook JE, MacDonald JS, Haller DG, Mayer RJ, Gunderson LL, Rich TA (Mayo Clinic and Found, Rochester, Minn; Temple Univ, Philadelphia; Univ of Pennsylvania, Philadelphia; et al)
N Engl J Med 331:502–507, 1994   119-95-48-9

Background.—Although rectal cancer is often diagnosed at a stage when complete resection is possible, only half the patients treated surgically are cured. Research has suggested that the combination of postoperative chemotherapy and radiation improves local tumor control and survival in stages II and III rectal cancer. The efficacy of protracted venous infusion of fluorouracil throughout the irradiation of the pelvis was compared with that of conventional bolus administration of fluorouracil. Continuous infusion was intended to prolong noncycling tumor cell exposure to fluorouracil.

Methods.—Six hundred sixty patients with TNM stage II or III rectal cancer were given intermittent bolus injections or protracted venous infusions of fluorouracil during postoperative radiation to the pelvis. Sys-

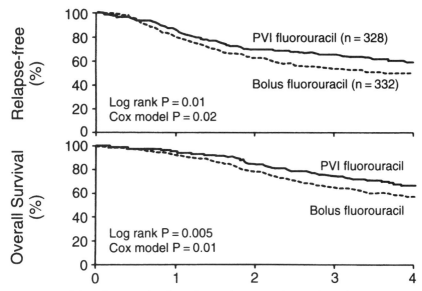

Fig 48–4.—Relapse-free interval and overall survival among patients with rectal cancer receiving fluorouracil by protracted venous infusion *(PVI)* or bolus injection during radiation. (Courtesy of O'Connell MJ, Martenson JA, Wieand HS, et al: N Engl J Med 331:502–507, 1994.)

temic chemotherapy with semustine plus fluorouracil or higher-dose fluorouracil alone was also administered before and after pelvic irradiation. The median follow-up was 46 months.

Findings.—Patients given a protracted infusion of fluorouracil had a significantly increased time to relapse and improved survival. No benefical effect was found in patients given semustine plus fluorouracil (Fig 48–4).

Conclusion.—Protracted infusion of fluorouracil during pelvic irradiation improved the effect of combined-treatment postoperative adjuvant therapy in patients with high-risk rectal cancer. Semustine plus fluorouracil was no more beneficial than higher-dose fluorouracil given alone.

▶ Rectal cancer is a common malignant disease in the United States, with an estimated 43,000 new cases in 1993. The risk of relapse and death is increased if the carcinoma has penetrated through the rectal wall (TNM stage II) or spread to regional lymph nodes (TNM stage III). The data provided by O'Connell et al. indicate that patients who had a protracted infusion of fluorouracil had a significantly increased time to relapse and improved survival. As the authors point out, more effective control of occult distant metastases remains the principal challenge in the curative treatment of rectal carcinoma.—N.J. Greenberger, M.D.

Antidepressant Therapy in 138 Patients With Irritable Bowel Syndrome: A Five-Year Clinical Experience

Clouse RE, Lustman PJ, Geisman RA, Alpers DH (Washington Univ, St Louis, Mo)

Aliment Pharmacol Ther 8:409–416, 1994   1 1 9-95-48–10

Objective.—Antidepressant drugs have long been used in the treatment of irritable bowel syndrome (IBS), but their efficacy remains unproven. The symptoms of IBS could be influenced by a number of specific and nonspecific properties of antidepressant agents, independent of their direct central actions against depression. Toward identification of important factors for the design of prospective trials, a 5-year clinical experience with antidepressant drugs in the outpatient treatment of IBS was reported.

Patients.—The review included 138 patients attending a university-based gastroenterology practice. The median age was 47 years, and 67% of the patients were female. The predominant symptom pattern was diarrhea in 42% of patients, constipation in 38%, and pain in 20%. Fifty-three percent of patients had identified psychiatric features. Fifty-seven

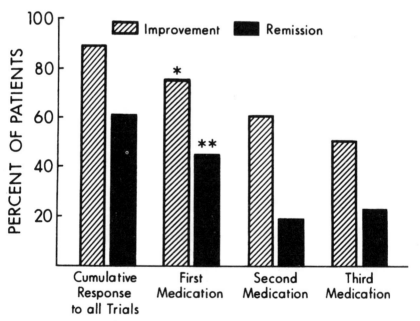

Fig 48–5.—Percentage of the 138 patients who were assessed as having improvement or complete remission of IBS symptoms during antidepressant treatment. (Improvement includes those who attained remission.) Cumulative response during all trials and during each of the first through third trials is shown. The improvement and remission rates decreased significantly after the first medication trial. *P <0.05 compared with the third trial. **P <0.01 compared with the second and third trials. (Courtesy of Clouse RE, Lustman PJ, Geisman RA, et al: *Aliment Pharmacol Ther* 8:409-416, 1994.)

percent received a single antidepressant; 18% were treated with 2 and 25% with 3 or more drugs consecutively. The antidepressants used were tricyclic antidepressants in 130 patients, newer antidepressants in 39, and anxiolytic antidepressants in 47.

Outcomes.—Eighty-nine percent of patients achieved improvement in their bowel symptoms, and 61% achieved complete remission. The median prescribed dosages in patients going into remission were less than those used in clinical psychiatry. The only clinical factor associated with remission of symptoms was a pain-predominant symptom pattern (Fig 48–5). Symptom remission was most likely to occur with the first antidepressant tried, although nearly half the patients who discontinued 1 drug achieved remission with an alternative antidepressant.

Conclusion.—An experience with antidepressant drug treatment for IBS is reviewed. Patients with a pain-predominant symptom pattern have the highest response rates. The drugs are effective in a low-dose range, and the presence of psychiatric symptoms does not affect outcome. The findings underscore the emerging recognition of visceral afferent mechanisms in functional gastrointestinal disorders, and refute the previous suggestion that anticholinergic activity is the sole mediator of beneficial antidepressant effects in IBS.

▶ I selected this article for inclusion in the 1995 YEAR BOOK OF MEDICINE for 2 reasons. First, an appreciable number of patients with (IBS) and a pain-predominant symptom pattern achieved a complete remission of symptoms with administration of 1 or 2 antidepressant medications. Second, the findings underscore the emerging recognition of the importance of visceral afferent mechanisms in functional gastrointestinal disorders such as IBS. The reader is referred to 2 articles (1, 2) that discuss the different mechanisms that, alone or in combination, may be responsible for the apparent *visceral hyperalgesia* observed in the great majority of patients with functional bowel disorders.—N.J. Greenberger, M.D.

References

1. Mayer EA, Gebhardt GF: Basic and clinical aspects of visceral hyperalgesia. *Gastroenterology* 107:271–293, 1994.
2. Camilleri M, Ford MJ: Functional gastrointestinal disease and the autonomic nervous system: A way ahead? *Gastroenterology* 106:1114–1117, 1994.

49 Liver

A Long-Term Follow-Up Study of Asymptomatic Hepatitis B Surface Antigen—Positive Carriers in Montreal
Villeneuve J-P, Desrochers M, Infante-Rivard C, Willems B, Raymond G, Bourcier M, Côté J, Richer G (Hôpital Saint-Luc, Montreal; Université de Montréal; McGill Univ, Montreal)
Gastroenterology 106:1000–1005, 1994   119-95-49–1

Objective.—Several studies from Taiwan, Japan, and Alaska have demonstrated an increased morbidity and mortality from liver disease among

Descriptive Features of the Cohort After 16 Years of Follow-Up

	Initial HBeAg status		
Initial HBeAg status Patients	anti-HBe–positive (n = 200)	HBeAg-negative, anti-HBe–negative (n = 7)	HBeAg-positive (n = 11)
Age (yr)[a]	46 ± 8	49 ± 8	47 ± 8
HBeAg status[b]			
anti-HBe–positive	198 (99.0%)	6 (86%)	10 (91%)
HBeAg-negative/ anti-HBe–negative	1 (0.5%)	1 (14%)	0 (0%)
HBeAg-positive	1 (0.5%)	0 (0%)	1 (9%)
HBsAg status[b]			
Positive	182 (91%)	6 (86%)	5 (45%)[c]
Negative	18 (9%)	1 (14%)	6 (55%)[c]
Serum AST-ALT[b]			
<40 IU/L	172 (86%)	5 (72%)	9 (82%)
40–100 IU/L	24 (12%)	2 (28%)	1 (9%)
>100 IU/L	4 (2%)	0 (0%)	1 (9%)
anti-HDV–positive[b]	1 (0.5%)	0	0
anti-HCV–positive[b]	1 (0.5%)	0	0

[a] Data include 218 cases with visit to the clinic.
[b] Data expressed as mean ±standard deviation.
[c] Data expressed as number of carriers with characteristic (percentage within group).
$P < 0.05$ compared with the anti–HBe-positive group.
(Courtesy of Villeneuve J-P, Desrochers M, Infante-Rivard C, et al: *Gastroenterology* 106:1000–1005, 1994.)

asymptomatic long-term carriers of hepatitis B virus (HBV). However, the magnitude of this risk in Western countries is unclear. The long-term outcome of apparently healthy Canadian hepatitis B surface antigen (HBsAg)-positive carriers was assessed.

Methods.—The analysis included 340 asymptomatic subjects who were identified as being HBsAg-positive by the Montreal Red Cross when they volunteered to donate blood, as well as 29 asymptomatic contacts of these subjects who were also HBsAg-positive. Sixteen years later, complete follow-up was achieved in 317 carriers; the mean age at this time was 46 years. Follow-up included a physician interview and examination and blood testing.

Results.—Most of the subjects were of French Canadian origin. Eighty-nine percent were positive for antibody to hepatitis B e antigen and negative for the antigen itself. Most had normal serum transaminase levels. The most important epidemiologic risk factor was institutionalization in an orphanage as an infant or child, indicating horizontal transmission of HBV during childhood. There were 13 deaths during follow-up: 3 of HBV-related cirrhosis, 1 of alcoholic cirrhosis, and 9 of causes unrelated to liver disease. There were no deaths resulting from hepatocellular carcinoma; had the risk of hepatocellular carcinoma been similar to that reported in the Far East and Alaska studies, 17 patients would have been expected to die of hepatocellular carcinoma. Eighteen subjects became HBsAg-negative during follow-up, for an annual negativation rate of .5% (table).

Conclusion.—Long-term follow-up of a cohort of asymptomatic North American HBV carriers suggests that most remain asymptomatic. There is a low risk of death resulting from HBV-related cirrhosis and/or hepatocellular carcinoma; the latter finding is at variance with the results of previous studies from the Far East and Alaska. Follow-up will continue in the relatively young study cohort.

▶ The finding by Villeneuve and colleagues that HBsAg carriers with normal liver tests have an excellent prognosis is supported by another recent study. (1) De Franchis et al. (1) followed 92 HbsAg-positive blood donors with normal liver tests for a mean of 130 months. At baseline, liver biopsy specimens showed normal findings or mild abnormalities in about 69 subjects, chronic persistent hepatitis in 18, and mild chronic active hepatitis in 5. Of 68 evaluable patients at follow-up, liver enzyme levels remained normal in 56 (85%), sustained elevation in serum aminotransferase levels were documented in 3 (4%), and in only 1 patient was there histologic deterioration to chronic active hepatitis. One patient had developed alcoholic cirrhosis. Ten patients had loss of HBsAg. Twenty-one patients with no biochemical change at follow-up consented to have repeat liver biopsy specimen taken, and none had histologic changes. In contrast to reports from Taiwan on the increased risk of HBsAg carriers developing hepatoma after 10–30 years, no patient had developed hepatocellular carcinoma. It should be noted, however, that the mean follow-up in the study by de Franchis et al. was only 11 years.—N.J. Greenberger, M.D.

Reference

1. de Franchis R, Meucchi G, Vecchi M: The natural history of asymptomatic hepatitis B surface antigen carriers. *Ann Intern Med* 118:191–194, 1993.

Hepatitis B Virus Persistence After Recovery From Acute Viral Hepatitis

Michalak TI, Pasquinelli C, Guilhot S, Chisari FV (Scripps Research Inst, La Jolla, Calif)

J Clin Invest 93:230–239, 1994   119-95-49–2

Background.—Most physicians consider that the disappearance of hepatitis B surface antigen (HBsAg) from serum, the development of anti-HBs antibodies and the normalization of liver function constitute complete virologic recovery from hepatitis B virus (HBV) infection. However, because HBV DNA can persist in the serum and liver long afterward, viral DNA may not be completely eradicated at the time of clinical, biochemical, and serologic recovery.

Methods.—The polymerase chain reaction was used to determine whether HBV persists in the circulation after serologic and clinical recovery. The serum and peripheral blood mononuclear cells (PBMCs) of 4 patients with a history of self-limited acute hepatitis B were examined.

Results.—Hepatitis B virus DNA persisted in the serum and PBMCs for up to 70 months after apparent complete recovery. The results indicated co-sedimentation of serum HBV DNA with HBsAg in sucrose gradients, with the DNA having the size and density of naked core particles and intact HBV virions, presumably contained within circulating immune complexes. Levels of HBV DNA did not decrease dramatically from the earliest to the last samples. Late convalescent samples from all 4 patients also showed HBV DNA in PBMCs, whereas 2 samples showed HBV RNA.

Conclusion.—It is suggested that HBV DNA, and perhaps even HBV virions, can persist in serum long after clinical and biochemical recovery. The viral genome may be able to persist in a transcriptionally active form in PBMCs for more than 5 years after apparent complete recovery. These findings may have important epidemiologic and pathogenetic implications, especially if the HBV DNA-containing particles are infectious.

▶ These results suggest that HBV DNA and possibly HBV viremia can be present in the serum and that the viral genome can persist as a transcriptionally active form in PBMCs for longer than 5 years after complete clinical and serologic recovery from acute hepatitis B. These findings are reminiscent of similar results reported in patients with hepatitis C in whom persistence of hepatitis viral RNA (HCV-RNA) was demonstrated as long as 15 years after a full recovery from hepatitis C. The risk of contracting viral hepatitis from asymptomatic patients with persistence of HBV DNA and HCV RNA remains incompletely defined. The much greater infectivity of HBV vs. HCV virions is recognized. It is likely, however, that the blood titer of HCV RNA and HBV DNA, as well as strain differences, may be additive factors that influence the likelihood of transmission of the infection.—N.J. Greenberger, M.D.

Hepatitis C Virus Infection in Spouses of Patients With Type C Chronic Liver Disease

Akahane Y, Kojima M, Sugai Y, Sakamoto M, Miyazaki Y, Tanaka T, Tsuda F, Mishiro S, Okamoto H, Miyakawa Y, Mayumi M (Yamanashi Med College, Japan; Iwaki Kyoritsu Gen Hosp, Japan; Japanese Red Cross Saitama Blood Ctr, Japan; et al)
Ann Intern Med 120:748–752, 1994   119-95-49-3

Introduction.—A defined parenteral exposure accounts for only half the reported cases of acute infection with the hepatitis C virus (HCV). Previous studies of sexual transmission of HCV have been done in settings where sexual contact was transient or in spouses married for a relatively short time. The risk for long-term spouses of patients with HCV-related chronic liver disease was studied.

Methods.—Male and female spouses of 154 patients with HCV viremia and chronic hepatitis, cirrhosis, or hepatocarcinoma completed questionnaires and underwent testing for HCV-associated antibodies. Second-generation enzyme immunoassay and assays with oligopeptides deduced from the HCV core gene were used. Hepatitis C virus RNA was detected by polymerase chain reaction.

Results.—Anti-HCV detected by enzyme immunoassay-II, anti-CP9 or anti CP10 was detected in 42 of the spouses (27%). Of these, 25 (16%) were also positive for HCV RNA. Two of the spouses without HCV-associated antibodies (2%) were also positive for HCV RNA. Among spouses with HCV RNA, 89% were infected with HCV genotypes identical to those of their spouses. In the group infected with the identical genotype to the spouse, 8 had previously noted liver disease and 2 more were found to have elevated transaminase levels and chronic hepatitis. The prevalence of HCV antibodies paralleled duration of marriage. No markers were found in spouses married for less than 10 years. In those married for less than 30 years, 9% had markers, for those married 30 years or longer, 24% were positive, and marriage for more than 50 years yielded 60% of spouses with markers for HCV.

Discussion.—Although discordance of HCV genotypes may disprove infection from a suspected source, concordance does not necessarily prove it. However, in a group of other spouses with known additional risk factors, the concordance rate was only 25%. The increased prevalence of HCV markers in those married for longer periods along with the lack of other risk factors in this group favors the possible transmission of HCV from patient to spouse. Although the length of the marriage is known, the actual exposure time is not known in this study, as the duration of HCV infection in the index patients was not determined. Prospective studies are indicated to examine this issue. The results of recent investigations, which found substantial evidence for heterosexual transmission of HCV, are corroborated. Many HCV-infected people have normal aminotransferase levels. Liver biopsies were not performed on those with normal aminotransferase levels. Therefore, some silent HCV-associated liver disease may have been missed among the infected spouses. Spouses of persons with demonstrable anti-HCV are at increasing risk over time of HCV infection. They should be screened at regular intervals to receive prompt care when indicated.

▶ Several studies have indicated that up to 50% of patients with hepatitis C have no defined parenteral exposure. This has prompted detailed investigations to determine the extent to which HCV can be transmitted sexually. Most studies have suggested that HCV is transmitted sexually only infrequently, the range being 0% to 5%. However, the risk may vary considerably depending on the HCV RNA titer in the infected individual, the HCV genotype, and the duration of exposure. In a study of 50 sexual partners of HCV-infected individuals, none of the partners were found to have evidence of HCV infection. (1) The author of this study ascribed this to low HCV RNA levels in the hepatitis C index individuals.

In contrast, the studies by Akahane et al. clearly document that spouses of patients with HCV viremia *and* chronic liver disease have an increased risk of acquiring HCV that is proportional to the duration of the exposure. That 16% of the spouses were positive for both HCV antibodies and HCV RNA indicates that the risk may be higher than previously believed. Finally, I should mention a recent study (2) that demonstrated that the incidence of spousal transmission after liver transplantation remains low (5%) and similar to chronic causes of HCV.—N.J. Greenberger, M.D.

References

1. Bresters D, Mauser-Brunschoten ER, Riseink HW: Sexual transmission of hepatitis C virus. *Lancet* 342:210–211, 1993.
2. McCashland TM, Wright TL, Donovan JP, et al: Spousal transmission of hepatitis C after liver transplantation. *Hepatology* 20:134A, 1994 (Abstract)

Transmission of Hepatitis C Virus From Mothers to Infants

Ohto H, Terazawa S, Sasaki N, Sasaki N, Hino K, Ishiwata C, Kako M, Ujiie N, Endo C, Matsui A, Okamoto H, Mishiro S, and the Vertical Transmission of Hepatitis C Virus Collaborative Study Group (Fukushima Med College, Japan; Gifu Kouseiren Gihoku Hosp, Japan; Jichi Med School, Tochigi, Japan; et al)
N Engl J Med 330:744–750, 1994   119-95-49-4

Background.—Although cases of vertical transmission of hepatitis C virus (HCV) have been reported in the literature, it is not known to what extent infected mothers transmit the virus to their infants. The transmission of HCV from infected mothers to their infants was investigated by analyzing HCV RNA in the blood.

Methods.—Three studies were performed independently. In the first, 53 of 7,698 parturient women tested for anti-HCV antibodies were found to be positive. Their 54 infants were then followed for 6 months or more and tested for HCV infection. In the second study, the infants of 6 women with known HCV disease were investigated prospectively. In the third study, the families of 3 HCV-infected infants were assessed retrospectively.

Findings.—Thirty-one of the 53 antibody-positive mothers were also found to be positive for serum HCV RNA. Three of the infants of these mothers, or 5.6%, became positive for HCV RNA during follow-up. None of the infants of women who were antibody-positive but HCV RNA–negative became positive for HCV RNA. The results of the second study showed that 1 of the 6 infants of infected mothers was HCV RNA–positive. In the third study, HCV RNA was found in the mothers of the 3 HCV-infected infants. In the 7 infected infants, the genomic sequence of HCV was nearly identical to that of the mother. These 7 mothers had significantly higher titers of HCV RNA than the mothers of infants with no evidence of infection.

Conclusion.—Hepatitis C virus is transmitted vertically from mother to infant. The risk of transmission is associated with the titer of HCV RNA in the mother.

▶ This study clearly demonstrates that HCV is vertically transmitted from mother to infant and the overall risk of transmission is approximately 6%. The risk of transmission is higher in mothers with higher HCV RNA titers and those with chronic liver disease. However, the latter may reflect the link between more advanced liver disease and higher circulating HCV RNA titers. Whether certain HCV genotypes are associated with increased risk of transmission remains an open question.—N.J. Greenberger, M.D.

Continuous Versus Intermittent Therapy for Chronic Hepatitis C With Recombinant Interferon Alfa-2a

Negro F, Baldi M, Mondardini A, Leandro G, Chaneac M, Manzini P, Abate

ML, Zahm F, Dastoli G, Ballaré M, Ryff J-C, Verme G, Bonino F (Ospedale Molinette, Torino, Italy; IRCCS De Bellis, Castellana Grotte, Italy; Hoffmann-La Roche, Basel, Switzerland; et al)
Gastroenterology 107:479–485, 1994   119-95-49–5

Introduction.—Although hepatitis C may remain asymptomatic, in approximately 10% to 25% of patients, it will progress toward fatal liver cirrhosis or carcinoma. The response rate to long-term interferon therapy has been high but the drug is poorly tolerated, and drug resistance may develop, with relapse after discontinuance. The efficacy of intermittent interferon therapy was compared with that of continuous treatment in patients with chronic hepatitis C.

Methods.—Of 135 patients with chronic hepatitis C, 69 were randomly assigned to receive two 3-month cycles of interferon-α-2a separated by 6 months, and 66 were assigned to receive continuous interferon-α-2a treatment for 9 months. Serum alanine aminotransferase levels were monitored to measure treatment efficacy at the end of each cycle, at the end of treatment, and at monthly follow-ups for 6 months after the end of treatment. Drug resistance was monitored through measurement of serum anti-interferon antibodies.

Results.—Of the original 135 patients, 114 completed the treatment regimen and follow-up (54, continuous therapy; 60, intermittent therapy). Complete response was realized in 46.3% of the continuous therapy group and 45% of the intermittent therapy group, whereas 22.2% of the continuous therapy group and 16.7% of the intermittent therapy group had a partial response. By the 6-month follow-up, 16.7% of the continuous therapy group and 10.1% of the intermittent therapy group

Characteristics of Response to Interferon Alfa-2a		
	Group 1	Group 2
Total no. of patients	66	69
Drop-outs	12 (1 bt)	9
Completing therapy and follow-up	54	60
Nonresponders	17 (31.5%) (3 bt)	23 (38.3%) (6 bt)
Complete responders at EOT	25 (46.3%)	27 (45%)
Partial responders at EOT	12 (22.2%) (6 bt)	10 (16.7%)
Relapsers (% of responders)	26 (70.3%)	31 (81.6%)
Sustained responders vs. all patients included	11 (16.7%)	7 (10.1%)

Abbreviations: bt, breakthrough; *EOT*, end of therapy.
(Courtesy of Negro F, Baldi M, Mondardini A, et al: *Gastroenterology* 107:479–485, 1994.)

had maintained a sustained response (table). Serum anti-interferon antibodies were evident in 1 of 7 and in 6 of 6 complete responders who relapsed during continuous and intermittent therapy, respectively.

Discussion.—Intermittent therapy with interferon-α-2a was effective in treating patients with chronic hepatitis C. Intermittent therapy is a more attractive option because of the high cost, poor tolerance, and development of drug resistance associated with long-term interferon therapy. All the patients receiving intermittent therapy who experienced breakthrough relapse had interferon-neutralizing antibodies, but continuous treatment was associated with other, more complex drug resistance mechanisms.

▶ Several papers presented at the 1994 meeting of the American Association for the Study of Liver Diseases dealt with the influence of the dose and duration of interferon treatment on the response to interferon therapy (1–3). Marcellin et al. (1) carried out a retrospective study suggesting that a 12-month course of interferon therapy is more effective than a 6-month course in patients with chronic hepatitis C with a hepatitis C virus genotype other than 1B. Ascione and colleagues (2) reported that the long-term response to interferon occurred significantly more frequently in patients receiving 6 million units 3 times weekly for 1 year compared to those receiving 3 million units 3 times weekly. Marcelles and colleagues (3) reported that in patients with chronic hepatitis C without cirrhosis, prolonging interferon therapy seemed to be useful only in those patients who had responded within the first 8 weeks of therapy.—N.J. Greenberger, M.D.

References

1. Marcellin P, Casteenan P, Milotava V: Influence of the dose and the duration of interferon treatment on the response to therapy according to HCV genotype in chronic hepatitis C. *Hepatology* 20:155A, 1994. (Abstract)
2. Ascione A, DeLuca M, Canestrini C, et al: Three versus six mm interferon (IFN) α26 in the therapy of HCV-related chronic liver disease: Randomized multicenter study. *Hepatology* 20:155A, 1994. (Abstract)
3. Marcelles P, Pauteau M, Boya N: Usefulness of prolonging interferon therapy according to the initial response in patients with chronic hepatitis C without cirrhosis. *Hepatology* 20:154A, 1994. (Abstract)

The Role of Hepatitis C Virus in Fulminant Viral Hepatitis in an Area With Endemic Hepatitis A and B

Chu C-M, Sheen I-S, Liaw Y-F (Chang Gung Mem Hosp, Taipei, Taiwan; Chang Gung Medical College, Taipei, Taiwan)
Gastroenterology 107:189–195, 1994   119-95-49–6

Background.—The many causes of acute liver failure include hepatotropic viruses, all of which have been associated with fulminant viral hepatitis, the most common form of acute liver failure worldwide. The hepatitis C virus (HCV) has been identified as a major etiologic agent in some forms of non-A and non-B hepatitis, and its role in fulminant hepatitis was investigated in Taiwan.

Methods.—During a 3-year period, 62 patients from Taiwan with fulminant viral hepatitis were studied retrospectively. None of the patients had preexisting liver conditions. Serologic markers of HCV were studied.

Results.—Of 62 patients, 5 had acute type B hepatitis and 11 had acute non-A, non-B hepatitis. The other 46 patients were positive for hepatitis B surface antigen, but negative for IgM antibody to hepatitis B core antigen. Of these 46, 11 were positive for IgM antibody to hepatitis D virus; 16 of 46 had high titered serum hepatitis B virus DNA and were suspected of having acute reactivation of hepatitis B virus; 19 of 46 had acute hepatitis of undetermined cause. Serum HCV RNA was positive in 5 of 11 patients with fulminant non-A, non-B hepatitis, and in 9 of 46 patients who were positive for hepatitis B surface antigen.

Conclusion.—In Taiwan, about 50% of cases of fulminant non-A, non-B hepatitis and about 20% of instances of hepatitis B surface antigen carriers with superimposed fulminant hepatitis could be attributed to HCV infection.

▶ The prevalence of HCV in fulminant hepatitis in Western countries appears to be very low. This study is one of the first to document a role for hepatitis C in fulminant viral hepatitis. Chia-Ming Chu and colleagues have demonstrated that nearly half of fulminant non-A, non-B hepatitis and about 20% of hepatitis B surface antigen carriers with superimposed fulminant hepatitis in Taiwan could be attributed to HCV infection.

Farci et al. (1) have reported for the first time the experimental transmission of HCV from a patient with fulminant hepatitis to a chimpanzee, thus providing further support for an etiologic role of HCV in fulminant hepatitis.

Kuwada et al. (2) carried out detailed virological studies in 8 patients with presumed viral non-A, non-B fulminant hepatitis. These investigators checked for HCV and HEV antibodies as well as HCV and HEV RNA and could not find evidence implicating either HCV or HEV in presumed viral non-A, non-B fulminant hepatitis, or as agents contributing to or causing fulminant hepatic failure in patients with autoimmune hepatitis, drug-induced hepatotoxicity, or halthene hepatotoxicity.—N.J. Greenberger, M.D.

References

1. Farci P, Munoz S, Alter H, et al: Hepatitis C virus (HCV) associated fulminant hepatitis and its transmission to a chimpanzee. *Hepatology* 20:265A, 1994. (Abstract)
2. Kuwada SK, Patel VM, Hollinger FB, et al: Non-A, non-B fulminant hepatitis is also non-E and non-C. *Am J Gastroenterol* 89:57–61, 1994.

Short-Term Prednisone Therapy Affects Aminotransferase Activity and Hepatitis C Virus RNA Levels in Chronic Hepatitis C

Fong T-L, Valinluck B, Govindarajan S, Charboneau F, Adkins RH, Redeker AG (Univ of Southern California, Downey)

Gastroenterology 107:196–199, 1994   119-95-49-7

Background.—Although the histopathology of chronic active hepatitis caused by the hepatitis C virus (HCV) has been well described, the mechanism of liver cell injury caused by hepatitis C is not known. Using the mechanism of liver cell injury caused by hepatitis B virus and the effects of corticosteroids on chronic hepatitis B as a model, the effects of prednisone on alanine aminotransferase and HCV RNA levels were investigated.

Methods.—A 7-week course of a tapering dose of prednisone was given to 10 patients with chronic hepatitis C with increased levels of alanine aminotransferase and with HCV RNA detectable in serum. Blood samples were taken every 2 weeks for the first 3 months, then once per month for the last 3 months.

Results.—Serum alanine aminotransferase levels decreased in 8 of the 10 patients. Mean levels of alanine aminotransferase decreased in all 10 patients from 184 units k/L before therapy to 84 units/L after therapy; after the prednisone was discontinued, these levels increased in 7 of the 8 patients and reached levels higher than in the pretreatment period in 7 of these 8 patients. Hepatitis C virus RNA was detectable by branched-chain DNA amplification in 9 of 10 patients, and these levels increased in all 9 patients. The mean serum HCV RNA levels increased from 40.9 before treatment to 414.3 during treatment. Using reverse transcription polymerase chain reaction, the geometric mean titer increased 1 log–fold in 8 of 10 patients. After prednisone was discontinued, levels of HCV RNA dropped to pretreatment values within a mean of 2.8 weeks.

Conclusion.—In chronic hepatitis C, the responses of alanine aminotransferase and HCV RNA before and after the administration of prednisone suggest the participation of an immune-mediated mechanism in liver cell injury.

▶ McHutchison and associates (1) carried out studies to determine whether prednisone priming prior to alpha-interferon therapy improves the response rate to interferon or alters the viral load. The main finding was that prednisone priming to interferon therapy in patients with chronic HCV infections did not improve the complete or sustained response rate. The therapy was also associated with a short-term increase in viral load and with significant morbidity.—N.J. Greenberger, M.D.

Reference

1. McHutchinson JG, Pockros PJ, Byland D, et al: Prednisone withdrawal followed

by alpha interferon for chronic HCV infection: Result of a randomized controlled trial. *Hepatology* 20:156A, 1994. (Abstract)

Discrepancy Between Biochemical and Virological Responses to Interferon-α in Chronic Hepatitis C

Lau JYN, Mizokami M, Ohno T, Diamond DA, Kniffen J, Davis GL (Univ of Florida, Gainesville; Nagoya City Univ, Japan)

Lancet 342:1208–1209, 1993   119-95-49–8

Objective.—Treatment with interferon-α(IFN-α) can normalize serum alanine aminotransferase activity in 40% of patients with chronic hepatitis C virus (HCV) infection, although at least half of the responders relapse after cessation of treatment. It remains to be seen whether patients with an alanine aminotransferase response also become negative for HCV RNA in serum and whether a sustained response is associated with sustained disappearance of HCV.

Observations.—Serial serum samples and pretreatment and post-treatment liver tissue from patients with chronic HCV infection were analyzed. The samples were tested for HCV RNA by reverse-transcription polymerase chain reaction and branched DNA signal amplification assays. Of 5 patients with no biochemical response to IFN-α, 4 were serologically positive for HCV RNA throughout treatment. Three of 5 patients with a complete response and relapse were persistently positive, whereas in the other 2, HCV RNA became undetectable during treatment; in 1 of the latter, HCV RNA returned before the end of treatment. In both of these groups, biopsy samples were positive in all pa-

Clinical, Biochemical, and Virologic Details of Study Patients

	No response (n=5)	Complete response with early relapse (n=5)	Complete and sustained response (n=5)
M/F	3/2	4/1	3/2
Age range (years)	40–68	37–63	37–72
Before IFNα			
Median (range) ALT (IU/L)	106 (73–144)	136 (68–184)	315 (115–503)
No + ve for anti-HCV*	5	5	5
No + ve for HCV RNA†	5	5	5
Median HCV RNA‡	$1 \cdot 0 \times 10^6$	$1 \cdot 5 \times 10^6$	bDNA-
No with HCV subtype[6]			
I	3	1	1
II	1	2	1
III	0	0	0
IV	0	2	3
Mixed	1	0	0

* By enzyme immunoassay 2.
† By reverse-transcription nested polymerase chain reaction.
‡ bDNA assay; unit is genome equivalents per mL.
(Courtesy of Lau JYN, Mizokami M, Ohno T, et al: *Lancet* 342:1208–1209, 1993.)

tients. In 5 patients with complete and sustained alanine aminotransferase responses, HCV RNA was undetectable after 12 weeks of IFN-α, although it reappeared before the end of therapy in 1 case. The biopsy specimen was negative in all 4 responders tested. Virologic relapse occurred within 6 months in all 5 patients (table).

Conclusion.—Patients with chronic HCV infection who have a biochemical response to IFN-α do not necessarily have complete eradication of the virus. Even patients with a persistent response are vulnerable to relapse and, thus, need long-term follow-up. Relapse could result from an extrahepatic reservoir of HCV.

▶ Several factors appear to influence the response to interferon in patients with chronic hepatitis C. Factors associated with an increased likelihood of response are as follows:

- Age < 40 years.
- Absence of cirrhosis.
- Histological features of chronic persistent rather than chronic active hepatitis.
- Low HCV RNA titers.
- Serum aminotransferase less than 3 × normal.
- Dosage schedule.
- HCV genotype

Several studies (1–3) have indicated that HCV genotype is particularly important. Zein et al. (1) noted an overall response to interferon in 24 of 76 (31%) patients with hepatitis C. They demonstrated that liver histology and HCV genotypes are 2 independent risk factors for interferon sensitivity. Specifically, HCV genotype 2b is more sensitive to interferon than HCV genotypes 1a and 1b. The presence of liver cirrhosis was an indicator of a poor response to interferon as only 4 of 27 (14%) patients responded.

Portal et al. (2) studied 40 patients with hepatitis C who received interferon and drew the following conclusions: first, that low HCV RNA viremia levels, as determined by bDNA testing before treatment, are predictive for a response to interferon but not a sustained response; second, that genotype 1 is associated with relapse or absence of response; and finally, that genotype 3a and low viremia level are associated with 75% of the complete and sustained responses in the patients studied.

Further evidence that the type 1 HCV genotype is associated with an inferior response to interferon therapy derives from the study by Swanson et al. (3) who studied 71 patients with chronic hepatitis C. These investigators demonstrated that the short- and long-term response rates in type 1 chronic hepatitis C were clearly inferior to those with type 3.—N.J. Greenberger, M.D.

References

1. Zein NN, Rakela J, Krawitt EC, et al: Response to interferon in patients with different HCV genotypes. *Hepatology* 20:156A, 1994. (Abstract)

2. Portal I, Bourliere M, Halfon PH, et al: Predictive value of serum HCV RNA levels and genotypes for response to interferon alfa therapy. *Hepatology* 20:156A, 1994. (Abstract)
3. Swanson NR, Larea RR, Reed WD, et al: An analysis of the influence of HCV genotype on short- and long-term responses to α-interferon therapy for chronic hepatitis C. *Hepatology* 20:157A, 1994. (Abstract)

Quantitation of Hepatitis C Virus RNA in Liver Transplant Recipients

Chazouilleres O, Kim M, Combs C, Ferrell L, Bacchetti P, Roberts J, Ascher NL, Neuwald P, Wilber J, Urdea M, Quan S, Sanchez-Pescador R, Wright TL (VA Med Ctr, San Francisco; Univ of California, San Francisco; Chiron Corp, Emeryville, Calif)
Gastroenterology 106:994–999, 1994   119-95-49-9

Background.—Hepatitis C virus infection is both a cause of liver disease before liver transplantation and a cause of chronic hepatitis after transplantation. In almost all patients with hepatitis C virus (HCV) infection before transplantation, the infection recurs post-transplant and is acquired during the peritransplant period as well. The effects of immunosuppression on HCV RNA levels and the relationship of these levels to hepatic damage were studied.

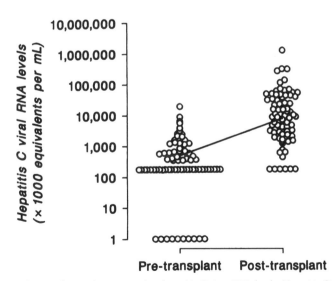

Fig 49–1.—Pretransplant and post-transplant hepatitis C virus RNA levels. Hepatitis C virus RNA levels determined by bDNA assay in 75 patients with recurrent infection are shown. Serum hepatitis C virus RNA was not detected by polymerase chain reaction or bDNA in 10 patients. The *line* indicates the evolution of the geometric mean in the remaining 65 patients with detectable hepatitis C virus RNA by polymerase chain reaction in pretransplant serum. There was a 16-fold increase from mean pretransplant levels of 496,000 to 7,935,000 Eq/mL (P < .0001 by paired *t* test). (Courtesy of Chazouilleres O, Kim M, Combs C, et al: *Gastroenterology* 106:994–999, 1994.)

Methods.—In 100 patients with HCV infection and undergoing liver transplantation, HCV RNA in serum was measured using polymerase chain reaction amplification and branched DNA assay. The relationship between liver histology and HCV RNA level was determined by drawing and testing serum before antiviral treatment and within 3 months of liver biopsy.

Results.—Mean post-transplant levels increased 16-fold from pretransplant levels (Fig 49-1); this increase was highly significant. The mean post-transplant levels were higher in patients with high pretransplant levels than in those with low pretransplant levels. In patients with recurrent and acquired infection, post-transplant levels were similar. Liver biopsy specimens were normal in 50% of patients with HCV infection; there was not strong correlation between the level of viremia and degree of hepatic damage.

Discussion.—A "carrier" state for hepatitis C virus with detectable HCV RNA in serum without histologic hepatitis clearly exists in nonimmunosuppressed patients. The absence of allograft damage in spite of high levels of viral RNA suggests that HCV infection may be tolerated in immunosuppressed patients without direct damage to liver cells.

▶ Several studies have indicated that recurrent HCV infection after transplantation does not seem to be related either to the level of viremia or to any HCV genotype. An interesting study (1) documented lower recurrence of HCV after liver transplantation in patients receiving hepatitis B immune globulin. This could be caused by either a decreased replication of HCV before liver transplantation (due to HBV) or by hepatitis B immune globulin containing anti-HCV.—N.J. Greenberger, M.D.

Reference

1. Feray C, Samuel D, Gigan M, et al: Reduced incidence of recurrent and acquired infection by HCV after liver transplantation in patients receiving immunoglobulin. *Hepatology* 20:131A, 1994. (Abstract)

Sclerotherapy for Male Alcoholic Cirrhotic Patients Who Have Bled From Esophageal Varices: Results of a Randomized, Multicenter Clinical Trial

Hartigan P, for the Veterans Affairs Cooperative Variceal Sclerotherapy Group (VA Med Ctr, West Haven, Conn)

Hepatology 20:618–625, 1994

119-95-49-10

Introduction.—Patients with alcoholic cirrhosis often have devastating episodes of bleeding esophageal varices. Studies have found that sclerotherapy reduced bleeding, but they have reported mixed survival benefits. In a 5-year Veterans Affairs cooperative study, the effect of sclerotherapy on variceal rebleeding and survival was examined.

Parameters	Major Outcomes Sham-therapy (N = 131)	Sclerotherapy (N = 122)	p Value
Rebleeding			
Ever rebled—overall	83	67	NS
Stratum I	15/24	11/25	NS
Stratum II	59/89	52/87	NS
Number of bleeds	210	137	
Total units of blood	1328	630	
Mean units per bleeding patient	16.0	9.4	0.002
Source of bleeds			
Esophageal varices	112	52	0.005
Esophageal ulcers	2	29	<0.001
Gastric varices	10	11	NS
Other	17	11	NS
Uncertain	32	23	NS
Endoscopy not done	37	11	0.01
Death			
Died			
Overall	74	77	NS
Stratum I	17/24	18/25	NS
Stratum II	46/89	55/87	NS
Primary cause of death			
Upper gastrointestinal bleeding	32	20	NS
Liver failure	15	18	NS
Infection	8	10	NS
Cardiac failure	8	5	NS
Respiratory failure	3	5	NS
Renal failure	2	4	NS
Other†	0	9	0.002
Unknown	6	4	NS

Note: Except where specified as a mean, values are given as numbers of patients, units, or episodes.
† Other causes of death included cancer (2), CVA (2), ischemic bowel, suicide, intraperitoneal bleed, aplastic anemia, and bleed after thoracentesis.
(Courtesy of Hartigan P, for the Veterans Affairs Cooperative Variceal Sclerotherapy Group: *Hepatology* 20:618–625, 1994.)

Methods.—Two hundred fifty-three male patients with alcoholic cirrhosis were stratified by the time of the last esophageal variceal bleeding episode: current, within 2 weeks, between 2 weeks and 1 year, and 1–4 years before the study. The patients in each stratum were randomly assigned to receive either endoscopy with sclerotherapy (122 patients) or endoscopy with sham sclerotherapy (131 patients) at 4–6 days, 9–11 days, 1 month, 3 months, and every 3 months for 2 years. The patients were followed for the rest of the 5-year study.

Results.—Patients in the sclerotherapy group experienced an upper gastrointestinal rebleeding rate of 66 per 100 person-years of follow-up, whereas the rate among patients in the sham-sclerotherapy group was 101 per 100 person-years of follow-up. The bleeding was significantly more likely to be caused by esophageal varices in the sham-sclerotherapy group. Seventy-four patients in the sham-sclerotherapy group (56%) and 77 patients in the sclerotherapy group (63%) died. Mortality was highest in the patients with current bleeding at baseline. Patients receiving sham-sclerotherapy were significantly more likely to require shunt surgery, transfusion, balloon tamponade, and vasopressin; patients receiving sclerotherapy were significantly more likely to have treatment complications, including esophageal ulcers. All major outcomes are listed in the table.

Discussion.—Sclerotherapy significantly reduced esophageal variceal bleeding and requirements for treatments of massive or uncontrolled bleeding, but it did not improve survival in patients with alcoholic cirrhosis and esophageal varices. Sclerotherapy was commonly associated with minor complications, including esophageal strictures requiring bouginage in 20% of the patients and 33 episodes of bleeding esophageal ulcers. These findings indicate that sclerotherapy should be used primarily for short-term treatment of acute variceal bleeding and not for long-term treatment to obliterate varices.

▶ A recent meta-analysis was carried out on 5 randomized, controlled trials dealing with the efficacy of endoscopic sclerotherapy on first variceal bleeding and mortality in cirrhosis with high-risk varices (1). The key findings were that endoscopic sclerotherapy in cirrhotics with high-risk varices is effective in preventing only the first variceal bleeding episodes that occur after 6 months and decreases the death rate through a 2-year period. This seeming discrepancy may be due to bleeding endoscopic sclerotherapy–related ulcers that frequently occur before variceal obliteration.

Two recent studies have compared the efficacy of endoscopic sclerotherapy (2) and transjugular intrahepatic portal systemic shunts (TIPS) in preventing variceal bleeding (3) and in patients with recurrent variceal hemorrhage. (2) Merli et al. (3) have reported that in 46 patients—half of whom received endoscopic sclerotherapy and half TIPS—bleeding varices and mortality were 30% and 9%, respectively, in the endoscopic sclerotherapy group and 13% and 3.7%, respectively, in the TIPS group. Although TIPS was associated with a lower rebleeding rate, the difference is not statistically significant because the numbers are still too small.

Rössle (2) reported that in 54 patients with prior variceal hemorrhage, recurrent bleeding occurred in 7 of 27 (26%) patients receiving sclerotherapy (6 ± 3 sessions) compared with 2 of 27 (8%) patients receiving TIPS. Thus, in this trial, recurrent bleeding was significantly lower in the shunted patients. However, comparison of mortality and survival will require a large number of patients followed over an extended follow-up period.—N.J. Greenberger, M.D.

References

1. Saringo R, Muia A, Bolandi L, et al: Meta-analysis of efficacy of endoscopic sclerotherapy (ES) on the first variceal bleeding (FVB) and mortality rate in cirrhotics with high risk varices. Hepatology 20:107A, 1994. (Abstract)
2. Rössle M, Deibert P, Hoog K, et al: TIPS vs sclerotherapy and β-blockade: Pulmonary results of a randomized study on patients with recurrent variceal hemorrhage. Hepatology 20:107A, 1994. (Abstract)
3. Merli M, Riggio O, Capocaccia L, et al:Transjugular intrahepaticportosystemic shunt (TIPS) vs endoscopic sclerotherapy (ES) in preventing variceal bleeding:

Pulmonary results of a randomized controlled trial. *Hepatology* 20:107A, 1994. (Abstract)

The Transjugular Intrahepatic Portosystemic Stent-Shunt Procedure for Variceal Bleeding

Rössle M, Haag K, Ochs A, Sellinger M, Nöldge G, Perarnau J-M, Berger E, Blum U, Gabelmann A, Hauenstein K, Langer M, Gerok W (Medizinische Universitätsklinik, Freiburg, Germany; Radiologische Universitätsklinik, Freiburg, Germany; Hôpital de Bon-Secours, Metz, France)
N Engl J Med 330:165–171, 1994   119-95-49-11

Purpose.—In patients with portal hypertension, a portosystemic shunt may be established by transjugular placement of an intrahepatic shunt. In this new technique, a puncture needle is placed via a catheter through the inferior vena cava into an hepatic vein. After the intrahepatic branch of the portal vein is punctured, the shunt is established by implanting an expandable stent of metallic mesh. The results with this procedure in 100 consecutive patients were reported.

Patients.—The patients, two thirds of whom were men, all had variceal bleeding caused by cirrhosis. The mean age was 57 years. The procedure was done electively in 90 cases and on an emergency basis in 10. Previous endoscopic sclerotherapy had failed in most of the patients. Ei-

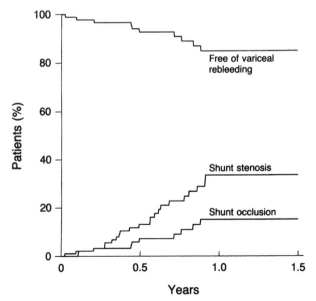

Fig 49–2.—Cumulative rates of shunt stenosis and shunt occlusion, and cumulative percentages of patients free of variceal rebleeding among 93 patients receiving stents (calculated by the Kaplan-Meier method). (Courtesy of Rössle M, Haag K, Ochs A, et al: *N Engl J Med* 330:165-171, 1994.)

ther endoscopic sclerotherapy or esophageal balloon tamponade was used to manage acute bleeding episodes. The patients were followed for a mean of 12 months.

Outcomes.—The procedure took a mean of 1.2 hours, and the mean shunt diameter was 9 mm. The technical success rate was 93%. The portal venous pressure gradient was immediately reduced by 57%, and portal flow velocity and portal blood flow increased 2.5-fold. Major complications were stent dislocation; bleeding, including intraperitoneal and biliary hemorrhage and hematoma of the liver capsule; and stent migration into the pulmonary artery. During follow-up, the hepatic encephalopathy rate increased from 10% to 25%. In 23 patients, hepatic encephalopathy appeared within the first 3 months of stent placement; 16 of these patients responded to medical treatment. The bilirubin concentration increased by more than 3mg/dL in 18 patients within 1 week of the procedure. Child–Pugh scores improved because of the reduction in ascites. Shunt insufficiency was related to reduction of flow to less than 1,000 mL/min and of portal flow velocity to less than 10 cm/sec. One third of patients had either stenosis or occlusion; these cases were treated successfully. Eighty-two percent of patients were free of variceal bleeding by 1 year (Fig 49–2). Early mortality was 30% in the emergency group. There were late deaths from hepatic failure but none from variceal bleeding. Overall, 1-year survival was 85%.

Conclusion.—Transjugular placement of an intrahepatic portosystemic stent is a safe and effective treatment for variceal hemorrhage in patients with portal hypertension. Hepatic encephalopathy may occur early because of stent endothelialization. This risk may be decreased by placing small caliber stents and embolizing the coronary veins in patients older than 60 years of age and in those with Child–Pugh class C cirrhosis. The stent–shunt procedure carries a much lower rate of variceal rebleeding than endoscopic sclerotherapy.

▶ Transjugular intrahepatic portal systemic shunts (TIPS) are a new technique for treatment of portal hypertension and variceal bleeding, especially after failure of endoscopic sclerotherapy. Although TIPS has proven effective in sharply reducing the likelihood of recurrent variceal bleeding, 2 major problems have emerged: an appreciable incidence of portal systemic encephalopathy (PSE) ranging from 10% to 25%, and shunt stenosis or occlusion. Two factors are associated with an increased risk of the development of PSE after TIPS, i.e., age greater than 60 years and a serum albumin less than 2.5 g/dL. The following article (Abstract 119-95-49–12) deals with shunt stenosis and occlusion. Finally, I would point out that in addition to decompression of esophageal and gastric varices, TIPS is also an effective method of decompressing intestinal varices (1).—N.J. Greenberger, M.D.

Reference

1. Haskel ZJ, Scott M, Rubin RA, et al: Intestinal varices: Treatment with the transjugular intrahepatic portosystemic shunt. *Radiology* 191:183–187, 1994.

Incidence of Shunt Occlusion or Stenosis Following Transjugular Intrahepatic Portosystemic Shunt Placement

Lind CD, Malisch TW, Chong WK, Richards WO, Pinson CW, Meranze SG, Mazer M (Vanderbilt Univ, Nashville, Tenn)
Gastroenterology 106:1277–1283, 1994   119-95-49–12

Background.—Treatment of recurrent variceal hemorrhage includes β-blocker therapy, endoscopic variceal sclerotherapy or banding, and portal decompressive shunt surgery. Transjugular intrahepatic portosystemic shunt (TIPS) placement has been used to treat patients with recurrent variceal hemorrhage who do not respond to endoscopic treatment. The incidence of shunt stenosis or occlusion within 1 year after TIPS placement was assessed prospectively, and color Doppler ultrasonography was evaluated as a technique to assess TIPS patency.

Methods.—Transjugular intrahepatic portosystemic shunt placement was done in 22 patients with recurrent variceal hemorrhage. All patients had clinical assessment, upper gastrointestinal endoscopy, portal angiography with pressure measurements, and Doppler ultrasonography before and after the procedure. Follow-up examinations were done after 3 and 12 months and when bleeding developed.

Results.—Transjugular intrahepatic portosystemic shunts were successfully placed in 21 patients. At 12-month follow-up, TIPS occlusion developed in 2 of 17 patients, shunt stenosis in 7, and no stenosis in 8. Color Doppler ultrasonography predicted shunt stenosis or occlusion with 100% sensitivity, 98% specificity, and 90% positive predictive value.

Discussion.—In 53% of these patients, shunt stenosis or occlusion developed within 1 year. Doppler ultrasonography accurately identifies shunt stenosis and should be used every 3 months as part of routine follow-up of all patients who have TIPS placement. Careful follow-up and shunt revision are a necessary part of long-term treatment of variceal hemorrhage.

▶ In addition to portal systemic encephalopathy and shunt occlusion, TIPS has the potential for other serious complications. Such complications include peritoneal bleeding, liver capsular bleeding, pulmonary embolism, disseminated intravascular coagulation, and shunt migration. A recent article (1) documents the development of hepatic infarction following TIPS, and the authors caution that TIPS should be performed only in centers with a liver transplant program nearby.—N.J. Greenberger, M.D.

Reference

1. Lim H, Abbitt PL, Kniffen JC, et al: Hepatic infarction complicating a transjugular intrahepatic portosystemic shunt. *Am J Gastroenterol* 88:2095–2097, 1994.

Screening for Hemochromatosis: A Cost-Effectiveness Study Based on 12,258 Patients

Balan V, Baldus W, Fairbanks V, Michels V, Burritt M, Klee G (Mayo Clinic and Found, Rochester, Minn)
Gastroenterology 107:453–459, 1994   119-95-49-13

Results of Screening

Criteria	Total no. of patients tested	Patients meeting criteria
Initial serum iron ≥180 μg/dL	12,258	127
Repeat iron ≥180 μg/dL Transferrin saturation ≥62% and ferritin ≥400 μg/L	127	44
No other explanation for abnormal iron test results	44	8

(Courtesy of Balan V, Baldus W, Fairbanks V, et al: *Gastroenterology* 107:453–459, 1994.)

Background.—Genetic hemochromatosis is a disorder of iron metabolism characterized by inappropriately high iron absorption for existing iron stores. Hepatocellular carcinoma develops in 30% of patients with hemochromatosis who have cirrhosis. However, cirrhosis and hepatic malignancy can be prevented if the disease is treated early. Patients with early hemochromatosis may not have any symptoms; early indicators are elevated values for transferrin saturation and/or ferritin. Screening has been limited to subsets of the general population, such as blood donors or those with an affected relative. Without systematic screening, only a fraction of affected individuals can be identified. To evaluate the feasibility of screening for hemochromatosis, unselected patients were prospectively screened.

Methods.—Blood samples were collected from 12,258 patients of the Mayo Clinic seeking medical care for a variety of conditions, and serum iron levels were determined. Data were recorded from each patient's medical record and included major and minor diagnoses, family history if relevant to iron overload, transfusion history, and use of medicinal iron.

Results.—An initial serum iron concentration ≥ 180 μg/dL was detected in 127 patients (table). Transferrin saturation ≥62% and a serum

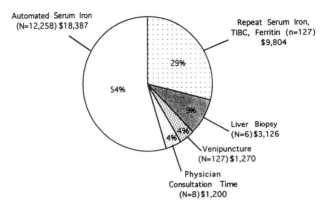

Fig 49–3.—Cost of tests and procedures (total cost, $33,787). (Courtesy of Balan V, Baldus W, Fairbanks V, et al: *Gastroenterology* 107:453–459, 1994.)

ferritin value ≥400 μg/L were detected in 8 patients with no other explanation for the abnormal results. A markedly elevated hepatic iron concentration and hepatic iron index indicative of homozygous hemochromatosis was found in 3 patients. One patient who refused liver biopsy had 7 g of iron removed via phlebotomy and was considered homozygous. Two patients had hepatic iron indices < 1.5 and were considered heterozygous. The genotype of 1 patient was uncertain. One patient who had a normal hepatic iron concentration and hepatic iron index had chronic active hepatitis. Figure 49–3 shows the results of cost analysis.

Discussion.—These patients with hemochromatosis would not have been identified without this study. Even at this yield of one tenth the predicted homozygote frequency, screening is cost-effective, especially because liver transplantation can be required for patients whose disease is diagnosed too late, and because early detection and treatment affords patients a normal life expectancy.

▶ The yield in this series, .33 cases of 1,000 screened, is approximately one tenth of the predicted homozygote frequency as judged by recent estimates. However, the authors believe that even at this yield screening appears cost-effective.

The Ca 19.9 antigen is mainly secreted by biliary and pancreatic cells, but its metabolism could also be modified in genetic hemochromatosis by hepatocyte iron accumulation. Deugnier et al. (1) tested this hypothesis by measuring Ca 19.9 levels in 84 patients with hemochromatosis before and after iron depletion therapy. The study demonstrated that Ca 19.9 was increased before treatment compared with the venesection period and correlated, before treatment, with the amount of iron excess, transaminases, fibrosis, and biliary iron deposits. The authors conclude that an unexplained finding of a mild increase in serum Ca 19.9 should lead, in a patient with no diagnosis, to a consideration of liver iron overload.—N.J. Greenberger, M.D.

Reference

1. Deugnier YN, Rabot AF, Guyader D, et al: Serum increase and liver overexpression for carbohydrate 19.9 antigen in patients with genetic hemochromatosis. *Gut* 35:1107–1111, 1994.

Ursodiol for the Long-Term Treatment of Primary Biliary Cirrhosis
Poupon RE, Poupon R, Balkau B, and the UDCA-PBC Study Group (INSERM Unité 21, Villejuif, France; Hôpital Saint-Antoine, Paris)
N Engl J Med 330:1342–1347, 1994   119-95-49–14

Introduction.—Ursodiol, or ursodeoxycholic acid, has no apparent hepatotoxicity in human beings and can lead to major improvement in patients with primary biliary cirrhosis. Long-term ursodiol therapy may displace treatment with endogenous bile acids, thus averting their suspected cytotoxicity. The benefits of long-term treatment are unproved, however.

Methods.—The benefits of 2 years of treatment with ursodiol in patients with biopsy-proved primary biliary cirrhosis were examined in a double-blind randomized study in which 145 patients received ursodiol, 13–15 mg/kg per day, or placebo. Patients were eligible regardless of the duration or stage of their disease; those with a serum level of bilirubin of more than 8.8 mg/dL or a serum level of albumin of less than 2.5 g/dL were exlcuded. After the double-blind period, all patients received ursodiol for a further 2 years. Treatment failure was the main end point for evaluation of efficacy.

Results.—Patients who received ursodiol for 4 years were significantly more likely to achieve a response to treatment than those who initially received placebo. Liver transplantation was also less likely in the group initially assigned to ursodiol. Mortality was about twice as high with placebo as with ursodiol (6% vs. 12%) (Fig 49–4). Factors predicting treatment failure were high levels of bilirubin and bile acids, low levels of albumin, and the clinical findings of hepatomegaly and splenomegaly.

Conclusion.—Long term treatment with ursodiol can slow the progression of primary biliary cirrhosis, thus decreasing the need for liver transplantation. The rate of treatment failure appears to be the same at 4 years as at 2 years. Histologic stage, already a controversial marker of prognosis, has no independent value in the prediction of a treatment response.

▶ Two other recent trials (1, 2) have also demonstrated that ursodiol slows the progression of primary biliary cirrhosis (PBC) and improves liver tests. Whether ursodiol ultimately reduces the need for liver transplantation remains an open question. Accordingly, the search continues for the optimal medical treatment regimen for PBC. Several controlled studies are now under way to determine whether the combination of ursodiol plus methotrexate

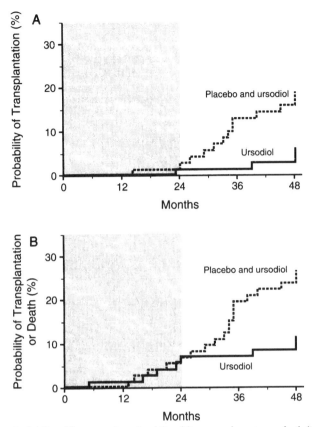

Fig 49–4.—Probability of liver transplantation (**A**) and liver transplantation or death (**B**) in patients treated with ursodiol. These probabilities were significantly lower in patients treated for 4 years with ursodiol than in those who first received placebo (for transplantation alone, P = .003; relative risk, .21; 95% confidence interval, .07 –.66; for transplantation or death, P =.005 relative risk, .32; 95% confidence interval, .14–.74). *Shaded area* indicates period of double-blind trial. Data on transplantation include referrals for liver transplantation. (Courtesy of Poupon RE, Poupon R, Balkau B, and the UDCA-PBC Study Group: *N Engl J Med* 330:1342–1347, 1994.)

or ursodiol plus colchicine will prove to be more effective than ursodiol alone (3–5).

Poupon et al. confirm that certain clinical findings portend a poor prognosis in PBC, i.e., hyperbilirubinemia, hypoalbuminemia, and hepatosplenomegaly.—N.J. Greenberger, M.D.

References

1. Lindor KD, Dickson ER, Baldus WP: Ursodeoxycholic acid in the treatment of primary biliary cirrhosis. *Gastroenterology* 106:1284–1290, 1993.
2. Heathcote EJG, Capuch K, Walker V: The Canadian Multicenter double blind randomized trial of ursodeoxycholic acid in primary biliary cirrhosis. *Hepatology* 19:1149–1156, 1994.

3. Lindor KR, Jorgenson MI, Anderson ELJ, et al: The combination of ursodeoxycholic acid (UDCA) and methotrexate (MTX) for patients with primary biliary cirrhosis (PBC): The results of a pilot study. *Hepatology* 20:202A, 1994. (Abstract)

4. Goddard CJR, Hunt O, Smith A, et al: A trial of ursodeoxycholic acid (UDCA) and colchicine in primary biliary cirrhosis (PBC). *Hepatology* 20:151A, 1994. (Abstract)

5. Poupon RE, Niard AM, Hunt PM, et al: A randomized trial comparing the combination of ursodeoxycholic acid (UDCA) and colchicine to UDCA alone in primary biliary cirrhosis. *Hepatology* 20:151A, 1994. (Abstract)

Hepatic Outflow Obstruction (Budd-Chiari Syndrome): Experience With 177 Patients and a Review of the Literature

Dilawari JB, Bambery P, Chawla Y, Kaur U, Bhusnurmath SR, Malhotra HS, Sood GK, Mitra SK, Khanna SK, Walia BS (Postgraduate Inst of Med Education and Research, Chandigarh, India)
Medicine 73:21–36, 1994   119-95-49–15

Introduction.—The structural and functional liver abnormalities seen in patients with Budd–Chiari syndrome (BCS) are caused by hepatic venous obstruction, which can result from numerous pathogenic conditions. The 25-year experience at 1 institution of 177 patients with BCS was reported.

Methods.—Budd–Chiari syndrome was confirmed radiologically in the 177 patients. Data regarding the clinical presentation, etiologic factors, natural course of the disease, vascular obstructions, treatment, and outcome were reviewed.

Results.—Of the 177 patients, 63 had acute BCS and came to the hospital within 6 months of symptom onset, and 114 had chronic BCS and came to the hospital after having symptoms for 1 to 10 years. Although there was significant overlap, the 2 types of BCS typically had different etiologic features and clinical presentations. Typically, pregancy- or puerperium-related BCS was diagnosed within 3 months of onset, whereas disease with other etiologic factors—tumors, hypercoagulable states, infections, and other miscellaneous disorders—was diagnosed later. Disease in patients with membranous obstruction of the inferior vena cava or idiopathic BCS was often diagnosed more than 120 months after onset (Table 1). Pregnancy-related acute BCS was usually fulminant, and 69% of these patients died soon after presentation; these patients represented 56% of the overall deaths. Patients with acute BCS were more likely to be seen with abdominal pain, distention, jaundice, hepatic encephalopathy, ascites, hyperbilirubinemia, and hypercoagulability, whereas patients with chronic BCS were more likely to be seen with upper gastrointestinal bleeding, splenomegaly, and distended veins (Table 2). Childhood BCS was rarely acute and predominantly affected males in a 3:2 ratio; these patients had a proportionally higher incidence of visibly

TABLE 1.—Etiologic Factors of BCS in Relation to Duration

Duration (mo.)	<1	1-3	4-6	7-12	13-59	60-119	>120	Total (%)
Cause								
Inferior vena cava membrane	0	6	4	9	13	9	13	54 (28.7)
Pregnancy	13	11	2	0	8	2	2	38 (20.2)
Tumors	3	1	0	2	0	1	4	11 (5.8)
Hypercoagulable states*	1	4	2	0	0	0	0	7 (3.7)
Infection	0	1	0	0	2	1	1	5 (2.6)
Others (see text)	0	0	1	0	4	3	0	8 (4.3)
Idiopathic	0	4	13	14	20	8	6	65 (34.6)

* Hypercoagulable states included 4 patients with polycythemia vera and 3 with paroxysmal nocturnal hemoglobinuria. Infections included amebic liver abscess and tuberculosis (1 each) and hydatid disease (3 cases). Six patients with inferior vena cava membrane also had hepatocellular carcinoma, and 5 with pregnancy-related BCS had inferior vena cava membranes.
(Courtesy of Dilawari JB, Bambery P, Chawla Y, et al: Medicine 73:21–36, 1994.)

dilated abdominal veins and splenomegaly and a lower incidence of encephalopathy.

Discussion.—These findings delineate 2 relatively distinct forms of BCS, with different etiologic features and clinical presentation. The acute form is always associated with extensive hepatic vascular blockage,

TABLE 2.—Acute and Chronic BCS: Clinical and
Etiologic Differentiation*

		Acute (<6 mo.) N = 63	Chronic (>6 mo.) N = 114
Male:Female		1:12	1.5:1
Abdominal pain	(p < 0.001)	50 (79)	50 (44)
Distension	(p < 0.001)	58 (92)	78 (68)
Jaundice	(p < 0.001)	23 (37)	9 (8)
Upper G.I. bleeding	(p < 0.005)	4 (6)	30 (26)
Distended veins†	(p < 0.001)	1 (2)	70 (61)
Hepatic encephalopathy	(p < 0.005)	13 (20)	7 (6)
Hepatomegaly	(NS)	55 (87)	104 (91)
Splenomegaly	(p < 0.01)	20 (31)	61 (54)
Ascites	(p < 0.001)	59 (94)	72 (63)
Edema	(NS)	21 (33)	37 (32)
Serum bilirubin > 1 mg/dl	(p < 0.001)	50 (77)	29 (25)
Serum albumin < 3 g/dl	(NS)	35 (55)	52 (47)
Hepatic vein block	(NS)	54/55	65/89
IVC block	(NS)	32/48	87/110
Pregnancy related	(p < 0.001)	26 (41)	12 (11)
Hypercoagulability	(p < 0.001)	7 (11)	0
IVC membrane	(p < 0.005)	10 (16)	44 (39)
Tumors & others (see text)	(NS)	6 (9)	18 (16)
Idiopathic	(p < 0.05)	17 (27)	48 (42)

Abbreviations: NS, not significant; IVC, inferior vena cava; G.I.,
gastrointestinal.
* Numbers in parentheses are percentages.
† These patients complained of abdominal venous distention as a symptom.
(Courtesy of Dilawari JB, Bambery P, Chawla Y, et al: *Medicine* 73:21-36,
1994.)

sometimes including occlusion of the inferior vena cava. Appropriate
therapy includes shunt placement. However, the long survival of patients
with chronic BCS recommends a more conservative approach, with
treatment of the primary pathologic entity. Budd–Chiari syndrome may
be a spectrum of hypercoagulation disease, and its expression is dependent on the individual balance between rate of formation and extent of
thrombosis and the rate of thrombolysis and recanalization.

▶ This study has substantiated the existence of 2 major clincial forms of
BCS. The authors believe that BCS represents a spectrum of disease caused
primarily by a hypercoagulable state and having a varied presentation, depending on the balance between rate of formation and the extent of fibrosis
and the subsequent site of thrombolysis and recanalization. Whereas a
French study (1) demonstrated an *occult* myeloproliferative syndrome in almost 80% of patients believed to have idiopathic BCS, a more recent German study (2) of 500 patients with established myeloproliferative syndromes
documented the development of BCS in only 6 patients (1%). These seem-

ingly disparate observations indicated the need for more detailed studies of occult myeloproliferative disorders to determine how often they progress to overt disease and clear-cut BCS. Other disorders leading to hypercoagulable state, i.e., protein C, protein S, plasminogen activator deficiency or inhibitors need to be evaluated in patients with BCS.—N.J. Greenberger, M.D.

References

1. Valla D, Csadevoll N, Lacombe C, et al: Primary myeloproliferative disorders and hepatic vein thrombosis. *Ann Intern Med* 103:329–333, 1985.
2. Anger BR, Seifred E, Scheppach J, et al: Budd-Chiari syndrome and thrombosis of other abdominal vessels in the chronic myeloproliferative diseases. *Klin Wochenschr* 67:818–825, 1989.

Hepatocyte Proliferation as an Indicator of Outcome in Acute Alcoholic Hepatitis

Fang JWS, Bird GLA, Nakamura T, Davis GL, Lau JYN (Univ of Florida, Gainesville; Gartnavel General Hosp, Glasgow, Scotland; Osaka Univ, Japan)
Lancet 343:820–823, 1994   119-95-49–16

Background.—Up to 60% of patients with acute alcoholic hepatitis (AAH) will die within 4 weeks of diagnosis, and over half of the survivors will go on to have cirrhosis. Treatment of AAH with hepatotropic agents decreases short-term mortality, suggesting that clinical outcome

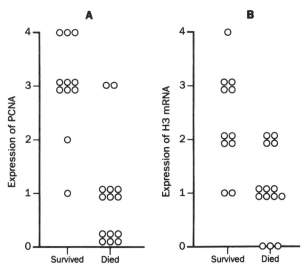

Fig 49–5.—Expression of proliferating cell nuclear antigen (PCNA) (**A**) and H3 mRNA (**B**) in hepatocytes in relation to clinical outcome at 6 months. $n = 25$; $P < .01$ for both cases. (Courtesy of Fang JWS, Bird GLA, Nakamura T, et al: *Lancet* 343:820–823, 1994.)

may be related to liver regeneration capacity. This hypothesis was tested in the biopsy results of 25 patients with AAH.

Methods.—Liver biopsy specimens taken at admission were studied for expression of messenger RNA for 2 proliferation markers: proliferating cell nuclear antigen and human histone. Also assessed were transforming growth factor-α (TGFα), transforming growth factor-β_1 (TGFβ_1), and hepatocyte growth factor (HGF), which regulate hepatocyte proliferation. Patients who survived were followed for at least 6 months.

Results.—Varying levels of proliferation markers were detected in 0% to 80% of hepatocytes and, occasionally, in sinusoidal cells and bile duct epithelium in 76% of patients. Expression of proliferation markers was greater in patients who survived for 6 months than in those who died. Hepatocytes and bile duct epithelium demonstrated TGFα; sinusoidal cells demonstrated TGFβ_1, which was associated with perivenular fibrosis. Survivors showed greater expression of TGFs than nonsurvivors. Seven patients demonstrated HGF in sinusoidal cells, which was also correlated with survival (Fig 49–5).

Conclusion.—In patients with AAH, hepatocyte proliferation, possibly related to the pattern of hepatotropic factor expression, appears to be a good indicator of outcome. Patients with low discriminant function have high-level expression of cell proliferation markers. The factors determining proliferative response are unclear.

▶ Several clinical parameters have proven useful as indicators of outcome in AAH. Factors associated with increased mortality include: an elevated blood urea nitrogen (BUN) greater than 25 mg/dL, portal systemic encephalopathy, oliguric hepatic failure, marked hyperbilirubinemia with serum bilirubin levels greater than 25 mg/dL, and prolongation of the prothrombin time to values greater than 6 seconds above controls. The latter 2 parameters have been incorporated into a discriminant function defined by the expression [4.6 × (prothrombin time − control prothrombin time) plus screen bilirubin]. A value greater than 32 is clearly associated with increased mortality.

I have listed below 3 interesting articles dealing with alcohol and the liver that all are worth reading.—N.J. Greenberger, M.D.

References

1. Lieber CS: Alcohol and the liver: 1994 update. *Ann Intern Med* 106:1085–1105, 1994.
2. Lumeing L, Crabb DW: Genetic aspects and risk factors in alcoholism and alcoholic liver disease. *Gastroenterology* 107:572–578, 1994.
3. Crabb DW, Dipple KH, Thomassom KR: Alcohol sensitivity, alcohol metabolism, risk of alcoholism, and the role of alcohol and aldehyde dehydrogenase genotypes. *J Lab Clin Med* 122:252–290, 1994.

50 Biliary Tract

Effects of Dietary Cholesterol on Cholesterol and Bile Acid Homeostasis in Patients With Cholesterol Gallstones
Kern F Jr (Univ of Colorado, Denver)
J Clin Invest 93:1186–1194, 1994   119-95-50-1

Introduction.—An association between cholesterol gallstones and diet is generally accepted but has not been definitively established. It was hypothesized that patients with and without gallstones would have different metabolic responses to dietary cholesterol.

Methods.—Cholesterol absorption and synthesis, biliary lipid composition and secretion rates, and bile acid kinetics were measured in 8 women with asymptomatic radiolucent gallstones and 8 control women without gallstones, first with intake of regular diets and again after 15–18 days with regular diets plus 5 eggs per day.

Results.—With regular diets, the 2 groups were similar for dietary intake, plasma lipids and apolipoproteins, and biliary lipids, but the gallstone group had lower cholesterol absorption, higher cholesterol synthesis, and a greater fractional turnover rate of the primary bile acid. With the high-cholesterol diet, both groups had similar responses in plasma lipids, with no changes in total or low-density lipoproteins and a slight decrease in plasma triglycerides. Cholesterol absorption decreased in both patients and controls, whereas cholesterol synthesis decreased significantly only in the gallstone patients. Biliary lipid composition and secretion were not significantly altered in the controls, but cholesterol secretion and the molar percent cholesterol in the bile was increased in the gallstone patients. Controls tended to have increased total bile acid and cholic acid synthesis and pool size. The gallstone patients experienced reductions in the cholic acid and total bile acid pools and synthesis rates.

Discussion.—Patients with and without gallstones had significantly different metabolic responses to a high-cholesterol diet. The increase in biliary cholesterol secretion and decrease in bile acid synthesis explain the presence of supersaturated bile seen in gallstone formers. These findings provide support for an association between dietary cholesterol and gallstones.

▶ This interesting paper demonstrates that in patients with gallstones, cholesterol and bile salt homeostasis is significantly altered and that increasing dietary cholesterol *increases* biliary cholesterol secretion and decreases bile acid synthesis and pool size, changes associated with cholesterol gallstone formation.

A recent study has provided useful data on the prevalence of gallstone disease in the United States (1). The conclusions are as follows: Approximately 12% of the adults in the United States have gallstone disease (GSD). The prevalence of GSD increases with age and is twice as common among women as men. Gallstone disease is more prevalent among Mexican Americans than non-Hispanic whites and is least common among non-Hispanic blacks.—N.J. Greenberger, M.D.

Reference

1. Khare M, Everhart JE, Maurer KR: Prevalence of gallstone disease in the United States. *Hepatology* 20:118A, 1994. (Abstract)

51 Pancreas

Comparison of Pancreatic Morphology and Exocrine Functional Impairment in Patients With Chronic Pancreatitis

Bozkurt T, Braun U, Leferink S, Gilly G, Lux G (Univ of Cologne, Solingen, Germany)
Gut 35:1132–1136, 1994   119-95-51–1

Introduction.—Chronic pancreatitis is generally diagnosed by endoscopic retrograde pancreatography (ERP), ultrasound, and CT. Additional pancreatic function tests are usually needed to establish the degree of exocrine insufficiency; these tests are associated with a number of method-related problems. Pancreatic morphology and exocrine function were compared prospectively in 48 patients with chronic pancreatitis.

Methods.—The patients were 39 men and 9 women (average age, 47 years). All had suspected or proved chronic pancreatitis but no clinical or biochemical evidence of acute pancreatitis. Each patient underwent transabdominal ultrasound, CT, ERP, and a secretin-caerulein test. The imaging studies were classified according to the Cambridge classification (Table 1). No pancreatic duct changes were detected on pancreatography in 10 patients; equivocal ductal changes were detected in 10 patients (Cambridge I); mild-to-moderate changes in 12 patients (Cambridge II); and considerable ductal changes in 16 patients (Cambridge III). Correlations between the morphological changes and the degree of functional

TABLE 1.—Revised Cambridge Classification of Chronic Pancreatitis

		ERP		Ultrasound and computed tomography
Normal		Visualisation of the whole gland without abnormal features		
Equivocal	(Cambridge I)	Fewer than three abnormal branches	one sign only	Main duct enlarged (less than 4 mm) Gland enlarged (up to twice normal) Cavities (less than 10 mm)
Mild Moderate	(Cambridge II)	More than three abnormal branches Abnormal main duct and branches	two or more signs	Irregular ducts Focal reduction in parenchymal echogenicity Echogenic foci in parenchyma Increased or irregular echogenicity of wall of main duct Irregular contour to gland, particularly focal enlargements
Considerable	(Cambridge III)	As above with one or more of: Large cavities (greater than 10 mm) Intraductal calculi Ductal obstruction with stricture Gross irregularity of main pancreatic duct		Large cavities (greater than 10 mm) Calculi Ductal obstruction (greater than 4 mm) Major ductal irregularity Gross enlargements (greater than 4 mm) Contiguous organ invasion

(Courtesy of Bozkurt T, Braun U, Leferink S, et al: *Gut* 35:1132–1136, 1994.)

TABLE 2.—Ultrasound and CT Findings (*n*) in Patients With Normal Pancreatic Duct Morphology and Chronic Pancreatitis Shown by ERP

Cambridge classification	Morphological changes	Ultrasound	Computed tomography
Normal (n = 10)	Normal	5	6
	Focal reduction in parenchymal echogenicity	3	2
	Irregular contour to gland	2	2
Cambridge I (n = 10)	Normal	5	5
	Focal reduction in parenchymal echogenicity	3	3
	Irregular contour to gland	2	2
Cambridge II (n = 12)	Focal reduction in parenchymal echogenicity	12	12
	Irregular contour to gland	4	6
	Echogenic foci in parenchyma	4	2
	Gland enlarged	2	2
Cambridge III (n = 16)	Focal reduction in parechymal echogenicity	16	16
	Irregular contour to gland	12	11
	Echogenic foci in parenchyma	7	6
	Gland enlarged	11	12
	Calculi	5	4
	Ductal obstruction (greater than 4 mm)	7	4
	Large cavities (greater than 10 mm)	6	4
	Major duct irregularity	4	2

(Courtesy of Bozkurt T, Braun U, Leferink S, et al: *Gut* 35:1132–1136, 1994.)

impairment were sought. Normal values on the functional study, as previously reported in healthy subjects, were volume secretion, over 300 mL/hr; bicarbonate, over 30 mmol/hr; amylase output, over 5,000 IU/hr; and lipase output, over 100,000 IU/hr. Patients with no more than 2 abnormal findings on the secretin-caerulein test were considered to have dissociated pancreatic insufficiency, whereas those with 3 or 4 abnormal parameters were considered to have global insufficiency.

Results.—The CT and ultrasound changes correlated in 40% to 50% of Cambridge I patients, 67% of Cambridge II patients, and 94% of Cambridge III patients (Table 2). None of the patients with a normal pancreatogram showed functional impairment. Of the patients with equivocal pancreatic duct changes, 70% had dissociated and 30% had global pancreatic insufficiency. Functional impairment was dissociated in 50% of patients with mild to moderate duct abnormalities and global in the other 50%. Global pancreatic insufficiency was present in all patients with considerable morphological changes (Fig 51–1).

Conclusion.—Normal ERP findings are extremely well correlated with normal pancreatic function and Cambridge III ductal changes with advanced functional insufficiency. In the evaluation of chronic pancreatitis, ultrasound and CT are as sensitive as ERP only in patients with considerable morphological abnormalities. Ultrasound and CT may overestimate normal pancreatic morphology in up to 50% of patients by demonstrating equivocal changes not detected by ERP.

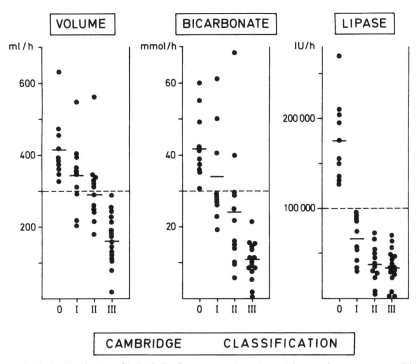

Fig 51–1.—Distribution of individualized parameters in patients with normal pancreatograms (0) and chronic pancreatitis (I–III). (Courtesy of Bozkurt T, Braun U, Leferink S, et al: *Gut* 35:1132–1136, 1994.)

▶ Pancreatic function tests such as the secretin-caerulein test are not generally available in either academic health centers or community hospitals. Consequently, the diagnosis of chronic pancreatic disease frequently rests on morphologic changes as demonstrated by ERP, CT scan, and ultrasound. Earlier studies had suggested that abnormalities in pancreatic function tests could occur with normal findings upon ERP and in CT scans. However, only a limited number of patients was studied. The well-designed study by Bozkurt and colleagues provides valuable information on the use of pancreatic function tests, ERP, CT scan, and ultrasound in the diagnosis of chronic pancreatitis. I would like to reiterate the key findings:

- In patients with a normal pancreatogram, no patient had evidence of functional impairment.
- Conversely, all patients with considerable pancreatic duct changes by ERP had evidence of "global" pancreatic exocrine insufficiency.
- Clearly abnormal pancreatic function tests were demonstrated in only 30% of patients with equivocal ERP findings.
- CT scan and ultrasound are comparably sensitive to ERP *only* in chronic pancreatitis with considerable morphologic changes.

From a clinical standpoint, the diagnosis of chronic pancreatitis and frank pancreatic exocrine insufficiency can be made if 3 findings are present: steatorrhea, diabetes mellitus, and pancreatic calcification. However, the vast majority of patients with chronic pancreatitis do not present with this diagnostic triad, and further studies such as ERP and CT scan are frequently ordered. The study by Bozkurt et al. provides important information as to the utility of these tests to assess pancreatic morphology and indirectly to assess pancreatic exocrine function.—N.J. Greenberger, M.D.

Pancreatitis in Patients With End-Stage Renal Disease
Padilla B, Pollak VE, Pesce A, Kant KS, Gilinsky NH, Deddens JA (Dialysis Clinic, Cincinnati, Ohio; Univ of Cincinnati, Ohio)
Medicine 73:8–20, 1994   119-95-51–2

Background.—Although renal failure affects nearly every organ system, the pancreas has not been well studied in patients with this disorder. The incidence of clinically evident pancreatitis was determined in one dialysis and transplant population. The natural history and prognosis of pancreatitis and its associated conditions were also investigated.

Methods and Findings.—Seven hundred sixteen patients with end-stage renal disease (ESRD) were included in the study. Forty-six, or 6.4%, had pancreatitis. This condition was significantly more common in patients who abused alcohol, in those with systemic lupus erythematosus, and in those with polycystic kidney disease. Pancreatitis was not significantly related to hyperlipidemia, biliary tract disease, or hypercalcemia. Acute pancreatitis that developed before ESRD was primarily alcohol-related and did not seem to be a significant risk factor for future episodes of pancreatitis during dialysis (Table 1). Chronic calcific pancreatitis diagnosed before ESRD was almost always the result of alcohol abuse. In such cases, it tended to be a marker for recurrent acute exacerbation after ESRD development, whether or not the patient continued to drink. Pancreatitis developing initially after ESRD in patients undergoing dialysis was generally benign; it was associated with an uneventful recovery and few recurrent episodes (Table 2). However, these patients had a significant increase in the calcium X phosphate product. In about half these patients, this increase occurred with no apparent precipitating factor. The occurrence of pancreatitis after kidney transplantation was associated with greater mortality and morbidity. Chronic calcific pancreatitis diagnosed after ESRD occurred only in patients with systemic lupus erythematosus and may have been a manifestation of long-standing disease and/or chronic steroid treatment.

Conclusion.—In this series, pancreatitis developed in 4.3% of patients after they had begun ESRD treatment. Pancreatitis unassociated with alcohol abuse occurred in 2.5% during maintenance dialysis.

TABLE 1.—Characteristics of 15 Patients With ESRD Who First Had Pancreatitis Before ESRD (Group 1)

Patient	Age at ESRD (yr)	Sex	Race	Primary Renal Disease	Precipitating Factor	Episodes of Pancreatitis Before ESRD	Episodes of Pancreatitis After ESRD
Acute pancreatitis							
1	40	M	W	HTN	Alcohol	1	0
2	33	M	B	Lupus nephritis	Alcohol	2	0
3	40	M	B	CGN	Alcohol	2	0
4	44	M	B	CGN	Alcohol	1	0
5	36	F	B	DM I	Alcohol	1	0
6	73	M	B	HTN	Alcohol	3	0
7	40	M	B	HTN	Alcohol	2	1
8	61	M	B	DM II	Alcohol and cholelithiasis	1	1
Chronic pancreatitis							
9*	67	F	B	HTN	Alcohol and cholelithiasis	6	0
10*	62	M	B	DM II	Alcohol	1	0
11*	58	F	B	HTN	Alcohol	1	0
12*	54	F	B	PKD, nephrolithiasis	Alcohol	4	3
13*	47	F	B	CGN	Alcohol	1	9
14*	28	F	B	Lupus nephritis	Hyperlipidemia	4	5
15*	44	F	B	PKD	None	1	1

* Pancreatic calcification was present.
Abbreviations: W, white; *B,* black; CGN, chronic glomerulonephritis; *HTN,* hypertensive nephrosclerosis; *PKD,* autosomal dominant polycystic kidney disease; *DM I,* diabetes mellitus type I; *DM II,* diabetes mellitus type II.
(Courtesy of Padilla B, Pollak VE, Pesce A, et al: *Medicine* 73:8–20, 1994.)

▶ In renal failure, the diagnosis of acute pancreatitis may be confounded by the fact that a proportion of patients may have elevated amylase levels in the absence of pancreatitis, although the values rarely exceed 3 times normal. Padilla devised a useful scoring system in which patients with ESRD were

TABLE 2.—Characteristics of 13 Patients With ESRD Who First Had Pancreatitis After Treatment for ESRD (Group 2)

Patient	Age (yr)	Sex	Race	Primary Renal Disease	Precipitating Factor	ESRD → Pancreatitis Interval (mo)	Episodes (n)	Dialysis Treatment When Pancreatitis Occurred
16	56	F	W	PKD	Hyperlipidemia and cholelithiasis	64	3	PD
17	40	M	W	Drug toxicity	Alcohol	115	1	HD
18	21	M	W	Membranous GN	Cholelithiasis	87	1	HD
19	26	M	B	HTN	Splenectomy	16	1	HD
20	41	F	W	PKD	Splenectomy	10	1	HD
21	33	F	W	PKD	Hypercalcemia	43	1	PD
22	37	M	B	Obstructive uropathy	None	27	1	HD
23	49	F	B	HTN	None	69	2	HD
24	57	F	B	Horseshoe kidney	None	21	1	HD
25	65	F	B	HTN	None	41	2	HD
26	49	F	B	Undocumented	None	9	1	HD
27	30	F	W	CGN	None	7	2	PD
28	19	F	W	Reflux nephropathy	None	32	1	PD

Abbreviations: PKD, autosomal dominant polycystic kidney disease; *HTN,* hypertensive nephrosclerosis; CGN, chronic glomerulonephritis; *PD,* peritoneal dialysis; HD, hemodialysis.
(Courtesy of Padilla B, Pollak VE, Pesce A, et al: *Medicine* 73:8–20, 1994.)

diagnosed as having acute pancreatitis if they obtained a total score of 3 or more points. The scoring system used can be found in Table 1 of the original article.—N.J. Greenberger, M.D.

Diabetes and the Risk of Pancreatic Cancer

Gullo L, Pezzilli R, Morselli-Labate AM, and the Italian Pancreatic Cancer Study Group (Univ of Bologna, Italy)
N Engl J Med 331:81–84, 1994   119-95-51–3

Background.—Although patients with pancreatic cancer are known to have an increased frequency of diabetes, the nature of this relationship is not understood. Authorities disagree on whether diabetes is a risk factor for pancreatic cancer.

Methods.—Seven hundred twenty patients with pancreatic cancer and 720 control patients from 14 centers in Italy were studied. All were interviewed in detail to elicit their clinical histories. The diagnosis of diabetes was based on American Diabetes Association criteria.

Findings.—Twenty-three percent of the patients with pancreatic cancer and 8% of the control patients had diabetes. In 56% of the patients with pancreatic cancer, diabetes was diagnosed concomitantly with the cancer or within 2 years before the diagnosis of cancer. Although the association between the 2 conditions was significant, when only patients with diabetes of 3 or more years' duration were included in the analysis, the relationship became nonsignificant (table). All the patients with pan-

DURATION (YR)	CASE PATIENTS		CONTROL PATIENTS		P VALUE
	NO. (%)	MALE/ FEMALE	NO. (%)	MALE/ FEMALE	
0	66 (40.2)	38/28	2 (3.3)	2/0	<0.001
1	15 (9.2)	8/7	2 (3.3)	1/1	0.177
2	11 (6.7)	6/5	4 (6.7)	1/3	0.875
3–4	11 (6.7)	6/5	7 (11.7)	5/2	0.162
5–6	13 (7.9)	9/4	6 (10.0)	4/2	0.490
7–9	14 (8.5)	9/5	7 (11.7)	2/5	0.364
10–14	17 (10.4)	10/7	9 (15.0)	2/7	0.254
≥15	17 (10.4)	10/7	23 (38.3)	13/10	<0.001
Total	164	96/68	60	30/30	

Clinical Duration of Diabetes in Case and Control Patients

Note: Interval between diagnosis of diabetes and the diagnosis of cancer or the date of interview.
(Courtesy of Gullo L, Pezzilli R, Morselli-Labate AM, and the Italian Pancreatic Cancer Study Group: *N Engl J Med* 331:81–84, 1994.)

creatic cancer whose diabetes had been diagnosed before the cancer and all but 1 of the diabetic control patients had the non–insulin-dependent form of the disease.

Conclusion.—Diabetes is significantly associated with pancreatic cancer. However, no association was found between diabetes and pancreatic cancer in patients with long-standing diabetes. The increased prevalence of diabetes in patients with pancreatic cancer appears to result mainly from diabetes of recent onset, presumably caused by the tumor.

▶ This paper prompted several letters to the editor of the *New England Journal of Medicine* (1) in which 3 groups presented data supporting the notion that diabetes *precedes* pancreatic cancer and, therefore, should be recognized as a risk factor. Gullo et al. counter these arguments by emphasizing that in a large number of patients with pancreatic cancer and diabetes (40%), the diabetes was diagnosed simultaneously with or after the tumor, and all of these patients were normoglycemic in prior examinations. Gullo also points out that pancreatic cancer is a frequent cause of impaired glucose metabolism. From the above 2 lines of reasoning, Gullo concludes that in these patients, diabetes was caused by the tumor rather than by a preceding long-standing undiagnosed disorder.

While there clearly is an *association* between diabetes and pancreatic cancer, Gullo's data do not support the concept that diabetes per se is a risk factor for this disorder. The following article (Abstract 119-95-51–4) provides further support for the concept that pancreatic cancer can cause diabetes.—N.J. Greenberger, M.D.

Reference

1. Correspondence. Pancreatic Cancer and Diabetes. N Engl J Med 331:1326–1328, 1994.

Islet Amyloid Polypeptide in Patients With Pancreatic Cancer and Diabetes

Permert J, Larsson J, Westermark GT, Herrington MK, Christmanson L, Pour PM, Westermark P, Adrian TE (Creighton Univ, Omaha, Neb; Univ of Linköping, Sweden; Univ of Uppsala, Sweden; et al)
N Engl J Med 330:313–318, 1994   119-95-51–4

Objective.—Whereas diabetes was once thought to predispose to pancreatic cancer, it is now known that pancreatic cancer can cause diabetes. Some specific diabetogenic factors have been suggested to exist. Islet amyloid polypeptide (IAPP), produced in the beta cells of the islets, is the main constituent of the pancreatic amyloid and pancreas in 90% of patients with non–insulin-dependent diabetes mellitus. Although IAPP is normally released along with insulin, the secretion of the 2 hormones is

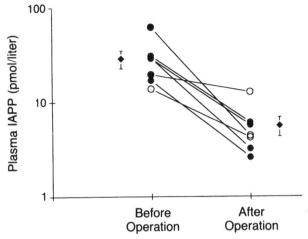

Fig 51–2.—Fasting plasma concentrations of IAPP in 7 patients with pancreatic cancer, before and 3 months after subtotal pancreatectomy. The IAPP concentrations were significantly decreased after the operation (P = 0.01) The *solid circles* denote patients with diabetes; the *open circles,* patients with normal glucose tolerance; and the *diamonds,* means ± SE. (Courtesy of Permert J, Larsson J, Westermark GT, et al: N Engl J Med 330:313–318, 1994.)

controlled independently. The association between IAPP and diabetes in patients with pancreatic cancer was studied.

Methods.—A radioimmunoassay was used to measure plasma IAPP in 30 patients with pancreatic cancer, 46 with other types of cancer, and 23

Fasting Plasma IAPP and C-Peptide Concentrations and the IAPP:C-Peptide Ratio in Normal Subjects and Subgroups of Patients With Pancreatic Cancer

GROUP	No.	IAPP	C PEPTIDE	IAPP:C PEPTIDE	IAPP >2 SD ABOVE NORMAL MEAN
		pmol/liter		*molar ratio ×100*	*no. (%)*
Normal subjects	25	8.0±5.0	497±205	2.0±1.7	1 (4)
Patients with pancreatic cancer					
Normal glucose tolerance	9	12.2±2.4 (P = 0.007)	472±144 (P = 0.87)	2.7±0.6 (P = 0.003)	0
Impaired glucose tolerance	3	11.7±5.5	452±223	2.2±0.9	1 (33)
Non-insulin-requiring diabetes	11	31.4±12.6 (P<0.001)	1052±464 (P<0.001)	3.1±1.0 (P = 0.005)	11 (100)
Insulin-requiring diabetes	7	25.0±8.7 (P<0.001)	459±127 (P = 0.75)	6.1±3.4 (P<0.001)	5 (71)
After subtotal pancreatectomy	7†	5.6±3.4 (P = 0.26)	283±11 (P = 0.008)	2.1±1.3 (P = 0.80)	0

Note: Plus-minus values are means ± SD. The P values refer to comparisons with the normal subjects.
† Among the 7 patients with resectable tumors, 1 patient had normal glucose tolerance, 2 had non-insulin-requiring diabetes, and 4 had insulin-requiring diabetes.
(Courtesy of Permert J, Larsson J, Westermark GT, et al: N Engl J Med 330:313–318, 1994.)

with diabetes. A control group of 25 normal individuals was also examined. Samples of pancreatic cancers and the tissue around them, as well as normal pancreatic tissue, were studied for IAPP immunoreactivity and IAPP messenger RNA.

Findings.—The patients with pancreatic cancer had higher fasting plasma IAPP concentrations than those in the control group because of increased concentrations in the patients with either insulin-requiring or non–insulin-requiring diabetes (Fig 51–2). Plasma IAPP concentrations normalized after surgery in 7 patients studied before and after subtotal pancreatectomy. The patients with pancreatic cancer, especially those with diabetes, had a significantly higher ratio of IAPP to C peptide (table). Again, this ratio normalized after surgery. Among patients who had non–insulin-dependent diabetes mellitus but not pancreatic cancer, plasma IAPP was reduced in those receiving insulin but normal in those receiving oral hypoglycemic drugs.

Normal pancreatic tissue had a significantly higher IAPP content than cancerous tissue. Islets surrounded by or immediately adjacent to tumor exhibited greatly reduced or even absent staining for IAPP. Islets in normal pancreatic tissue and those adjacent to tumor tissue that were negative for IAPP on immunohistochemical evaluation were strongly positive for IAPP messenger RNA on in situ hybridization.

Conclusion.—Plasma IAPP concentrations increased in patients with pancreatic cancer and diabetes, particularly those with insulin-requiring diabetes. The increase appears to result from elevated secretion of IAPP, rather than from production by the tumor or decreased degradation. Overproduction of IAPP, which can cause insulin resistance, may contribute to the diabetes that occurs in patients with pancreatic cancer. Islet amyloid polypeptide measurement might prove useful in the early diagnosis of pancreatic cancer among patients with newly diagnosed non–insulin-dependent diabetes mellitus who have experienced weight loss.

▶ This study demonstrates that plasma IAPP concentrations are elevated in patients with pancreatic cancer who have diabetes. Furthermore, because IAPP may cause insulin resistance, its overproduction may contribute to the diabetes that occurs in these patients. Finally, as the authors point out, measurement of plasma IAPP could prove valuable in the diagnosis of pancreatic cancer in the small subgroup of patients with newly diagnosed non–insulin-dependent diabetes mellitus who present with *weight loss* rather than obesity.—N.J. Greenberger, M.D.

Frequent Alterations of the Tumor Suppressor Genes *p53* and *DCC* in Human Pancreatic Carcinoma

Simon B, Weinel R, Höhne M, Watz J, Schmidt J, Körtner G, Arnold R (Philips

Univ, Marburg, Germany; Univ Giessen, Germany)
Gastroenterology 106:1645–1651, 1994   119-95-51–5

Purpose.—The pathogenesis of pancreatic cancer is largely unknown; it is usually diagnosed late, so it is usually studied only in its advanced stages. The mechanisms involved in tumor development might be clarified through analysis of various accumulated genetic changes. Activated c-Ki-*ras* oncogene is one common finding, but additional alterations of tumor suppressor genes are expected as well. Pancreatic carcinoma cell lines and primary tumors were analyzed for concomitant genetic changes of *p53* and the putative tumor suppressor gene deleted in colon carcinoma (DCC).

Methods and Results.—Immunocytochemistry and immunohistochemistry, immunoassay, and Northern blot analysis were used to study *p53* protein and transcript expression in 12 cell lines and 6 primary pancreatic carcinomas. A reverse-transcription polymerase chain reaction was used to assess *DCC* expression. Seventy-five percent of the cell lines showed *P53* overexpression. Seven of the 9 cell lines that overexpressed *p53* had *p53* point mutations. Most cell lines had concomitant alter-

p53 Alterations and Loss of DCC Gene Expression in Primary Pancreatic Carcinomas

	Overexpression of *p53*	Loss of *DCC* expression
Pancreatic carcinoma tumors		
722		
N	−	+
T	+	−
927		
N	−	+
T	−	+
228		
N	−	+
T	+	−
323		
N	−	+
T	+	−
AS		
T	−	+[a]
BE		
T	+	−[a]
M	+	−[a]

Abbreviations: T, primary tumor; N, normal tissue; M, metastasis.
[a] Obtained from previous work.
(Courtesy of Simon B, Weinel R, Höhne M, et al: *Gastroenterology* 106:1645–1651, 1994.)

ations in *p53* and *DCC*. Overexpression of *p53* and loss of *DCC* expression were also found in 67% of primary tumors (table).

Conclusion.—Pancreatic cancer and the frequently activated c-Ki-*ras* oncogene appear to be associated with *p53* and *DCC* genetic changes. The findings support the relevance of the multihit model in the carcinogenesis of pancreatic cancer. Mutational alterations of the *ras* and *p53* genes are now documented in colorectal, gastric, and pancreatic cancers, suggesting a common set of genetic changes with these tumors that might be relevant for tumor development and progression.

▶ For an excellent brief review of the role of *p53* and tumor suppression through the cell cycle, see the editorial by Kern (1). He presents a very clear schematic model of *p53* and its ability to suppress the cell cycle and details how a mutant *p53* can lead to uncontrolled tumor growth.—N.J. Greenberger, M.D.

Reference

1. Kern JE: *p53*: Tumor suppression through control of the cell cycles. *Gastroenterology* 106:1708–1710, 1994.

PART SIX

ENDOCRINOLOGY, DIABETES, AND METABOLISM

ROBERT D. UTIGER, M.D.

Introduction

The 48 articles chosen for this section of the 1995 YEAR BOOK OF MEDICINE represent an attempt to obtain a balance among material covering the pathophysiology, diagnosis, and management of many of the common problems in endocrinology and metabolism, with an occasional article on basic mechanisms of disease. There was no report last year of any large clinical trial to match the report of the Diabetes Control and Complications Trial that was published in 1993 and covered in the 1994 YEAR BOOK OF MEDICINE, but several smaller trials providing useful therapeutic information—for example, for the treatment of patients with diabetic nephropathy or osteoporosis—are included that should have some impact on clinical practice.

The chapter on the pituitary gland includes an article on the occurrence of apparent pituitary adenomas seen on MRI of the head in normal subjects and an article on the diagnosis of growth hormone deficiency in adults with pituitary disease. The former article serves as a reminder that powerful imaging procedures cannot be used for diagnosis, but only for localization, and the latter reminds us that testing for growth hormone deficiency in adults remains difficult (and a bit hazardous), notwithstanding the increasing interest in growth hormone replacement therapy for adults with hypopituitarism.

The chapter on adrenal glands includes 2 articles that demonstrate that pituitary-adrenal function is nearly always normal in patients with acute pulmonary tuberculosis, which is welcome information in view of the resurgence of the disease in recent years. An article on Cushing's syndrome in children and adolescents points out the similarities in the clinical manifestations of glucocorticoid excess in these groups and in adults, except for growth retardation in the former. Another article documents the safety of inhaled glucocorticoid therapy in children with asthma, a finding that can be extrapolated directly to adults.

The availability of more sensitive serum thyrotropin (TSH) assays in the last decade has unquestionably made the diagnosis of hyperthyroidism easier. The first article in the chapter on the thyroid gland indicates that so-called third-generation assays with even greater sensitivity are not a large further advance. Several articles in this chapter concern subclinical hyperthyroidism (low serum TSH and normal serum free thyroxine values), its frequency and its consequences. It is a rather common problem and, if persistent, can have both cardiovascular and skeletal effects. It is most often caused by overzealous thyroxine therapy and thus can be avoided by proper monitoring of therapy; when caused by thyroid disease, therapy is more problematic. The management of hyperthyroidism caused by Graves' disease continues to receive attention, in part because of the unresolved debate about whether an antithyroid drug or radioactive iodine is the best therapy. One article describes a study in which older patients had more rapid responses to treatment with methimazole and were more likely to have remissions of Graves' disease than younger patients. Another demonstrates that assays for TSH receptor antibodies have little value in identifying whether a patient with Graves' hyperthyroidism has had a remission of the Graves' disease during antithyroid drug therapy, and thus in guiding the duration of therapy. The last article in this chapter concerns the use of analysis of DNA to identify germline mutations in affected members of families with multiple endocrine neoplasia or medullary thyroid carcinoma, and equally important to identify those family members who are not affected and thus do not need periodic surveillance for the components of these syndromes.

The chapter on the reproductive system focuses on hirsutism, secondary amenorrhea, and the menopause in women and the possibility of declining fertility in men. Hirsutism is a common problem among young women, and many hirsute women have polycystic ovaries, but few have important disturbances in ovarian or adrenal function, and extensive evaluation is rarely indicated. Attention is given to a search for risk factors for secondary amenorrhea, which is also common. After women with well-known causes (prolactinoma, drugs) were excluded, relatively few risk factors could be identified. There are articles that examine the risk factors for hot flashes and the relationship between both premenstrual symptoms and hot flashes and postmenopausal osteoporosis. The question of whether sperm concentrations in men are declining is also considered. There are data both supporting and denying the existence of a decline. The debate to some extent concerns procedural and analytic issues, but if there has in fact been a decline and it is continuing, the implications for the future are substantial.

The first article in the chapter on the parathyroid glands and bone concerns a study from Australia indicating that the genotype for the vitamin D receptor might be a very important determinant of osteoporosis. Although this relationship has not been confirmed in some other populations, this topic is sure to be investigated intensively in the near future because it might provide a new way to identify persons at risk for osteoporosis. Several articles in this chapter concern the prevention and treatment of osteoporosis, a subject that continues to attract much attention. One is about the ability of alkali administration to increase bone formation and decrease bone resorption, based on the premise that bone mineral is lost in the process of buffering acid produced in the process of metabolism of dietary protein. Other articles provide further evidence of the benefit of calcium supplementation and information about the durability of the benefit of estrogen or etidronate therapy on the skeleton in postmenopausal women. The final article in this chapter describes a careful study of pamidronate, now the best pharmacologic treatment for severe hypercalcemia.

The topics of the articles in the chapter on carbohydrate metabolism and diabetes mellitus include the importance of both insulin secretion and action in the maintenance of glucose tolerance in normal subjects and the efficacy of caloric restriction—as opposed to weight reduction—in ameliorating hyperglycemia in patients with non–insulin-dependent diabetes mellitus (NIDDM). Other articles concern the diagnosis of diabetes mellitus—a measurement of fasting plasma glucose is adequate—and a comparison of glipizide and glyburide, now easily the most widely used oral hypoglycemic drugs, in patients with NIDDM. Several selections concern the ability of antihypertensive drugs to slow the progression of diabetic nephropathy, even in normotensive patients. This topic has attracted much interest because diabetic nephropathy is such a common cause of end-stage renal disease.

This brief listing of many of the articles selected for this section of the 1995 YEAR BOOK OF MEDICINE is meant only to highlight what questions are being pursued by investigators in this area. I hope that readers who look further into the next 7 chapters will find the articles and the comments both informative and useful.

Robert D. Utiger, M.D.

52 The Pituitary Gland

Pituitary Magnetic Resonance Imaging in Normal Human Volunteers: Occult Adenomas in the General Population
Hall WA, Luciano MG, Doppman JL, Patronas NJ, Oldfield EH (Natl Inst of Neurological Disorders and Stroke, Bethesda, Md; NIH, Bethesda, Md)
Ann Intern Med 120:817–820, 1994   119-95-52-1

Introduction.—The prevalence of focal pituitary lesions consistent with an adenoma was determined in 100 normal persons (70 women and 30 men aged 18 to 60 years). MR images of the pituitary fossa acquired in the coronal and sagittal planes, before and after the IV administration of gadolinium-diethylenetriaminepentaacetic acid were evaluated by 3 experienced reviewers.

Observations.—All 3 reviewers agreed that 59 of the 100 persons had normal pituitary glands. At least 1 reviewer noted a focus of low signal intensity consistent with a pituitary microadenoma in 21 persons before contrast administration. The abnormality was detected by all 3 reviewers in 1 person, by 2 reviewers in 7 persons, and by 1 reviewer in 13 persons. After contrast injection, 41 sites of abnormal signal intensity were found in 34 persons, 10 of whom had changes interpreted as representing a pituitary adenoma by at least 2 of the reviewers. These 10 persons all had normal endocrine studies.

Patient Review.—Of 50 patients with Cushing's disease who had an adenoma identified operatively, 56% had focal areas of low signal intensity on MRI after contrast administration. In 4 patients, however, the site of the adenoma was incorrectly read on the MRI study.

Conclusion.—Approximately 10% of normal adults have MRI changes in the pituitary that are consistent with pituitary microadenoma.

▶ Magnetic resonance imaging with gadolinium enhancement is the best radiologic procedure for evaluating patients suspected to have hypothalamic and pituitary disease, especially pituitary tumors. In this careful study of normal subjects, abnormalities consistent with a pituitary microadenoma were found by 1 reviewer in nearly half, and the proportion was 10% when the images were evaluated by several persons. (The results of CT of normal subjects are similar). It is important to note that the subjects studied by Hall et al. not only had a normal history and physical examination, but also normal basal growth hormone, prolactin, and thyrotropin secretion; why pituitary-adrenal and pituitary-gonadal hormone secretion was not evaluated is not mentioned, but they are likely to have been normal (all the young women had normal menstrual cycles). Another commendable aspect of the study is the wide age range of the study subjects; an excess of women was recruited because they have pituitary microadenomas more often than men. Most of the MRI abnormalities probably indicate the presence of a nonsecreting pituitary microadenoma, because microadenomas are found in 5% to 25% of pituitary glands at autopsy, figures far, far higher than the frequency of clinical pituitary hyperfunction. (I know of no study of pituitary MRI or CT and postmortem examination of the pituitary gland in the same persons.)

What should be done in a patient who undergoes MRI for some nonendocrine reason and is found to have a pituitary microadenoma? The patient's clinical status should be reevaluated for evidence of Cushing's syndrome, hyperthyroidism, prolactin excess (amenorrhea, galactorrhea, hypogonadism), and acromegaly. Microadenomas rarely cause deficiency syndromes, except for microprolactinomas, because of the ability of prolactin excess to cause gonadotropin deficiency. In the absence of any clinical abnormalities, I would measure serum cortisol, thyroxine, prolactin, and testosterone (in men). Some would add serum growth hormone or insulin-like growth factor-1 to this list, but I would just look closely for evidence of acromegaly. If all are normal, MRI should be repeated yearly for 2 years and then, assuming no change, at less frequent intervals (1).

The identification of microadenomas in normal subjects means that imaging should not be used to diagnose a functioning pituitary tumor, but only to determine whether a patient who has clinical and biochemical evidence of pituitary hormone hypersecretion has a pituitary tumor. As noted by the authors' and others' (2), only 50% to 60% of patients with Cushing's disease have CT or MRI evidence of a pituitary tumor. The proportion of patients with pituitary tumors secreting other hormones who have detectable tumors is higher, but still not 100%. Furthermore, although MRI identification of a pituitary tumor in a patient with, for example, Cushing's disease, does not guarantee that the tumor is the source of the excess adrenocorticotropin, the conclusion seems sufficiently reasonable that no further study, e.g., petrosal sinus sampling, is indicated.—R.D. Utiger, M.D.

References

1. Molitch ME: Evaluation and treatment of the patient with a pituitary incidentaloma. *J Clin Endocrinol Metab* 80:3–6, 1995.
2. Kaye TB, Crapo L: The Cushing syndrome: An update on diagnostic tests. *Ann Intern Med* 112:434–444, 1990.

Diagnosis of Growth-Hormone Deficiency in Adults
Hoffman DM, O'Sullivan AJ, Baxter RC, Ho KKY (St Vincent's Hosp, Sydney, Australia; Royal Prince Alfred Hosp, Sydney, Australia)
Lancet 343:1064–1068, 1994 119-95-52–2

Background.—The optimal method for diagnosing growth hormone (GH) deficiency in adults has not been defined. Current cutoff values for

GH deficiency are either arbitrary or based on studies of children and have no statistical basis because a normal range has never been established. The diagnostic merits of serum GH responses to a provocative stimulus, 24-hour GH concentration (IGHC), insulin-like growth factor I (IGF-I), and IGF-binding protein 3 (IGFBP-3) were investigated in adults with suspected GH deficiency.

Methods.—Serum GH responses to insulin-induced hypoglycemia, the mean serum IGHC derived from 20-minute blood sampling, and serum IGF-I and serum IGFBP-3 concentrations were measured in 23 patients with extensive organic pituitary disease considered GH-deficient and in 35 normal controls matched for sex, age, and body mass index.

Results.—The peak serum GH response to hypoglycemia clearly differentiated the hypopituitary patients from the normal subjects. The hypopituitary patients also had significantly lower mean serum IGHC, IGF-I, and IGFBP-3 values. To overcome the age-related decline in spontaneous GH secretion that occurs in normal persons, the diagnostic value of serum IGHC and IGF-I were analyzed by stratifying persons by age. Using the upper limit of serum IGHC in the hypopituitary patients would have wrongly classified 5 of 15 young and 4 of 16 elderly normal individuals as having hypopituitarism. Use of an undetectable serum IGHC value (less than 2 ng/mL) as an indicator of GH deficiency would have correctly identified 16 of 20 patients and 26 of 31 normal subjects. Thus, the overall predictive value of an undetectable serum IGHC value was 70%, and for the elderly, 84%. Using the upper limit of serum IGF-I values in the young and elderly hypopituitary patients as a diagnostic cutoff would have correctly classified 10 of 35 normal individuals; the lower limit of serum IGF-I values in normal subjects would have identified correctly only 9 of 23 hypopituitary patients. Combining serum IGF-I and IGFBP-3 measurements did not improve the diagnostic accuracy achieved with either measurement alone.

Conclusion.—GH deficiency in adults is most reliably identified by measurements of serum GH during hypoglycemia, and serum IGF-I and IGFBP-3 measurements are poor diagnostic tests for adult GH deficiency.

▶ No one has paid much attention to GH deficiency in adults, for several reasons. First, most of the symptoms and signs that occur in these patients can be attributed to other deficiencies, and until recently, suspected changes in body composition were poorly documented and of uncertain clinical importance. Second, most provocative tests of GH secretion are cumbersome and even dangerous, e.g., inducing hypoglycemia, and certainly in children and probably also in adults the results of these tests may not mirror endogenous secretion. Third, replacement therapy was not available until recent years, and although available now, it is inconvenient and extremely expensive ($20,000/year). So I, and I suspect many others, consider evaluating adults for GH deficiency an academic exercise.

This view may prove to be misplaced, for reasons mentioned below, and therefore the biochemical diagnosis of GH deficiency in adults may become important. As demonstrated by Hoffman et al., neither of the methods to detect GH deficiency based on a single blood sample—determination of serum IGF-I or IGFBP-3, both of which are GH-dependent—is satisfactory. They are insensitive and nonspecific and must be compared with age-based norms. Multiple sampling is little better and is very impractical. The likelihood of GH deficiency in a patient with hypopituitarism increases with an increasing number of other pituitary hormone deficiencies, to be sure, but that is guilt by association (1). Other tests of GH reserve are available, for example stimulation with L-dopa or vasopressin, and synthetic GH-releasing substances may become available fairly soon, but for now I think that the insulin-induced hypoglycemia test, notwithstanding its limitations and the charge that it is normal in all but the most severely GH-deficient patients, must be done if one really wants to know anything about GH secretory status in an adult. This test, despite the hazard of hypoglycemia, has the advantage of allowing simultaneous testing of pituitary-adrenal reserve.

The availability of recombinant GH has prompted a closer look at the manifestations of GH deficiency in adults. Symptoms attributed to GH deficiency (and that improve with GH therapy) include lack of vigor, poor exercise tolerance, and poor social functioning (2). More objective abnormalities are decreases in lean body mass and bone density, an increase in adipose mass, and impaired cardiovascular function; these too can be reversed by GH therapy (3, 4). Finally, there is evidence of increased cardiovascular mortality in hypopituitarism (5). The ultimate benefit, if any, of GH replacement therapy in adults with GH deficiency is certainly far from established, but at least the thought of treatment seems somewhat less far-fetched than it did a few years ago.—R.D. Utiger, M.D.

References

1. Toogood AA, Beardwell CG, Shalet SM: The severity of growth hormone deficiency in adults with pituitary disease is related to the degree of hypopituitarism. *Clin Endocrinol* 41:511–516, 1994.
2. Vance ML: Hypopituitarism. *N Engl J Med* 330:1651–1662, 1994.
3. Bengtsson B-A, Eden S, Lonn L, et al: Treatment of adults with growth hormone (GH) deficiency with recombinant GH. *J Clin Endocrinol Metab* 76:309–317, 1993.
4. O'Halloran DJ, Tsatsoulis A, Whitehouse RW, Holmes SJ, Adams JE, Shalet SM: Increased bone density after recombinant human growth hormone (GH) therapy in adults with isolated GH deficiency. *J Clin Endocrinol Metab* 76:1344–1348, 1993.
5. Rosen T, Bengtsson B-A: Premature mortality due to cardiovascular disease in hypopituitarism. *Lancet* 336:285–288, 1990.

Arginine Vasopressin and Osmolality in the Elderly

Johnson AG, Crawford GA, Kelly D, Nguyen TV, Gyory AZ (St Vincents Hosp, Darlinghurst, Australia; Royal North Shore Hosp, St Leonards, Australia; Univ

of Sydney, Australia)
J Am Geriatr Soc 42:399–404, 1994   119-95-52–3

Objective.—Young and elderly healthy subjects were compared to evaluate the influence of age on plasma arginine vasopressin (AVP) secretion. In the elderly, the effect of sex on plasma concentrations of AVP and the impact of prostaglandin blockade on renal responsiveness to AVP were assessed.

Methods.—Forty-five healthy younger adults with a mean age of 35 years and 41 healthy elderly adults (29 men, 12 women) aged 75 years or older with a mean age of 79 years were studied. Blood samples were drawn from both groups at study entry. The elderly were randomly selected to receive indomethacin or placebo for 1 month; the alternative was administered for an additional month after a 1- to 2-week washout period. At entry and at the end of each treatment period, the elderly

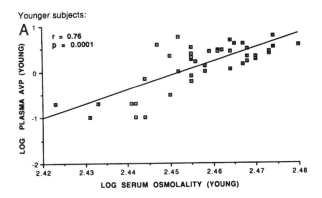

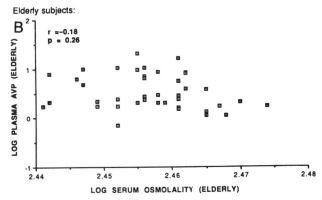

Fig 52–1.—Plasma AVP compared with serum osmolality (logarithm-transformed) in (**A**) younger adults and (**B**) elderly subjects. (Courtesy of Johnson AG, Crawford GA, Kelly D, et al: *J Am Geriatr Soc* 42:399-404, 1994.)

subjects had repeat plasma and serum studies and completed a 24-hour urine collection for measurement of urinary osmolality.

Results.—The mean baseline plasma concentration of AVP was significantly higher in the elderly group (4.7 pg/mL [4.3 pmol/L]) than in the younger group (2.1 pg/mL [1.9 pmol/L]). Their mean baseline serum osmolality, however, was similar (elderly, 286; younger, 287 mOsm/kg). There was a strong correlation between baseline plasma AVP and serum osmolality in young adults but no apparent correlation between these measures in the elderly (Fig 52–1). Plasma AVP did not differ between elderly men and women, and indomethacin treatment did not significantly alter the plasma AVP/urine osmolality ratio. The changes in plasma AVP after indomethacin therapy did not correlate with changes in serum osmolality.

Conclusion.—In both men and women, aging was associated with an increase in plasma concentrations of AVP. Serum osmolality and plasma AVP were strongly correlated in younger adults but not in the elderly. Indomethacin treatment did not affect renal responsiveness to plasma AVP. The cause of the apparent loss of osmotic regulation of plasma AVP in healthy, elderly individuals is not known.

▶ Vasopressin secretion and action are essential for the maintenance of normal osmolality in the extracellular fluid compartment and water balance. Usually, as exemplified by part A of Figure 52–1, there is a close relationship between plasma vasopressin and serum osmolality, so that small increases or decreases in serum osmolality result, respectively, in small increases or decreases in vasopressin secretion and therefore in retention or excretion of free water. An additional, often overlooked component of this system is thirst, which varies similarly in response to equally small variations in serum osmolality and is as important as vasopressin in defending against hyperosmolality and volume depletion. These relationships are less evident in elderly persons, even very healthy ones, as in this study. As shown in part B of Figure 52–1, plasma vasopressin was not correlated with serum osmolality in them, and in other studies, elderly subjects had less thirst when their serum osmolality was increased (1).

What accounts for the higher plasma vasopressin concentrations and lack of positive correlation between plasma vasopressin and serum osmolality in elderly subjects? Some nonosmotic stimulus must be involved, most likely hypovolemia, perhaps occurring as a result of diminished thirst and an age-related decline in both renal-concentrating capacity and sodium reabsorption. The practical importance of these observations relates to the risk of volume depletion in elderly subjects, a particular risk in a person with impaired thirst whose access to fluid is limited by some other infirmity.

With respect to this study, it is important to note that these were (apparently) random measurements, done while the subjects were eating and drinking according to their usual preferences; therefore, the results represent the net effect of the factors that determine fluid and solute intake in everyday life. The portion of the study in which indomethacin was given was done to determine whether inhibition of prostaglandin production might alter vaso-pressin action. No effect was noted, but one wonders what would have happened had the measurements been repeated after a period of fluid restriction.—R.D. Utiger, M.D.

Reference

1. Phillips PA, Rolls BJ, Ledingham JGG, et al: Reduced thirst after water deprivation in healthy elderly men. *N Engl J Med* 311:753–759, 1984.

53 The Adrenal Glands

Plasma Corticotrophin Releasing Hormone, Vasopressin, ACTH and Cortisol Responses to Acute Myocardial Infarction
Donald RA, Crozier IG, Foy SG, Richards AM, Livesey JH, Ellis MJ, Mattioli L, Ikram H (Christchurch Hosp, New Zealand)
Clin Endocrinol 40:499–504, 1994   119-95-53–1

Introduction.—Although an association has been clearly established between myocardial infarction and an increase in plasma cortisol concentrations, the response of the hypothalamic-pituitary-adrenal axis hormones to this stress has not been established. The interrelation of hormonal responses was studied by measuring plasma cortisol, adrenocorticotropin (ACTH), vasopressin (AVP), and corticotropin-releasing hormone (CRH) concentrations in patients with acute myocardial infarction who were or were not treated with angiotensin-converting enzyme inhibitors.

Methods.—Thirty-four patients (24 men, 10 women) who were examined within 6 hours of the onset of chest pain and had ECG or biochemical evidence of an acute myocardial infarction were randomly assigned to 1 of 3 groups: 1 group received placebo, 1 group receive captopril, and 1 group received enalapril. Most patients also received thrombolytic therapy. Plasma cortisol, ACTH, AVP, and CRH concentrations were measured at baseline; 10, 30, and 60 minutes; and 4, 8, 12, 24, 48, and 72 hours.

Results.—At baseline, the mean plasma concentrations of cortisol, AVP, and CRH were significantly elevated in the patients, whereas ACTH was significantly lower as compared with reference means. With time, plasma cortisol, AVP, and CRH decreased significantly and ACTH increased (Fig 53–1). The 3 treatment groups did not significantly differ in the responses of any of the hormones, indicating that angiotensin-converting enzyme inhibitors do not affect the secretion of these hormones.

Discussion.—The normal relations between the hypothalamic-adrenal-pituitary axis hormones are disturbed in patients with acute myocardial infarction. If the heart, like the peripheral vasculature, responds to AVP with vasoconstriction, vasopressin V_1 receptor antagonists may have a role in improving myocardial perfusion.

▶ I chose this study especially for the figure showing the changes in plasma cortisol concentrations for several days after an uncomplicated acute myo-

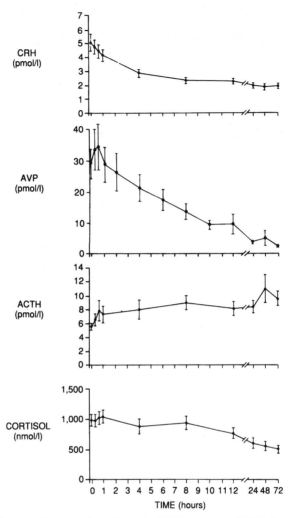

Fig 53–1.—Plasma corticotropin-releasing hormone (CRH), vasopressin (AVP), adrenocorticotropin (ACTH), and cortisol (mean values from all 34 patients in groups 1-3 ± SEM) in the 72 hours after hospital admission. (Courtesy of Donald RA, Crozier IG, Foy SG, et al: *Clin Endocrinol* 40:499–504, 1994.)

cardial infarction. The initial mean plasma cortisol concentration was 34.8 μg/dL (960 nmol/L), and it declined by about 50% during the 3-day study period. The initial value is only about 2 times that of most normal subjects in the morning, leading to the conclusion that the "stress" was moderate and subsided rather promptly.

The unusual aspect of the results is that the plasma ACTH concentrations were low-normal at the time of admission. Plasma AVP and CRH concentrations, both of which stimulate ACTH secretion, were high, and the plasma cortisol concentrations were not so high that they would be expected to inhibit ACTH secretion in the presence of the large amounts of AVP and CRH. The ACTH secretion presumably had increased soon after the myocardial infarction, which had occurred up to 6 hours earlier (why else would plasma cortisol be elevated?), but I cannot think of anything other than these cortisol elevations to explain why plasma ACTH concentrations were relatively low at the time of admission. This explanation is supported by the results of studies of patients undergoing elective surgery in whom in an initial increase in ACTH secretion was attenuated by persistently increased plasma cortisol concentrations or exogenous glucocorticoid administration (1, 2). That is, whatever the mediators of stress-induced increases in ACTH secretion are, their action can be overcome by a lot of glucocorticoid.

The initial plasma AVP concentrations approached those capable of raising blood pressure, and they were certainly high enough for the first several days to cause inappropriate water retention. The pattern of AVP secretion is similar during and soon after surgery (3). Awareness that large amounts of AVP are secreted under these circumstances should minimize the likelihood of overzealous fluid administration and the attendant risks of volume expansion and hyponatremia.—R.D. Utiger, M.D.

References

1. Raff H, Flemma RJ, Findling JW, Nelson DK: Fast cortisol-induced inhibition of the adrenocorticotropin response to surgery in humans. *J Clin Endocrinol Metab* 67:1146–1148, 1988.
2. Naito Y, Fukata J, Tamai S, et al: Biphasic changes in hypothalamo-pituitary-adrenal function during the early recovery period after major abdominal surgery. *J Clin Endocrinol Metab* 73:111–117, 1991.
3. Donald RA, Perry EG, Wittert GA, et al: The plasma ACTH, AVP, CRH and catecholamine responses to conventional and laparoscopic cholecystectomy. *Clin Endocrinol* 38:609–615, 1993.

The Spectrum of Endocrine Dysfunction in Active Pulmonary Tuberculosis

Post FA, Soule SG, Willcox PA, Levitt NS (Univ of Cape Town, South Africa; Groote Schuur Hosp, South Africa)
Clin Endocrinol 40:367–371, 1994   119-95-53-2

Introduction.—Reports of the prevalence of hypoadrenalism in patients with pulmonary tuberculosis have varied widely, from 0 to 55%. A prospective study was undertaken to determine the prevalence of hypoadrenalism in tuberculous patients, using several accepted criteria for diagnosing hypoadrenalism. Thyroid and gonadal dysfunction was also assessed.

Methods.—Fifty patients (41 men, 9 women) hospitalized with active pulmonary tuberculosis were evaluated for hypoadrenalism on the day after their admission. Serum cortisol and plasma adrenocorticotropin

(ACTH) concentrations were measured before and 20 and 60 minutes after IV ACTH (cosyntropin) administration. Basal thyroid and gonadal function was also assessed.

Results.—The patients' mean basal (8:30–10 A.M.) serum cortisol concentration was 22.6 µg/dL (625 nmol/L), and it was elevated (more than 25.4 µg/dL [700 nmol/L]) in 15 patients. After IV ACTH stimulation, the mean increment in serum cortisol was 9.3 µg/dL (256 nmol/L) and did not correlate with the basal concentration. All patients had a peak serum cortisol concentration exceeding 19.9 µg/dL (550 nmol/L). The basal plasma ACTH concentration was normal in 17 patients, low in 32, and high in 1 patient. The basal plasma ACTH and serum cortisol concentrations were not correlated. Most (92%) of the patients had low serum free triiodothyronine concentrations, and 20% had low serum free thyroxine (T_4) concentrations. Twenty percent of the patients had minor increases in serum thyrotropin, including 4 with low serum free T_4 values. Thirty of the 41 men had biochemical evidence of hypogonadism.

Discussion.—All 50 patients with active pulmonary tuberculosis had adequate adrenal function, although more than 90% had abnormalities of thyroid function and more than 70% had abnormalities of gonadal function indicative of nonendocrine illness.

A Hormonal and Radiological Evaluation of Adrenal Gland in Patients With Acute or Chronic Pulmonary Tuberculosis

Kelestimur F, Ünlü Y, Özesmi M, Tolu I (Erciyes Univ, Kayseri, Turkey)
Clin Endocrinol 41:53–56, 1994   119-95-53-3

Introduction.—Active tuberculosis may involve the adrenal glands, although the precise frequency and extent of adrenal involvement are unknown. Most studies of this issue have not included adequate endocrinologic and radiologic tests. Adrenal function and structure of patients with acute and chronic pulmonary tuberculosis were assessed, and the results were compared with those of normal subjects.

Methods.—The study sample comprised 20 patients (16 men, 4 women) with acute pulmonary tuberculosis, 41 patients (29 men, 12 women) with chronic (longer than 3 years) pulmonary tuberculosis, and a total of 20 normal men and women. All participants underwent CT imaging of the adrenals. Endocrine testing included measurements of basal plasma cortisol concentrations and cortisol responses to adrenocorticotropin (ACTH), 250 µg IV.

Results.—Basal (8–9 A.M.) plasma cortisol concentrations were normal to high in the patients with acute tuberculosis (mean, 28.0 µg/dL [772 nmol/L]), 20.1 µg/dL (554 nmol/L) in the patients with chronic tuberculosis, and 20.2 µg/dL (557 nmol/L) in the normal controls. Similarly, the controls and patients with chronic tuberculosis had similar values 60 minutes after ACTH administration (36.6 μg/dL [1,011 nmol/L] and 37.7 μg/dL [1,040 nmol/L], respectively, at 30 minutes). In contrast, the plasma cortisol responses were 41.5 μg/dL (1,146 nmol/L) at 30 min and 53.1 μg/dL (1,466 nmol/L) at 60 min in the acute tuberculosis group. Two patients in the chronic tuberculosis group were found to have Addison's disease. On CT imaging, the length and thickness of both adrenal glands were increased in patients with acute tuberculosis.

Conclusions.—Patients with acute pulmonary tuberculosis have enlarged adrenal glands, but the glands become smaller in chronic tuberculosis. The functional capacity of the adrenal glands tends to parallel their size.

▶ The patients with acute pulmonary tuberculosis in both of these studies (Abstracts 119-95-53–2 and 119-95-53–3) had extensive disease. The findings are described better in the study of Post et al.; 40 of their 50 patients had bilateral disease and 27 had cavitary disease, and all had sputum smears positive for acid-fast bacilli. All were probably quite sick, judged not only from these findings, but also the high frequency of abnormalities in thyroid and gonadal function. The patients of Keleştimur et al. are described only as having typical x-ray changes and positive sputum smears. Considering their illness, all these patients with acute pulmonary tuberculosis had normal cortisol secretion, as indicated by both the slightly elevated basal values and the responses to ACTH. In addition, plasma ACTH values when measured were nearly all normal as well. The finding of slightly enlarged adrenal glands in patients who had been sick for a few weeks (not stated but likely), during which ACTH secretion was undoubtedly increased during part of the day or night, is expected, because of its trophic properties. I suppose that the adrenals could have been enlarged because they contained multiple small granulomas, with plenty of surrounding normal adrenal cortex, but that seems unlikely. The patients' aldosterone secretion was probably normal, although it can be diminished during acute illness as a result of diversion of common precursors to production of cortisol (1). (Some of the patients in the study of Post et al. did have hyponatremia, which the authors reasonably attributed to inappropriate vasopressin secretion.) These results indicate that acute pulmonary tuberculosis must rarely be associated with adrenal insufficiency. I suppose, however, that it could happen, either as a result of hematogenous spread or adrenal hemorrhage. Patients with both HIV infection and tuberculosis may be at increased risk, because they have abnormal adrenal secretion anyway (2).

Adrenal insufficiency is a well-known sequel of tuberculosis and is often, although not invariably, associated with adrenal calcification. On the other hand, some patients with adrenal calcification do not have adrenal insufficiency (3), although I would look for it in any patient with calcified adrenal glands. (A thorough review of laboratory evaluation of patients suspected of having adrenal insufficiency was recently published [4].)—R.D. Utiger, M.D.

References

1. Findling JW, Waters VO, Raff H: The dissociation of renin and aldosterone during critical illness. *J Clin Endocrinol Metab* 64:592–595, 1987.
2. Findling JW, Buggy BP, Gilson IH, Brummitt CF, Bernstein BS, Raff H: Longitudinal evaluation of adrenocortical function in patients infected with the human immunodeficiency virus. *J Clin Endocrinol Metab* 79:1091–1096, 1994.
3. Hoeldtke RD, Donald RA, Nicholls MG: Functional significance of idiopathic adrenal calcification in the adult. *Clin Endocrinol* 12:319–325, 1980.
4. Grinspoon SK, Biller BMK: Laboratory assessment of adrenal insufficiency. *J Clin Endocrinol Metab* 79:923–931, 1994.

Effect of Glucocorticoid Replacement Therapy on Bone Mineral Density in Patients With Addison Disease

Zelissen PMJ, Croughs RJM, van Rijk PP, Raymakers JA (Univ Hosp, Utrecht, The Netherlands)
Ann Intern Med 120:207–210, 1994   119-95-53–4

Background.—Glucocorticoids cause osteoporosis, but little is known about the occurrence of osteoporosis during glucocorticoid replacement therapy in patients with Addison's disease. The bone mineral density in a large group of patients with Addison's disease was examined to determine the relationship between their drug regimen and the development of osteoporosis.

Methods.—Ninety-one patients with Addison's disease (31 men and 60 women) who had been receiving glucocorticoid replacement therapy for a mean of 10.6 years participated in the study. Bone mineral density of the lumbar spine and both femoral necks was measured by dual-energy x-ray absorptiometry. Bone mineral density was considered to be decreased if it was less than 2 SDs of the mean value of the control population in at least one region.

Results.—Decreased bone mineral density was found in at least 1 of the measured regions in 10 of the 31 men and in 4 of the 60 women. Five men had low bone mineral density in 3 regions, 4 in the lumbar spine only, and 1 in the right femoral neck only. One woman had decreased bone mineral density in 3 regions, 1 in 2 regions (both femoral necks), and 2 in 1 region (lumbar spine). There was a significant inverse correlation between age and bone mineral density of the lumbar spine, left femoral neck, and right femoral neck. No significant differences were found between the men and women with regard to age, duration of glucocorticoid treatment, or dose. However, men with decreased bone mineral density were taking a significantly higher dose of hydrocortisone per kilogram of body weight than men with normal bone mineral density. After correction for possible confounding variables, a significant linear correlation was confirmed between the hydrocortisone dose per kilogram of body weight and bone mineral density of the lumbar spine in men, but not in women.

Conclusion.—Decreased bone mineral density occurred in 32% of men with Addison's disease who were receiving long-term glucocorticoid replacement therapy. The men receiving higher daily doses of hydrocortisone per kilogram of body weight had a significantly greater decrease in bone mineral density.

▶ These results are rather odd, in that more men had low bone density of the lumbar spine and femoral neck than women, despite the similarity of the mean daily doses of hydrocortisone per kilogram body weight in the 2 groups. In several other studies of patients with Addison's disease who had received hydrocortisone or prednisone for many years, only postmenopausal women had evidence of excessive bone loss (1–3), as would be expected. The yearly rate of bone loss is little increased, and so-called replacement doses of hydrocortisone do not affect biochemical markers of bone formation and resorption. The lack of abnormal findings in the women in this study may be explained by the fact that about 75% were premenopausal or taking estrogen.

The low bone density in some treated patients with Addison's disease could be due to overreplacement or to deficiency of adrenal androgens (more likely the former). Most patients are treated with 20 mg of hydrocortisone in the morning and 10 mg in the evening, a practice historically based largely on subjective responses to therapy (as is the usual prednisone regimen of 5 mg in the morning and 2.5 mg in the afternoon). These doses of hydrocortisone raise plasma cortisol concentrations to peak values that are often higher than are those in normal subjects both in the morning and afternoon. The increases often last longer (4) too, and 24-hour urine cortisol excretion is often in the upper part of the normal range. Most patients are also given a mineralocorticoid (9a-fluorohydrocortisone), which, in conjunction with hydrocortisone, may predispose them to hypertension.

I think that the "usual" doses of hydrocortisone or prednisone may provide too much glucocorticoid. Although the clinical consequences of slight overtreatment do not appear to be large, they are rather easily avoided. We should pay more attention to the dose given to a particular patient and rely less on generally recommended doses.—R.D. Utiger, M.D.

References

1. Devogelaer JP, Crabbe J, Nagant de Deuxchaisnes C: Bone mineral density in Addison's disease: Evidence for an effect of adrenal androgens on bone mass. BMJ 294:798–800, 1987.
2. Florkowski CM, Holmes SJ, Elliott JR, Donald RA, Espiner EA: Bone mineral density is reduced in female but not male subjects with Addison's disease. N Z Med J 107:52–53, 1994.
3. Valero M-A, Leon M, Ruiz Valdepenas MP, et al: Bone density and turnover in Addison's disease: Effect of glucocorticoid treatment. Bone Miner 26:9–17, 1994.
4. Feek CJ, Ratcliffe JG, Seth J, Gray CE, Toft AD, Irvine WJ: Patterns of plasma cortisol and ACTH concentrations in patients with Addison's disease treated with conventional corticosteroid replacement. Clin Endocrinol 14:451–458, 1981.

Cushing's Syndrome in Children and Adolescents: Presentation, Diagnosis, and Therapy

Magiakou MA, Mastorakos G, Oldfield EH, Gomez MT, Doppman JL, Cutler GB Jr, Nieman LK, Chrousos GP (Natl Inst of Child Health and Human Development, Bethesda, Md; Natl Inst of Neurological Disorders and Stroke, Bethesda, Md; Natl Insts of Health, Bethesda, Md)
N Engl J Med 331:629–636, 1994   119-95-53–5

Introduction.—The diagnosis of Cushing's syndrome in children can be challenging. The findings of a retrospective review of the clinical presentation, diagnostic tests, and treatment of a large group of children and adolescents with hypercortisolism were reported.

Methods.—Cushing's syndrome was diagnosed in 59 children and adolescents. Diagnostic tests and imaging scans were done to identify the cause of the hypercortisolism. Surgery, pathologic analysis, and treatment response established the final diagnosis.

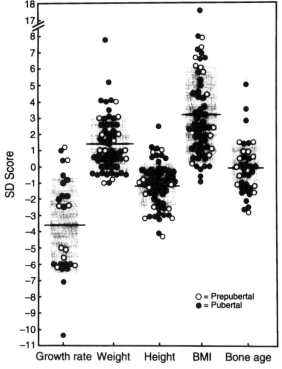

Fig 53–2.—Growth rate, weight, height, body-mass index (BMI), and bone age of 59 children and adolescents with Cushing's syndrome as compared with expected values for age and sex. *Horizontal lines* and *shaded bars* indicate the means ± SD. (Courtesy of Magiakou MA, Mastorakos G, Oldfield EH, et al: *N Engl J Med* 331:629–636, 1994)

Results.—Hypercortisolism was caused by a pituitary adenoma in 50 patients, primary adrenal disease in 4, and ectopic adrenocorticotropin (ACTH) secretion in 5. Development of the disease was insidious. The most common initial signs were weight gain (in 90% of the patients) and growth retardation (83%), although bone age was generally not retarded. Growth retardation was more pronounced in prepubertal than in pubertal patients (Fig 53-2). The high-dose dexamethasone suppression test identified 68% of the patients with pituitary adenomas, in all of the patients with primary adrenal disease, but in none of the patients with ectopic ACTH secretion. The corticotropin-releasing hormone (CRH) stimulation test detected 80% of the patients with pituitary adenomas and in 1 of the patients with ectopic ACTH secretion. Magnetic resonance imaging identified pituitary tumors in 52% of the patients with Cushing's disease. Computed tomography identified enlarged adrenal glands in 28 patients. With bilateral inferior petrosal sinus sampling, all of the patients with Cushing's disease had a maximal central-to-peripheral ratio of plasma ACTH of at least 2.5, whereas the ratio was no more than 2.2 in all other patients. Forty-nine patients with Cushing's disease had transsphenoidal resection of a pituitary adenoma; urinary cortisol excretion decreased to normal in 48 of them by the third postoperative day.

Discussion.—The following differential diagnostic and treatment protocol is suggested for patients with documented hypercortisolism. Plasma ACTH measurements and CRH test results should be obtained. Patients with ACTH-dependent hypercortisolism should have pituitary MRI scans. Unequivocally positive results on both the CRH test and MRI should be followed by transsphenoidal surgery. Inferior petrosal sinus sampling should be done in patients with negative or equivocal MRI scans and in patients with CRH test results suggesting ectopic ACTH secretion. These patients should also have CT or MRI scans of the chest and abdomen. The adrenal glands should be scanned with CT or MRI in patients with ACTH-independent Cushing's syndrome.

▶ I included this study to remind readers that Cushing's syndrome occurs at all ages. Its clinical manifestations in children and adolescents are similar to those in adults, with the exception of growth retardation. Glucocorticoid excess inhibits bone formation directly and also decreases growth hormone and insulin-like growth factor-I production. After treatment, there is some catch-up growth, but adult height is less than predicted from parental height (1). With respect to sexual development, young children may have premature sexual development and accelerated epiphyseal maturation, as a result of increased adrenal androgen secretion, whereas older children and adolescents tend to have delayed puberty, as a result of glucocorticoid-induced hypogonadism. These latter abnormalities do not seem to affect growth much, because most of the patients had normal skeletal maturation at the time of diagnosis.

Children and adolescents with Cushing's syndrome should be studied in the same way as are adults. First, determine whether the hypercortisolism is ACTH-dependent or -independent by measuring plasma ACTH and adrenal responsiveness to dexamethasone (the authors recommend a CRH test for this purpose, but I disagree). Second, perform pituitary, adrenal, or other imaging as appropriate. Third, if necessary, perform petrosal sinus catheterization and measure plasma ACTH before and after CRH administration in petrosal and peripheral venous blood.

As in adults, most children and adolescents with Cushing's syndrome have Cushing's disease. The ectopic ACTH syndrome is less common, because its most common cause—small-cell lung cancer—is rare in this age group, and adrenal tumors are more common. The latter was not true in this study, probably because it was from a referral center where the proportion of patients with equivocal biochemical and radiologic test results is high. In contrast, in patients with adrenal tumors, the results of these studies tend to be less equivocal, e.g., plasma ACTH concentrations are low and adrenal secretion decreases little if at all in response to any regimen of exogenous glucocorticoid administration, and adrenal imaging studies nearly always reveal an abnormality.—R.D. Utiger, M.D.

Reference

1. Magiakou MA, Mastorakos G, Chrousos GP: Final stature in patients with endogenous Cushing's syndrome. *J Clin Endocrinol Metab* 79:1082–1085, 1994.

Growth and Pituitary–Adrenal Function in Children With Severe Asthma Treated With Inhaled Budesonide

Volovitz B, Amir J, Malik H, Kauschansky A, Varsano I (Golda Med Ctr, Petach-Tiqva, Israel)
N Engl J Med 329:1703–1708, 1993   119-95-53-6

Objective.—Concern about the safety of inhaled corticosteroids in children with asthma prompted a long-term study of inhaled budesonide treatment in 15 children 2–7 years of age with severe perennial asthma. These patients had not been adequately controlled by cromolyn sodium combined with terbutaline sulfate, sustained-release theophylline, and occasional oral prednisone therapy.

Study Plan.—In the open trial, budesonide was instituted after a 1-month run-in period in a dosage of 100 μg twice a day for 3–5 years. Respiratory symptoms and the need for other medication were monitored, and serial estimates were made of growth velocity, bone age, and pituitary-adrenal function.

Clinical Response.—Asthmatic control improved in the first month of budesonide therapy, during which time the number of symptomatic days decreased by 58% and the use of other drugs decreased by 75%. Wheezing scores declined 71%, and the mean peak expiratory flow rates increased 17% in the 12 children evaluated. Improvement was sustained throughout the observation period. Asthmatic exacerbations and emergency room visits decreased, as did the need for hospitalization. Withdrawal of budesonide was possible in only 2 children.

Safety.—All children grew and gained body weight normally during budesonide treatment. Their bone age advanced in accord with chronologic age. Urinary cortisol excretion remained normal. No child had a cataract or oral candidiasis develop.

Conclusion.—Long-term use of inhaled budesonide in a daily dose of 200 μg is an effective and safe treatment for children with severe asthma.

▶ I am not competent to discuss the treatment of asthma, but I thought an example and brief discussion of the lack of systemic effects of inhaled glucocorticoid therapy might be worthwhile. Glucocorticoid therapy is very effective in patients with asthma, and it is now given earlier in the course of the disease than in the past. This is all well and good, so long as the side effects of glucocorticoid therapy are minimized. Inhaled glucocorticoid therapy, usually with either beclomethasone or budesonide (the latter is not available in the United States), accomplishes this goal. These drugs are administered by aerosol or as a dry powder, using a variety of devices, but pharmacokinetic data are sparse, and most of what data are available were obtained in single-dose studies in normal subjects, not asthmatic patients with abnormal airways. Suffice it to say that a relatively low proportion of the drug reaches the lung and a lot is swallowed, and that the amount absorbed through the lungs or absorbed by the gut and passing through the liver to reach the systemic circulation is sufficiently small that inhibition of pituitary-adrenal function and iatrogenic Cushing's syndrome are almost unheard of (1). This is nicely documented by the results of this study, in which a group of children treated with 200 μg of budesonide (roughly equivalent to 200 μg of beclomethasone) daily had no pituitary-adrenal suppression and also no growth retardation. The latter is a prominent manifestation of iatrogenic and spontaneously occurring Cushing's syndrome in children (see the preceding article [Abstract 119-95-53–5]), and its absence in the budesonide-treated children is very reassuring.

The usual dose of either inhaled glucocorticoid in adults is 800 μg daily. This dose is roughly equivalent systemically to 4 to 6 mg of prednisone (2), amounts that are not effective therapeutically in patients with asthma. Doses of inhaled budesonide or beclomethasone up to 1000 μg daily are very safe. Larger doses may inhibit pituitary-adrenal function slightly and have been associated with decreases in bone density, but many, if not all, of the patients also had received prednisone orally for varying intervals (3).—R.D. Utiger, M.D.

References

1. Barnes PJ, Pedersen S: Efficacy and safety of inhaled corticosteroids in asthma. *Am Rev Respir Dis* 148:1S–26S, 1993.
2. Toogood JH, Baskerville J, Jennings B, Lefcoe NM, Johansson S-A: Bioequiva-

lent doses of budesonide and prednisone in moderate and severe asthma. *J Allergy Clin Immunol* 84:688–700, 1989.

3. Packe GE, Douglas JG, McDonald AF, Robins SP, Reid DM: Bone density in asthmatic patients taking high dose inhaled beclomethasone propionate and intermittent systemic corticosteroids. *Thorax* 47:414–417, 1992.

The Efficacy of Iodine-123 MIBG as a Screening Test for Pheochromocytoma

Mozley PD, Kim CK, Mohsin J, Jatlow A, Gosfield III E, Alavi A (Univ of Pennsylvania, Philadelphia)
J Nucl Med 35:1138–1144, 1994   119-95-53-7

Objective.—Because there is no consensus regarding which form of iodine-labeled meta-iodobenzylguanidine (MIBG) is preferable in screening for pheochromocytoma, the performance of ^{123}I-MIBG was examined in 130 consecutive patients in a 4-year period. A final diagnosis was established in 120 of them.

Imaging.—After withdrawing sympathomimetic drugs that might interfere with MIBG uptake, the patients were given Lugol's solution approximately an hour before a 10-mCi dose of ^{123}I-MIBG. Scanning was per-

	Intensity of Adrenal Activity		
Intensity of adrenal uptake	Adrenal glands with pheochromocytoma (m = 24)	Adrenal glands without pheochromocytoma (m = 214)*	PPV
Grade 0	0	148	0%
Grade 1			
Bilateral (n = 21)	0	42	0%
Asymmetric[†]	0	5	0%
Solitary[‡] (n = 17)	2	15	13.3%
Grade 2			
Bilateral (n = 1)	0	2	0%
Unilateral (n = 3)	1	2	33%
Grade 3			
Bilateral (n = 1)	2	0	100%
Unilateral (n = 19)	19	0	100%

Notes: *m* indicates the number of adrenal glands; *n*, the number of patients
* Based on the sum of 182 adrenal glands in 91 patients without pheochromocytoma and 32 adrenal glands in the 29 patients with pheochromocytoma that were not involved with the disease.
† Patients with a solitary pheochromocytoma who had grade 3 uptake in the tumor and grade 1 uptake in the normal gland of the other side.
‡ Includes 1 patient with extra-adrenal pheochromocytoma who had faint uptake in an uninvolved gland, 14 patients without pheochromocytoma, and 2 patients with grade 1 uptake in a surgically proven tumor.
(Courtesy of Mozley PD, Kim CK, Mohsin J, et al: *J Nucl Med* 35:1138–1144, 1994.)

formed 18 hours later, using a gamma camera and a low-energy, large-field parallel-hole collimator to record images of the entire body. Two experienced observers compared the intensity of adrenal MIBG uptake with that in the liver.

Findings.—Twenty-nine patients received a final diagnosis of pheochromocytoma, including 23 with a total of 24 intramedullary tumors. All the tumors were visualized by imaging with ^{123}I-MIBG (table). A mild-to-moderate increase in activity was noted in 31% of adrenal glands without pheochromocytoma. Urinary catecholamine excretion did not distinguish these patients from those with pheochromocytomas that took up a small portion of injected radioactivity. Four of 5 patients with multifocal extra-adrenal disease had at least 2 tumors exhibiting uptake.

Conclusion.—Adrenal scintigraphy with ^{123}I-labeled MIBG allows a confident diagnosis of pheochromocytoma in most cases. A single set of delayed images suffices, and no special processing or quantification is necessary. A negative study will usually preclude the need for further imaging.

▶ Meta-iodobenzylguanidine is an analogue of norepinephrine that is taken up selectively by chromaffin tissue. Iodine-131 MIBG has been used for over a decade for imaging in patients suspected to have pheochromocytomas or other chromaffin tumors. It reveals most adrenal pheochromocytomas and does not reveal normal adrenal medullary tissue (1). Meta-iodobenzylguanidine labeled with ^{123}I would be expected to yield higher-quality images with lower radiation exposure, allowing a larger dose to be administered. In this large study of consecutive patients, some simply with hypertension and others with biochemical evidence of pheochromocytoma, ^{123}I-MIBG imaging was falsely positive in a number of patients, but in them, uptake was usually bilateral and faint. That normal adrenomedullary tissue should be visualized with a sensitive imaging technique that reflects normal function is not surprising; indeed one might wonder why uptake was not detected in everyone with normal adrenal medullas. I don't know whether ^{123}I-MIBG will in time replace ^{131}I-MIBG; sensitivity may be better, but specificity is poorer and it is more costly.

From the clinical perspective, the important question is, When is MIBG imaging indicated? As in most endocrinopathies, the diagnosis should be based on clinical and biochemical findings, including elevated plasma catecholamine and urinary catecholamine, metanephrine and vanilylmandelic acid values, and not on anatomical studies. Of these biochemical tests, the best combination is probably urinary catecholamines and metanephrines. If both are elevated, MRI is indicated. Magnetic resonance imaging is somewhat superior to CT because pheochromocytomas can often be distinguished from adrenocortical tumors by their brightness on T2-weighted MR image (2). Imaging with MIBG should be reserved for patients likely to have a pheochromocytoma but have normal adrenal glands on MRI or CT scan.—R.D. Utiger, M.D.

References

1. Bravo EL: Pheochromocytoma: New concepts and future trends. *Kidney Int* 40:544–556, 1991.
2. Doppman JL, Reining JW, Dwyer AJ, et al: Differentiation of adrenal masses by magnetic resonance imaging. *Surgery* 102:1018–1026, 1987.

54 The Thyroid Gland

Comparison of Second and Third Generation Methods for Measurement of Serum Thyrotropin in Patients With Overt Hyperthyroidism, Patients Receiving Thyroxine Therapy, and Those With Nonthyroidal Illness
Franklyn JA, Black EG, Betteridge J, Sheppard MC (Univ of Birmingham, England)
J Clin Endocrinol Metab 78:1368–1371, 1994   119-95-54–1

Background.—The development of assays for serum thyrotropin (TSH) with improved sensitivity has been a major advance in the assessment of thyroid status. The clinical usefulness of a further increase in sensitivity was investigated by comparing serum TSH results determined in second- and third-generation assays in patients with overt hyperthyroi-

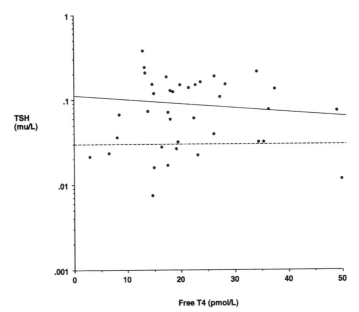

Fig 54–1.—Plot of serum thyrotropin (TSH) concentrations determined with a third-generation assay against measurements of free T$_4$ in 38 hospital inpatients with NTIs and serum TSH values below normal (< .5 mU/L). *Dashed line,* functional or clinically applicable limit of sensitivity of the TSH assay (.03 mU/L). (Courtesy of Franklyn JA, Black EG, Betteridge J, et al: *J Clin Endocrinol Metab* 78:1368–1371, 1994.)

dism before and during treatment, in patients receiving thyroxine (T_4) therapy, and in patients with nonthyroidal illnesses.

Methods.—Serum samples were obtained from 19 patients with untreated overt hyperthyroidism and from 12 patients studied serially at monthly intervals for as many as 7 months after commencing antithyroid drug (carbimazole) treatment. Samples were also obtained from 153 patients receiving long-term T_4 therapy and from 300 inpatients with nonthyroidal illnesses. Serum TSH was measured in all samples using a second-generation immunometric assay (functional sensitivity 0.2 mU/L) together with free T_4 and free triiodothyronine (T_3), and samples with TSH values less than 0.5 mU/L were reassayed using a third-generation chemiluminescent immunometric method (functional sensitivity less than 0.03 mU/L).

Results.—Serum TSH concentrations were undetectable in both assays in 18 of the 19 patients with overt hyperthyroidism. Similarly, the values were undetectable in the patients who were being treated for hyperthyroidism, 11 of whom had normal serum free T_4 and T_3 concentrations. Most of the T_4-treated patients also had undetectable serum TSH values as concentrations in both assays, as did many of those with nonthyroidal illness. However, use of the more sensitive assay resulted in a reduction in the number of patients with undetectable serum TSH values as compared with the results of second-generation assays (T_4-treated, 55 vs. 77 patients; nonthyroidal illness, 13 vs. 19 patients). There was a significant inverse correlation between serum TSH and free T_4 in the T_4-treated patients but not in the patients with nonthyroidal illnesses (Fig 54–1).

Conclusion.—When more sensitive (third generation) serum TSH assays are used, serum TSH concentrations are more often detectable in T_4-treated patients and patients with nonthyroidal illness than when a less sensitive assay is used, but nearly all patients with overt hyperthyroidism have undetectable values.

▶ Second-generation assays for serum TSH are—or should be—available everywhere now. The analytic sensitivity of these assays varies from 0.05 to 0.1 mU/L, about 1/10th or 1/20th that of the original (first generation) assays. The functional sensitivity, defined as the lowest values for which the coefficient of variation of repeated measurements is less than 10 or 20%, is about twofold higher. Few laboratories report either of these values, but give only the normal range (which is usually about 0.5–4 mU/L).

The great advantage of the second-generation assays is that TSH can be detected in the serum of all normal subjects. Serum TSH determinations, therefore, can be used to detect not only primary hypothyroidism (and distinguish primary from secondary hypothyroidism), but also to detect hyperthyroidism, because of the sensitivity of TSH secretion to inhibition by T_4 and T_3. In fact, a determination of serum TSH is the single best test of thyroid function.

It became evident soon after the second-generation assays were introduced that some patients, in addition to those with overt hyperthyroidism, have undetectable serum TSH concentrations. These patients have either subclinical hyperthyroidism, whether spontaneously occurring or caused by exogenous thyroid hormone therapy, or nonthyroidal illness. The former have serum T_4 and T_3 concentrations in the upper reaches of the normal range, whereas in the latter serum T_4 and T_3 concentrations are low or normal. These 2 groups of patients can usually be distinguished from those with overt hyperthyroidism on the basis of history, physical examination, serum T_4 concentrations, and clinical context, e.g., is the patient being seen in the office or is he or she in the hospital for other problems?

This study by Franklyn et al. demonstrates that measuring serum TSH using an assay with even more sensitivity (third generation, 10-fold greater sensitivity) doesn't help much in differentiating between the several causes of low serum TSH concentrations. Yes, more of the patients with subclinical hyperthyroidism have detectable values, and the expected inverse relationship between serum TSH and free T_4 concentrations is evident (Fig 54–1). More of the patients with nonthyroidal illness also have detectable values, but they correlate poorly with serum free T_4 concentrations (lower panel). Laboratories are now offering third-generation assays (fourth-generation ones are on the way!), but the gain in information or clinical value is very small, if there is any, and the test costs more. It is far better to use one's clinical skills, serum T_4 measurements, and a second-generation TSH assay.—R.D. Utiger, M.D.

The Clinical Evaluation of Patients With Subclinical Hyperthyroidism and Free Triiodothyronine (Free T_3) Toxicosis

Figge J, Leinung M, Goodman AD, Izquierdo R, Mydosh T, Gates S, Line B, Lee DW (Albany Med College, NY; Samuel S Stratton VA Med Ctr, Albany, NY; Park Med Group, Rochester, NY)
Am J Med 96:229–234, 1994　　　　　　　　　　　　119-95-54–2

Background.—Sensitive assays for serum thyrotropin (TSH) have provided an excellent means of screening for thyroid dysfunction. A low serum TSH value, in conjunction with an elevated serum free thyroxine (T_4) value, confirms a diagnosis of hyperthyroidism. However, in certain patients with hyperthyroidism, the serum free T_4 value is normal, but the patient has an elevated serum triiodothyronine (T_3) value (T_3-toxicosis). A means of evaluating patients with low serum TSH concentrations was developed to identify those with free T_3 toxicosis and those with subclinical hyperthyroidism (normal serum free T_3).

Methods.—The records of ambulatory patients who had determinations of serum TSH between October 1, 1991, and August 31, 1992 were reviewed retrospectively. The serum TSH concentrations were measured by second- or third-generation assays, and each patient had a simultaneous measurement of serum free T_4. A subgroup of patients who had serum TSH concentrations less than or equal to 0.1 mU/L but

Diagnoses in 140 Patients With Normal Free T_4 and
Subnormal Serum Thyrotropin Levels

1. Patients on Exogenous Levothyroxine:	
(a) For treatment of central hypothyroidism;	23 patients
(b) For treatment of primary hypothyroidism,	
radioiodine-induced,	18
autoimmune & other;	21
(c) For suppression of thyroid cancer;	13
(d) For suppression of benign nodular thyroid disease and/or goiter	25
2. Patients undergoing treatment or follow-up for pre-existing hyperthyroidism	32
3. Pregnancy-related*	1
4. Classical T_3 toxicosis	1
5. Free T_3 toxicosis	3
6. Subclinical hyperthyroidism (endogenous)	3
TOTAL	140

*Serum thyrotropin (TSH) suppressed secondary to increased hCG at week 10-12 of pregnancy.
(Courtesy of Figge J, Leinung M, Goodman AD, et al: *Am J Med* 96:229–234, 1994.)

normal serum free T_4 concentrations was then identified. The records of these patients were reviewed. Patients were excluded from the group if they had active, concurrent nonthyroidal illness, psychiatric disease, or known hypothalamic or pituitary lesions, or were receiving treatment for hyper- or hypothyroidism, were taking drugs known to affect TSH secretion, or were pregnant. Patients without exclusions were diagnosed as having free T_3-toxicosis according to the following criteria: markedly subnormal serum TSH, normal serum free T_4, normal serum T_3, evidence of a primary thyroid abnormality, and elevated serum T_3 by equilibrium dialysis. Patients who met the first 4 conditions, but who had normal serum free T_3 values, were considered to have subclinical hyperthyroidism.

Results.—A total of 1,025 patients underwent screening. Of these 148 had subnormal serum TSH but normal free T_4 concentrations. Of the 140 patients for whom information was available, 100 were receiving exogenous T_4 for a variety of indications, 32 patients were receiving treatment for hyperthyroidism, and 1 patient was pregnant (table). Of the remaining 7 patients, 1 patient had an elevated serum total T_3 concentration, 3 patients satisfied the criteria for free T_3-toxicosis, and 3 patients had normal serum total and free T_3 concentrations and were therefore given a diagnosis of subclinical hyperthyroidism.

Conclusion.—Apparently healthy ambulatory patients with subnormal serum TSH concentrations should have measurements of serum free T_4 and total T_3. If these are normal, serum free T_3 should be measured to distinguish subclinical hyperthyroidism from free T_3-toxicosis. In some patients with these conditions, treatment can be beneficial.

► As serum TSH measurements become used more widely for the initial evaluation of patients suspected of having thyroid dysfunction, more patients with low values will be encountered, both in and out of the hospital (see Abstract 119-95-54–1). When the serum TSH concentration is low, the serum free T_4 should be measured. If it is high, we conclude that the patient has overt hyperthyroidism and usually recommend some treatment, even in the absence of symptoms. If the serum free T_4 value is normal, and the patient does not have a major nonthyroidal illness, we call it subclinical hyperthyroidism. Strictly speaking, that diagnosis can be made only if the patient has a normal serum free T_3 value as well, but in practice, a serum free T_3 measurement is not necessary, even if the test was widely available, and it is not.

A sizable proportion of adults seeking medical care, in this case in an endocrine clinic, and elderly adults in the community have subclinical hyperthyroidism (1). Most of them are receiving thyroid hormone therapy, but some have a multinodular goiter, a solitary thyroid adenoma, or Graves' disease. Others have no obvious thyroid disease, and serum TSH is normal when measured again several weeks or more later (2, 3). The abnormality can persist, but few patients have overt hyperthyroidism develop during follow-up for several years.

Figge et al. took the next step and measured serum T_3 concentrations in their patients with low serum TSH and normal free T_4 values. Three had elevated serum free T_3 values, leading to the diagnosis of free T_3-thyrotoxicosis. Some patients in both groups had a few symptoms of hyperthyroidism, such as tremor, weight loss, or tachycardia, and were treated. These findings reinforce the point I made above; in a patient with a low serum TSH concentration who has a normal serum free T_4 value, the real importance is not whether the serum T_3 is elevated but whether the patient has any symptoms or signs of hyperthyroidism. The latter will undoubtedly be modest, but if present, treatment is indicated. If not present, periodic reevaluation is all that is indicated, because of the very low risk of overt hyperthyroidism and the low risk of atrial fibrillation (4).—R.D. Utiger, M.D.

References

1. Utiger RD: Subclinical hyperthyroidism: A low serum thyrotropin concentration, or something more? *N Engl J Med* 331:1302–1303, 1994.
2. Eggertsen R, Petersen K, Lundberg P-A, Nystrom E, Lindstedt G: Screening for thyroid disease in a primary care unit with a thyroid-stimulating hormone assay with a low detection limit. *BMJ* 297:1586–1592, 1988.
3. Parle JV, Franklyn JA, Cross KW, Jones SC, Sheppard MC: Prevalence and follow-up of abnormal thyrotropin (TSH) concentrations in the elderly in the United Kingdom. *Clin Endocrinol* 34:77–83, 1991.
4. Sawin CT, Geller A, Wolf PA, et al: Low serum thyrotropin concentrations as a risk factor for atrial fibrillation in older persons. *N Engl J Med* 331:1249–1252, 1994.

Changes in Bone Mass During Prolonged Subclinical Hyperthyroidism Due to L-Thyroxine Treatment: A Meta-Analysis

Faber J, Galløe AM (Frederiksberg Hosp, Denmark; Herlev Univ, Denmark)
Eur J Endocrinol 130:350–356, 1994   119-95-54–3

Introduction.—Subclinical hyperthyroidism is defined as low serum thyrotropin (TSH) but normal thyroxine and triiodothyronine values. It may adversely affect bone mass and increase the risk of osteoporosis. Several recent studies, however, fail to show such a detrimental effect. A meta-analysis was performed to determine whether L-thyroxine (T_4) in doses large enough to suppress serum TSH concentrations reduces bone mass in treated patients relative to normal subjects.

Methods.—Thirteen studies were identified in which bone mass was measured in the distal forearm, femoral neck, or lumbar spine in a cross-sectional manner. For each study, the differences in the reductions in bone mass at these sites were calculated for either pre- or postmenopausal women because of the protective role of preserved estrogen production.

Results.—The combined studies yielded 441 measurements performed in premenopausal women treated for an average of 8.5 years with an average dose of T_4 of 164 μg/day; 317 measurements were performed in postmenopausal women treated for an average of 9.9 years with an average dose of 171 μg/day. The excess loss of bone mass at the 3 sites in the T_4-treated premenopausal women relative to normal premenopausal women was not significant. The measurements at the 3 sites obtained in the premenopausal women were used to construct a theoretical bone. A premenopausal woman at an average age of 39.6 years, with a duration of treatment of 8.5 years and a low serum TSH concentration, would have an excess loss of bone mass of 2.7% or 0.3% annually as compared with a normal premenopausal woman. The excess loss of bone mass for postmenopausal women, however, proved to be significant. The theoretical bone in a postmenopausal woman with an average age of 61.2 years and a low serum TSH concentration during 9.9 years of treatment would have an excess loss of mass of 9.0%, or 0.9% annually as compared with bone in a healthy postmenopausal woman.

Conclusion.—Low serum TSH concentrations in premenopausal women receiving T_4 are not detrimental to bone mass. In contrast, among similarly treated postmenopausal women, excess bone loss is significant and probably clinically important.

Thyroid Hormone Use and Bone Mineral Density in Elderly Women: Effects of Estrogen

Schneider DL, Barrett-Connor EL, Morton DJ (Univ of California–San Diego,

La Jolla)
JAMA 271:1245–1249, 1994   119-95-54–4

Background.—The extent to which thyroid hormone therapy affects bone mineral density remains unresolved. The effect of long-term thyroid hormone therapy on bone mineral density and the possible mitigating effect of estrogen replacement therapy were examined in a cross-sectional study.

Methods.—The study included 991 white women aged 50-98 years who participated in a study of osteoporosis. Bone mineral density was measured at the ultradistal and midshaft radius, the hip, and the lumbar spine. The results in 196 women who had taken thyroid hormone for a mean duration of 20 years were compared with those of 795 women who were not taking thyroid hormone.

Results.—Bone mineral density correlated inversely with the thyroid hormone dose but not with the duration of therapy. The bone mineral density was lower at all sites in women receiving 200 μg of thyroxine daily compared with lower doses, with statistically significant differences at the midshaft radius and hip. Women taking estrogen and thyroid hormone had significantly denser bones at all 4 sites than women taking thyroid hormone but not estrogen (Fig 54-2). The bone mineral density was 17.7% higher at the ultradistal radius, 12.9% higher at the midshaft

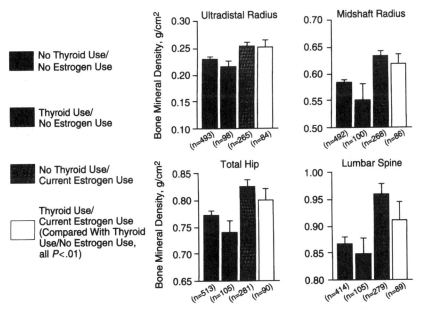

Fig 54–2.—Mean bone mineral densities (95% confidence intervals) by current thyroid hormone use and estrogen use adjusted for age, body mass index, smoking, and use of thiazide diuretics and oral corticosteroids in women, Rancho Bernardo, California, 1988 to 1991. (Courtesy of Schneider DL, Barrett-Connor EL, Morton DJ: *JAMA* 271:1245-1249, 1994.)

radius, 8.1% higher at the hip, and 7.8% higher at the lumbar spine. When adjusted for age, body mass index, smoking status, and thiazide and oral corticosteroid therapy, the bone mineral density in women taking estrogen and thyroid hormone was comparable to that of women taking estrogen but not thyroid hormone.

Conclusion.—High doses of thyroid hormone increase the risk of osteopenia in women who are postmenopausal. Estrogen therapy appears to mitigate thyroid hormone–associated bone loss, even with higher thyroid hormone doses.

▶ The extent to which thyroid hormone excess increases the rate of bone loss has been a contentious issue in the last few years (1). Notwithstanding the debate about bone loss, there is no evidence for an increase in the risk of fracture either in women taking thyroxine (T_4) or women with spontaneously occurring subclinical hyperthyroidism.

To summarize very briefly the results of the meta-analysis of Faber and Galløe (Abstract 119-95-54–3), the rate of bone loss seems to be increased in postmenopausal women, but not premenopausal women, mostly at sites composed primarily of cortical bone, when the thyroid hormone excess is substantial. The data on which the authors base this conclusion are derived entirely from cross-sectional studies of heterogenous patients in whom bone density was measured at different sites using different methods, and with individually variable results. Some of the patients were receiving T_4 to treat hypothyroidism. Others were being treated to shrink a goiter, and still others were being treated for thyroid carcinoma, the situation for which the largest doses are given. The duration of therapy varied from 5 to 12 years, and it is likely that the dosage was not constant. In the cumulative analysis, the excess loss of bone density was greatest in the radius, intermediate in the hip, and least in the lumbar spine. The amalgamation of the results into a theoretical bone composed of varying proportions of radial, femoral, and lumbar spine bone allows one to simplify data presentation but doesn't have much biological validity. The difference in the rates of bone loss in the pre- and postmenopausal women is remarkable and suggests that the ability of excess T_4 to stimulate bone resorption is prevented by normal quantities of estrogen.

This latter point is supported by the results of Schneider et al (Abstract 119-95-54–4). Their study subjects were postmenopausal women (mean age, 73 years) living in a retirement community who had taken T_4 for a long time, and they had information not only about estrogen therapy but also thiazide therapy, smoking, and exercise. Figure 54–2 shows lower bone density at all sites in those taking T_4 (or T_4 equivalents of other preparations) and normal or increased bone density in the women taking T_4 and estrogen. In a further analysis in which the women were divided according to the dose of T_4, the benefit of estrogen was apparent only in those women taking daily doses of T_4 of 1.6 μg/kg or more (80 μg or more for a 50-kg woman).

These studies further define the risk of osteoporosis associated with T_4 therapy and demonstrate that it can be ameliorated by estrogen. Because nearly all hypothyroid patients can be adequately treated with daily doses of 75 to 100 μg of T_4, they should have little risk for increased bone loss. Suppressive therapy is indicated only in patients with thyroid carcinoma, and even in them, reduction in serum TSH concentrations to 0.1 mU/L (lower limit of normal, 0.5 mU/L) or just below (which should require no more than 25% to 50% above the replacement dose in most patients) should be safe with respect to the skeleton and yet adequately minimize the likelihood of tumor recurrence (2). In managing these patients, it is important to remember that T_4 clearance slows gradually with age and, therefore, that whatever the goal of therapy, the dose may need to be reduced as time passes. —R.D. Utiger, M.D.

References

1. Ross DS: Hyperthyroidism, thyroid hormone therapy, and bone. *Thyroid* 4:319–326, 1994.
2. Marcocci C, Golia F, Bruno-Bossio G, Vignali E, Pinchera A: Carefully monitored levothyroxine suppressive therapy is not associated with bone loss in premenopausal women. *J Clin Endocrinol Metab* 78:818–823, 1994.

Control of Adrenergic Overactivity by β-Blockade Improves the Quality of Life in Patients Receiving Long Term Suppressive Therapy With Levothyroxine
Biondi B, Fazio S, Carella C, Sabatini D, Amato G, Cittadini A, Bellastella A, Lombardi G, Sacca L (Federico II Univ, Naples, Italy; Second Univ, Naples, Italy)
J Clin Endocrinol Metab 78:1028–1033, 1994   119-95-54–5

Background.—The palpitations reported by many patients receiving thyroxine (T_4) therapy for thyroid carcinoma or nontoxic multinodular goiter are strongly related to increases in heart rate, frequency of atrial arrhythmias, and myocardial contractility. β-Adrenergic blocking drugs are frequently used to relieve these symptoms in patients with spontaneously occurring hyperthyroidism. The effects of a β-adrenergic blocking drug on these signs and symptoms in patients receiving T_4 suppressive therapy were evaluated.

Methods.—Eleven patients with thyroid carcinoma or nontoxic multinodular goiter received bisoprolol, 2.5–5 mg/day, a cardioselective β-adrenergic blocking drug, in addition to L-T_4 suppressive therapy. A symptom rating scale (range 0 to 40) was used to assess quality of life. Twenty age and sex-matched normal subjects served as controls.

Results.—Before the addition of bisoprolol, the mean symptom rating scale score in the patient group was significantly greater than that in the control group. The difference was primarily the result of a higher incidence of palpitations, nervousness, tremor, heat intolerance, and sweating in the patient group. After 6 months of bisoprolol therapy, the patient group's mean score decreased significantly from 11.1 to 5.4 (Fig

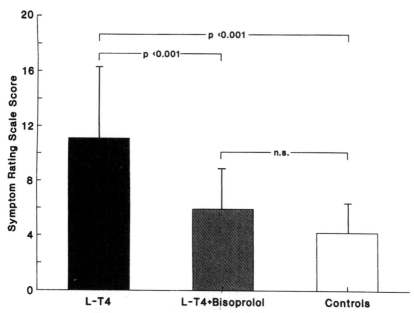

Fig 54–3.—The mean score of the symptom-rating scale is significantly higher in the patients than in the control group during treatment with L-T$_4$; the addition of bisoprolol to L-T$_4$ therapy reduces this score to a range comparable to that in the control group. (Courtesy of Biondi B, Fazio S, Carella C, et al: *Clin Endocrinol Metab* 78:1028–1033, 1994.)

54-3); 9 patients reported considerable relief of their symptoms. The heart rate, frequency of atrial premature contractions, and several measures of cardiac systolic function were increased before bisoprolol in the patients, as compared with the normal subjects, and decreased during its administration.

Conclusion.—The addition of a β-adrenergic blocking drug in patients receiving L-T$_4$ suppressive therapy improves the quality of life and diminishes the signs and symptoms of hyperkinetic cardiac activity.

▶ These thyroid cancer or goiter patients had been treated with T$_4$ in a dose (mean, 160 μg/day) sufficient to reduce their serum thyrotropin (TSH) concentrations to undetectable levels for from 2 to 7 years. No serum TSH values are given in this paper, but the patients were part of a larger group of 20 patients (1) in which the serum TSH values were less than 0.05 mU/L (the sensitivity limit of the assay, normal range, 0.2–3 mU/L). All had serum T$_4$ and triiodothyronine concentrations within the normal range, although the values were higher than in normal subjects, fulfilling the biochemical criteria for subclinical hyperthyroidism. These patients might be said to be at the extreme end of the spectrum of this disorder, because they had some symptoms of hyperthyroidism and their serum TSH concentrations were more than a little low.

The results of the studies done before the bisoprolol was given indicate that patients with subclinical hyperthyroidism can have some symptoms of hyperthyroidism. Their mean symptom score was 11; that of a group of patients with overt hyperthyroidism in the paper describing this scoring system was more than 20 (2). They also had evidence of increases in heart rate and cardiac contractility and in left ventricular mass similar to but less marked than the increases that occur in patients with overt hyperthyroidism. The amelioration of symptoms with bisoprolol would be expected, and the amelioration of the cardiac abnormalities provides evidence that many of the cardiac effects of hyperthyroidism are a physiologic response to increased cardiac work (3).

The long-term effects of these changes in cardiovascular physiology are mostly unknown, but we do know that the risk of atrial fibrillation is increased several-fold among patients with low serum TSH values followed for up to 10 years (4). Because it is difficult to assume any of the changes would be beneficial, the study provides more evidence, not that any is needed, that doses of T_4 that reduce TSH secretion a lot should not be given without good reason. High-dose treatment to reduce the size of a goiter is certainly not a good reason, nor is prevention of recurrence of thyroid carcinoma in patients who have no evidence of the disease.—R.D. Utiger, M.D.

References

1. Biondi B, Fazio S, Carella C, et al: Cardiac effects of long term thyrotropin-suppressive therapy with levothyroxine. *J Clin Endocrinol Metab* 77:334–338, 1993.
2. Klein I, Trzepacz P, Roberts M, et al: Symptom rating scale for assessing hyperthyroidism. *Arch Intern Med* 148:387–390, 1988.
3. Klein I, Ojamaa K: Thyroid hormone and the cardiovascular system: From theory to practice. *J Clin Endocrinol Metab* 78:1026–1027, 1994.
4. Sawin CT, Geller A, Wolf PA, et al: Low serum thyrotropin concentrations as a risk factor for atrial fibrillation in older patients. *N Engl J Med* 331:1249–1252, 1994.

Age-Related Therapeutic Response to Antithyroid Drug in Patients With Hyperthyroid Graves' Disease

Yamada T, Aizawa T, Koizumi Y, Komiya I, Ichikawa K, Hashizume K (Kashiwa City Hosp, Japan; Shinshu Univ, Matsumoto, Japan; Shinonoi Gen Hosp, Nagano, Japan)
J Am Geriatr Soc 42:513–516, 1994   119-95-54-6

Purpose.—Among patients with Graves' hyperthyroidism, those in the second decade of life have the highest serum thyroid hormone concentrations, and the values decline progressively with age. Elderly patients often have mild and sometimes atypical symptoms. No studies have addressed the degree to which these age-related differences affect the therapeutic response to antithyroid drugs. This issue was examined in a retrospective study.

Methods.—The analysis included 222 patients with Graves' hyperthyroidism who regained triiodothyronine (T_3) suppressibility within 4 years of methimazole treatment. The patients, who ranged in age from 7 to 81 years, were divided into 6 age groups (younger than 20 years, 21–30, 31–40, 41–50, 51–60, older than 61 years) for comparison of serum thyroid hormone concentrations, serum thyrotropin receptor antibody titers (measured by receptor assay), and thyroidal radioiodine uptake values.

Results.—Younger patients required a longer period of methimazole treatment to normalize serum thyroid hormone concentrations and restore normal thyroidal T_3 suppressibility, at which time methimazole was discontinued. For the latter end point, the mean duration of treatment varied from 29 months in patients aged 21 to 30 years to 17 months in those aged 61 years or older. Regardless of age, restoration of thyroidal T_3 suppressibility lagged an average of 10 months behind normalization of thyrotropin receptor antibody values. Young patients were less likely to achieve normal thyroid suppressibility during methazole therapy and more likely to have a recurrence of hyperthyroidism after discontinuing methimazole.

Conclusions.—Among patients with Graves' hyperthyroidism, treatment failure and recurrence after treatment are both more common in younger patients.

▶ At the time of diagnosis, serum thyroid hormone concentrations are higher in younger than older patients with hyperthyroidism caused by Graves' disease. For example, in this study, the mean serum thyroxine (T_4) and T_3 concentrations were 23.7 μg/dL (305 nmol/L) and 547 ng/dL (8.4 nmol/L), respectively, in the 21–30-year age group, and they declined progressively in the older groups, to 18.8 μg/dL (242 nmol/L) and 364 ng/dL (5.6 nmol/L), respectively, in the patients who were 61 years of age or older. Although not documented, younger patients probably have more symptoms of hyperthyroidism but tolerate them better and therefore seek medical care later, thus perhaps explaining their higher serum T_4 and T_3 concentrations. The pattern of symptoms and signs is known to change with age; hyperactivity, irritability, heat intolerance, increased appetite, and goiter are more common in younger patients, and weight loss, weakness, arrhythmia, and heart failure are more common in older patients (1). These differences are as or more likely to be related to variations in age-related sensitivity of different organ systems to T_4 and T_3 excess than to the biochemical severity of hyperthyroidism, although the latter is likely a contributing factor. The serum thyrotropin receptor antibody (TRAb) values were on average higher in the younger patients, indicating that their Graves' disease as well as their degree of biochemical hyperthyroidism was more severe.

The average 10-month lag in the time from when the patients' TRAb values fell into the normal range to the time of restoration of normal T_3 suppressibility is a reflection of the limitations of TRAb receptor assays. If TRAb production had indeed ceased the first time that serum TRAb values were in the normal range, T_3 suppressibility should also have been normal, e.g., the thyroid iodine-131 (^{131}I) uptake value during T_3 administration should have been low, because thyroid function would be dependent only on thyrotropin secretion. Thus, despite having "normal" serum TRAb values, the patients surely continued to produce small amounts of TRAb for up to 10 months on average (normal subjects produce none, of course, but their serum has a small nonspecific effect in the TRAb assay). In other words, the patients with Graves' disease have falsely normal values, because the normal range is artefactually broad. (The use of TRAb measurements to predict the likelihood of persistent remission or relapse in patients with Graves' disease is discussed in Abstract 119-95-54–7.)

In contrast to the differences in the rates of normalization of TRAb and T_3 suppression tests in the younger vs. the older groups, the time to euthyroidism (serum T_4 and T_3 concentrations within the normal range) after initiation of methimazole therapy varied much less in the different age groups. It was 3.9 months in the youngest group, 2.8 months in the oldest group, and varied from 3.1 to 4.3 months in the other groups. The intervals from euthyroidism to normal T_3 suppressibility varied from 22 months in the youngest to 14 months in the oldest age group. These results suggest that reducing thyroid secretion is not a very important determinant of the rate of improvement of Graves' disease, as compared with hyperthyroidism, although information about the mean serum T_4 and T_3 concentrations at regular intervals during the early months of treatment might reveal greater differences between the groups and weaken this conclusion. Antithyroid drugs are thought to affect Graves' disease as well as thyroid secretion (because the remission rate is higher than occurs in patients treated with β-adrenergic antagonist drugs), but whether the anti–Graves' disease action is caused by a decline in T_4 and T_3 production, some other actions of the drugs on thyroid cells, or immunosuppressive actions of the drugs is debated (2, 3). The poor relationship between time to euthyroidism and appearance of T_3 suppressibility (as a proxy for remission) provides some support for the latter possibility.

The practical lessons from this study are that older patients are more likely to have a remission of Graves' disease during methimazole therapy (the best antithyroid drug [4]) and that they are less likely to have recurrent hyperthyroidism after it is discontinued. Among the 54 patients in the two youngest age groups treated for as long as 4 years, 12 (22%) did not have a remission, as compared with 2 of 57 patients (4%) in the 2 oldest age groups. The respective recurrence rates in the 4 years after methimazole was discontinued were 24% (13 of 54) and 4% (2 of 57). These are low failure and recurrence rates and may not be achievable in the United States, because for reasons I have never understood most physicians here are not willing to give methimazole (or propylthiouracil) for a prolonged period. For the patient who can be managed with a small dose of either drug, but who becomes hyperthyroid when it is discontinued—say once a year—prolonged treatment is quite appropriate and safe. If Yamada et al. are correct, and I know of no data to the contrary, it is even more appropriate for older patients, the group that is even more often treated with ^{131}I in the United States.—R.D. Utiger, M.D.

References

1. Nordyke RA, Gilbert Jr FI, Harada ASM: Graves' disease: Influence of age on clinical findings. *Arch Intern Med* 148:626–631, 1988.
2. Volpe R: Evidence that the immunosuppressive effects of antithyroid drugs are mediated through actions on the thyroid cell, modulating thyrocyte-immunocyte signalling: A review. *Thyroid* 4:217–223, 1994.
3. Weetman AP: The immunomodulatory effects of antithyroid drugs. *Thyroid* 4:145–146, 1994.
4. Cooper DS: Which anti-thyroid drug? *Am J Med* 80:1165–1168, 1986.

Meta-Analysis Evaluation of the Impact of Thyrotropin Receptor Antibodies on Long Term Remission After Medical Therapy of Graves' Disease

Feldt-Rasmussen U, Schleusener H, Carayon P (Univ Hosp, Copenhagen; Freie Universität Berlin; Univ d'Aix-Marseille, Marseille, France)
J Clin Endocrinol Metab 78:98–102, 1994   119-95-54–7

Introduction.—Relapse is common among patients treated with antithyroid drugs for hyperthyroidism caused by Graves' disease. The risk of relapse is higher when thyrotropin (TSH) receptor antibodies (TRAbs) are present when therapy is discontinued, but it is not known whether the presence of TRAb can be used to determine the duration of treatment. A meta-analysis was performed to assess the use of TRAb as a predictor of long-term (at least 1 year) relapse after antithyroid drug therapy.

Methods.—Data on antithyroid drug therapy and measurements of TRAbs in patients with Graves' hyperthyroidism were obtained in a MEDLINE search for the years 1975–1991. The reference lists of these articles were used to gather additional information. The publications were divided into prospective and retrospective studies and according to the method used for measurement of TRAbs, either thyroid-stimulating antibodies (TSAbs) or TSH-binding inhibiting immunoglobulins (TBII).

Results.—For inclusion in the meta-analysis, 18 publications (1,524 patients) fulfilled the 4 criteria: availability of TRAb assay data at the end of antithyroid drug treatment; at least 1 year of follow-up after therapy was discontinued; data presentation in a suitable form (numbers of patients in all groups, etc); and no thyroid-related treatment during follow-up. There were 10 prospective studies, in which TBII was measured in 5 and TSAbs were measured in 5. Of the 8 retrospective studies, TBII was measured in 5 and TSAbs in 3. The overall relapse rate was 49%. Although only 10 of the 18 studies had statistical significance when TRAb status and relapse were examined, the meta-analysis revealed the risk of relapse to be significantly decreased in patients without detectable TRAb

(78% less risk) as compared with patients with detectable TRAbs when therapy was discontinued. The relationship between TRAb and relapse rate was clearer in the retrospective studies (92 vs. 65% risk reduction).

Conclusion.—The absence of TRAbs in patients treated with an antithyroid drug for hyperthyroidism caused by Graves' disease when therapy is discontinued is significantly protective against relapse. However, if a positive test for TRAbs at the end of the treatment was used to prolong therapy, 25% of TRAb-positive patients would be treated unnecessarily. Thus, TRAb assays are not highly reliable predictors of relapse or remission after discontinuation of antithyroid drug therapy.

▶ The theory behind the proposition that patients with hyperthyroidism caused by Graves' disease who have no TRAbs in their serum when antithyroid drug therapy is discontinued should remain euthyroid is sound. If TRABs cause the hyperthyroidism, and they are gone, the Graves' disease is much better or even gone away completely, so the patient should remain euthyroid at least for a while. Conversely, if the patient still has TRAbs, then hyperthyroidism should recur fairly soon, although perhaps not immediately if the quantity of TRAbs is low and the patient's thyroid gland has been severely depleted of iodide.

Despite the rather impressive reduction in the risk of relapse associated with a negative test at the conclusion of therapy that was calculated from these 18 studies, the overall results provide a picture that makes the theory look less strong. Among the TRAb-positive patients, 29% remained in remission, and among the TRAb-negative patients, 31% relapsed. One might expect that the results would be closer to expectation if TRAb were measured by bioassay, in which a positive test indicates TSAbs, than by measuring TBII, which does not discriminate between antibodies that activate TSH receptors and antibodies that inhibit the action of TSH. However, the results based on TBII assays were somewhat more predictive. These are not simple, highly specific, or reproducible (or cheap or widely available) assays, however, so some discrepancy between the methods is not surprising. Also, the assays aren't very sensitive, as noted in the preceding abstract (Abstract 119-95-54-6) of a study of treatment of patients with Graves' hyperthyroidism in whom the values of TRAb (measured as TBII) fell to normal many months before the results of triiodothyronine suppression tests became normal.

It is worth noting that the studies accepted for this meta-analysis came from 4 continents. Most patients had been treated with methimazole, in doses ranging from 5 to 120 mg/day; the duration of treatment varied from 4 to 48 months; and the duration of follow-up varied from 12 to 90 months. The relationship of all these variables with the likelihood of TRAbs being absent when treatment is discontinued or, more importantly, the likelihood of relapse is not clear. Although longer treatment and possibly larger doses may reduce the likelihood of relapse, there is plenty of contradictory evidence (1, 2).

As a practical matter, it is not worth measuring either TSAbs or TBII either to decide when to discontinue antithyroid drug therapy or to determine the likelihood of relapse when therapy is discontinued. In addition, no other test of pituitary-thyroid function (thyrotropin-releasing hormone [TRH] stimulation test, suppression test, serum thyroglobulin measurement) or of thyroid auto-immunity (antithyroid peroxidase antibodies) is useful (3). Assuming the patient is euthyroid while taking a low dose of antithyroid drug, just stop, and see what happens.—R.D. Utiger, M.D.

References

1. Feldt-Rasmussen U, Glinoer D, Orgiazzi J: Reassessment of antithyroid drug therapy of Graves' disease. *Annu Rev Med* 44:323–334, 1993.
2. Franklyn JA: The management of hyperthyroidism. *N Engl J Med* 330:1731–1738, 1994.
3. Schleusener H, Schwander J, Fischer C, et al: Prospective multicentre study on the prediction of relapse after antithyroid drug treatment in patients with Graves' disease. *Acta Endocrinol* 120:689–701, 1989.

Does Early Administration of Thyroxine Reduce the Development of Graves' Ophthalmopathy After Radioiodine Treatment?

Tallstedt L, Lundell G, Blomgren H, Bring J (Huddinge Hosp, Stockholm; Karolinska Hosp, Stockholm; Univ of Uppsala, Sweden)
Eur J Endocrinol 130:494–497, 1994   119-95-54–8

Background.—Graves' ophthalmopathy develops more frequently in patients treated with iodine-131 (^{131}I) therapy for hyperthyroidism than in patients treated with an antithyroid drug or thyroidectomy, but the ^{131}I-treated patients are more likely to be hypothyroid for several weeks or months. The effects of early thyroxine (T_4) administration after ^{131}I treatment for hyperthyroidism caused by Graves' disease were retrospectively analyzed.

Methods.—Records from patients with Graves' hyperthyroidism treated with ^{131}I were reviewed. Two hundred forty-eight patients (group A) received T_4 when their serum TSH or T_4 concentration indicated the presence of hypothyroidism; in group B (244 patients), T_4, 0.05 mg/day, was initiated 2 weeks after ^{131}I therapy with a dose increase to 0.1 mg after 2 weeks. The patients were examined periodically for 18 months after ^{131}I therapy.

Results.—Ophthalmopathy developed or worsened after treatment in 45 patients (18%) in group A and 27 patients (11%) in group B (relative risk, 1.64; P = 0.03). The average increases in exophthalmometer readings were comparable in the two groups: 3.5 mm in group A and 3.2 mm in group B. Twenty-six patients in group A and 11 in group B required treatment for progressive ophthalmopathy, including an antithyroid drug, corticosteroids, orbital irradiation, or orbital decompression.

Conclusion.—Early administration of T_4 after ^{131}I treatment reduces the occurrence or worsening of ophthalmopathy in patients with hyperthyroidism caused by Graves' disease.

▶ The risk of progressive eye disease is a major concern of patients with Graves' hyperthyroidism, especially if they have some ocular abnormalities at the time of diagnosis. Factors that are associated with an increased risk of clinically important ophthalmopathy include older age, male sex, smoking, and poor control of hyperthyroidism (1).

A much-debated issue is whether the type of antithyroid therapy influences the later development or worsening of ophthalmopathy. These same authors, in a randomized trial (2), found that among patients aged 35 to 55 years, ophthalmopathy developed or worsened in 10% of those treated with methimazole, 16% of those treated by thyroidectomy, and 33% of those treated with ^{131}I. The methimazole- and surgically treated patients were given T_4 very soon, whereas the ^{131}I-treated patients were not given any T_4 until they became hypothyroid, although none were hypothyroid for more than 3 months.

This difference led to the notion that the hypothyroidism was somehow responsible for the development or worsening of ophthalmopathy, possibly because of thyrotropin (TSH) stimulation of expression of some thyroid antigen that is shared with orbital muscle cells or fibroblasts (3, 4). This notion led these same investigators to change their policy of giving T_4 to patients with Graves' hyperthyroidism treated with ^{131}I only when they became hypothyroid to giving it routinely soon after ^{131}I administration. The change in management—albeit known to the physicians and not prospectively or randomly assigned—was accompanied by a moderate decrease in ophthalmopathy (most of the difference was accounted for by a decrease in the frequency of development rather than in worsening of ophthalmopathy). Thus, the results do provide support for the view that hypothyroidism is not good for the eyes, but whether the effect is mediated via TSH actions on thyroid follicular cells or via an effect of T_4 deficiency or TSH excess on ocular muscle cells or fibroblasts is entirely speculative.

Notwithstanding these results, the role of hypothyroidism in ophthalmopathy surely is not fundamental, because the ophthalmopathy usually appears concomitantly with hyperthyroidism (5). Whatever the fundamental pathogenesis of ophthalmopathy, the practical impact of the results of this study, however imperfectly it was done, is clear and not difficult to accomplish. No matter how a patient with Graves' hyperthyroidism is treated, care should be taken to avoid hypothyroidism.—R.D. Utiger, M.D.

References

1. 1994 Year Book of Medicine, pp 582–583.
2. 1993 Year Book of Medicine, pp 534–535.
3. Tallstedt L, Lundell G, Torring O, et al: Occurrence of ophthalmopathy after treatment for Graves' hyperthyroidism. N Engl J Med 326:1733–1738, 1992.
4. Utiger RD: Pathogenesis of Graves' ophthalmopathy. N Engl J Med 326:1772–1773, 1992.

5. Burch HB, Wartofsky L: Graves' ophthalmopathy: Current concepts regarding pathogenesis and management. *Endocr Rev* 14:747–793, 1993.

Radioiodine Treatment of Multinodular Non-Toxic Goitre
Nygaard B, Hegedüs L, Gervil M, Hjalgrim H, Søe-Jensen P, Hansen JM (Herlev Univ, Denmark; Odense Univ, Denmark)
BMJ 307:828–832, 1993   119-95-54–9

Background.—Among patients with nontoxic multinodular goiter, the standard therapy has been subtotal thyroidectomy. An effective nonoperative means of reducing the size of the thyroid gland would be helpful.

Patients and Treatment.—The value of radioiodine therapy for decreasing goiter size was examined in 69 patients (62 women and 7 men with a median age of 57 years) who had a multinodular goiter. The indications for treatment were an enlarging goiter that caused compressive symptoms or was cosmetically displeasing. The patients received iodine-131 in a dose of 100 μCi per gram of total thyroid mass, to a maximum of 30 mCi.

Results.—Fifty-six patients were followed for a median of 5 years after receiving a single dose of radioiodine. Forty-five of them remained euthyroid during follow-up. The median thyroid volume decreased by 60% in 2 years in the 39 evaluable patients, and in 49% of the patients the thyroid decreased to normal size (Fig 54–4). Nine patients became hypothyroid a median of 6 months after treatment, and 2 became hyperthyroid. Nine of 12 patients given a second dose of radioiodine, mainly to reduce thyroid volume further, remained euthyroid. In 2 patients, permanent hypothyroid developed after the second dose. The overall rate of

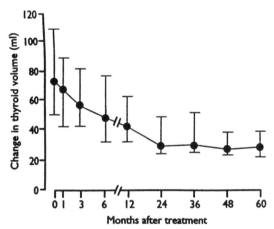

Fig 54–4.—Median changes in thyroid volume alterations after iodine-131 treatment in 39 patients with nontoxic multinodular goiter who remained euthyroid after a single dose. Bars are quartiles. (Courtesy of Nygaard B, Hegedüs L, Gervil M, et al: *BMJ* 307:828–832, 1993.)

hypothyroidism was 16%, and the risk of hypothyroidism developing 5 years after treatment was 22%.

Conclusion.—Radioiodine is an effective treatment for patients with nontoxic multinodular goiter and does not usually result in hypothyroidism.

▶ The natural history of nontoxic multinodular goiter is one of very gradual enlargement. Concomitantly, the goiters gradually become autonomous, e.g., less dependent on thyrotropin (TSH) secretion, and serum TSH concentrations decline (1). This evolution occurs as a result of growth of nodules that may be either monoclonal or polyclonal (2) and results ultimately in first subclinical (normal serum thyroid hormone concentrations) and later overt hyperthyroidism. The process is very gradual, so that the patients with the larger goiters—which are more likely to compress the larynx, trachea, or esophagus, be deemed cosmetically bothersome, and cause hyperthyroidism—are usually elderly.

The usual treatment is thyroxine (T_4), but it presupposes that the goiters are TSH-dependent, which may be true initially but is less so as time passes. The T_4 therapy reduces goiter size in about 50% of patients (3), but rarely by more than 25% to 50%, and many of the reported studies included young patients and patients with small non-nodular goiters. In patients whose goiters are largely autonomous, T_4 therapy may cause hyperthyroidism. The simplest way to estimate the degree of autonomy is by measuring serum TSH; the lower the value, the greater the degree of autonomy.

In the absence of local symptoms or a patient's insistence that something be done to decrease the size of the goiter, I do not think any therapy is indicated. If the patient desires treatment (or has minor local symptoms) and cannot be dissuaded from it, I recommend T_4 only if the serum TSH is well above the lower limit of the normal range, and not with much hope of benefit. Patients with definite laryngeal or tracheal compression require a treatment that is likely to be more effective than T_4, usually thyroidectomy. Based on this study and others (4, 5), iodine-131 (^{131}I) is a reasonable, although obviously slower and less uniformly effective, alternative. The decrease in goiter size, although gradual, relieves compressive symptoms; it is safer than an operation; and up to 30 mCi of ^{131}I can be given without hospitalization in the United States. The benefit in patients in the United States might not be as great as in this study, which was done in Denmark, because the iodine intake here is higher and therefore radioiodine uptake would be on average lower. Nevertheless, this therapy probably ought to be used more often.—R.D. Utiger, M.D.

References

1. Berghout A, Wiersinga WM, Smits N, Touber JL: Interrelationships between age, thyroid volume, thyroid nodularity, and thyroid function in patients with sporadic nodular goiter. *Am J Med* 89:602–608, 1990.
2. Kopp P, Kimura ET, Aeschimann S, et al: Polyclonal and monoclonal thyroid

nodules coexist within human multinodular goiters. *J Clin Endocrinol Metab* 79:134–139, 1994.

3. Ross DS: Thyroid hormone suppressive therapy of sporadic nontoxic goiter. *Thyroid* 2:263–269, 1992.
4. Kay TWH, d'Emden MC, Andrews JT, Martin FIR: Treatment of non-toxic multinodular goiter with radioactive iodine. *Am J Med* 84:19–22, 1988.
5. Huysmans DAKC, Hermus ARMM, Corstens FHM, Barentsz JO, Kloppenborg PWC: Large, compressive goiters treated with radioiodine. *Ann Intern Med* 121:757–762, 1994.

Clinical Screening as Compared With DNA Analysis in Families With Multiple Endocrine Neoplasia Type 2A

Lips CJM, Landsvater RM, Höppener JWM, Geerdink RA, Blijham G, van Veen JMJ-S, van Gils APG, de Wit MJ, Zewald RA, Berends MJH, Beemer FA, Brouwers-Smalbraak J, Jansen RPM, van Amstel HKP, van Vroonhoven TJ MV, Vroom TM (Univ Hosp Utrecht, The Netherlands; Westeinde Hosp, The Hague, The Netherlands; Clinical Genetics Ctr, Utrecht, The Netherlands)

N Engl J Med 331:828–835, 1994   119-95-54–10

Introduction.—Multiple endocrine neoplasia type 2A (MEN-2A), an inherited disease with an autosomal dominant pattern, is characterized

Clinical Results for Subjects with MEN-2A in Four Families Diagnosed by Biochemical, Radiologic, and Pathologic Studies and DNA Analysis

Family	No. of Subjects with MEN-2A	MTC PROVED	Medullary Thyroid Carcinoma (MTC)					Pheochromocytoma	Hyperparathyroidism
			POSITIVE CALCITONIN TEST BEFORE SURGERY*		NEGATIVE CALCITONIN TEST, BUT *RET* MUTATION PRESENT				
			group 1	group 2	group 3	MTC proved	not yet operated on		
				no. operated on (no. cured)					
A	30†	27	3 (0)	17 (6)	4 (4)	3	3†	15	1
B	19†	18	4 (0)	5 (1)	4 (3)	5	1†	12	2
C	16	16	4 (1)	9 (4)	3 (3)	—	—	6	—
D	15	13	3 (1)	8 (4)	2 (2)	—	2	6	—
All	80	74	14 (2)	39 (15)	13 (12)	8	6	39	3

* Group 1 included subjects initially examined because of symptoms or signs; group 2, first-degree relatives of subjects in group 1 who were found to be affected at the time of the initial screening; and group 3, subjects originally testing negative who later became positive

† Two subjects (Family A, Subject VI-4, and Family B, Subject V-14) who were operated on for pheochromocytoma had no signs of medullary thyroid carcinoma (MTC) at this writing, but total thyroidectomy was scheduled to be performed shortly.

(Courtesy of Lips CJM, Landsvater RM, Höppener JWM, et al: *N Engl J Med* 331:828–835, 1994) by medullary thyroid carcinoma, pheochromocytoma, and parathyroid adenoma. Screening for the biochemical signs of medullary thyroid carcinoma has allowed early surgical treatment and improved survival. It is also possible to identify carriers of the MEN2A gene by DNA analysis. Four large families with MEN-2A were screened to compare the reliability of biochemical tests with that of DNA analysis.

Methods.—Three hundred members of the 4 families were repeatedly studied since 1974. Screening was carried out annually starting between the ages of 5 and 10 years; after age 35, testing was performed every 3 years. The tests were measurements of basal and stimulated plasma calcitonin concentrations, urinary excretion of catecholamines and catecholamine metabolites, and serum calcium concentrations. Carrier status was assessed by linked genetic markers until 1993 and, more recently, by analysis of mutations in the RET proto-oncogene on chromosome 10.

Results.—Biochemical and radiologic tests, pathologic examinations, and DNA analysis identified 80 MEN2A gene carriers. Sixty-six had abnormal plasma calcitonin values and medullary thyroid carcinoma. Eight of 14 young carriers, as determined by DNA analysis, with normal plasma calcitonin values were found to have small foci of medullary thyroid carcinoma at thyroidectomy; the other 6 carriers have not had surgery (table). Sixty-eight of the remaining 220 family members were found by DNA analysis not to carry the MEN2A gene. Six of these 68 individuals had elevated plasma calcitonin concentrations and underwent thyroidectomy but had only C-cell hyperplasia.

Conclusions.—Analysis of DNA is more accurate than biochemical tests in identifying MEN2A gene carriers. There have been no false positive or false negative results in the families studied, which thereby allows unaffected family members to discontinue screening for the disease.

▶ About 10% of thyroid carcinomas are medullary thyroid carcinomas, which are tumors of the calcitonin-secreting thyroid parafollicular cells (C cells). Twenty five percent of these carcinomas occur as part of 1 of 3 familial tumor syndromes: familial medullary thyroid carcinoma; MEN-2A—medullary thyroid carcinoma, pheochromocytoma, and primary hyperparathyroidism (the most common); and MEN-2B—medullary thyroid carcinoma, pheochromocytoma, and mucosal neuromas. All three syndromes are inherited as autosomal dominant traits. In the 2 MEN syndromes, the penetrance of medullary thyroid carcinoma approaches 100%, and about half of the cases appear by adolescence. The penetrance of pheochromocytomas is lower; they appear later and are often bilateral but are rarely malignant. In short, it is the medullary thyroid carcinomas that are life-threatening.

Among families with these syndromes, medullary thyroid carcinomas are preceded by hyperplasia of the C cells. C-cell hyperplasia is associated with elevated plasma calcitonin concentrations or supernormal increases in plasma calcitonin after administration of pentagastrin or calcium, which has made it possible to identify subjects at high risk for medullary thyroid carcinoma. As a result of regular testing starting at an early age in affected families, medullary thyroid carcinoma can be detected at a very early, microscopic stage. This type of screening, in use for over 20 years, has resulted in greatly improved survival (table; [1]). Biochemical screening, which despite its value has transient side effects, causes anxiety, and can be hard to interpret or falsely positive, can now be replaced by DNA analysis.

Both MEN syndromes and familial medullary thyroid carcinoma are associated with germline mutations of the *RET* proto-oncogene on chromosome 10. Based on this and other studies (2), the results of DNA analysis in affected families are 100% specific and sensitive. The question now is at what age an affected family member should undergo thyroidectomy. Because the thyroid carcinoma may appear as early as age 3 years, and about half appear by adolescence, I think that thyroidectomy should be done at an early age (3). Screening for pheochromocytoma—by clinical examination and urinary catecholamine measurements—should begin at an early age, but adrenalectomy should not be done until a tumor is identified, because the lifetime penetrance of these tumors is only about 50%.

Some broader questions are whether patients with a solitary thyroid nodule should be evaluated biochemically for medullary thyroid carcinoma and whether a patient found to have a seemingly sporadic medullary thyroid carcinoma could in fact have one of the familial syndromes. Among patients with solitary thyroid nodules, about 5% have thyroid carcinoma and 0.5% (or less) have medullary thyroid carcinoma. In a recent study in Italy (4) in which 1,385 patients with thyroid nodular disease had measurements of basal plasma calcitonin concentrations as part of their initial evaluation, 8 (0.6%) had elevated values; all 8 were operated on and proved to have medullary thyroid carcinoma, but fine-needle aspiration biopsy was positive for carcinoma in only 4 of the patients. I don't known whether these figures apply in the United States, and am not ready to recommend routine plasma calcitonin measurement as part of the initial evaluation of patients with a solitary thyroid nodule.

The possibility of one of the familial medullary thyroid carcinoma syndromes should be considered in any patient found to have a medullary thyroid carcinoma. Although the familial tumors usually occur at young ages, this is not always the case, and biochemical testing of other family members of patients presumed to have a sporadic medullary thyroid carcinoma has revealed other affected family members (5). Now that germline mutations can be identified in persons with familial tumors, this type of testing should be done in all patients with medullary thyroid carcinoma.—R.D. Utiger, M.D.

References

1. Gagel RF, Tashjian AH Jr, Cummings T, et al: The clinical outcome of prospective screening for multiple endocrine neoplasia type 2a: An 18-year experience. N Engl J Med 318:478–484, 1988.
2. Quadro L, Panariello L, Salvatore D, et al: Frequent RET protooncogene mutations in multiple endocrine neoplasia type 2A. J Clin Endocrinol Metab 79:590–594, 1994.
3. Utiger RD: Medullary thyroid carcinoma, genes, and the prevention of cancer. N Engl J Med 331:870–871, 1994.

4. Pacini F, Fontanelli M, Fugazzola L, et al: Routine measurement of serum calcitonin in nodular thyroid diseases allows the preoperative diagnosis of unsuspected sporadic medullary thyroid carcinoma. *J Clin Endocrinol Metab* 78:826–829, 1994.
5. Ponder BA, Finer N, Coffey R, et al: Family screening in medullary thyroid carcinoma presenting without a family history. *Q J Med* 67:299–308, 1988.

55 The Reproductive System

A Prospective Study of the Prevalence of Clear-Cut Endocrine Disorders and Polycystic Ovaries in 350 Patients Presenting With Hirsutism or Androgenic Alopecia

O'Driscoll JB, Mamtora H, Higginson J, Pollock A, Kane J, Anderson DC (The Skin Hosp, Salford, England; Hope Hosp, Salford, England; Chinese Univ, Hong Kong; et al)

Clin Endocrinol 41:231–236, 1994   119-95-55–1

Introduction.—Hirsutism and androgenic alopecia in women are caused by androgen excess, but identifying the source of the excess androgen is often difficult. The usefulness of several serum androgen measurements and of ultrasound imaging of the ovaries was evaluated in detecting an endocrine disorder in a prospective study of women with hirsutism or androgenic alopecia.

Methods.—Two baseline blood samples were collected on separate days in 350 consecutive women seen with hirsutism and/or androgenic alopecia for measurements of serum testosterone, androstenedione, and 17-hydroxyprogesterone (17-OHP). High-resolution pelvic ultrasonography was performed on 282 women. Findings suggestive of endocrine

Menstrual History and Results of Ultrasound Scanning

Menstrual cycle	Patients	PCO on scan (%)	Normal scan	Not scanned/ visualized
Regular periods	161	68 (52)	62	31
Irregular periods	112	77 (81)	18	17
Amenorrhoea	9	8 (89)	1	0
Contraceptive pill	26	11 (50)	11	4
Hysterectomy	14	4 (44)	5	5
Post-menopausal	28	2 (12)	15	11
Total	350	170 (60%)	112	68

(Courtesy of O'Driscoll JB, Mamtora H, Higginson J, et al: *Clin Endocrinol* 41:231–236, 1994.)

disorders were confirmed with urinary steroid profiles and CT imaging of the adrenal glands and ovaries.

Results.—Of the 282 women who underwent ultrasonography, 170 (60%) had polycystic ovaries (PCOs) (10 or more cysts 2–8 mm in diameter in each ovary). Of the women with PCOs, 12% were post-menopausal (table). The mean serum testosterone concentration was higher in the women with than in those without PCOs. Eight women had definite endocrine disorders: 1 acromegaly, 1 prolactinoma, 3 adrenal 21-hydroxylase deficiency, 1 a hepatic 11-reductase deficiency, 1 a virilizing adrenal carcinoma, and 1 an ovarian tumor. The serum testosterone concentration was unequivocally elevated (145 ng/dL greater than 5 nmol/L) in 13 women; 6 of them had a definite endocrine disorder and 6 of the remaining 7 had PCOs. The serum androstenedione concentration was elevated in 19 women, 5 of whom had an endocrine disorder. Although 18 women had serum 17-OHP concentrations greater than 165 ng/dL (5 nmol/L), only the 3 women with 21-hydroxylase deficiency had 17-OHP concentrations greater than 660 ng/dL (20 nmol/L).

Discussion.—Women with hirsutism or androgenic alopecia should be initially screened with a measurement of serum testosterone, and those whose values exceed 140 ng/dL (5 nmol/L) should undergo more complete endocrine evaluation. Although ultrasonographic findings of PCOs are very common among women with hirsutism or androgenic alopecia, they do not exclude other pathology.

▶ Hirsutism is very common among premenopausal women, most of whom have little in the way of menstrual abnormalities or infertility. Although many of these women have PCOs (table), so do as many as 20% of normal women (1, 2). It is, therefore, difficult to ascribe hirsutism to PCOs in most women with the latter, even if no other abnormality is detected. We do so mainly because most women with PCOs have slightly higher serum testosterone concentrations than those without PCOs; in this study, the mean serum testosterone concentrations were 71 ng/dL (2.47 nmol/L) in the women with PCOs and 59 ng/dL (2.04 nmol/L) in those without. Both of these means are well within the normal range in most laboratories, but, curiously, the authors did not indicate the normal range in their laboratory.

Hirsutism is not often caused by a readily definable abnormality in androgen production and, in fact, is not often associated with unequivocal increases in serum testosterone. The important, well-definable causes are late-onset congenital adrenal hyperplasia, ovarian tumors, and adrenal tumors, a few of which are carcinomas. All are rare, especially in women with few menstrual abnormalities. The extent to which hirsute women should be studied to rule out these disorders is controversial. In younger women who have had hirsutism for more than 1–2 years and who have no other clinical manifestations of androgen excess (acne, frontal balding, deep voice, clitoromegaly, or unequivocal menstrual disturbances) and little or no elevation in serum testosterone, further studies are rarely rewarding and are not indicated (3). —R.D. Utiger, M.D.

References

1. Polson DW, Adams J, Franks S, et al: Polycystic ovaries: A common finding in normal women. *Lancet* 1:870–872, 1988.
2. Clayton RN, Ogden V, Hodgkinson J, et al: How common are polycystic ovaries in normal women and what is their significance for the fertility of the population. *Clin Endocrinol* 37:127–134, 1992.
3. McKenna TJ: Screening for sinister causes of hirsutism. *N Engl J Med* 331:1015–1016, 1994.

Risk Factors for Secondary Amenorrhea and Galactorrhea
Gold EB, Bush T, Chee E (Univ of Calif, Davis; Johns Hopkins Univ, Baltimore, Md)
Int J Fertil 39:177–184, 1994   119-95-55–2

Introduction.—Secondary amenorrhea is a common cause of reproductive dysfunction and may have an impact on the long-term health of women. Factors known to be associated with the condition probably explain only a small proportion of cases. In addition, little is known about the risk factors for galactorrhea without amenorrhea. Data gathered by the Pituitary Adenoma Study Group were examined for differences in clinical and demographic characteristics between cases of secondary amenorrhea or galactorrhea and matched normal women.

Methods.—The multicenter study was originally designed to determine whether a relationship existed between oral contraceptive use and the occurrence of pituitary adenomas. Of 364 women with secondary amenorrhea (for 6 or more months) or galactorrhea, 253 were interviewed for the study. The women were assigned to 1 of 3 study groups: 114 (group 1) had secondary amenorrhea, with or without galactorrhea, and normal serum prolactin (PRL) concentrations; 85 (group 2) had secondary amenorrhea, with or without galactorrhea, and elevated serum PRL concentrations; and 53 (group 3) had galactorrhea and were menstruating. About half (52%) of the women in group 3 had elevated serum PRL concentrations at diagnosis. Neighborhood women were matched to each case.

Results.—The 3 patient groups differed only slightly from each other in clinical presentation. The women in group 1 were significantly more educated and older at menarche than their controls. The women in groups 2 and 3 did not differ significantly from their controls in these variables. The group 3 women had significantly longer menstrual periods than their controls and weighed more than their controls 2 years before diagnosis. There were significantly fewer smokers among the amenorrhea groups than their control groups. Overall, the study patients and their controls did not differ significantly in history or duration of oral contraceptive use.

Conclusions.—The low frequency of smoking in the women with secondary amenorrhea suggests that the antiestrogenic effect of smoking is not a prominent factor in their amenorrhea. Increased weight may be a risk factor for galactorrhea.

▶ Women with all the well-established causes of either secondary amenorrhea, galactorrhea, or hyperprolactinemia were excluded from this study. Specifically, women were excluded if they were perimenopausal or had a prolactinoma; ovarian failure, as determined by elevated serum follicle-stimulating hormone concentrations; identifiable gynecologic disease; anorexia nervosa; thyroid disease; or various other medical problems. Women taking any drug that might cause hyperprolactinemia, which can itself cause secondary amenorrhea, galactorrhea, or both, also were excluded. No mention was made about excessive physical activity.

Most of the women were in their 20s or 30s, and the differences between the 3 study groups and their respective control groups were very small. There were no differences in weight at the time of the study or 2 years earlier in the 2 groups of women with amenorrhea and their respective control groups. Unlike these investigators, others have found a relationship between smoking and secondary amenorrhea (1). In short, with respect to the information collected in this study, no new clues to the causes of secondary amenorrhea with or without hyperprolactinemia in women were obtained.

Women with secondary amenorrhea should be evaluated clinically, hormonally, and, at times, radiologically for the disorders mentioned above and others, such as a nonsecreting pituitary tumor. The diagnoses of exclusion are hypothalamic amenorrhea and idiopathic hyperprolactinemia, either of which may be due to as yet unrecognized psychological factors or subtle nutritional abnormalities (2). In either case, the prognosis is for persistence (3, 4), so that consideration should be given to estrogen replacement therapy if fertility is not desired.—R.D. Utiger, M.D.

References

1. Pettersson F, Fires H, Nillius SJ: Epidemiology of secondary amenorrhea. I: Incidence and prevalence rates. *Am J Obstet Gynecol* 1973:80–86, 1973.
2. Warren MP, Holderness CC, Lesobre V, Tzen R, Vossoughian F, Brooks-Gunn J: Hypothalamic amenorrhea and hidden nutritional insults. *J Soc Gynecol Invest* 1:84–88, 1994.
3. 1992 YEAR BOOK OF MEDICINE, pp 502–503.
4. Schlecthe J, Dolan K, Sherman B, et al: The natural history of untreated hyperprolactinemia: A prospective analysis. *J Clin Endocrinol Metab* 68:412–418, 1989.

Risk Factors for Menopausal Hot Flashes

Schwingl PJ, Hulka BS, Harlow SD (Univ of North Carolina, Chapel Hill)
Obstet Gynecol 84:29–34, 1994   119-95-55–3

Background.—Between 50% and 85% of women have hot flashes during their menopause, and approximately 75% of these women seek medical attention and are prescribed estrogens for symptom relief. The potential risk factors for hot flashes were investigated in a population-based sample of black and white women who were within 20 years of menopause.

Methods.—A total of 1,571 women were interviewed in their homes. Of these, 908 had stopped menstruating at least 12 months before the interview and 527 were naturally menopausal. Because the proportion of women reporting hot flashes at the time of menopause declined both with the number of years since the menopause and with age at interview, only the 334 women who were interviewed within 20 years of their reported age at the time of natural menopause were included in the study (table). The interview comprised questions on demographic variables, menstrual history, reproductive events, medical history, menopausal status and symptoms, history of estrogen and oral contraceptive administration, smoking and alcohol use, and family history of cancer. The women were also asked when hot flashes started.

Selected Characteristics of 334 Naturally Postmenopausal Women.

	Mean	SD	Range	Percent
Age at interview (y)	58.4	6.0	41–75	
Years since menopause	9.2	5.5	1–20	
Age at menopause (y)	49.1	3.9	40–59	
Age at menarche (y)	13.3	1.6	9–19	
Age at first pregnancy (y)	22.5	5.1	12–40	
Age at last pregnancy (y)	32.9	7.4	16–49	
Body mass index	26.7	5.8	16.3–56.7	
Hot flashes				71
Black race				24
Education < 12 y				65
Nulliparous				12
Parity ≥ 3				51
BMI ≥ 27.1				40
Smoked at or around the time of menopause				26
Ever drank alcohol				33
Periods usually irregular				8

(Courtesy of Schwingl PJ, Hulka BS, Harlow SD: *Obstet Gynecol* 84:29–34, 1994.)

Results.—Seventy-one percent of the women reported having hot flashes at the time their menses stopped. The most important predictors of hot flashes were menopause before the age of 53 years and fewer than 12 years of education. Age at menarche after 11 years and regular menstrual periods were also significantly correlated with the incidence of hot flashes at menopause. Thin women who smoked were also likely to have hot flashes. Among nonsmokers, weight was not a significant factor.

Conclusion.—The incidence of hot flashes is related to demographic and life-style factors as well as reproductive events. The hypothesis that a pattern of estrogen depletion plays a significant role in the etiology of hot flashes at menopause was supported.

▶ Hot flashes are the most characteristic feature of cessation of ovarian function and the symptom most likely to cause menopausal women to seek medical care. Subjective hot flashes are associated with elevations of skin temperature, cutaneous vasodilatation, and perspiration that occur as a result of activation of hypothalamic thermoregulatory centers. Although hot flashes clearly have some relation to decreased ovarian function, and more specially decreased estrogen production (1), the correlation can be poor. For example, whereas hot flashes may begin within a week after bilateral ovariectomy, some women begin to have hot flashes while still having regular menstrual cycles. The hot flashes usually subside within a few years after cessation of menses, but they persist for 5 years in about 25% of women.

The finding in this study that 71% of the women no more than 20 years post cessation of menses had hot flashes at some time may be an underestimate, because of loss of remote memory. There was no difference among black and white women. The difference in likelihood of hot flashes according to age at the time of menopause was rather striking: 78% of the 85 women aged 40 to 46 years at menopause had hot flashes, as compared with 73% of the 180 women aged 47 to 52 years and 56% of the 69 women aged 53 to 59 years. The greater frequency of hot flashes in the younger age group may relate to more rapid cessation of menses and more rapid decline in estrogen production. Both thinness and smoking are associated with lower plasma estrogen concentrations; the former because thin women produce less estrogen at extragonadal (adipose tissue) sites than heavier women, and the latter because smoking accelerates clearance of estrogen from plasma. In this study, however, either alone was not associated with a higher frequency of hot flashes, but the combination was. Other findings associated with a higher frequency of hot flashes were fewer than 12 years of education (76 vs. 64%), menarche at age 12 or older (73 vs. 57%), and regular menstrual periods (72% vs. 55%). I don't know why any of these factors should be important.

I found these results interesting, even though their impact on practice may be small. The occurrence of hot flashes, or their absence, cannot be used to make inferences about the degree of estrogen deficiency in an individual postmenopausal woman (but see Abstract 119-95-55-4 next). Hot flashes are certainly one indication for estrogen therapy, but others—psychological symptoms (fatigue, insomnia), treatment of urogenital atrophy, prevention of osteoporosis, and prevention of ischemic heart disease (2)—may warrant estrogen replacement even if the woman has no hot flashes.—R.D. Utiger, M.D.

References

1. Erlik Y, Meldrum DR, Judd HL: Estrogen levels in postmenopausal women with hot flashes. *Obstet Gynecol* 59: 403–407, 1982.
2. Belchetz PE: Hormonal treatment of postmenopausal women. N *Engl J Med* 330:1062–1071, 1994.

An Association Between Osteoporosis and Premenstrual Symptoms and Postmenopausal Symptoms

Lee SJ, Kanis JA (Univ of Sheffield, England)
Bone Miner 24:127–134, 1994   119-95-55–4

Background.—Estrogen deficiency, a well-documented risk factor for osteoporosis as well as vasomotor symptoms, may be a feature of premenstrual tension in the decade before menopause. Bone density at maturity, which may be affected by estrogen status, may influence the development of postmenopausal osteoporosis. The relationship between premenstrual symptoms and risk for osteoporosis, as well as a possible relationship between menopausal vasomotor symptoms and the development of vertebral osteoporosis, were studied.

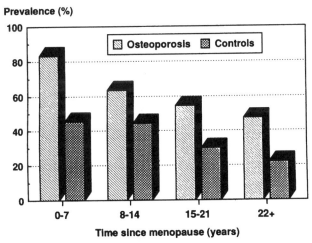

Fig 55–1.—Prevalence of vasomotor symptoms in 69 osteoporotic (*hatched*) and 67 control women (*crosshatched*) as a function of menopausal age. Women with hysterectomy and ovarian conservation were not included. (Courtesy of Lee SJ, Kanis JA: *Bone Miner* 24:127–134, 1994.)

Methods.—Seventy-five postmenopausal women aged 55–70 years with confirmed vertebral osteoporosis, as determined by vertebral fractures or low lumbar spine bone density measurements, and 77 age-matched women recruited from an ophthalmologic clinic were interviewed to determine their history of premenstrual symptoms and present and past history of postmenopausal vasomotor symptoms.

Results.—Premenstrual symptoms, cycle irregularity, and history of menopausal vasomotor symptoms were significantly more frequent among the osteoporotic women than the control women, and the former were more likely than the latter to describe their menopausal symptoms as severe and persistent. Although vasomotor symptoms did not correlate with premenstrual symptoms, the co-existence of both types of symptoms had an additive effect on the relative risk for vertebral osteoporosis. Grouping the osteoporotic and control women by menopausal age revealed a significantly greater prevalence of vasomotor symptoms among women who are osteoporotic at each time interval (Fig 55–1).

Conclusion.—A history of premenstrual symptoms may indicate a low peak bone mass, and severe menopausal vasomotor symptoms may predict excessive bone loss.

▶ No one questions that estrogen deficiency is the major cause of postmenopausal bone loss. If estrogen deficiency began before the menopause, while menstrual cycles continued, then bone loss should begin then. Furthermore, if women with more menopausal symptoms are more estrogen-deficient, then they should have more bone loss.

Those suppositions are supported by the results of this study, with caveats about the uncertainties of memory of events many years ago and the lack of bone density measurements in the control group. The women with osteoporosis and the control group were well matched for age, age at menarche, and age at menopause. As shown in Figure 55–1, more women in the osteoporosis group had postmenopausal vasomotor symptoms. In addition, their symptoms had been more severe and lasted longer. More also had premenstrual symptoms and oligomenorrhea. They therefore probably started to lose bone earlier and, after the menopause, more rapidly. There is evidence that premenopausal women with ovulatory disturbances have decreased bone density (1) and that lower serum estrogen concentrations equate with lower bone density in the perimenopausal period (2). After the menopause, even soon after it, the correlation between measurements of estrogen production, menopausal symptoms, and bone density is poor, probably due to the difficulties of measuring estrogen production when it is very low and the inability to account for estrogen production from androgen in estrogen-target tissues (3).

The practical message of these results is to pay heed to complaints of estrogen deficiency and consider recommending replacement—for the sake of the bones—even if a woman doesn't think she needs it for symptom relief. There are, of course, lots of other risk factors for postmenopausal osteoporosis—low weight, tall height, smoking, late menarche—but few more amenable to correction than estrogen deficiency.—R.D. Utiger, M.D.

References

1. Prior JC, Vigna YM, Schechter MT, Burgess AE: Spinal bone loss and ovulatory disturbances. N Engl J Med 323:1221–1227, 1990.
2. Steinberg KK, Freni-Titulaer LW, DePuey EG, et al: Sex steroids and bone density in premenopausal and perimenopausal women. J Clin Endocrinol Metab 69:533–539, 1989.
3. Spector TD, Thompson PW, Perry LA, McGarrigle HH, Edwards AC: The relationship between sex steroids and bone mineral content in women soon after the menopause. Clin Endocrinol 34:37–41, 1991.

Decline in Sperm Counts: An Artefact of Changed Reference Range of "Normal"?
Bromwich P, Cohen J, Stewart I, Walker A (Midland Fertility Services, Adlridge, England; Univ of Warwick, Coventry, England)
BMJ 309:19–22, 1994   119-95-55–5

Introduction.—A decline in sperm concentration between 1938 and 1990 has been reported, with a decline in the lower reference value defining a normal sperm concentration from 60×10^6/mL to 20×10^6/mL in this interval. However, the decrease in the lower reference value may have confounded the results of comparison studies, as men with sperm concentrations between 20 and 60×10^6/mL would have been excluded from studies during the 1940s but included in more recent studies. The effect of the change in reference value on sperm concentration data was explored.

Methods.—Sperm concentrations were measured in 235 men participating in an in vitro fertilization program and in 20 ejaculates each from 5 other men in the same program. The probability distribution was then analyzed, excluding those men with a sperm concentration lower than 60×10^6/mL first, and then those whose sperm concentration was lower than 20×10^6/mL.

Results.—When a sperm concentration of 60×10^6/mL was used as the lower reference value, the percentage in the highest range (greater than 190×10^9/L) was 55%. When a concentration of 20×10^6/mL was used as the lower reference value, the proportion of men with a sperm concentration in the highest range was 28%. In addition, there was wide variability in multiple ejaculates from a group of 5 men tested repeatedly; in them, the concentrations varied by as much as sixfold.

Discussion.—The finding of a decline in sperm count may be invalidated by changing the lower reference value. In addition, the wide individual variations in sperm concentration suggest that averages may not predict fertility.

▶ This paper is what I would call a rather arcane analysis of how the results of semen analyses done in the last several decades in presumably normal men should be evaluated. This study was precipitated by an analysis of 61 sets of data that suggested that mean sperm concentrations in normal men in industrialized countries had decreased from 113×10^6/mL to 66×10^6/mL during the last 5 decades, a decline of 40% (semen volume decreased by 18%) (1). I am not sure that arguments about what constitutes normal values enlighten the debate, unless values from supposedly normal men were arbitrarily eliminated from some studies. This does not seem to have been the case, but I looked at only a small minority of the 61 studies. In a very recent study of about 1,300 men in Paris (2), the mean sperm concentration decreased from 89×10^6/mL in 1973 to 60×10^6/mL in 1992 (2).

What is clear about sperm concentrations is that they vary a great deal, even in an individual man. Some of this variation can be explained by the frequency of ejaculation; sperm concentrations increase after a few days of abstinence but decrease if it is prolonged. Furthermore, there is much interindividual variation, and most of the reported data are from men about to undergo vasectomy, men who are volunteer sperm donors, or men who with their partners are attending fertility clinics—all of whom may differ from the general population of men. Measurement methods also may have varied over the years.

Notwithstanding these caveats, maybe sperm concentrations have deceased in the last several decades in some places. If the trend is real and the rate of decline continues relentlessly, the pessimist can conclude that concentrations will reach 0 by some time during the next century. That seems unlikely, but the possibility that there has been a decline should force us to look more carefully at the problem and to consider the possibility that environmental factors may have widespread effects on spermatogenesis.—R.D. Utiger, M.D.

References

1. Carlsen E, Giwercman A, Keiding N, Skakkebaek NE: Evidence for decreasing quality of semen during the past 50 years. *BMJ* 305:609–612, 1992.
2. Auger J, Kunstmann JM, Czyglik F, Jouannet P: Decline in semen quality of fertile men in Paris during the last 20 years. *N Engl J Med* 332:281–285, 1995.

Risk of Gynaecomastia Associated With Cimetidine, Omeprazole, and Other Antiulcer Drugs

Garcia Rodríguez LA, Jick H (Boston Univ, Lexington, Mass)
BMJ 308:503–506, 1994

119-95-55-6

Objective and Methods.—Because various antiulcer medications have been implicated in causing gynecomastia, a large population-based cohort study was undertaken to examine this possible association. The study group was 81,535 men 25 to 84 years of age who were cared for in 478 general practices in the United Kingdom and who received at least 1 prescription for an antiulcer drug (cimetidine, misoprostol, omeprazole, or ranitidine) during a 2.7 year period.

Findings.—Gynecomastia developed in 138 men. Only those men who received cimetidine had a substantially increased risk for gynecomastia developing (relative risk, 7.2) as compared with men who received none of these antiulcer drugs. The risk appeared to be highest after 7–12 months of cimetidine therapy, and most of the risk was associated with a daily dose of 1 g or more. The effects of the dose and duration of therapy were strongly synergistic. The only other drugs associated with a comparable risk of gynecomastia were spironolactone and verapamil, with respective relative risk values of 9.3 and 9.7.

Conclusion.—Cimetidine treatment is associated with a significant risk of idiopathic gynecomastia.

▶ Ascertainment of gynecomastia and drug therapy in this study was based on physician entry of data from office visits into standardized computerized files to which the investigators had access. The sources of error in studies like this include the extent of adherence to therapy and the care with which the men were examined. For example, men taking drugs reasonably well known to cause gynecomastia may be questioned or examined more carefully, increasing the likelihood of detection and so increasing the relative risk. Of the men with gynecomastia, 86 were taking cimetidine, 1 misoprostol, 1 omeprazole, 26 ranitidine, and 24 no antiulcer drug, but the relative risk of gynecomastia exceeded 1 significantly only in those men receiving cimetidine. Further information about 80 of the 153 men in this study with gynecomastia was obtained from their physicians. The gynecomastia was self-reported by 67 of the men (84%), detected incidentally on physical examination in 11 (14%), and the method of detection was not known in 2 (2%); it was bilateral in 38 men (47%), unilateral in 34 (43%), and unknown in 8 (10%). The gynecomastia subsequently regressed in most of the men, but 5 underwent mastectomy.

The list of drugs that have been associated with gynecomastia is long (1), but what I would call the real list is much shorter, and for the most part includes drugs that are known to have estrogenic effects or alter endogenous estrogen production. Besides, I believe that gynecomastia is overdiagnosed, especially when I see incidence figures as high as 65% (2). When I examine men, I have a great deal of difficulty deciding whether a circular mass of tissue beneath the nipple is fat or mammary tissue, and I confess that my conclusion is based as much on ancillary findings (Is the breast changing, and is it tender?) and the clinical setting (Is the man taking a drug reasonably well known to cause gynecomastia, or does he have a disease known to cause it?). The key question, of course, is, Could the man have a breast tumor, a rare occurrence and an unlikely possibility in a man with bilateral gynecomastia; or unilateral gynecomastia in the absence of a discrete mass.—R.D. Utiger, M.D.

References

1. Braunstein GD: Gynecomastia. N Engl J Med 328:490–495, 1993.
2. Niewoehner CB, Nuttall FQ: Gynecomastia in a hospitalized male population. Am J Med 77:633–638, 1984.

Relations of Endogenous Anabolic Hormones and Physical Activity to Bone Mineral Density and Lean Body Mass in Elderly Men
Rudman D, Drinka PJ, Wilson CR, Mattson DE, Scherman F, Cuisinier MC, Schultz S (Med College of Wisconsin, Milwaukee; VA Med Ctr, Milwaukee, Wis; Wisconsin Veterans Home, King)
Clin Endocrinol 40:653–661, 1994   1 19-95-55–7

Introduction.—Bone mineral density (BMD), total body bone mineral content (TBBMC), and lean body mass (LBM) steadily diminish in aging men, together with declines in serum growth hormone, insulin-like growth factor (IGF-I) and testosterone, hormones that influence body composition. The age-related losses of BMD and LBM have been attributed in part to declining growth hormone, IGF-I, or testosterone secretion or to a sedentary life-style. These hypotheses were tested in 2 groups of older men.

Methods.—Of 98 men ranging in age from 58 to 95 years, half were independent and community dwelling (group I), and half lived in VA extended-care facilities (group II). The group I men were in good general health, and none had diabetes mellitus or were substantially overweight; 77% were retired. Those in group II had no acute illness, diabetes, or obesity, but most had chronic medical conditions and were receiving various medications. All the men had measurements of serum IGF-I and testosterone, and LBM and bone status were measured at 9 skeletal sites by dual x-ray absorptiometry. Physical activity and mobility were also recorded.

Results.—The men in both groups were similar in mean age (69 and 73 years) and body mass index (24.5 and 26.4 kg/m²). The community-dwelling men (group I) had BMD and TBBMC values that were 4% to 20% higher than those of the institutionalized men (group II). In group I, serum testosterone was the strongest predictor of BMD and TBBMC, and age was the only predictor of LBM. Age, body weight, and immobility were the strongest predictors of body composition in group II; serum testosterone concentrations were correlated only with femoral neck BMD in the institutionalized men.

Conclusion.—The most influential predictor of bone status in independent elderly men was serum testosterone. In institutionalized elderly men, the relation of predictor variables to body composition was more complex; very old age and immobility appeared to be stronger risk factors for osteopenia than was hypogonadism. Exogenous testosterone might improve bone status in healthy older men, whereas weight gain and greater mobility might benefit men in nursing homes.

▶ Growth hormone (GH), IGF-I, and testosterone secretion decline in aging men. So do BMD and muscle mass (and strength). This study can be considered an attempt to determine the extent to which these changes can be attributed to normal hormonal events during aging as compared with the effects of chronic illness. The results suggest that the key factors are declining serum testosterone concentrations—yes, there is a male menopause—and illness, which among other things inhibits pituitary-gonadal secretion. Partial correction of these deficits can be obtained by proper management of the chronic illness.

The hormonal and metabolic changes that occur in aging or sick men have already led to trials of GH and testosterone therapy (1, 2). Each of these treatments has benefits in terms of increased muscle (LBM) and bone density, or at least decreased bone resorption, and a variety of subjective findings (increased well-being and increased libido [see Abstract 119-95-52–2]). Growth hormone is hugely expensive and will quite appropriately remain an experimental therapy for a while. The situation with respect to testosterone is somewhat different. It is not very expensive and can be given at several week intervals, but it has not been demonstrated to have any long-term benefit with respect to longevity, lower fracture rate, fewer falls, etc. Furthermore, it stimulates prostatic growth and therefore could not only exacerbate benign prostatic hyperplasia, but also stimulate the growth of prostatic carcinoma. It also raises serum low-density lipoprotein cholesterol concentrations. Given these considerations, GH or testosterone replacement therapy for older men is a far different proposition than estrogen replacement for older women.—R.D. Utiger, M.D.

References

1. Rudman D, Feller AG, Nagraj HS, et al: Effect of human growth hormone in men over 60 years old. N Engl J Med 323:1–6, 1990.
2. Tenover JS: Effects of testosterone supplementation in the aging male. J Clin Endocrinol Metab 75:1092–1098, 1992.

56 The Parathyroid Glands and Bone

Prediction of Bone Density From Vitamin D Receptor Alleles

Morrison NA, Qi JC, Tokita A, Kelly PJ, Crofts L, Nguyen TV, Sambrook PN, Eisman JA (St Vincent's Hosp, Sydney, Australia)
Nature 367:284–287, 1994   119-95-56-1

Purpose.—Osteoporotic fracture risk in later life is largely determined by an individual's peak bone density in early adulthood. Peak bone density is at least in part under genetic control via effects on bone turnover.

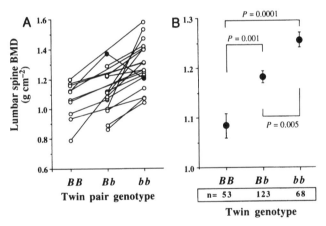

Fig 56–1.—Higher bone density is associated with the *b* allele of the vitamin D receptor gene. Lumbar spine bone densities of dizygotic twins discordant for vitamin D receptor alleles ($n = 22$) are plotted as twin and co-twin according to genotype, with lines joining each twin pair (**A**). In 21 of 22 associated twin pairs, the twin carrying 1 or 2 extra copies of the *b* allele has the higher bone density. A single pair of young male twins exhibited the reverse situation. Bone mineral density (mean ± SEM) is shown for all twins according to genotype, regardless of zygosity (**B**). It is clear that the *BB* genotype is associated with lower mean bone density. The magnitude of the effect can be seen in relation to the standard deviation of an age-matched population of $\sim$ .11 g/cm^{-2}. The significance of difference between groups was calculated by the mixed-model analysis of variance, incorporating a fixed effect for genotype and random effects for other twin pair-specific factors. At the lumbar spine, the effect of genotype was significant at $P = .000054$, and at the femoral neck, $P = .038$. The *P* values displayed are for pairwise Student's *t*-tests between the genotypes. A similar significant effect was observed for the Ward's triangle ($P = .033$) but not the trochanteric region ($P = .1$) by mixed model random effect analysis of variance. When the analysis was limited to females, *P* values were: lumbar spine, $P = .0000036$; femoral neck, $P = .06$; Ward's triangle, $P = .05$; trochanteric region, $P = .019$. (Courtesy of Morrison NA, Qi JC, Tokita A, et al: *Nature* 367:284–287, 1994.)

Common allelic variants in the gene encoding the vitamin D receptor (VDR) were shown to predict differences in bone density.

Findings.—In a study of 70 white monozygotic and 55 white dizygotic twin pairs in Australia, the VDR genotype was a strong predictor of bone density at both the lumbar spine, femoral neck, and Ward's triangle (Fig 56–1). Among 311 unrelated white Australian women, those with femoral neck bone densities more than 2 SD below the values of normal young women had overrepresentation of the BB genotype associated with lower bone density. On average, women with the BB genotype reached this level of bone density at age 63 years, as compared with age 71 years for those with the bb genotype. The results were similar with respect to vertebral bone density. Women with the Bb genotype reached this level of vertebral bone density at an intermediate age (data for femoral neck bone density in this group were not reported).

Conclusion.—Allelic variants in the VDR gene may account for as much as three fourths of the total genetic effect on bone density in healthy individuals. Identification of this genetic marker may have important ramifications for early intervention in persons at increased risk of osteoporosis and understanding of the mechanisms of variability in bone density.

▶ Peak bone density is strongly influenced by genetic factors (1, 2), and if Morrison et al. are correct, one factor is genetic polymorphism of the vitamin D receptor (VDR). How might this occur? The VDR is a cytoplasmic protein that translocates calcitriol to cell nuclei, in which the VDR complex regulates gene transcription. The key target organs are the gut, in which the complex acts to stimulate calcium absorption, and the bone, in which it stimulates bone formation, mineralization, and resorption. Vitamin D stimulation of osteoblast function, leading to increased bone formation, is associated with increased serum concentrations of osteocalcin, a marker of osteoblast activity, which the same group has found to be related to polymorphism of the VDR (3). These observations lead to the conclusion that the b allele codes for a VDR protein that is a better activator of osteoblast function than the B allele, and thus is associated with formation of more bone and higher peak bone density.

The clinical implications of these findings are substantial, especially if they are applicable to racial groups other than white Australians. Identification of persons with the higher-risk B allele could lead to targeting not only of efforts to slow bone loss—the major component of risk of fracture among the elderly—but also of efforts to maximize bone formation in early life. Something as simple as an increase in vitamin D intake, thereby increasing the occupancy of the less favorable B form of the receptor, might increase calcium absorption and bone formation.

Other investigators have moved quickly to confirm, with very mixed success, that different alleles of the gene for the VDR are related to bone density. Specifically, the results were confirmed in studies in England and Japan, but not in the United States and Sweden (4–7). It may well be that the importance of VDR status as a determinant of bone density varies among different populations, but even so, it offers an exciting way to look at bone disease risk.—R.D. Utiger, M.D.

References

1. Evans RA, Marel GM, Lancaster EK, Kos S, Evans M, Wong SYP: Bone mass is low in relatives of osteoporotic patients. *Ann Intern Med* 109:870–873, 1988.
2. Seeman E, Hopper H, Bach LA, et al: Reduced bone mass in daughters of women with osteoporosis. *N Engl J Med* 320:554–558, 1990.
3. Morrison NA, Yeoman R, Kelly PJ, Eisman JA: Contribution of trans-activating factor alleles to normal physiological variability: Vitamin D receptor gene polymorphism and circulating osteocalcin. *Proc Natl Acad Sci U S A* 89:6665–6669, 1992.
4. Spector TD, Keen RW, Arden NK, et al: Vitamin D receptor gene (VDR) alleles and bone density in postmenopausal women: A UK twin study. *J Bone Miner Res* 9:143S, 1994.
5. Yamagata Z, Miyamura T, Iijima S, et al: Vitamin D receptor gene polymorphism and bone mineral density in healthy Japanese women. *Lancet* 344:1027, 1994.
6. Melhus H, Kindmark A, Amer S, Wilen B, Lindh E, Ljunghall S: Vitamin D receptor genotypes in osteoporosis. *Lancet* 344:949–950, 1994.
7. Hustmyer FG, Peacock M, Hui S, Johnston CC, Christian J: Bone mineral density in relation to polymorphism at the vitamin D receptor gene locus. *J Clin Invest* 94:2130–2134, 1994.

Walking is Related to Bone Density and Rates of Bone Loss
Krall EA, Dawson-Hughes B (Tufts Univ, Boston)
Am J Med 96:20–26, 1994   119-95-56–2

Introduction.—Walking is frequently recommended to slow bone loss. Bone density was examined in 239 healthy white postmenopausal women, aged 43 to 72 years, who participated in a 1-year placebo-controlled trial of supplemental vitamin D to determine whether walking is related to bone mineral density.

Methods.—Time spent in current and historical walking and 14 non-walking activities was recorded for all participants. Quadriceps muscle strength was assessed, and lumbar spine and whole body bone density was measured by dual-energy absorptiometry (Fig 56–2).

Results.—Walking was not independent of other activities. Women who walked more than 7.5 miles per week had a significantly higher whole body, leg, and trunk (including ribs, spine, and pelvis) bone mineral density than did women who walked less than 1 mile per week. Past walking activities were good indicators of present walking activities. The weekly number of miles walked correlated inversely with loss of bone density in the legs during the 1-year follow-up.

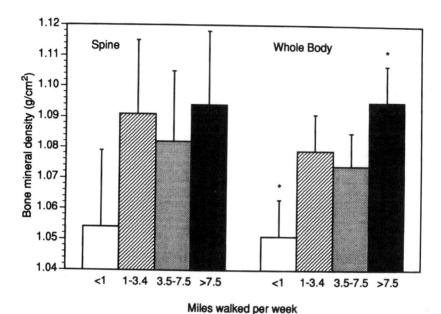

Fig 56–2.—Mean (± SE) bone density of the whole body and lumbar spine at study baseline by quartiles of current miles walked per week. (Courtesy of Krall EA, Dawson-Hughes B: *Am J Med* 96:20-26, 1994.)

Comments.—Walking has long-term positive effects on bone density. Walking at least 1 mile a day may help postmenopausal women to reduce bone loss.

▶ The data for current walking and other activities (e.g., aerobics, golf, jogging, skating) in these women were collected twice, in the spring and fall, each questionnaire covering the preceding 1 month. There were some differences in the spring and fall results, which perhaps is not surprising for women living in Boston. For example, the mean walking distance was 6.1 miles per week in the fall and 4.4 miles per week in the spring. The legs region (both lower extremities) was the only region in which less bone was lost in the women who walked more during the 1-year interval between bone density measurements. Although the accuracy of such self-reports can always be challenged, and there were differences in the results at different skeletal sites, the results agree with those of other, smaller studies, including some prospective studies of not only special training using treadmills and other devices, but also of walking (1–3). Many of these training programs are unrealistic for the vast majority of women, so it is good to see data documenting that walking alone is beneficial. Walking ought to be encouraged from an early age, because it probably augments bone mass in early years as well as slowing it in later years. Maybe the vast spaces of modern shopping malls have some hidden benefits.—R.D. Utiger, M.D.

References

1. Dalsky GP, Stocke KS, Ehsani AA, Slatopolsky E, Lee WC, Birge Jr SJ: Weight-bearing exercise training and lumbar bone mineral content in postmenopausal women. *Ann Intern Med* 108:824–828, 1988.

2. Martin D, Notelovitz M: Effects of aerobic training on bone mineral density of postmenopausal women. *J Bone Miner Res* 8:931–936, 1993.

3. Hatori M, Hasegawa A, Adachi H, et al: The effects of walking at the anaerobic threshold level on vertebral bone loss in postmenopausal women. *Calcif Tissue Int* 52:411–414, 1993.

Improved Mineral Balance and Skeletal Metabolism in Postmenopausal Women Treated With Potassium Bicarbonate

Sebastian A, Harris ST, Ottaway JH, Todd KM, Morris Jr RC (Univ of California, San Francisco)

N Engl J Med 330:1776–1781, 1994 119-95-56-3

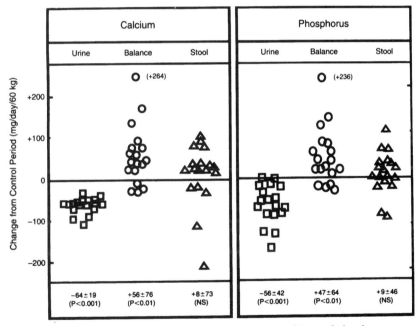

Fig 56–3.—Effect of potassium bicarbonate supplementation on calcium and phosphorous excretion in urine, external calcium and phosphorous balance, and calcium and phosphorous excretion in stool in 18 postmenopausal women. The values shown at the bottom of the figure are the average (± SD) potassium bicarbonate—induced changes from the control period (before supplementation). To convert calcium values to millimoles per day per 60 kg, divide by 40; to convert phosphorous values to millimoles per day per 60 kg, divide by 31. *Abbreviation:* NS, not significant. The P values are for the comparisons between the control period and the supplementation period. (Courtesy of Sebastian A, Harris ST, Ottaway JH, et al: *N Engl J Med* 330:1776–1781, 1994.)

Background.—The skeleton serves as a reservoir of calcium and also of labile base, in the form of alkaline calcium salts, that may be mobilized to defend the blood pH and plasma bicarbonate. Age-related osteoporosis may result, at least in part, from the cumulative mobilization of skeletal calcium salts to balance the endogenous acid formed from dietary precursors. Normal individuals maintain a low level of metabolic acidosis and a positive acid balance.

Objective and Methods.—The role of endogenous acid in the aging-related decrease in bone was studied in 18 postmenopausal women. The women ingested a constant daily diet containing 652 mg (16 mmol) of calcium and 96 g of protein per 60 kg of body weight. After a 6-day control period, potassium bicarbonate was given orally in a daily dose of 60 to 120 mmol for 18 days to neutralize endogenous acid, followed by a 12-day recovery period. Mineral and hydrogen ion balance was determined daily.

Results.—Calcium balance remained negative but became less negative when potassium bicarbonate was given. Net intestinal calcium absorption did not change, but urinary calcium excretion decreased (Fig 56–3). The phosphorus balance changed in a similar manner. The potassium balance became positive during the period of supplementation. The plasma potassium and bicarbonate concentrations and blood pH all increased significantly. There were no significant changes in plasma ionized calcium or phosphorus. There was a significant increase in the serum osteocalcin and a decrease in the urinary hydroxyproline excretion, indicative of increased bone formation and decreased bone resorption, respectively. The net renal acid excretion declined promptly when potassium bicarbonate supplementation began and returned to baseline when it was discontinued.

Implications.—The reduction in bone mass associated with advancing age may result, at least in part, from ongoing skeletal buffering of diet-derived endogenous acid. Long-term supplementation with potassium bicarbonate might help prevent osteoporosis in women who are postmenopausal.

▶ This study raises the possibility that postmenopausal bone loss may be minimized or even treated with alkali, assuming that the decrease in urinary calcium and hydroxyproline excretion and increase in serum osteocalcin concentration mean that bone formation will increase and bone resorption will decrease with long-term therapy. Note that the protein content of the diet was high (1.6 g/kg body weight) and so the acid load was high, but these investigators have found that a diet containing 0.8 g of protein/kg also reduces urinary calcium excretion substantially (1). There is, however, conflicting evidence on the amount and type (animal, vegetable, or both) of protein that increases calcium excretion and on whether sodium as well as potassium bicarbonate are effective in decreasing calcium excretion (2). All these questions are definitely worth pursuing, because there is strong epidemio-

logic evidence relating dietary intake of animal protein to hip fracture (3).
—R.D. Utiger, M.D.

References

1. Sebastian A, Morris RC Jr: Mineral balance in postmenopausal women treated with potassium bicarbonate. N Engl J Med 331:1312–1313, 1994.
2. Kraut JA, Coburn JW: Bone, acid, and osteoporosis. N Engl J Med 330:1821–1822, 1994.
3. Abelow BJ, Holford TR, Insogna KL: Cross-cultural association between dietary animal protein and hip fracture: A hypothesis. Calcif Tissue Int 50:14–18, 1992.

Calcium Supplementation With and Without Hormone Replacement Therapy to Prevent Postmenopausal Bone Loss

Aloia JF, Vaswani A, Yeh JK, Ross PL, Flaster E, Dilmanian FA (Winthrop-Univ Hosp, Mineola, NY; Brookhaven Natl Lab, Upton, NY)
Ann Intern Med 120:97–103, 1994   119-95-56-4

Objective.—A randomized parallel-design, placebo-controlled study was carried out in healthy white women within 6 years of a natural menopause to determine whether increasing dietary calcium intake prevents early postmenopausal bone loss, or whether hormonal replacement is also necessary.

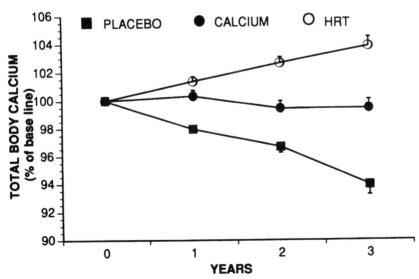

Fig 56–4.—The change in total body calcium with time. Calcium augmentation remained intermediate in effect between placebo and estrogen-progesterone-calcium throughout the 3 years of the study. *Abbreviation:* HRT, hormone replacement therapy. (Courtesy of Aloia JF, Vaswani A, Yeh JK, et al: *Ann Intern Med* 120:97–103, 1994.)

Study Plan.—A total of 118 white women who were 3–6 years post-menopausal were randomly assigned to receive 1,700 mg of elemental calcium (as calcium carbonate) daily, a placebo, or hormonal treatment combined with 1,700 mg of elemental calcium daily for 2.9 ± 1.1 (mean ± SD) years. Hormonal therapy consisted of 0.625 mg of conjugated equine estrogens, given on cycle days 1–25, and 10 mg of medroxyprogesterone on days 16 to 25. All women received vitamin D in a daily dose of 400 IU. Total body calcium was measured by delayed gamma neutron activation analysis. Bone mineral density was measured by photon absorptiometry in the spine, femur, and distal radius. The women's dietary calcium intake was approximately 500 mg daily.

Results.—The total body calcium in the women in the calcium group decreased by 0.5% per year, as compared with 2% per year in the placebo group and an increase of 0.9% per year in the calcium plus hormone group (P < 0.01) (Fig 56–4). The bone mineral density of the femoral neck declined less in the calcium group (0.8% per year) than in the placebo group (2% per year, P < 0.05), but more than in the calcium plus hormone group (0.1% per year). The patterns of change in the 3 groups were similar in the lumbar spine, trochanter and Ward's triangle.

Implications.—In early postmenopausal women, calcium supplementation improves overall calcium balance substantially and limits the decline in bone density of the femoral neck.

▶ This study provides further evidence, if anyone still has any doubt, that increasing calcium intake minimizes bone loss in postmenopausal women. Bone loss was slowed at all sites, albeit to varying degrees at different sites, but did not increase as it did in the women treated with calcium plus estrogen. The patterns of changes in bone density at other sites during the 3-year study were similar to those in total body calcium content (Fig 56–4), but there was more fluctuation, so the lines were not as straight. The daily dose of calcium was rather large, 1,500 mg, but only 1 woman dropped out of the study because of side effects of calcium; a daily supplement of 1,000 mg proved effective in another study (1).

All the women in this study received 400 IU of vitamin D daily. How much it contributed to the benefit of calcium or calcium and estrogen is unknown. It probably had little effect in the control group; at least the rate of bone loss in this group was similar to that in other studies of women who received no supplements of anything. Nevertheless, because vitamin D intake among older women is so often marginal, vitamin D supplementation should be routine. Indeed, to my knowledge, in prospective treatment studies, only the combination of calcium and vitamin D has been proved to reduce fracture rate (2), although in epidemiologic and case-control studies of women with hip fracture, calcium supplements were protective (3, 4). I agree with the view expressed by Heaney (5) that postmenopausal women should receive supplements of at least 1,000 mg of calcium and 400 IU of vitamin D each day.—R.D. Utiger, M.D.

References

1. 1994 YEAR BOOK OF MEDICINE, pp 604–606.
2. YEAR BOOK OF MEDICINE, pp 607–609.
3. Holbrook TL, Barrett-Connor E, Wingard D: Dietary calcium and risk of hip fracture: 14-year prospective population study. *Lancet* 2:1046–1049, 1988.
4. YEAR BOOK OF MEDICINE, pp 602–604.
5. Heaney RP: Thinking straight about calcium. N *Engl J Med* 328:503–505, 1993.

The Effect of Postmenopausal Estrogen Therapy on Bone Density in Elderly Women

Felson DT, Zhang Y, Hannan MT, Kiel DP, Wilson PWF, Anderson JJ (Boston Univ; Hebrew Rehabilitation Ctr for Aged, Boston; Framingham Study, Mass)
N *Engl J Med* 329:1141–1146, 1993   119-95-56-5

Introduction.—Little is known about the effects of estrogen, given early in the postmenopausal period, on bone density much later in life. It would be helpful to know the minimal duration of treatment that is needed to ensure a lasting effect on bone density.

Study Plan.—The effects of postmenopausal estrogen treatment on bone density were reviewed in elderly women participating in the Framingham Osteoporosis Study. Bone mineral density was measured in the lumbar spine, femur, and 2 radial sites during the 20th biennial examina-

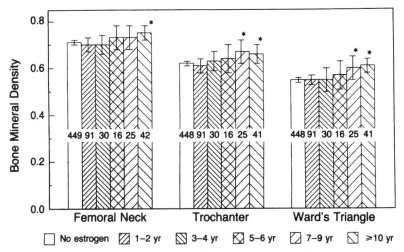

Fig 56–5.—Bone mineral density at the proximal femur, according to the duration of estrogen therapy in postmenopausal women in the Framingham Study. The results, shown in gm/cm², have been adjusted for age, age at menopause, weight, height, and cigarette smoking. The number of women in each group is shown within each bar. These numbers do not total 670 because bone assessments were not obtained at all sites in some women. The *asterisks* indicate P < 0.5 for the comparison with women not treated with estrogen. The *I bars* show the 95% confidence interval. (Courtesy Felson DT, Zhang Y, Hannan MT, et al: N *Engl J Med* 329:1141–1146, 1993.)

tion in 1988 or 1989. Of 670 white women, whose mean age was 76 years, 212 had received estrogen therapy in the past.

Results.—The bone density of both the radial shaft and the ultradistal radius was higher in the women who received more prolonged estrogen therapy. Women who had taken estrogen for 7 years or longer generally had higher femoral bone density than those who had not taken estrogen (Fig 56–5). Similar results were noted in the spine. A marginal effect on bone density appeared after 5–6 years of estrogen treatment. A large majority of women aged 75 and older had discontinued using estrogen many years before the study. In women younger than 75 years of age, bone mineral density correlated positively with the duration of estrogen therapy, but even prolonged earlier treatment had a comparatively small effect on bone density in older women.

Implications.—Estrogen therapy for at least 7 years is required to ensure that increased bone density will be maintained. Even prolonged treatment may fail to protect women aged 75 years and older.

▶ These women ranged in age from 68 to 96 years. They had taken estrogen for varying periods of time starting soon after menopause, but only 10% had taken it for 7 or more years, and all had ceased treatment well before bone density was measured. It is evident from Figure 56–5 that prolonged therapy is needed if an effect is to be demonstrated in later years, but if the interval from cessation to measurement is prolonged, as in the women aged 75 years and older, prolonged earlier treatment has no residual effect.

Estrogen is most effective within the first 5 years after the menopause, when it prevents the accelerated bone loss (about 2% per year) that occurs normally during this period. When given later, at a time when bone loss is normally slower (about 1% per year), it slows but does not prevent bone loss for as long as it is given. Because discontinuation of estrogen is accompanied by accelerated ("catch-up") bone loss, the benefit wanes and ultimately disappears, as reported by Felson et al.

The data with respect to a major end point—hip fracture—are similar; postmenopausal estrogen therapy reduces the risk of fracture among younger women, but not among those over 75 (1), and current therapy is much more protective than past therapy (2, 3). Because most of these fractures occur in the latter group, we are going to have to give estrogen for a lot longer if it is to have a large impact on this problem.—R.D. Utiger, M.D.

References

1. Ettinger B, Grady D: The waning effect of postmenopausal estrogen therapy on osteoporosis. *N Engl J Med* 329:1192–1193, 1993.
2. Kiel DP, Felson DT, Anderson JJ, Wilson PWF, Moskowitz MA: Hip fracture and the use of estrogens in postmenopausal women: The Framingham Study. *N Engl J Med* 317:1169–1174, 1987.
3. Cauley JP, Seeley DG, Ensrud K, et al: Estrogen replacement therapy and fractures in older women. *Ann Intern Med* 122:9–16, 1995.

Four-Year Study of Intermittent Cyclic Etidronate Treatment of Post-menopausal Osteoporosis: Three Years of Blinded Therapy Followed By One Year of Open Therapy

Harris ST, Watts NB, Jackson RD, Genant HK, Wasnich RD, Ross P, Miller PD, Licata AA, Chestnut III CH (Univ of California, San Francisco; Emory Univ, Atlanta, Ga; Ohio State Univ, Columbus; et al)
Am J Med 95:557–567, 1993   119-95-56-6

Background.—Currently, the only 2 drugs approved in the United States for the treatment of osteoporosis are estrogen and synthetic salmon calcitonin. The effect of long-term intermittent cyclic etidronate on spinal bone density and vertebral fracture rates was investigated.

Methods.—Four hundred twenty-three white and Asian women with postmenopausal osteoporosis were enrolled in the 2-year, double-blind, randomized, multicenter trial. Three hundred fifty-seven women continued treatment for a third year and 277 for a fourth year. In the first 3 years, the women were given double-blind treatment with phosphate, 1 g, or placebo twice a day for 3 days; etidronate, 400 mg, or placebo daily for 14 days; and calcium, 500 mg/day for the rest of each 91-day treatment cycle. In the fourth year, all the women received open-label intermittent cyclic etidronate without preceding phosphate.

Findings.—The significant increases in spinal bone mineral density that had occurred during the first 2 years of etidronate therapy were maintained during the third year (Fig 56-6). Proximal femur bone density also increased in women given etidronate during the 3-year period. Three years of etidronate significantly reduced the vertebral fracture rate in women at greater risk for fracture (low spinal bone density and vertebral fractures at study entry) as compared with no etidronate therapy. During year 4 of open-label therapy, women previously given etidronate

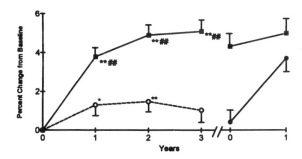

Fig 56–6.—Mean changes (± SEM) in spinal bone mineral density in non–etidronate-treated patients (*open circles*) and etidronate-treated patients (*filled squares*) during 3 years of blinded treatment and a subsequent year of open-label intermittent cyclic etiodronate treatment (4 years of etidronate, *filled squares*; 1 year of etidronate, *filled circles*). The *asterisks* indicate a significant change from baseline (*P < .05, **P < .01); the *pound signs* indicate a significant difference from the nonetidronate group (## P < .01). No statistical comparisons of Year 4 data were performed. (Courtesy of Harris ST, Watts NB, Jackson RD, et al: *Am J Med* 95:557–567, 1993.)

maintained bone mass, and the vertebral fracture rates in all groups were lower than during any other study period. There were no serious side effects.

Conclusions.—Three years of intermittent cyclic etidronate treatment significantly increased spinal and hip bone density, with a significant decrease in vertebral fracture rates in women at higher risk of fracture. When etidronate was continued for another year, bone mass and the low fracture rate were maintained.

▶ The reports of beneficial effects of intermittent disphosphonate (etidronate) therapy in women with postmenopausal osteoporosis in 1990 were viewed by many as opening a new chapter in the treatment of this disorder, particularly because etidronate not only increased bone density in the spine and femur, but also reduced the rate of vertebral fractures (1, 2). In years 3 and 4 of one of these studies (1) described in this new report, the increase in bone density in the etidronate-treated women was maintained, although bone density did not increase further (nor was there resumption of bone loss). Some continued benefit was seen with respect to the decreased rate of vertebral fracture, but only in those women at higher risk for fractures (the same group that benefited most during the first 2 years of the study). Figure 56–6 also shows clearly that the women who received etidronate during year 4, after receiving placebo for 3 years, had about the same 1-year increase in vertebral bone density as occurred in the women who received etidronate initially.

The major action of etidronate (and other diphosphonates) is to inhibit bone resorption. It is given intermittently because constant administration may inhibit bone formation. Because it accumulates in the skeleton, intermittent administration may be as effective in inhibiting bone resorption as constant administration. There has as yet been no evidence of impaired bone formation or osteomalacia—an effect of high-dose chronic etidronate therapy—in women receiving intermittent lower-dose therapy.

Some of the women in this study received phosphate, which had no effect, and thus need not be included in an etidronate regimen. All received supplemental calcium, which may explain why the women who did not receive etidronate during the randomized part of the trial (years 0–3) had a slight increase in bone density. All these women were in their mid-60s, an age when bone turnover is slower than in the immediate postmenopausal years. We still don't know whether etidronate would be effective soon after the menopause, when the rate of bone turnover is higher, but another diphosphonate compound, tiludronate, is effective at that time (3).

What is the role of intermittent etidonate therapy in women with postmenopausal osteoporosis (and assuming that it and other regimens are equally effective whatever the age of the woman)? Its beneficial effects on bone are roughly similar to those of estrogen, calcium and vitamin D, and calcitonin, but, as yet, it has not been compared directly with another regimen. It has none of the extraskeletal benefits of estrogen, is less physiologic than calcium and vitamin D, and is cheaper and more convenient than calcitonin (whether the latter is given intranasally or parenterally). I think that its major value is in women who cannot tolerate estrogen or large doses of calcium, with supplemental vitamin D. Etidronate also probably increases bone density in postmenopausal women who do not have osteoporosis, but estrogen or calcium and vitamin D are preferable for this purpose as well.—R.D. Utiger, M.D.

References

1. Watts NB, Harris ST, Genant HK, et al: Intermittent cyclic etidronate treatment of postmenopausal osteoporosis. *N Engl J Med* 323:73–79, 1990 (Abstract 43-4, 1991 YEAR BOOK OF MEDICINE).
2. Storm T, Thamsborg G, Steiniche T, Genant HK, Sorensen OH: Effect of intermittent cyclical etidronate therapy on bone mass and fracture rate in women with postmenopausal osteoporosis. *N Engl J Med* 322:1265–1271, 1990.
3. Reginster JY, Lecart MP, Deroisy R, et al: Prevention of postmenopausal bone loss by tiludronate. *Lancet* 2:1469–1471, 1989.

Risk Factors for Hip Fracture in Black Women
Grisso JA, Kelsey JL, Strom BL, O'Brien LA, Maislin G, LaPann K, Samelson L, Hoffman S, Northeast Hip Fracture Study Group (Univ of Pennsylvania, Philadelphia; Stanford Univ, Calif; Columbia Univ, New York)
N Engl J Med 330:1555–1559, 1994   119-95-56–7

Background.—More than 1% of black women 80 years or older sustain hip fractures each year, and postfracture mortality and disability are higher among black women than among white women. Nevertheless, little is known about risk factors for hip fracture in black women. Risk factors for hip fracture in black women were identified in a case-control study.

Methods.—One hundred forty-four black women hospitalized for first hip fracture, 218 age- and hospital-matched black women living in the community and 181 black women matched for age and hospital were interviewed. Information was gathered regarding alcohol consumption, smoking, medications, body mass index, prefracture lower limb function, visual impairment, and co-existing neurologic disease.

Results.—Multivariate analysis revealed low body mass index, no estrogen therapy, use of ambulatory aids, high alcohol consumption, and history of stroke as independent predictors of hip fracture in the case women as compared with the community control women (table) and also the hospital control women.

Conclusion.—Thinness, previous stroke, use of ambulatory aids, and alcohol consumption are important risk factors for hip fracture in black women.

▶ The incidence of hip fracture among postmenopausal black women is about half that of white women. The risk factors for hip fracture in this group

Multivariable Analysis of Risk Factors for Hip Fractures in Black Women

VARIABLE	ADJUSTED ODDS RATIO (95% CONFIDENCE INTERVAL)*
Body-mass index†	
≤22.6	13.5 (4.2–43.3)
22.7–24.4	4.2 (1.3–14.0)
24.5–27.2	3.5 (1.2–10.3)
27.3–31.5	1.5 (0.4–5.3)
≥31.6	1.0
Estrogen therapy lasting ≥1 yr‡	
Women <75 yr old	0.1 (<0.1–0.5)
Women ≥75 yr old	1.1 (0.2–6.3)
Alcohol consumed, past yr — drinks/wk§	
≤1	1.0
2–6	2.0 (0.8–5.0)
≥7	4.6 (1.5–14.1)
History of stroke (vs. none)	3.1 (1.2–8.1)
Use of ambulatory aids (vs. none) ‖	5.6 (2.7–11.5)
Chronic illnesses — no ¶	
0	1.0
1	1.8 (0.9–3.7)
2–6	0.9 (0.3–2.4)

* Ratios were based on conditional logistic-regression models, with control for age category, ZIP code or telephone exchange, age as a continuous variable, and all other variables shown in the table. Odds ratios (ORs) of 1 were assigned to reference groups.

† Expressed in quintiles based on the distribution in community controls.

‡ Estrogen effect varied with age ($P = .03$). Age-specific ORs and 95% confidence intervals were calculated with age used as dichotomous variable.

§ Based on assumption that 1 bottle of bear, 1 glass of wine, and 1 drink of spirits each contain 28 g (1 oz) of alcohol.

‖ Includes women who used a cane, walker, wheelchair, artificial leg, or who were confined to bed.

¶ Expressed as a categorical variable and includes following 6 conditions: diabetes mellitus, coronary heart disease, epilepsy, kidney disease, Parkinson's disease, and cancer.

(Courtesy of Grisso JA, Kelsey JL, Strom BL, and the Northeast Hip Fracture Study Group: N Engl J Med 330: 1555-1559, 1994.)

of black women are those that would be expected to be associated with either low bone density or falls: no estrogen therapy, low body weight, history of stroke, need for ambulatory aids, and heavy alcohol consumption. Several of these factors, not surprisingly, were identified as risk factors for falls leading to hip fracture in white women by the same investigators several years ago (1).

Bone density was not measured in either of the studies by these authors, but there is little doubt that low bone density is a predictor of hip fracture, particularly low femoral bone density (2). Although peak bone density at all sites is higher among black than white women (3), rates of loss after the menopause are similar, as are the factors associated with rapid loss. Therefore, bone density in black women may be expected to reach the threshold (2 SD below the mean for age) where fracture risk rises sharply later than white women, but reach it they will, unless preventive measures are taken.

This study reminds us—it should not be necessary—that preventing falls and the conditions that lead to falls are of paramount importance in preventing hip fracture (4). We can do many simple things—for example, improve vision, ensure the availability and proper use of ambulatory aids, minimize use of drugs that may impair coordination, provide protective padding for those at risk for falls—to minimize the chance of a fall or the likelihood of a fracture if a patient does fall. Estrogen, calcium, vitamin D, etc., are fine, but attention to these details is surely as important.—R.D. Utiger, M.D.

References

1. Grisso JA, Kelsey JL, Strom BL, et al: Risk factors for falls as a cause of hip fracture in women. *N Engl J Med* 324: 1326–1331, 1991.
2. Cummings SR, Black DM, Nevitt MC, et al: Bone density at various sites for prediction of hip fractures. *Lancet* 341:72–75, 1993.
3. Liel Y, Edwards J, Shary J, Spicer KM, Gordon L, Bell NH: The effects of race and body habitus on bone mineral density of the radius, hip and spine in premenopausal women. *J Clin Endocrinol Metab* 66:1247–1250, 1988.
4. Greenspan SL, Myers ER, Maitland LA, Resnick NA, Hayes WC: Fall severity and bone mineral density as risk factors for hip fracture in ambulatory elderly. *JAMA* 271:128–133, 1994.

Parathyroid Hormone-Related Protein and Life Expectancy in Hypercalcemic Cancer Patients
Pecherstorfer M, Schilling T, Blind E, Zimmer-Roth I, Baumgartner G, Ziegler R, Raue F (Lainz Hosp, Vienna; Univ of Heidelberg, Germany)
J Clin Endocrinol Metab 78:1268–1270, 1994   119-95-56-8

Background.—Hypercalcemia is a common metabolic disorder in patients with cancer. It is most often caused by tumoral secretion of parathyroid hormone–related protein (PTHrP), which stimulates both bone resorption and renal calcium reabsorption. Both actions lead to elevated serum calcium concentrations. The effects of increased serum concentrations of PTHrP on life expectancy in cancer patients with a first presentation of hypercalcemia were investigated.

Methods.—Fifty-nine patients with histologically proven cancer and first occurrence of hypercalcemia were studied. The patients were stratified according to their serum PTHrP concentrations after fluid repletion. Twenty-nine patients with serum PTHrP concentrations equal to or less than 21 pmol/L composed group N (normal), and 30 patients with serum PTHrP concentrations greater than 21 pmol/L composed group E (elevated).

Results.—The proportion of patients with breast cancer was higher in group N, whereas squamous cell cancers predominated in group E. In addition, more patients with low serum PTHrP concentrations had evidence of bone metastases, whereas patients with raised serum PTHrP concentrations tended to have a higher incidence of visceral metastases.

There were no significant differences in serum PTHrP concentrations with regard to age, sex, extent of tumor involvement, and World Health Organization performance status. The duration of the hypercalcemia-free interval after diagnosis of cancer was 250 days in group N and 86 days in group E. Six patients with normal serum PTHrP concentrations achieved remission with chemotherapy, whereas no patient in group E had an objective response. Calculated from day 0, the median survival of the entire study group was 47 days. Patients in group N had a median life expectancy of 66 days, as compared with 33 days in group E. After bisphosphonate therapy on day 0, 96% of the patients with normal serum PTHrP concentrations became normocalcemic within 1 week, as compared with only 70% of the group with elevated serum PTHrP concentrations.

Conclusion.—In cancer-related hypercalcemia, increased serum concentrations of PTHrP indicate a reduced hypocalcemic response to bisphosphonate therapy, a more advanced tumor state, and, subsequently, an extremely poor prognosis.

▶ Life expectancy is poor among cancer patients who have hypercalcemia; the median survival in this group of patients after the onset of hypercalcemia was 47 days. The longer survival in the patients who had normal serum PTHrP concentrations is probably related more to tumor type than hypercalcemia, serum PTHrP production, or efficacy of antihypercalcemic therapy. Specifically, in this group, the most common tumor was breast cancer (10 patients), whereas the most common tumor in the high serum PTHrP group was squamous cell cancer of the lung (17 patients). But there were patients in each group with each of these tumors, as well as renal tumors, adenocarcinomas, and multiple myeloma. So PTHrP is produced by virtually all types of tumors. Although just more than half the patients had elevated serum PTHrP concentrations, the proportion in most series is about 80% (1).

Whatever the frequency of elevated values, I don't think the distinction between elevated and normal serum PTHrP concentrations in hypercalcemic patients is clinically important, because we have no specific ways to prevent its secretion or action, and therapy of hypercalcemia is empirical. Besides, many cancers contain PTHrP and undoubtedly secrete it locally, so that if there are bony metastases, the patient may have hypercalcemia due to local action of PTHrP yet normal serum PTHrP concentrations (2, 3).

Serum PTHrP concentrations need not be measured in a patient with hypercalcemia who is known to have metastatic cancer. It is important to remember, however, that hypercalcemia may be the first manifestation of a cancer, so that serum PTHrP should be measured in a hypercalcemic patient who has a low serum parathyroid hormone concentration and no obvious evidence of other nontumor causes of hypercalcemia.—R.D. Utiger, M.D.

References

1. Walls J, Ratcliffe WA, Howell A, Bundred NJ: Parathyroid hormone and para-

thyroid hormone-related protein in the investigation of hypercalcemia in two hospital populations. *Clin Endocrinol* 41:407–413, 1994.

2. 1993 YEAR BOOK OF MEDICINE, pp 548–550.
3. Dunne FP, Lee S, Ratcliffe WA, Hutchesson AC, Bundred NJ, Heath DA: Parathyroid hormone-related protein (PTHrP) gene expression in solid tumours associated with normocalcemia and hypercalcemia. *J Pathol* 171:215–221, 1993.

Treatment of Cancer-Associated Hypercalcemia: Double-Blind Comparison of Rapid and Slow Intravenous Infusion Regimens of Pamidronate Disodium and Saline Alone

Gucalp R, Theriault R, Gill I, Madajewicz S, Chapman R, Navari R, Ahmann F, Zelenakas K, Heffernan M, Knight RD (Univ of Texas, Houston; Univ of Southern California, Los Angeles; State Univ of New York, Stony Brook; et al)
Arch Intern Med 154:1935–1944, 1994   119-95-56–9

Background.—Among patients with cancer who have symptomatic hypercalcemia, the standard initial treatment is hydration with 0.9% sodium chloride hydration to restore intravascular volume and enhance renal calcium excretion. Pamidronate disodium, the most potent bisphosphonate agent clinically available, shows promise as an effective and lasting treatment of cancer-associated hypercalcemia. The therapeutic efficacy of IV pamidronate was evaluated in a prospective, double-blind study.

Patients and Methods.—Sixty-nine patients were enrolled from 12 centers. All had a malignant tumor and a corrected serum calcium concentration of 12 mg/dL (3 mmol/L) or higher after adequate hydration. The patients were randomly assigned to receive a single infusion of pamidronate (60 mg) for either 4 or 24 hours or continued infusion of 0.9% saline alone. Corrected serum calcium concentrations were measured daily for 7 days.

Results.—All patients, 23 per treatment group, were included in the analysis, although 27 were dropped from the study because of death, unsatisfactory response, or unacceptable concomitant medication. There were complete responses to treatment, defined as normalization of corrected serum calcium concentration, in 78% of patients who received a 4-hour infusion of pamidronate, 61% of those who received a 24-hour infusion of the drug, and 22% of those who received saline alone (Fig 56–7). The median duration of complete response in the 3 groups was 6, 11, and 6 days, respectively. Differences between the 2 pamidronate infusions were not significant, and the drug was well tolerated in both groups.

Conclusion.—Patients with cancer-associated hypercalcemia who remained hypercalcemic despite adequate hydration responded to both 4- and 24-hour infusions of pamidronate. A single IV infusion of the drug was significantly more efficacious than infusion of saline alone. The 4-

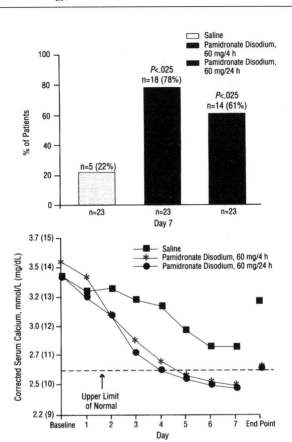

Fig 56–7.—Mean corrected serum calcium concentrations and percentages of patients with a complete, response (normal serum calcium concentration) after infusion. *P* values are for the difference between either pamidronate disodium infusion and saline (Fisher's Exact Test, overall α level adjusted for multiple comparisons). (Courtesy of Gucalp R, Theriault R, Gill I, et al: *Arch Intern Med* 154:1935–1944, 1994.)

hour infusion of pamidronate is recommended because of its convenience and duration of response.

▶ Pamidronate is the treatment of choice for patients with hypercalcemia in whom the serum concentration remains above 11.5–12 mg/dL (2.5–3 mmol/L) after IV administration of several liters of isotonic saline and furosemide for 24–48 hours. It probably should be given immediately to severely symptomatic patients with serum calcium concentrations above 14 mg/dL (3.5 mmol/L). The efficacy of the 4-hour infusion, as demonstrated both in this and another study (1), makes it the preferable regimen. Besides, the goal of treatment is not normocalcemia, but simply reduction in the serum calcium to a concentration that causes few symptoms, because most, if not all, patients who require treatment for severe hypercalcemia have metastatic cancer. In a study in which 24-hour infusions of 30, 60, or 90 mg of pami·

dronate were given to hypercalcemic cancer patients, the proportions who became normocalcemic were 40%, 61%, and 100%, respectively (2). Most patients relapse (serum calcium greater than 11.5 mg/dL [2.9 mmol/L]) after a week or two, and treatment can be repeated as often as needed.

Pamidronate, like other diphosphonates, inhibits bone resorption. It has few side effects—fever, infusion-site reactions, transient increases in serum creatinine, hypocalcemia, hypomagnesemia, and hypophosphatemia (the latter not so much side effects as indicators of the drug's antiresorptive potency). It is far more effective than etidronate as a treatment for hypercalcemia, and use of etidronate for this purpose should be abandoned. So too should calcitonin, because of its lack of potency and short duration of action. Plicamycin (mithramycin) should be reserved for patients who do not respond to pamidronate. Another potent antiresorptive drug—gallium nitrate—is available but has to be given daily for 5 days and is more nephrotoxic than pamidronate (3).—R.D. Utiger, M.D.

References

1. Sawyer N, Newstead C, Drummond A, Cunningham J: Fast (4-h) or slow (24-h) infusions of pamidronate disodium (aminohydroxypropylidene diphosphonate [APD]) as single shot treatment of hypercalcemia. *Bone Miner* 9:121–128, 1990.
2. Nussbaum S, Younger J, Vandepol CJ, et al: Single-dose intravenous therapy with pamidronate for the treatment of hypercalcemia of malignancy: Comparison of 30-, 60-, and 90-mg dosages. *Am J Med* 95:297–304, 1993.
3. Warrell Jr RP, Israel R, Frisone M, Snyder T, Gaynor JJ, Bockman RS: Gallium nitrate for acute treatment of cancer-related hypercalcemia: A randomized, double-blind comparison to calcitonin. *Ann Intern Med* 108:669–674, 1988.

57 Carbohydrate Metabolism and Diabetes Mellitus

Insulin Resistance and Insulin Secretion Are Determinants of Oral Glucose Tolerance in Normal Individuals
Reaven GM, Brand RJ, Chen Y-DI, Mathur AK, Goldfine I (Stanford Univ, Palo Alto, Calif; Dept of Veterans Affairs Med Ctr, Palo Alto, Calif; Mount Zion Hosp and Med Ctr, San Francisco; et al)
Diabetes 42:1324–1332, 1993   119-95-57–1

Introduction.—Insulin secretion and action are both defective in patients with non–insulin-dependent diabetes mellitus. However, although plasma insulin concentrations vary widely in nondiabetic patients after oral glucose administration, there has been little study of insulin resistance in normal subjects. The relative importance of insulin secretion and insulin action as determinants of glucose metabolism was studied in nonobese, nondiabetic subjects.

Methods.—Plasma glucose and insulin concentrations were measured in the 74 subjects (27 men and 47 women, mean age, 44 years) before and 30, 60, 120, and 180 minutes after oral administration of 75 g of glucose. As a measure of insulin resistance, the steady-state plasma glucose concentration was determined by measuring plasma glucose and insulin during continuous infusion of insulin, somatostatin, and glucose for 3 hours. The relationships between the glucose response and 6 predictive variables—age, sex, obesity, insulin resistance, insulin secretion, and fasting plasma glucose concentration—were examined by multiple regression analysis.

Results.—Both plasma glucose and insulin concentrations varied widely after oral glucose administration, as did plasma glucose concentrations during the steady-state plasma glucose test. The increase in plasma insulin after oral glucose was a negative predictor and the steady-state plasma glucose concentration was a positive predictor of the plasma glucose response to oral glucose.

Discussion.—The increase in plasma glucose concentrations after oral glucose administration in normal individuals indicates variations in both insulin secretion and action.

▶ Plasma glucose concentrations vary a lot in subjects considered to have normal glucose tolerance. In these subjects, who ranged in age from 19 to 71 years and were within 20% of ideal body weight, the fasting plasma glucose concentrations ranged from 67 to 112 mg/dL (3.7 to 6.2 mmol/L) and the 2-hour postprandial plasma glucose concentrations ranged from 43 to 133 mg/dL (2.4 to 7.4 mmol/L). The variations in both the plasma insulin responses after oral glucose administration and the steady-state plasma glucose concentration were likewise large. The latter—a measure of insulin sensitivity—is simply the mean of 4 plasma glucose measurements near the end of a 3-hour infusion of insulin, glucose, and somatostatin (to inhibit endogenous insulin and glucagon secretion). For example, the plasma insulin concentrations 2 hours after oral glucose administration ranged from 7 to 213 uU/mL (43 to 1,277 pmol/L), and the steady-state plasma glucose concentrations ranged from 41 to 300 mg/dL (2.3 to 16.7 mmol/L). In some of these subjects, insulin sensitivity was no better than that in patients with non–insulin-dependent diabetes mellitus, confirming the results of an earlier study (1). The normal subjects with poor insulin sensitivity are not diabetic because their insulin secretion is robust. These results nicely demonstrate that variations in both insulin secretion and insulin sensitivity are important determinants of glucose homeostatis in normal subjects. They also indicate why a small decrease in insulin sensitivity—caused for example by a small increase in weight or a little glucocorticoid excess—can sometimes precipitate diabetes.—R.D. Utiger, M.D.

Reference

1. Hollenbeck CB, Reaven GM: Variations in insulin-stimulated glucose uptake in healthy individuals with normal glucose tolerance. *J Clin Endocrinol Metab* 64:1169–1173, 1987.

Weight Loss in Severely Obese Subjects Prevents the Progression of Impaired Glucose Tolerance to Type II Diabetes: A Longitudinal Interventional Study
Long SD, O'Brien K, MacDonald Jr KG, Leggett-Frazier N, Swanson MS, Pories WJ, Caro JF (East Carolina Univ, Greenville, NC; Thomas Jefferson Univ, Philadelphia)
Diabetes Care 17:372–375, 1994   119-95-57–2

Introduction.—Impaired glucose tolerance (fasting plasma glucose concentration less than 140 mg/dL and plasma glucose concentrations of 140–200 mg/dL [7.8–11.1 mmol/L] 2 hours after 75-g oral glucose) is estimated to be present in 11% of the United States population between

20 and 74 years of age, and may be as high as 23% in the oldest age group. Patients with impaired glucose tolerance are at increased risk of macrovascular disease and non–insulin-dependent diabetes (NIDDM). The prevalence of NIDDM and impaired glucose tolerance is increased in the presence of obesity. Weight loss can improve glucose tolerance, but whether weight loss can prevent the progression of impaired glucose tolerance to NIDDM is unknown.

Procedures.—A total of 136 patients with severe obesity (45 kg or more above ideal weight) and impaired glucose tolerance who underwent gastric bypass surgery and 27 similarly obese patients with impaired glucose tolerance who chose not to have surgery were followed for a minimum of 2 years (mean, 5.8 years). Progression of diabetes in both groups was based on World Health Organization criteria of 2 fasting plasma glucose values greater than 140 mg/dL (7.8 mmol/L) or 1 random value greater than 200 mg/dL (11.1 mmol/L) plus classic symptoms of diabetes.

Results.—Of the surgical patients (about 50% weight loss), only 1 had NIDDM develop during the third year of follow-up, for an incidence rate of 0.15 cases per 100 person-years. In contrast, 6 of the 27 patients in the control group (no sustained weight loss) progressed to NIDDM in 1 to 6 years, for an incidence rate of 4.7 cases per 100 person-years.

Conclusion.—Weight loss from gastric bypass surgery resulted in a greater than 30-fold reduction in the risk of NIDDM developing in patients with impaired glucose tolerance.

▶ Among obese persons in general and obese persons with impaired glucose tolerance in particular, the risk of NIDDM is high, and the risk is proportional to the degree of obesity. Comparing obese subjects with normal-weight persons, insulin secretion is increased in those with normal glucose tolerance and increased even more in those with impaired glucose tolerance. However, NIDDM is associated with declining insulin secretion, and ultimately may be lower than in normal subjects, despite severe hyperglycemia. The deterioration of insulin secretion is variously attributed to hyperglycemia-induced injury of the β-cells (glucose toxicity) and environmental and genetic factors affecting β-cell function (1).

Halting the progression to NIDDM requires that insulin sensitivity be improved, so that the demand for insulin secretion is reduced. This can be done by weight reduction, no matter how achieved, and increased physical activity. Even among obese persons, the risk is lower in those who are more physically active (2). Finally, drugs that improve insulin sensitivity are on the horizon (3).—R.D. Utiger, M.D.

References

1. Yki-Jarvinen H: Pathogenesis of non-insulin-dependent diabetes mellitus. *Lancet* 434:91–95, 1994.
2. Helmrich SH, Ragland DP, Leung RW, Paffenbarger Jr RS: Physical activity and

reduced occurrence of non-insulin-dependent diabetes mellitus. *N Engl J Med* 325:147-152, 1991.

3. Nolan JJ, Ludvik B, Beerdsen P, Joyce M, Olefsky J: Improvement in glucose tolerance and insulin resistance in obese subjects treated with troglitazone. *N Engl J Med* 331:1188-1193, 1994.

Comparison of Tests for Glycated Haemoglobin and Fasting and Two Hour Plasma Glucose Concentrations as Diagnostic Methods for Diabetes

McCance DR, Hanson RL, Charles M-A, Jacobsson LTH, Pettitt DJ, Bennett PH, Knowler WC (Natl Inst of Diabetes and Digestive and Kidneys Diseases, Phoenix, Ariz; Natl Inst of Arthritis and Musculoskeletal and Skin Diseases, Phoenix, Ariz)
BMJ 308:1323-1328, 1994   119-95-57-3

Introduction.—Current diagnostic criteria for diabetes mellitus are based on hyperglycemia, either fasting or as assessed by an oral glucose tolerance test. The inconvenience of this test, however, suggests that an alternative screening method would be desirable. A group of subjects known to have a high frequency of diabetes was screened using measurements of plasma glucose and glycated hemoglobin.

Methods.—About half of Pima Indians older than age 35 years who live in the Gila River Indian Community in Arizona have diabetes. All community residents participate in a standardized medical examination every 2 years starting in childhood. The participants in this study were 960 Pima Indians aged 25 years or older who were not receiving insulin or oral hypoglycemic treatment. Each examination included measurements of glycated hemoglobin and plasma glucose concentrations before and 2 hours after oral administration of 75 grams of glucose. A physician unaware of the results of these tests examined the participants for retinopathy and nephropathy.

Results.—The frequency distribution of each test variable in the cross-sectional study was bimodal. The cutoff points that minimized overlap were 227 mg/dL (12.6 mmol/L) for 2-hour plasma glucose, 167 mg/dL (9.3 mmol/L) for fasting plasma glucose, and 7.8% for glycated hemoglobin. Longitudinally, each of these 3 measures of glycemia significantly predicted the development of retinopathy (Fig 57-1) and nephropathy. The 2-hour plasma glucose concentration was more accurate than the fasting plasma glucose concentration for identifying prevalent cases of retinopathy. Otherwise, no measured variable had a significant advantage for detecting incident or prevalent cases of retinopathy or nephropathy.

Conclusion.—For each of these tests, membership in the upper component of the distribution could be equated with having diabetes. For diagnostic purposes, measurement of glycated hemoglobin or fasting plasma glucose is more convenient and as useful as measurement of 2-hour plasma glucose.

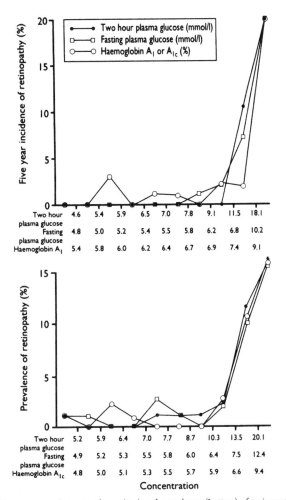

Fig 57–1.—Five-year cumulative incidence (**top**) and prevalence (**bottom**) of retinopathy in relation to tenths of 2-hour plasma glucose, fasting plasma glucose, and glycated haemoglobin A_1 and A_{1c} concentrations. (Courtesy of McCance DR, Hanson RL, Charles M-A, et al: *BMJ* 308:1323–1328, 1994.)

▶ The cross-sectional part of this study confirms that fasting and postprandial hyperglycemia and increased glycated hemoglobin values each can be considered as a discrete abnormality (that is not to say that they are unrelated), rather than being the high end of a continuous variation. There is no reason to doubt that these observations apply to other populations as well, but the proportion with abnormalities would be smaller because of the extraordinarily high frequency of abnormal glucose metabolism among Pima Indians.

The longitudinal part of the study included slightly fewer subjects, because those with retinopathy or nephropathy (proteinuria greater than 1 g/day) initially were excluded. None were being treated for hyperglycemia at baseline, but they could have received therapy thereafter. Overall, 3.6% of the subjects had retinopathy develop and 2.7% had nephropathy develop during the 1.4–8.3-year follow-up. As I hope is evident from Figure 57–1, the cutoff points separating normal and abnormal glucose metabolism from the cross-sectional study strongly predict the risk of retinopathy. The figure for nephropathy is similar, but the lines do not rise quite so steeply at the high values for plasma glucose or glycated hemoglobin. I should point out that, as compared with the glucose cutoff values from this study, the generally accepted criteria (World Health Organization and National Diabetes Data Group) for diabetes are a fasting plasma glucose concentration of 140 mg/dL (7.8 mmol/L) or more or a plasma glucose concentration 2 hours after an oral 75-g glucose load of 200 mg/dL (11.1 mmol/L).

Of the 3 tests, surely measurement of fasting plasma glucose is the simplest and least expensive. The question is, Who among the general population should be tested? Other than pregnant women, this is a contentious issue. As in other debates about screening, this one revolves primarily around benefits and risks (in this instance money). I don't much favor screening, at least in the community (for an example of its low yield, see reference 1), but refer the reader to the 2 recently published commentaries on the topic by people far more knowledgeable than I (2, 3).—R.D. Utiger, M.D.

References

1. Newman WP, Nelson R, Scheer K: Community screening for diabetes. Low detection rate in a low-risk population. *Diabetes Care* 17:363–365, 1994.
2. Harris MI, Modan M: Screening for diabetes: Why is there no national screening program? *Diabetes Care* 17:440–444, 1994.
3. Knowler WC: Screening for diabetes: Opportunities for detection, treatment, and prevention. *Diabetes Care* 17:445–450, 1994.

Caloric Restriction Per Se Is a Significant Factor in Improvements in Glycemic Control and Insulin Sensitivity During Weight Loss in Obese NIDDM Patients

Wing RR, Marcus MD, Blair EH, Watanabe R, Bononi P, Bergman RN (Univ of Pittsburgh, Pa; Univ of Southern California, Los Angeles)
Diabetes Care 17:30–36, 1994   119-95-57-4

Background.—Caloric restriction rather than actual weight loss may be responsible for improved glycemic control and insulin sensitivity in obese patients with non–insulin-dependent diabetes mellitus (NIDDM). However, the differential effects of caloric restriction vs. weight loss are difficult to evaluate because calorie restriction automatically leads to weight loss. The independent effects of caloric restriction on glycemic control, fasting serum insulin, and insulin sensitivity were examined in a randomized, prospective study.

Methods.—Changes in fasting serum glucose and insulin concentrations and insulin sensitivity as determined by an IV glucose tolerance test were compared in 53 obese patients with NIDDM who had lost 11% of body weight after eating either a 400- or 1,000-kcal diet daily. These parameters were reassessed in all patients after a 1,000-kcal/day regimen for an additional 15 weeks.

Results.—The patients in the 400-kcal group had significantly greater improvement in both glycemic control and insulin sensitivity as compared with the patients in the 1,000-kcal group. The mean fasting serum glucose concentration was 137 mg/dL (7.6 mmol/L) in the 400-kcal group and 182 mg/dL (10.1 mmol/L) in the 1,000-kcal group (P < .03). The mean insulin sensitivity value was greater in the 400-kcal group than the 1,000-kcal group (1.79 vs 1.13, P = .04). The groups did not differ in fasting serum insulin concentrations, although the values in both groups declined during weight loss. Fifteen weeks later, the fasting serum glucose concentrations increased to 153 mg/dL (8.5 mmol/L) despite continued weight loss in the patients who had increased their caloric intake from 400 to 1,000 kcal/day. In contrast, those who had maintained the 1,000-kcal diet had a further decrease in fasting serum glucose concentration to 151 mg/dL (8.4 mmol/L).

Conclusion.—The degree of caloric restriction and magnitude of weight loss independently impact fasting glucose and insulin sensitivity in patients with NIDDM.

▶ Fifty three of the 93 patients who entered this study were able to lose 11% of their body weight within the initial weeks of the program. The breakdown was 36 of 45 in the 400-calorie group and 17 of 48 in the 1,000-calorie group. There were some differences among the patients who were and were not able to lose this amount of weight in each group, but there were none among the patients who succeeded. The results of the studies after weight loss should therefore be comparable, but perhaps not generalizable. I doubt that the greater effect of the 400-calorie diet on glucose tolerance and insulin sensitivity—measured here by determination of plasma glucose and insulin concentrations after IV glucose administration (and some complicated mathematics)—was due to differences in any particular dietary component or eating behavior (1). Physiologically, the effect of the greater caloric restriction was probably to reduce hepatic glucose output by decreasing glycogen stores (2, 3).

The beneficial effect of caloric restriction is rapid. For example, among a group of 30 obese patients with NIDDM, the mean fasting plasma glucose concentrations fell progressively from 297 mg/dL (16.5 mmol/L) to 158 mg/dL (8.8 mmol/L) after 10 days of a 330-caloric diet and were a little lower (138 mg/dL [7.7 mmol/L]) after 40 days (2). Severe caloric restriction, therefore, can be useful in the short-term treatment of hyperglycemia in patients with NIDDM, even if it cannot be sustained. Those who might benefit, even as other hypoglycemic therapy is undertaken, are patients with newly diagnosed marked polyuria or polydipsia or symptomatic vaginitis, or patients with hyperglycemia induced by some medication—a thiazide or glucocorticoid—that will be discontinued. Calories count in the short term as well as the long term!—R.D. Utiger, M.D.

References

1. Beebe CA, Van Cauter E, Shapiro ET, et al: Effect of temporal distribution of calories on diurnal patterns of glucose levels and insulin secretion in NIDDM. *Diabetes Care* 13:748-755, 1990.
2. Henry RR, Schaeffer L, Olefsky JM: Glycemic effects of intensive caloric restriction and isocaloric refeeding in non-insulin-dependent diabetes mellitus. *J Clin Endocrinol Metab* 61:917-925, 1985.
2. Kelley DE, Wing R, Buonocore C, Sturis J, Polonsky K, Fitzsimmons M: Relative effects of caloric restriction and weight loss in noninsulin-dependent diabetes. *J Clin Endocrinol Metab* 77:1287-1293, 1993.

Glucocorticoids and the Risk for Initiation of Hypoglycemic Therapy

Gurwitz JH, Bohn RL, Glynn RJ, Monane M, Mogun H, Avorn J (Harvard Med School, Boston)
Arch Intern Med 154:97–101, 1994   119-95-57-5

Introduction.—Glucocorticoid excess increases hepatic glucose production; inhibits insulin-stimulated glucose use in adipocytes, thymocytes, and muscle; and increases the availability of gluconeogenic amino acids. The risk of hyperglycemia severe enough to warrant treatment among patients receiving glucocorticoid therapy has not previously been quantified. A case-control study of Medicaid patients in whom hypoglycemic therapy was newly initiated addressed that question.

Methods and Patients.—From 1981 to 1990, 11,855 patients aged 35–99 years enrolled in the New Jersey Medicaid program filled a first prescription for an oral hypoglycemic drug or insulin. For each study patient, a similar Medicaid control patient was selected who had not filled

Univariate Odds Ratios for the Initiation of Hypoglycemic Therapy According to Average Daily Glucocorticoid Dose

	No.			
Dose, mg/d*	Cases (n=11 855)	Controls (n=11 855)	Odds Ratio	95% Confidence Interval
0	11 080	11 461	1.0	. . .
1-39	589	345	1.77	1.54-2.02
40-79	111	38	3.02	2.09-4.37
80-119	45	8	5.82	2.74-12.35
120+	30	3	10.34	3.16-33.90

* Hydrocortisone equivalents.
(Courtesy of Gurwitz JH, Bohn RL, Glynn RJ, et al: *Arch Intern Med* 154:97-101, 1994.)

a prescription for hypoglycemic therapy. Medicaid and hospital records were the sources of data. The date of the first prescription for a hypoglycemic agent served as the index date.

Results.—Nonwhites were more likely than whites to begin hypoglycemic therapy. Of the hypoglycemic therapy group, 7.1% had received glucocorticoids (most often prednisone) during the 120 days preceding the index date, as compared with 3.8% of the control group (relative risk, 1.93). The risk increased with recency of glucocorticoid use. The relative risk of requiring hypoglycemic therapy in patients who received glucocorticoids within 45 days before the index date was 2.23 and it was 1.64 in those who received glucocorticoids 46–90 days before the index date. The lowest relative risk, 1.23, was associated with glucocoticoid use during the 91–120 days before the index date. With glucocorticoid treatment within 90 days before the index date, the odds ratio for initiation of hypoglycemic therapy for 39 mg of hydrocortisone or less per day or its equivalent was 1.77. For doses of 40–79 mg/day, the odds ratio was 3.02, for 80–119 mg/day it was 5.82, and for 120 mg/day or more it was 10.34 (table). The increasing glucocorticoid dose was directly related to the risk of initiation of hypoglycemic therapy whether the average daily dose was examined as a continuous term in the model or as a range of categoric variables.

Comment.—Patients treated with glucocorticoids have a substantial risk of glucose intolerance that requires treatment developing. The magnitude of the risk is related to the glucocorticoid dose.

▶ Most patients with spontaneously occurring Cushing's syndrome have impaired glucose tolerance or diabetes mellitus, and virtually all have insulin resistance. The same abnormalities occur in patients receiving exogenous glucocorticoids, but seemingly less often. The results of this study indicate that patients receiving glucocorticoids have an increase in risk of having hyperglycemia sufficient to warrant treatment with an oral hypoglycemic drug or insulin, and, as shown in the table, the risk is very strongly dose-related. Recall that 80–119 mg of hydrocortisone, for which the odds ratio of hypoglycemic therapy was 5.82, is equivalent to 20–30 mg of prednisone, a fairly commonly used dose.

Several limitations of the data should be noted. First, the indications for glucocorticoid therapy are not known, and it is possible that some patients at risk for diabetes, such as those with obesity or a family history of diabetes, were not treated with glucocorticoids. Second, hyperglycemia had to have been noted and acted on by a physician, and the patient had to have filled a new prescription for hypoglycemic therapy. Third, diabetes might have been noted but was treated with diet alone or reduction or discontinuation of glucocorticoid therapy. These factors would result in underestimation of the risk of diabetes and would have reduced the likelihood of demonstrating a relationship between glucocorticoid and hypoglycemic therapy. On the other hand, patients given a glucocorticoid may have been followed for the development of hyperglycemia more closely than other patients, thereby increasing the estimated risk of diabetes.

Notwithstanding the lack of detailed medical information about these patients, it seems clear that the risk of diabetes in patients taking large doses of glucocorticoids is substantial. Alternative drugs may not always be available, but at least the risk should be kept in mind when glucocorticoids are given.—R.D. Utiger, M.D.

Long-Term Randomized Placebo-Controlled Double-Blind Therapeutic Comparison of Glipizide and Glyburide: Glycemic Control and Insulin Secretion During 15 Months

Birkeland KI, Furuseth K, Melander A, Mowinckel P, Vaaler S (Aker Hosp, Oslo, Norway; Ullensaker Med Ctr, Jessheim, Norway; Univ of Lund, Malmö, Sweden; et al)
Diabetes Care 17:45–49, 1994   119-95-57-6

Objective.—The long-term effects of 2 second-generation sulfonylurea drugs, glipizide and glycuride, on control of blood glucose was studied in 46 patients with non–insulin-dependent diabetes mellitus (NIDDM).

Patients.—The patients, 24 women and 22 men (mean age, 59 years) were known to have had diabetes for 3.5 years on average. Their mean body mass index was 26.4 kg/m^2. All the patients had considerable residual β-cell function as indicated by an increase in serum C-peptide concentrations after glucagon injection. Their baseline hemoglobin A_{1c} (HbA$_{1c}$) values ranged from 7% to 11% (normal range, 4% to 6%).

Treatment.—Using a double-blind, placebo-controlled design, the patients received glipizide or glyburide starting with 1 morning tablet containing 2.5 and 1.75 mg, respectively. The dose was adjusted at weekly intervals to a maximum of 6 tablets per day to achieve a fasting plasma glucose concentration less than 144 mg/dL (8 mmol/L) and a HbA$_{1c}$ values less than 7.5% without hypoglycemia. The duration of the study was 15 months.

Results.—Both drugs reduced HbA$_{1c}$ initially, but in time, the values increased in both groups. The mean daily dose of glipizide at 15 months was 9.4 mg, and that of glyburide was 5.5 mg. The mean fasting plasma glucose concentration was significantly lower than at baseline after 3 and 15 months of glipizide therapy, but with glyburide only at 3 months. Fasting and postprandial serum insulin concentrations at 15 months were significantly higher than before treatment in both groups of drug-treated patients.

Conclusion.—Both glipizide and glyburide improve glycemic control to similar degrees over the long term in patients with NIDDM.

▶ Glipizide (Glucotrol) and glyburide (Dia-beta, Glynase, Micronase) are now virtually the only sulfonylurea drugs in use. They are considerably more potent and perhaps safer than the original drugs of this type (tolbutamide, chlorpropamide) (1). There is some evidence that they may not only augment insulin secretory responses to glucose, but also improve peripheral insulin responsiveness. However, the former is clearly the important action of these newer drugs, and like the older drugs, they have little activity in patients with insulin-dependent diabetes. As demonstrated in this study, the longest comparative study of the 2 drugs of which I am aware, their potency and efficacy of the 2 are quite similar, as are their side effects. Glipizide is absorbed and cleared more quickly and has usually been given in divided doses when larger doses were used. It is now available in an extended-release formulation (GlucotrolXL). Glynase is a micronized form of glyburide that is absorbed somewhat better than the standard formulation (Micronase).

In this study, no drug-treated patient had to withdraw from the study because of sustained hyperglycemia (HbA_{1c} value greater than 11%), as compared with 4 of the 16 patients in the placebo group. The rise in HbA_{1c} values that occurred in all 3 groups suggests that hyperglycemia increased because of increasing insulin resistance, especially in the drug treatment groups in which both fasting plasma insulin concentrations and insulin responses to a test meal increased during treatment. We are not told whether there were appreciable changes in weight in these normal-weight or slightly obese patients. As is so often the case, one can anticipate that most of these patients will eventually require insulin.

The final doses of glipizide or glyburide administered in this study were well below those often cited as maximal doses (glipizide, 20 to 40 mg; glyburide, 14 to 20 mg; the lower doses are for the sustained-release or micronized preparations). Smaller doses may have been adequate because the patients did not have severe diabetes (the mean fasting blood glucose concentrations in the 3 groups ranged from 162 to 182 mg/dL (9 to 10.1 mmol/L). However, there is little evidence that larger doses are better than moderate doses (2).—R.D. Utiger, M.D.

References

1. Gerich JE: Oral hypoglycemic agents. N *Engl J Med* 321:1231–1244, 1989.
2. Stenman S, Melander A, Groop P-H, Groop LC: What is the benefit of increasing the sulfonylurea dose? *Ann Intern Med* 118:169–172, 1993.

Oral Contraceptives and Renal and Retinal Complications in Young Women With Insulin-Dependent Diabetes Mellitus

Garg SK, Chase HP, Marshall G, Hoops SL, Holmes DL, Jackson WE (Univ of Colorado, Denver)
JAMA 271:1099–1102, 1994   119-95-57–7

Objective.—Diabetes mellitus is now the leading cause of new cases of renal failure and loss of vision in adults, and the use of oral contraceptives (OCs) may affect these complications. The effects of OCs on the occurrence of diabetic renal and retinal complications in young women with insulin-dependent diabetes mellitus (IDDM) were evaluated in a retrospective, case-control study.

Patients.—From among 295 young women with IDDM who were followed for a mean of 11.8 years, 43 had taken an OC containing a low dose of estrogen for 1 year or longer (mean, 3.4 years). As a control group, 43 women matched for race, age, and duration of diabetes who had not taken an OC were studied. The mean age was 23 years for the study patients and 22 years for the controls. The mean duration of diabetes was 14 years for both groups.

Results.—The mean longitudinal glycosylated hemoglobin values did not differ significantly between the study and control groups. The mean final albumin excretion rates as a measure of diabetic renal disease and the mean retinopathy scores were similar in both groups. Blood pressure and serum cholesterol concentrations were also similar in both groups. Among the women with renal or retinal damage initially, progression of these complications did not differ significantly between the 2 groups.

Summary.—Oral contraceptives are important for not only contraception but also pregnancy planning in young women with diabetes, because OC administration until excellent glycemic control is achieved lessens the risk of fetal malformations. The use of OCs in these women does not pose an additional risk for the development or progression of diabetic retinopathy or nephropathy.

▶ These are reassuring results. Oral contraceptive agents can impair glucose tolerance and insulin action slightly, depending both on the amount of estrogen and the particular progestin in them (1), and can also raise blood pressure. Higher blood glucose concentrations and higher blood pressure are both risk factors for the complications of diabetes (certainly including retinopathy). The women in the 2 groups were similar not only at the end of the study, as noted in the abstract, but they also had similar grades of retinal disease, glycosylated hemoglobin values, and rates of albumin excretion on repeated examinations during follow-up periods of up to 18 years. The duration of oral contraceptive administration ranged from 1 to 7 years, and I think the women were taking the oral contraceptive when the last studies were done; at least none (in either group) had ever been pregnant.

There is now substantial evidence that close blood glucose regulation before conception reduces the risk of fetal malformations (2, 3). Therefore, women with diabetes will benefit from contraception and a planned pregnancy more than other women. However desirable near-normalization of blood glucose all the time may be, it is not easily achieved. Knowledge of the value of normoglycemia for their offspring should motivate young women with diabetes to undertake more careful-than-usual glycemic control, and by taking an oral contraceptive, the woman can plan better both for the pregnancy.—R.D. Utiger, M.D.

References

1. Godsland IF, Walton C, Felton C, Proudler A, Patel A, Wynn V: Insulin resistance, secretion, and metabolism in users of oral contraceptives. *J Clin Endocrinol Metab* 74:64–70, 1991.
2. Rosenn B, Miodovnik M, Combs CA, et al: Pre-conception management of insulin-dependent diabetes: Improvement of pregnancy outcome. *Obstet Gynecol* 77:846–849, 1991.
3. 1992 YEAR BOOK OF MEDICINE, 518–520.

Effect of Captopril on Progression to Clinical Proteinuria in Patients With Insulin-Dependent Diabetes Mellitus and Microalbuminuria

Viberti G, for the European Microalbuminuria Captopril Study Group (United Medical and Dental Schools, London)
JAMA 271:275–279, 1994   119-95-57–8

Objective.—A randomized, double-blind, placebo-controlled, multicenter trial was performed to determine whether administration of the angiotensin-converting enzyme inhibitor captopril for 2 years delays the development of overt nephropathy in normotensive patients with insulin-dependent diabetes mellitus and persistent microalbuminuria (urinary albumin excretion 20–200 µg/min).

Study Plan.—The 92 patients, seen at 12 hospital-based diabetes centers, were aged 18–55 years at the time of the study and had had diabetes for 4–28 years. The patients received either captopril in a dose of 50 mg twice daily or a placebo.

Observations.—The patients in the captopril and placebo groups were well-matched. Four patients in the captopril group and 12 patients in the placebo group had clinical proteinuria (urinary albumin excretion rate

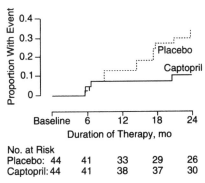

Fig 57–2.—Probability of progression to clinical proteinuria after treatment with captopril (*solid line*) or placebo (*broken line*) in patients with insulin-dependent diabetes mellitus who had microalbuminuria. The difference between the 2 treatments was statistically significant ($P = .03$ by log-rank test). (Courtesy of Viberti G, for the European Microalbuminuria Captopril Study Group: JAMA 271:275–279, 1994.)

persistently above 200 µg/min and at least 30% above baseline) during follow-up, a significant difference (Fig 57–2). The mean rate of albumin excretion increased in the placebo group but declined in the captopril group. The mean blood pressure did not change in the placebo group but declined significantly (by 3–7 mm Hg) in the captopril group. Both glomerular filtration rates and glycosylated hemoglobin values remained stable in both groups.

Conclusion.—The use of captopril to retard the progression of renal disease in patients with both insulin-dependent diabetes mellitus and microalbuminuria is supported.

Captopril and Atenolol Are Equally Effective in Retarding Progression of Diabetic Nephropathy: Results of a 2-Year Prospective, Randomized Study

Elving LD, Wetzels JFM, van Lier HJJ, de Nobel E, Berden JHM (Univ Hosp Nijmegen, The Netherlands)
Diabetologia 37:604–609, 1994   119-95-57–9

Introduction.—Antihypertensive treatment is an important component of the therapy for patients with diabetic nephropathy. Because dilation of afferent renal arterioles has been implicated in intraglomerular hypertension, angiotensin-converting enzyme (ACE) inhibitors may be more effective than conventional antihypertensive agents in controlling blood pressure in patients with diabetic nephropathy. The effects of an ACE inhibitor were compared with the effects of a β-blocker on the glomerular filtration rate (GFR) and on albuminuria in a prospective, randomized, controlled study.

Methods.—Twenty-nine patients with insulin-dependent diabetes and overt nephropathy (urinary protein excretion greater than 300 mg/day on 3 occasions) were randomly assigned to receive either captopril (15 patients) or atenolol (14 patients) for 2 years. The patients had measurements of blood pressure; urinary creatinine, albumin, total protein, and sodium; serum sodium, potassium, and creatinine; and hemoglobin A_{1c} every 6 weeks. Plasma renin activity, serum albumin, and hemoglobin were measured every 3 months and the GFR was measured every 6 months.

Results.—Baseline hemodynamic and renal function values were similar in the 2 treatment groups. Blood pressure was consistently controlled at the same level in both groups. The GFR significantly decreased in both groups, with the largest decline during the first 6 months of either treatment regimen. Both treatments decreased overall proteinuria and albuminuria equally. Neither treatment affected glycemic control, and there were no major side effects. However, patients taking captopril had significantly lower hemoglobin concentrations.

Discussion.—The ACE inhibitors and β-blockers appear to be equally effective in lowering blood pressure and urinary albumin and total protein excretion in patients with insulin-dependent diabetes and nephropathy, but neither prevents a decline in GFR.

▶ Nephropathy is the single most important complication of both insulin-dependent and non–insulin-dependent diabetes, and diabetic nephropathy is the single most important cause of end-stage renal disease. It is first manifest as microalbuminuria (defined as urinary albumin excretion of 20–200 μg/min [30–300 mg/day]). Among patients with microalbuminuria, about 25% have macroalbuminuria (called clinical proteinuria by Viberti et al.) develop in 5 to 10 years (1, 2), but it may simply persist or even subside. Macroalbuminuria is eventually followed by renal insufficiency and end-stage renal disease.

Among the risk factors for persistence or progression of microalbminuria are blood pressure, hyperglycemia, family history of diabetic nephropathy, and smoking (1, 3). Improved control of diabetes and treatment of hypertension slow the rate of progression (4). With respect to antihypertensive drug therapy, most attention has focused on ACE inhibitors. Drugs of this type slow the increase in urinary albumin excretion in not only hypertensive but also normotensive patients with either insulin-dependent or non–insulin-dependent diabetes (the study by Viberti et al. [Abstract 119-95-57–8]; 5, 6). The study by Elving et al. (Abstract 119-95-57–9) suggests that a β-adrenergic antagonist drug will do just about as well. The effects of these therapies on GFR have been more variable, although, in general, ACE drug therapy has been associated with stabilization or at least slowing of the decline in renal function. The benefit has been ascribed to both a small reduction in blood pressure and a more specific effect on glomerular permeability because of the ability of these drugs to reduce efferent arteriolar pressure. Most of these studies have lasted 2 to 3 years. Although the long-term impact of early treatment of microalbuminuria is not known, I think it will be substantial.

The question is not whether, but when, therapy should be initiated in normotensive patients with either insulin-dependent or insulin-independent diabetes. Urinary albumin excretion should be measured periodically in all diabetic patients. If microalbuminuria is detected and is confirmed on several occasions within several months (especially if urinary albumin excretion is in the 150–300-mg/day range), then therapy with an ACE inhibitor should be initiated. The drug given in most studies was captopril, in doses of 50–100 mg/day, but any ACE inhibitor is likely to be effective.

Two caveats: not all proteinuria in patients with diabetes is due to diabetic nephropathy, and the possibility of other renal disease should be considered. Also, if a young woman with diabetes is treated with an ACE inhibitor, the drug should be discontinued immediately if she becomes pregnant. These drugs cause fetal and neonatal injury, including renal failure and growth retardation, and should not be given to pregnant women.—R.D. Utiger, M.D.

References

1. Microalbuminuria Study Group, United Kingdom: Risk factors for development of microalbuminuria in insulin dependent diabetic patients: A cohort study. *BMJ* 306:1235–1239, 1993.
2. Almdal T, Feldt-Rasmussen B, Norgaard K, Deckert T: The predictive value of microalbuminuria. *Diabetes Care* 17:120–125, 1994.
3. Mogensen CE: Prediction of clinical diabetic nephropathy in IDDM patients: Alternatives to microalbuminuria. *Diabetes* 39:761–767, 1990.
4. 1994 YEAR BOOK OF MEDICINE, pp 628–631.
5. Lewis EJ, Hunsicker LG, Bain RP, Rohde RD, for the Collaborative Study Group: Effect of angiotensin-converting-enzyme inhibition on diabetic nephropathy. *N Engl J Med* 329:1456–1462, 1993.
6. Ravid M, Savin H, Jutrin I, Bental T, Katz B, Lishner M: Long-term stabilizing effect of angiotensin-converting enzyme inhibition on plasma creatinine and on proteinuria in normotensive type II diabetic patients. *Ann Intern Med* 118:577–581, 1993.

Counterregulatory Hormone Responses to Hypoglycemia in the Elderly Patient With Diabetes

Meneilly GS, Cheung E, Tuokko H (Univ of British Columbia, Vancouver, Canada; Univ Hosp, Vancouver, BC, Canada)
Diabetes 43:403–410, 1994   119-95-57–10

Introduction.—In patients with non–insulin-dependent diabetes mellitus (NIDDM), the risk of severe or fatal hypoglycemia with oral hypoglycemic drugs and insulin therapy increases with age. The increased susceptibility to hypoglycemia in elderly patients with diabetes may be caused by alterations in the release of counterregulatory hormones, lack of symptomatic awareness of hypoglycemia, and alterations in psychomotor performance during hypoglycemia.

Methods.—Ten healthy, nonobese, elderly individuals (mean age, 74 years) and 10 elderly patients with NIDDM (mean age, 72 years) underwent paired hyperinsulinemic glucose clamp studies. In the control study, plasma glucose was maintained at 90 mg/dL (5 mmol/L) for 5 hours. In the hypoglycemic study, plasma glucose was kept at this concentration for 1 hour and then lowered to 80 mg/dL (4.4 mmol/L), 68 mg/dl (3.8 mmol/L), 60 mg/dL (3.3 mmol/L), and 50 mg/dL (2.8 mmol/L) for each subsequent hour. A hypoglycemic symptom questionnaire and neuropsychological tests were administered at regular intervals. Plasma counterregulatory hormones were measured serially.

Results.—Compared with the age-matched normal individuals, the patients with NIDDM had impaired plasma glucagon and growth hormone responses and increased cortisol and epinephrine responses to hypoglycemia. Although the overall trend was toward an increase in autonomic and neuroglycopenic symptom scores as hypoglycemia progressed in both groups, no significant difference and no significant group-time interaction were noted between the normal individuals and diabetic pa-

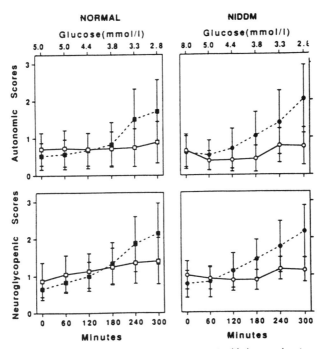

Fig 57–3.—Autonomic and neuroglycopenic symptom scores in elderly normal patients and patients with non–insulin-dependent diabetes mellitus (NIDDM) during control (*open circles and squares*) and hypoglycemic (*filled circles and squares*) studies. (Courtesy of Meneilly GS, Cheung E, Tuokko H: *Diabetes* 43:403–410, 1994.)

tients (Fig 57–3). The patients with NIDDM had a greater impairment on both simple and choice reaction time tests at a plasma glucose concentration of 50 mg/dL (2.8 mmol/L).

Summary.—Elderly patients with NIDDM have significant impairment in the release of counterregulatory hormones in response to hypoglycemia and impaired psychomotor speed and attention in response to low plasma glucose concentrations.

▶ As plasma glucose concentrations fall, older diabetic patients may not have either autonomic or neuroglycopenic symptoms develop more slowly than normal subjects of the same age (Fig 57–3), but their impaired ability to release counterregulatory hormones, especially glucagon and epinephrine, however, means that their ability to mobilize glycogen stores to defend against hypoglycemia is reduced. The risk of occurrence of hypoglycemia in the elderly may be increased because of lower clearance of oral hypoglycemic drugs or insulin (1) and physical limitations that could make it difficult to obtain food in an emergency. Furthermore, elderly patients are vulnerable to other (nonhypoglycemic) symptoms or potentially catastrophic events—angina, stroke, seizures, myocardial infarction, falls—during hypoglycemia. The obvious conclusions are that elderly diabetic patients should be treated less vigorously than younger ones and that more care should be taken to ensure that treatment is available should hypoglycemia occur.—R.D. Utiger, M.D.

Reference

1. Marker JC, Cryer PE, Clutter WE: Attenuated glucose recovery from hypoglycemia in the elderly. *Diabetes* 41:671–678, 1992.

58 Obesity and Lipid Metabolism

The Impact of Cigarette and Alcohol Consumption on Weight and Obesity: An Analysis of 1911 Monozygotic Male Twin Pairs
Eisen SA, Lyons MJ, Goldberg J, True WR (Washington Univ, St Louis, Mo; Harvard Med School, West Roxbury, Mass; Boston Univ; et al)
Arch Intern Med 153:2457–2463, 1993   119-95-58-1

Introduction.—The patterns of cigarette and alcohol use carry contradictory health risks. Although smoking cessation offers clear health benefits, these benefits may be diminished by the weight gain that often follows smoking cessation. Similarly, although there are cardiovascular benefits associated with moderate drinking, alcohol consumption may also cause weight gain. The relationships between weight and cigarette and alcohol consumption were examined in twins.

Methods.—Members of the Vietnam Era Twin Registry were surveyed to determine their zygosity, current height and weight, and cigarette and alcohol consumption. The data from 1,911 monozygotic twin pairs were analyzed.

Results.—Of the 3,822 respondents, 39% smoked regularly and 63% drank regularly; the mean age was 38 years. Analysis of weight differences in pairs with different smoking habits revealed that twins who had stopped smoking weighed 3.5 kg more than current smokers and that twins who had never smoked weighed 3.1 kg more than current smokers. Past smokers were more likely to be obese (26.5%) than were current smokers (19.9%). The relative risk of obesity was 1.8 in former smokers and 1.5 in twins who had never smoked as compared with the risk in heavy smokers. There was no difference in weight in twin pairs with different drinking habits. Multivariate regression analyses of the various degrees of cigarette and alcohol consumption revealed smoking but not alcohol consumption to be a significant determinant of weight.

Discussion.—The results of this twin study indicate that cigarette but not alcohol consumption significantly affects weight and the risk of obesity. Therefore, smoking cessation programs should include a weight-management component.

▶ The individual response rate in this study was 74%, and for both twins, it was 67%. These are good response rates for this type of study and suggest that the results are likely generalizable to the population, at least the twin population, at large. The twin study design eliminates confounding from inherited factors and minimizes differences in factors such as diet and physical activity, but it cannot ensure the validity of self-reports of smoking and alcohol consumption. Notwithstanding these caveats, these results provide further support for the notion that smoking is associated with lower weight and that cessation of smoking results in weight gain (1). As the authors note, any smoking cessation program must consider the problem of weight gain, whereas there are no implications for weight gain associated with cessation of alcohol intake.

This study also provides information concerning the genetic propensity for smoking and drinking alcohol. Among the 1,911 monozygotic twin pairs, 1,252 were concordant for smoking and 1,253 were concordant for drinking alcohol. The concordant pairs obviously provided no information about the questions regarding cessation of smoking and drinking asked by the investigators, but the high frequency of these behaviors (65%) among the twin pairs serves as a reminder of the genetic influence on these behaviors.—R.D. Utiger, M.D.

Reference

1. Williamson DF, Madans J, Anda RF, Kleinman JC, Giovino GA, Byers T: Smoking cessation and severity of weight gain in a national cohort. *N Engl J Med* 324:739–745, 1991.

Do Cholesterol-Lowering Agents Affect Brain Activity? A Comparison of Simvastatin, Pravastatin, and Placebo in Healthy Volunteers
Harrison RWS, Ashton CH (The Univ, Newcastle upon Tyne, England)
Br J Clin Pharmacol 37:231–236, 1994   119-95-58-2

Introduction.—Some studies have found an association between low plasma cholesterol concentrations and an increased rate of depression,

---

Sleep, HAD, and DSST Parameters of 25 Subjects After 4 Weeks Treatment on Simvastatin, Pravastatin, and Placebo

	Pravastatin	Simvastatin	Placebo
Leeds Sleep Questionnaire			
(Hard to sleep score) (mm)	51.4 (48.4–54.6)	47.0 (44.9–49.1)	50.1 (46.4–53.8) *
HAD (Depression scale)	1.5 (0.6–2.4)	1.6 (0.7–2.5)	1.5 (0.8–2.5)
HAD (Anxiety scale)	3.2 (2.0–4.4)	2.5 (1.7–3.3)	3.1 (2.2–4.0)
DSST	74.3 (70.3–78.3)	74.6 (70.3–78.9)	74.6 (70.9–78.3)

Figures are expressed as means (95% confidence intervals).
* Pravastatin va. simvastatin difference is significant $P = 0.05$.
No other Leeds Sleep Questionnaire variables showed significant differences.
(Courtesy of Harrison RWS, Ashton CH: *Br J Clin Pharmacol* 37:231–236, 1994.)

alcohol-related diseases, and suicide. Concerns that drugs used to lower plasma cholesterol might affect CNS activity prompted a placebo-controlled study of simvastatin and pravastatin.

Methods.—Twenty-five normal volunteers, 17 men and 8 women (mean age, 24 years), were studied. None had a personal or family psychiatric history or evidence of depression. In a crossover design, participants took 40 mg of simvastatin per day, 40 mg of pravastatin per day, or placebo in separate 4-week treatment phases, each separated by a 4-6-week washout phase during which placebo was taken. Measures used to detect drug effects on the CNS included electroencephologram (EEG)-evoked potentials, power spectral analysis, the Leeds Sleep Questionnaire, the Hospital Anxiety Depression (HAD) Scale, and the Digit Symbol Substitution Test (DSST). Biochemical measures recorded were plasma cholesterol, liver enzymes, and creatine kinase.

Results.—Both drugs significantly lowered plasma cholesterol concentrations relative to placebo, and the effect was greater with simvastatin than with pravastatin. There were no differences in EEG parameters between the treatment and placebo periods. Similarly, the HAD Scale and DSST scores were equivalent during all phases of the trial. Participants reported more trouble falling asleep while taking simvastatin than pravastatin, but neither was different from placebo (table). There were no significant correlations between sleep ratings and either plasma cholesterol concentrations or EEG-evoked potentials.

Conclusion.—Neither cholesterol-lowering agent had any effects on EEG-evoked potentials, indicating that pravastatin and simvastatin have no acute effects on brain activity. During the 4-week study, lowered plasma cholesterol concentrations did not influence mood in these normal subjects.

▶ All the studies I know of in which lower plasma cholesterol concentrations were associated with increased numbers of violent deaths (suicide and accident) preceded the introduction of the drugs (lovastatin, simvastatin, pravastatin, etc.) that lower plasma cholesterol by inhibiting 3-hydroxy-3-methylglutaryl coenzyme A (HMG Co A) reductase. Besides, the meaning of those data is much contested, and many view the relationship, if there is one, as indicating that the subject's low plasma cholesterol concentration was simply a marker of chronic illness, including psychiatric illness.

Still, it's worth determining whether the drugs that inhibit HMG CoA reductase have CNS actions that can be identified by detailed prospective study. Apparently they do not. They are not free of side effects, however. A small percentage of patients has a three-fold or greater increase in plasma aminotransferase concentrations. Others have small increases in plasma creatine kinase concentrations, a few have myalgia or myopathy, and severe rhabdomyolysis has been reported. Despite their ability to inhibit cholesterol synthesis, these drugs do not impair either adrenal or gonadal hormone secretion (1, 2).

Use of this class of cholesterol-lowering drugs can only increase. Prolonged safety has been demonstrated repeatedly, the drugs are much better tolerated than other hypocholesterolemic drugs (niacin and bile acid sequestering agents), and they have proven beneficial in slowing progression or even reversing coronary artery disease in secondary prevention trials and recently in a primary prevention trial (3). With more of them on the market, their cost should diminish, and smaller doses are just about as effective as larger ones (4).—R.D. Utiger, M.D.

References

1. Mol MJTM, Stalenhoef AFH, Stuyt PMJ, Hermus ARMM, Demacker PNM, Van'T Laar A: Effects of inhibition of cholesterol synthesis by simvastatin on the production of adrenocortical steroid hormones and ACTH. *Clin Endocrinol* 31:679–689, 1989.
2. Farnsworth WH, Hoeg JM, Maher M, Brittain EH, Sherins RJ, Brewer Jr HB: Testicular function in type II hyperlipoproteinemic patients treated with lovastatin (mevolin) or neomycin. *J Clin Endocrinol Metab* 65:546–550, 1987.
3. MAAS Investigators: Effect of simvastatin on coronary atheroma: The Multicentre Anti-Atheroma Study (MAAS). *Lancet* 344:633–638, 1994.
4. Illingworth DR, Erkelens DW, Keller U, Thompson GR, Tikkanen MJ: Defined daily doses in relation to hypolipidaemic efficacy of lovastatin, pravastatin, and simvastatin. *Lancet* 343:1554–1555, 1994.

PART SEVEN

KIDNEY, WATER, AND ELECTROLYTES

FRANKLIN H. EPSTEIN, M.D.

Introduction

The causes of the most common forms of the nephrotic syndrome—minimal-change disease and its treatment-resistant cousin, focal glomerulosclerosis—remain mysterious. An exciting new advance, however, is contained in the report of a circulating factor in the plasma of patients with recurrent focal sclerosis causing nephrotic syndrome after renal transplantation (Abstract 119-95-59–1). Adsorption of the protein factor from the plasma produced remission of the proteinuria in nephrotic patients, and injection of the adsorbed material into rats induced proteinuria. Cyclosporine A, for some years a first-line immunosuppressive drug in the treatment of transplant patients, turns out to be remarkably useful in treating resistant patients with the nephrotic syndrome (Abstract 119-95-59–2), suggesting that the mystery protein factor in plasma may be synthesized by the immune system. Collapsing glomerulopathy, a new clinicopathological entity that is usually seen in HIV-positive patients with nephropathy, has been described in patients who have no serological evidence of HIV infection (Abstract 119-95-59–3). The propensity to clotting, observed in many patients with heavy proteinuria, finds its explanation in the dysproteinemia that characterizes the nephrotic syndrome, which encourages coagulation and inhibits fibrinolysis (Abstract 119-95-59–4). Finally, this year's chapter on glomerular diseases closes with a comprehensive review of the most common cause of glomerulonephritis around the world—IgA nephropathy.

The chapter on other diseases of the kidney includes an interesting and puzzling account of the gradual decline of diabetic nephropathy in Sweden (Abstract 119-95-60–1) and a reminder that in patients with vasculitis, interstitial damage in the kidney may rival or even overshadow the signs of glomerular injury (Abstract 119-95-60–2). There is a detailed description of the peculiar nephropathy, associated with chronic intravascular hemolysis, that occurs as a late complication of bone marrow transplantation (Abstract 119-95-60–3). A remarkable syndrome with which few internists are familiar, produced by ovarian hyperstimulation, is summarized in Abstract 119-95-60–4. A practical note on urinary eosinophils (forget them!) (Abstract 119-95-60–5) completes the chapter.

Clinicians who treat patients with acute renal failure nurse the hope that some day a powerful and specific renal vasodilator will come along that will unlock the tight renal vasoconstriction that seems a part of this syndrome and, thereby, induce an increase in the glomerular filtration rate (GFR) and urine flow without causing unacceptable systemic vasodilatation and shock. Atrial natriuretic factor seemed ideal for this purpose, at least in theory, but thus far results with it have been disappointing (Abstract 119-95-61–1). Less dramatic attempts to reduce morbidity in patients with established acute renal failure look more promising, and they center on a reduction in cytokine release when dialysis is carried out with membranes that are less reactive (though more expensive) than cuprophane (Abstract 119-95-65–1 in the chapter on dialysis). Two unusual causes of acute renal failure are discussed in this year's chapter on acute renal failure: the hemolytic uremic syndrome caused by cyclosporine A (Abstract 119-95-61-2) and the proximal tubular toxicity sometimes seen as a byproduct of treatment with ifosfamide for malignancy (Abstract 119-95-61-3).

The chapter on chronic renal failure includes the results of two massive trials of therapy in chronic progressive renal disease (Abstracts 119-95-62-1 and 119-95-62-2). Restriction of dietary protein for 2–3 years had a negligible effect on the slow progression of renal insufficiency (Abstract 119-95-62-1). By contrast, angiotensin-converting enzyme inhibitors definitely reduced the rate of increase in serum creatinine in diabetics with moderate renal impairment who were followed for a median of 3 years (Abstract 119-95-6-2). Other papers in this chapter deal with systemic manifestations of dialysis-related amyloidosis (mainly in the vasculature) (Abstract 119-95-62-3), the nature of uremic cardiomyopathy (Abstract 119-95-62-4), and the epidemiology of end-stage renal disease (Abstract 119-95-62-5).

Although some rare forms of high blood pressure are clearly genetic in origin (e.g., familial pheochromocytoma, inherited disorders of adrenal steroid metabolism, and Liddle's syndrome), we call the most common varieties of hypertension "essential" because we have as yet no real clue as to their cause. Abstracts 119-95-63-1 and 119-95-63-2 report some of the first, halting steps toward the identification of a gene that may possibly be related to essential hypertension; it codes for an isoform of angiotensinogen. An unusual cause of labile hypertension, mimicking pheochromocytoma, is described in Abstract 119-95-63-3. Renal artery stenosis, often bilateral, is an increasingly frequent cause of resistant hypertension coupled with renal failure in an aging population. Abstract 119-95-63-4 describes the results of balloon angioplasty in such patients. The significant role of alcohol consumption in predisposing the patient to hypertension is documented by Abstract 119-95-63-5, and a possible mechanism for glucocorticoid-induced high blood pressure (an increase in vascular angiotensin-II receptors) is reported in Abstract 119-95-63-6. Two reassuring reports complete this chapter on hypertension. Abstract 119-95-63-7 shows that a trial of withdrawal of antihypertensive medication can be safely carried out in elderly patients, and Abstract 119-95-63-8 demonstrates that renal failure is exceedingly rare as a complication of mild essential hypertension, at least in white patients without diabetes. Antihypertensive therapy is probably more important for the prevention of kidney failure in diabetics and in blacks.

In the world of renal transplantation, the powerful technique of the polymerase chain reaction (PCR), which permits accurate detection and even quantification of minuscule amounts of genetic material, is being applied to biopsies of transplanted kidneys, with important theoretical and practical results. Early cellular rejection is characterized by the appearance of the message for certain cytokines specific for T cells (Abstract 119-95-64-6) and, further, by a special class of T lymphocytes (CTLs) (Abstract 119-95-64-4). Gamma-interferon is still another intragraft cytokine, activated early in the course of rejection, that is easily detected in biopsy specimens of kidneys with incipient acute rejection (Abstract 119-95-64-5). Attempts are now being made to standardize criteria for the histological diagnosis of rejection from renal biopsy specimens processed by conventional means (Abstract 119-95-64-3); such standard definitions may have to be modified in the future to take account of the alterations that can be detected through the use of molecular biology. Despite the well-known renal toxicity of cyclosporine overdosage (Abstract 119-95-64-1), this drug remains the backbone of standard immunosuppressive treatment for transplanted organs. The majority of renal transplant patients tolerate long-term cyclosporine therapy without evidence of progressive toxic nephropathy, and graft failure is most often due to rejection (Abstract 119-95-64-1). Other strategies for preventing T-cell–mediated rejection and inducing graft tolerance are in the wings; among them is the blockade of a cell surface molecule (CD28) necessary for T-cell activation, used in combination with donor-specific transfusion. Immunotherapy has its price, however, and one of the costs of chronic immunosuppression is an increased risk of malignancy, especially non-Hodgkin's lymphoma, reviewed in Abstract 119-95-64-2.

In addition to the report of the benefit of more biocompatible hemodialysis membranes, the chapter on dialysis discusses two alternatives to hemodialysis that deserve consideration in certain circumstances. Continuous venovenous hemodiafiltration may be preferable to intermittent "classical" hemodialysis for critically ill patients with acute renal failure (Abstract 119-95-65-2). Continuous ambulatory peritoneal dialysis (CAPD) often permits better nutrition and more independence than standard hemodialysis for patients with chronic renal failure, but for reasons still obscure, it appears to be associated with a higher mortality rate in diabetic patients (Abstract 119-95-65-3). Regardless of the form of treatment, in the United States, African-Americans and Hispanics with end-stage renal disease seem to have better survival rates than non-Hispanic white patients (Abstract 119-95-65-4). Two complications of long-term dialysis are also discussed in this chapter. Dialysis-related amyloidosis can be treated and perhaps prevented by adsorption of retained β_2-microglobulin on a column incorporated in the extracorporeal dialysis circuit (Abstract 119-95-65-5). Infection with the hepatitis C virus has a relatively high prevalence, especially in patients with other signs of liver disease, but it can be missed with commercially available antibody tests—a better but more difficult test is one for the viral RNA (Abstract 119-95-65-6). The last paper in this chapter summarizes what we know about the outcomes of pregnancy in women undergoing dialysis, which is not so rare an occurrence as you might think (Abstract 119-95-65-7).

The first abstract in this year's chapter on sodium, potassium, water, and acid-base addresses the age-old question of how we manage to excrete the excess sodium when our intake of salt is increased (Abstract 119-95-66-1). A major factor, it appears, is a reduction in circulating angiotensin-II (ANG-II). You may protest that you knew that, but I, at least, did not know that the main effect of the reduction in ANG-II is not the associated fall in circulating aldosterone but, rather, the decreased *direct effect* of ANG-II on renal tubular reabsorption of sodium. Abstract 119-95-66-2 strengthens the prevailing tendency to give potassium-sparing diuretics like triamterene whenever thiazides are prescribed, in order to avoid hypokalemia. The incidence of sudden death (presumably owing to arrhythmias) was significantly reduced by this maneuver. A variant of nephrogenic diabetes insipidus has been described, in which the genetic defect lies not within the vasopressin receptor but in the water channel of the collecting duct (Abstract 119-95-66–3). Renal tubular acidosis and, more rarely, other renal tubular abnormalities, all reversible, may complicate alcoholism (Abstract 119-95-66–4). A simplified test for distal renal tubular acidosis is reported in Abstract 119-95-66–5: just test 2 first-morning urines—the pH should normally be less than 6.1.

The chapter on calcium and phosphorus leads off with a remarkable report of a single unusual case with important implications for normal physiology (Abstract 119-95-67–1). Tumor-induced osteomalacia seems to be caused by a circulating peptide hormone, synthesized by the tumor, that induces the kidneys to excrete phosphate and might therefore play a key role in the control of phosphorus balance by normal kidneys. The treatment of uremic osteodystrophy with oral and intravenous calcitriol is described in Abstract 119-95-67–2 (no important difference between the two was detected). Finally, a severe, unexpected, and (fortunately) reversible complication of phosphate therapy—vocal cord paralysis—was encountered in a uremic patient whose calcium transiently plummeted when hypophosphatemia was overvigorously treated (Abstract 119-95-67–3).

Franklin H. Epstein, M.D.

59 Glomerular Diseases

Effect of Plasma Protein Adsorption on Protein Excretion in Kidney-Transplant Recipients With Recurrent Nephrotic Syndrome

Dantal J, Bigot E, Bogers W, Testa A, Kriaa F, Jacques Y, de Ligny BH, Niaudet P, Charpentier B, Soulillou JP (Centre Hospitalier Régional et Universitaire, Nantes, France; Hôpital de Bicêtre, Le Kremlin Bicêtre, France; Hôpital Necker Enfants Malades, Paris; et al)
N Engl J Med 330:7–14, 1994   119-95-59–1

Background.—In a subset of patients with idiopathic nephrotic syndrome, proteinuria is either resistant to treatment with corticosteroids or recurs rapidly when these are stopped. Such patients often have focal glomerulosclerosis, progress to chronic renal failure, and have a recurrence of the nephrotic syndrome soon after renal transplantation because the transplanted kidney develops glomerular proteinuria. There is evidence that these recurrences result from some unknown plasma factor that increases glomerular permeability. The effects were examined of plasma protein adsorption on proteinuria in patients with recurrent nephrotic syndrome.

Methods.—The subjects were 8 patients with recurrent heavy proteinuria within 1 week of renal transplantation. Six patients had steroid-resistant minimal-change glomerulonephritis, and 2 had focal and segmental

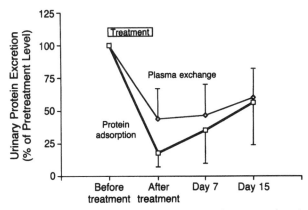

Fig 59–1.—Mean (± SD) changes in urinary protein excretion after protein adsorption in the 8 patients, 3 of whom also underwent plasma exchange. The results of single sessions of treatment are excluded. The box indicates the period when treatment was administered. (Courtesy of Dantal J, Bigot E, Bogers W, et al: *N Engl J Med* 330:7–14, 1994.)

glomerulosclerosis. The mean urinary protein excretion averaged 10 g per day. All underwent 1–3 cycles of 2–7 one-day sessions of plasma protein adsorption onto protein A. The patients, whose immunosuppressive treatment was not altered during treatment, underwent repeated measures of urinary protein excretion. In a further experiment, the investigators eluted the adsorbed proteins from the protein A cartridge, injected them into rats, and observed the effects on the animals' urinary albumin excretion.

Results.—Plasma protein adsorption reduced urinary protein excretion by an average of 82% at the end of each cycle (Fig 59–1). One patient had complete disappearance of proteinuria, and in another urinary protein excretion remained below 2.5 g/day with repeated cycles of treatment. The effects of treatment were time limited in all patients but 1; by 2 months, protein excretion returned to pretreatment levels. When the eluted material was administered to rats, their urinary albumin excretion increased by 2.9- to 4.6-fold. Analysis of the eluted proteins demonstrated that the active fraction had a molecular weight of less than 100,000, suggesting that immunoglobulin was not directly involved.

Conclusions.—For patients with recurrent nephrotic syndrome after renal transplantation, adsorption of plasma protein onto protein A can reduce urinary protein excretion consistently and significantly. This result suggests the possible role of a circulating protein in this disorder. Further studies of the adsorbed proteins from patients with recurrent nephrotic syndrome may shed light on its pathogenetic mechanism.

▶ Patients with steroid-resistant focal glomerulosclerosis that recurs in a transplanted kidney with return of the nephrotic syndrome provide one of the most frustrating and tragic dilemmas in nephrology. This fascinating paper provides the most convincing evidence to date that a circulating plasma factor is responsible for the increased glomerular permeability to protein that is at the root of this clinical entity. By extension, the same mechanism is probably at work in those patients whose idiopathic, minimal-change nephrotic syndrome responds to steroid treatment—but we do not yet know that. Earlier, these and other workers reported moderate but variable success in producing temporary remission in nephrosis by plasma exchange. The effect of plasma adsorption on proteinuria is much more pronounced, presumably because more of the plasma factor is removed from the circulation. Though dramatic, remissions were temporary, the longest one lasting 6 months after plasma adsorption was stopped. It seems possible that the efficacy of plasma adsorption in these renal transplant recipients may have been enhanced by concomitant antirejection therapy with cyclosporine, which, at least in theory, might have partially suppressed the production of factor X by the immune system. YEAR BOOK subscribers will recall that cyclosporine can induce substantial improvement in perhaps two thirds of patients with idiopathic nephrotic syndrome thought to be resistant to steroids (1).—F.H. Epstein, M.D.

Reference

1. Ponticelli C, Rizzoni G, Edefonte A, et al: A randomized trial of cyclosporine in steroid-resistant idiopathic nephrotic syndrome. *Kidney Int* 43:1377–1384, 1994 (abstracted in the 1994 YEAR BOOK OF MEDICINE, pp 662–664).

Long-Term Renal Tolerance of Cyclosporin A Treatment in Adult Idiopathic Nephrotic Syndrome

Meyrier A, Noël L-H, Auriche P, Callard P, and the Collaborative Group of the Société de Néphrologie (Hôpital Avicenne, Bobigny, France; INSERM U 90, Hôpital Necker, Paris; Hôpital Tenon, Paris)
Kidney Int 45:1446–1456, 1994   119-95-59–2

Objective.—Thirty-six adult patients who were treated for steroid-dependent or steroid-resistant idiopathic nephrotic syndrome with cyclosporine A (CsA) were evaluated forthe long-term renal tolerance of CsA therapy. Because of the well documented nephrotoxic potential of the drug, its long-term effects in patients with nephrosis is a critical issue.

Patients and Methods.—The study enrolled 112 patients who were either resistant to conventional treatment for nephrotic syndrome, corticosteroid dependent with unacceptable side effects, or had a contraindication to corticosteroids. The initial CsA dosage was 5 mg/kg/day, which was subsequently adjusted to a range of 4 to 7.8 mg/kg/day. Response was defined as complete remission, partial remission, or failure. The 36 patients selected for this phase of the study underwent renal biopsy before and after CsA treatment and were treated for at least 6 months. The initial biospy specimen identified the primary renal disease as minimal glomerular changes (MCD) or focal segmental glomerulosclerosis (FSGS).

Results.—Pre-CsA renal biopsy specimens taken at a mean of 11.6 months before treatment showed MCD in 22 patients and FSGS in 14. The mean pretreatment serum creatinine levels were 97.6 μmol/L, and were higher in FSGS (117.1 μmol/L) than in MCD (85.2 μmol/L). Repeat renal biopsies were performed at a mean of 19.6 months after the start of CsA treatment. Seven of the 22 patients with MCD at the first biopsy now showed FSGS. Serum creatinine was significantly higher at the time of the repeat biopsy in patients with FSGS both before and after CsA therapy than in those with MCD. The 3 most important predictors of tubulointerstitial insult after long-term CsA treatment of idiopathic nephrotic syndrome were the percentage of pretreatment glomeruli with lesions of FSGS, abnormal renal function before CsA treatment, and a dosage greater than 5.5 mg/kg/day. Eight patients were treated continuously with CsA for 3 to 7 years; another 8 stopped CsA because of rapidly declining renal function and required chronic hemodialysis; 3 were failures of CsA treatment and returned to conventional corticosteroid treatment; and 14 were able to taper CsA, stopping treatment after a mean of 26 months with the disease in remission. Two patients died during the study.

Conclusion.—A subset of patients with idiopathic nephrotic syndrome, MCD, and normal renal function can benefit from CsA treatment, up to 5.5 mg/kg/day. Especially for those with steroid toxicity, CsA is a promising treatment, but CsA can be relatively hazardous in patients with FSGS, preexisting incipient renal insufficiency, and tubulointerstitial lesions. A repeat renal biopsy should be performed after 1 year of CsA treatment. When prolonged remission has been obtained with CsA treatment of more than one year, a stable remission often persists when the drug is tapered and stopped.

▶ Cyclosporine A has been shown to be useful in the treatment of children with nephrotic syndrome (1), and this article summarizes an extensive French experience with CsA in adults. All 36 patients were resistant to glucocorticoids given for at least 4 months, and they were biopsied both before and after CsA was administered. The bottom line is that CsA was very good for patients with minimal-change disease (19 of 22 went into complete remission), but (as expected) it was not as reliable for focal glomerular sclerosis, where the 60% rate of progression resembled the behavior of untreated patients with this pathological picture. Most important was the fact that 14 patients (4 with FSGS and 10 with MCD) were able to stop CsA entirely and remained in stable remission after an average of 26 (ranging from 12–60) months of following the CsA regimen. Interstitial fibrosis, a toxic side effect of CsA treatment, was minimal if the dose was kept below 5.5 mg/kg/day. The authors emphasize, however, that a stable (and normal) serum creatinine did not rule out the development of interstitial fibrosis detected by a second renal biopsy carried out after prolonged treatment.—F.H. Epstein, M.D.

Reference

1. Niaudet P, et al: Comparison of cyclosporin and chlorambucil in the treatment of steroid-dependent idiopathic nephrotic syndrome: A multicentre randomized controlled trial. *Pediatr Nephrol* 6:1–3, 1992.

Collapsing Glomerulopathy: A Clinically and Pathologically Distinct Variant of Focal Segmental Glomerulosclerosis
Detwiler RK, Falk RJ, Hogan SL, Jennette JC (Univ of North Carolina, Chapel Hill)
Kidney Int 45:1416–1424, 1994   119-95-59–3

Introduction.—Collapsing glomerulopathy is a newly described entity characterized by renal biopsy findings of extensive focal glomerular capillary collapse, visceral epithelial cell swelling and hyperplasia, and variable degrees of tubulointerstitial injury. When discovered in patients with HIV infection, similar glomerular findings comprise the condition

Presenting Clinical Features of Patients With Collapsing
Glomerulopathy ($n = 16$)

Hypertension	56%
Peripheral edema	56%
Anorexia/weight loss	44%
Fever (subjective)	25%
Dyspnea	25%
Diarrhea	19%
Ascites	19%
Pleural effusion	19%
Dementia	13%
Arthralgias/myalgias	13%
Rash	13%
Polyuria	6%

(Courtesy of Detwiler RK, Falk RJ, Hogan SL, et al: *Kidney Int* 45:1416–1424, 1994.)

known as HIV nephropathy. The patients described in one study, however, had no evidence of HIV infection or known HIV risk factors.

Patients and Methods.—Sixteen patients were prospectively identified from a series of 849 consecutive nontransplant renal biopsy specimens evaluated during a 2-year period. The exclusion criteria included HIV seropositivity, a history of IV drug abuse, and any evidence of other HIV risk factors. A comparison group consisted of 25 randomly selected patients with noncollapsing focal segmental glomerulosclerosis (FSGS). The clinical and pathologic characteristics of the 2 groups were analyzed and compared.

Results.—Collapsing glomerulopathy was identified by the presence of focal, segmental, or global glomerular collapse. Noncollapsing FSGS lesions had a predilection for perihilar segments and had more hyalinosis. Other pathologic findings in collapsing glomerulopathy were hypertrophy and hyperplasia of visceral epithelial cells and interstitial infiltration of mononuclear leukocytes. The most common clinical features of collapsing glomerulopathy were hypertension, peripheral edema, and anorexia/weight loss (table). There were more black patients in the group with collapsing glomerulopathy (13 of 16) than in the group with FSGS (11 of 25). Both the mean serum creatinine level at entry and the 24-hour urine protein excretion rate were significantly higher in patients with collapsing glomerulopathy than in those with FSGS. Renal survival, as determined by life-table analysis, was significantly worse in the group with collapsing glomerulopathy. The difference in survival remained after controlling for entry serum creatinine and race.

Conclusion.—Collapsing glomerulopathy was found to be a distinct entity that differs clinically, pathologically, and epidemiologically from noncollapsing FSGS. In collapsing glomerulopathy there is a predominance of black patients, massive proteinuria, and relatively rapid progressive renal insufficiency. In contrast to HIV nephropathy, there is a lack of endothelial tubuloreticular inclusions.

▶ The clinical picture in patients with collapsing glomerulopathy is similar to that seen in patients with HIV nephropathy. It consists of the nephrotic syndrome with or without hypertension, usually associated with some degree of azotemia and renal insufficiency, which progresses inexorably over a period of months. The renal biopsy findings are identical to those of HIV nephropathy, except for the absence (in 15 of 16 specimens) of the endothelial tubuloreticular inclusions seen in many—but not all—cases of HIV nephropathy. Also, of course, there is no serological evidence of HIV infection or hepatitis (which also produces glomerulonephritis). Furthermore, these patients all denied IV drug abuse. The suspicion is strong that there is an unrecognized virus at work here, but thus far that hypothesis lacks any evidence.—F.H. Epstein, M.D.

Lipoprotein(a) in Nephrotic Syndrome

Stenvinkel P, Berglund L, Heimbürger O, Pettersson E, Alvestrand A (Huddinge Univ Hosp, Sweden)
Kidney Int 44:1116–1123, 1993
119-95-59-4

Introduction.—Hyperlipidemia, usually characterized by increases in total and low-density-lipoprotein cholesterol levels and normal or reduced high-density-lipoprotein cholesterol, is a defining feature of nephrotic syndrome (NS). Lipoprotein(a)—Lp(a)—, a plasma lipoprotein, may act as a competitive inhibitor of plasminogen activation, thereby promoting thrombosis rather than fibrinolysis. Increased levels of Lp(a) have recently been reported in patients with NS. The relationship between plasma Lp(a) levels and serum lipid and lipoprotein levels in NS was evaluated.

Methods.—Thirty-one patients, 18 men and 13 women, were enrolled in the study. A diagnosis of NS was based on a finding of urinary protein excretion > 3 g/24 hours and serum albumin ≤ 30 g/L in the presence or absence of clinically overt edema. The median duration of NS was 8 months. These patients, 24 patients with IgA nephropathy, and 43 healthy controls provided blood samples for measurement of Lp(a) levels and levels of serum cholesterol and triglycerides.

Results.—The median levels of Lp(a) were significantly elevated in patients with NS (49 mg/dL) compared with patients with IgA nephropathy (7 mg/dL) and healthy controls (9.7 mg/dL). All 10 patients with NS who achieved remission showed a marked fall in plasma Lp(a) levels. There was a direct correlation between Lp(a) levels and serum cholesterol in NS patients and an indirect correlation with plasma orosomucoid levels. Patients with NS tended to have higher Lp(a) levels when edema was present (median 54.3 mg/dL) than when edema was absent (median 19 mg/dL). Plasma levels of Lp(a) correlated directly with atrial natriuretic peptide and indirectly with urinary sodium excretion in the 9 patients with NS who underwent these additional evaluations.

Conclusion.—Patients with NS of diverse etiologies were found to have markedly increased plasma levels of Lp(a) and other lipid abnormalities. Plasma concentrations of Lp(a) were not affected by underlying renal pathology or glomerular filtration rate. Correlations between Lp(a), very-low-density lipoprotein (VLDL) cholesterol, and VLDL triglycerides suggest a close link between Lp(a) and triglyceride-rich lipoproteins in nephrosis.

▶ Thrombosis in both the arterial and the venous circulation is a serious and relatively frequent complication of the nephrotic syndrome. Its precise mechanism is not clear, but it probably has to do with the dysproteinemia that characterizes the nephrotic state. The concentration of some pro-coagulant factors are increased in nephrotic plasma, whereas that of certain regulator proteins that prevent clotting, such as antithrombin III and protein S, are decreased. Lipoprotein(a) is a small component of low-density lipoproteins, which are generally increased in the plasma of nephrotic patients. Its significance is that it can act as a competitive inhibitor of plasminogen activation (which lyses clots), and it thus promotes thrombosis rather than fibrinolysis. Therefore, a by-product of the lipemia of nephrosis is that vascular thrombosis is encouraged. We do not know how inhibiting cholesterol synthesis with lovastatin or similar drugs (as has been suggested for nephrotic hypercholesterolemia) would affect lipoprotein (a) levels.—F.H. Epstein, M.D.

IgA Nephropathy: Analysis of the Natural History, Important Factors in the Progression of Renal Disease, and a Review of the Literature
Ibels LS, Györy AZ (Univ of Sydney, Australia; Royal North Shore Hosp, St Leonards, Australia)
Medicine 73:79–102, 1994   119-95-59–5

Background.—The prognosis of patients with immunoglobulin A (IgA) nephropathy is still controversial. The important factors in the progression of renal impairment in these patients have not been established definitively. An analysis of the natural history of IgA nephropathy was presented.

Methods and Findings.—One hundred twenty-one patients were followed for a median of 92 months. The cumulative probability of renal survival was .87 15 years after the first onset of symptoms and .86 10 years after presentation and biopsy. Eight percent of patients progressed to end-stage renal failure. Twelve percent had a greater-than-20% decline in renal function. Twelve percent had complete remission of disease activity, and 68% had stable renal function. Several factors were found to affect renal outcome when the final serum creatinine was expressed as a percentage of the initial serum creatinine for each patient and compared with all other factors. In a univariate analysis, the presenting features associated with an adverse outcome were increased age, family history of nephritis, longer duration of symptoms, and presence of either nephrotic-range proteinuria or hypertension. A history of recurrent macroscopic hematuria and infection-related exacerbations of disease activity were related to a favorable outcome. In a multivariate analysis, nephrotic-range proteinuria had an independent adverse effect. In a univariate analysis of initial laboratory findings, number of hyaline casts, degree of renal function impairment, degree of proteinuria, increased β-globulins on serum protein electrophoresis, and serum C4 levels were related to an adverse outcome. Severity of initial hematuria and pyuria were associated with favorable outcomes. Also in a univariate analysis, renal biopsy results associated with adverse outcomes were percentage of glomeruli with global sclerosis or segmental sclerosis or adhesions, the degree of tubular atrophy or interstitial fibrosis, interstitial inflammation, and blood-vessel thickening on light microscopy and intensity of IgA deposition on immunofluorescence. In a multivariate analysis, global glomerulosclerosis, segmental glomerulosclerosis or adhesions, and a combined mesangial and capillary wall deposition of IgM had independent adverse effects on renal outcome. At final assessment or during follow-up, the number of hyaline casts, degree of renal function impairment, degree of proteinuria, reduced serum IgG and IgM levels, decreased final IgA expressed as a percentage of initial IgA concentration, transient reductions in creatinine clearance of more than 10% or 20% during follow-up, and persistence or development of hypertension were associated with adverse outcomes in a univariate analysis. Favorable outcomes were associated with infection-related exacerbations of disease activity. Factors with independent adverse effects in a multivariate analysis were the degree of persistent microscopic hematuria, degree of renal function impairment, degree of proteinuria, reduced serum IgG levels, decreased final serum IgA expressed as a percentage of the initial IgA, and serum C3 levels.

Conclusions.—In general, IgA nephropathy appears to be a benign disease process. Progression to end-stage renal failure occurs infrequently. Initial clinical and laboratory findings, renal biopsy findings, and the disease course during follow-up can be used to predict progressive renal disease.

▶ Immunoglobulin A nephropathy is the most common cause of glomerulonephritis worldwide and a leading cause of renal failure in all countries. This scholarly review of its natural history, from the University of Sydney, Australia, reminds us that, in the main, the disease is benign and indolent. After a median of 8 years, 70% of patients had unimpaired renal function, though hematuria usually persisted and only 10% entered a sustained remission. Nephrotic-range proteinuria (as in other forms of glomerulonephritis) was associated with a worse prognosis, as was persistent hypertension and glomerular or interstitial scarring seen in the renal biopsy. Thirteen patients were treated with immunosuppressive drugs, but no benefit was discerned. In a recent publication, however, patients with IgA nephropathy and heavy proteinuria were reported to do better when treated with fish oil (1). We will have more on this next year.—F.H. Epstein, M.D.

Reference

1. Donadio JV Jr, et al: A controlled trial of fish oil in IgA nephropathy. *N Engl J Med* 331:1194–1199, 1994.

60 Other Diseases of the Kidney

Declining Incidence of Nephropathy in Insulin-Dependent Diabetes Mellitus

Bojestig M, Arnqvist HJ, Hermansson G, Karlberg BE, Ludvigsson J (Univ Hosp, Linköping, Sweden; Eksjö Hosp, Sweden)

N Engl J Med 330:15–18, 1994

119-95-60–1

Introduction.—Diabetic kidney disease is the main reason for the high relative mortality of patients with insulin-dependent diabetes mellitus. From 1950 to the early 1980s, the cumulative incidence of nephropathy among patients with a 25-year history of diabetes remained relatively stable—25% to 30%. However, some important changes in diabetes man-

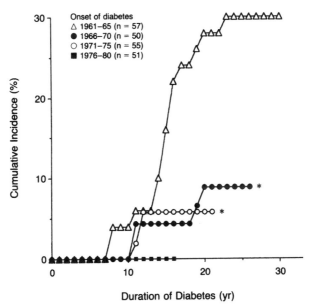

Fig 60–1.—Cumulative incidence of persistent albuminuria among patients in whom insulin-dependent diabetes began before the age of 15 years, according to the year of onset. Each *asterisk* denotes a significant difference in incidence ($P = .01$) between the group indicated and the group with onset of diabetes from 1961 to 1965. (Courtesy of Bojestig M, Arnqvist HJ, Hermansson G, et al: *N Engl J Med* 330:15–18, 1994.)

agement have occurred in recent years, including self-monitoring, better education, and better adjustment of treatment to the patient's lifestyle.

Methods.—A prospective, population-based, follow-up study examined recent trends in the incidence of diabetic nephropathy. The study included 213 Swedish patients with a diagnosis of insulin-dependent diabetes mellitus between 1961 and 1980. One hundred ninety-seven of these patients were followed up from the onset of their diabetes until 1991 or until they died. Diabetic nephropathy was considered present in patients with persistent albuminuria, as indicated by a positive Albustix test. Beginning in 1980, all patients had periodic measurement of glycosylated hemoglobin.

Findings.—For patients with a 25-year history of diabetes, the cumulative incidence of persistent albuminuria fell from 30% in those with a diagnosis between 1961 and 1965 to 8.9% for those with a diagnosis from 1966 to 1970. For patients with a 20-year history, the cumulative incidence was 28% for those with a diagnosis between 1961 and 1965 vs. 5.8% for those with a diagnosis between 1971 and 1975. None of the study patients with a diagnosis in 1976 or after had had persistent albuminuria by 1991 (Fig 60–1). The average glycosylated hemoglobin measurement fell from 7.4% in 1980–1985 to 7% in 1986–1991. The mean values for patients with and without persistent albuminuria were 8.1% vs. 7.1%, respectively.

Conclusions.—For patients with long-standing insulin-dependent diabetes mellitus, the cumulative incidence of diabetic nephropathy appears to have fallen dramatically in the last decade. The difference appears to be the result of improvements in glycemic control and not related to antihypertensive treatment.

▶ Dramatic changes seem to have occurred over a period of 15 years in the late development of proteinuria in Swedish children with diabetes, as illustrated in Figure 60–1. The authors ascribe this to improved glycemic control. I am skeptical because glycosylated hemoglobin levels were identical in the 1961–1965 and the 1971–1975 cohorts, whereas persistent proteinuria was detected in 14 or 50 patients in the earlier group of patients and only 3 of 53 in the later one, as shown in Figure 60–1. I wonder, for example, whether there might have been a parallel decrease in nondiabetic albuminuria during this period of time in Sweden. Because microalbuminuria precedes the macro variety, it seems peculiar that the prevalence of *microal*-buminuria (20 to 200 μg/min)—unlike that of "persistent albuminuria" (detected by Albustix)—did *not* decline from 1961–1965 to 1976–1980.

If these findings were borne out by other studies, one would have the sense of a vast, poorly understood sea-change in disease epidemiology, comparable to the slow disappearance of tuberculosis prior to the introduction of streptomycin or to the decline over the past 50 years in the incidence of rheumatic heart disease. Somehow, I doubt it.—F.H. Epstein, M.D.

Necrotizing Medullary Lesions in Patients With ANCA Associated Renal Disease

Bonsib SM, Goeken JA, Fandel T, Houghton DC (The Univ of Iowa Hosp and Clinics, Iowa City; The Oregon Health Sciences Univ, Portland)
Mod Pathol 7:181–185, 1994   119-95-60–2

Introduction.—Antineutrophil cytoplasmic antibody (ANCA)-associated disease is a common and grave renal injury that most frequently is associated with necrotizing arteritis or necrotizing glomerulonephritis. However, examination of renal biopsy specimens revealed that ANCA-associated injury may also affect the renal medulla.

Methods.—Fifty-six specimens from renal biopsies, nephrectomies, and autopsies containing portions of the renal medulla were examined for necrotizing medullar lesions. The lesions were characterized, and medullary inflammation was graded. The cortical compartments were also examined for necrotizing lesions. Serologic analysis determined the presence of ANCA.

Results.—Eight of the 56 specimens had necrotizing lesions in the medulla; all 8 had ANCA-associated kidney disease. None of the specimens with antiglomerular basement membrane antibody-associated disease or combined antiglomerular basement membrane/ANCA-associated disease had necrotizing lesions in the medulla. The 8 patients had 4 types of necrotizing medullary lesions: medullary capillaritis (7 patients), necrotizing arteriolitis (2), pathergic granulomas (3), and papillary tip necrosis (1). The lesions in the 7 patients with medullary capillaritis contained leukocytoclastic neutrophils. Seven of the 8 patients also had glomerular capillaritis in the cortical tissue, which contained no immune deposits. Activity seen in the cortical lesions did not correlate with the severity of the medullar lesions.

Discussion.—Necrotizing medullary lesions developed in 2 major types of renal sites—vascular and stromal—and were always associated with ANCA-associated renal disease. Although cortical injury was also seen, there was marked discordance between the extent and sites of cortical and medullary lesions. Because severe glomerular disease was also present, it is unclear how much the medullar involvement contributed to the renal dysfunction.

▶ The message here is that interstitial and medullary damage may be prominent in the kidneys of patients with vasculitis, accompanying and even overshadowing the signature lesion of this disease: crescentic glomerulonephritis. The authors, all pathologists, do not mention the clinical correlations of these remarkable medullary lesions, but polyuria and polydipsia probably were present in some of their patients, in association with a disproportionate reduction in concentrating ability, as expected in selective medullary lesions. Nephrogenic diabetes insipidus was, in fact, reported as a complication of

polyarteritis nodosa by Hugh deWardener and his colleagues in 1955 (1).
—F.H. Epstein, M.D.

Reference

1. Darmady EM, Griffiths WJ, Mattingly D, Spencer H, Stranek F, DeWardener HE: Renal tubular failure associated with polyarteritis nodosa. *Lancet* 1:371–383, 1955.

Clinical Course of Late-Onset Bone Marrow Transplant Nephropathy

Cohen EP, Lawton CA, Moulder JE, Becker CG, Ash RC (Med College of Wisconsin, Milwaukee)

Nephron 64:626–635, 1993

119-95-60-3

Background.—Late-onset renal insufficiency occurs between 6 and 12 months after bone marrow transplantation. It is an increasingly recognized complication of bone marrow transplantation, and in this study, it occurred in 25% of 2-year survivors. It is characterized by azotemia, hypertension, and anemia. Late-onset renal insufficiency is labeled bone marrow transplantation nephropathy; its pathogenesis, clinical features, and evolution were described.

Methods.—The patients described survived more than 100 days after bone marrow transplantation. Fifteen patients received related-donor bone marrow, and 4 received unrelated-donor bone marrow. Cases were defined by azotemia, hypertension, and severe anemia occurring between 6 and 12 months after transplantation.

Results.—Of 149 patients who survived more than 100 days after transplantation, 19 had bone marrow nephropathy develop. Acute nephropathy developed in 4 patients who had a hemolytic-uremic–like syndrome. Nephropathy developed more slowly in 15 patients, with no ongoing hemolysis. In one third of the patients, stabilization of function occurred. Mesangial and endothelial cell dropout with widening of glomerular capillary loops was revealed by light microscopy and was similar in 11 cases. Electron microscopy revealed endothelial cell injury and extreme subendothelial expansion of the glomerular basement membrane.

Discussion.—This syndrome resembles acute radiation nephritis. If bone marrow transplantation nephropathy is a form of renal radiation injury, then other expressions of the injury may develop in other long-term survivors of bone marrow transplantation who receive total body irradiation. These patients will require life-long follow-up and periodic monitoring of kidney function and blood pressure.

▶ Late bone marrow transplant nephropathy is best understood as a form of radiation nephritis in which the injurious agent is not necessarily x-radiation but, rather, the radiomimetic cytotoxic drugs given to suppress the immune response. As in radiation nephritis, vascular endothelial cells are the susceptible target, and the clinical picture resembles accelerated vascular disease of the kidneys, not unlike scleroderma, that is apparent 6–12 months after the transplant and is characterized by disproportionate anemia and signs of intravascular hemolysis, including low or falling platelets and a high level of lactic dehydrogenase in the serum, derived from hemolyzing erythrocytes. In these respects, it is like the hemolytic-uremic syndrome associated with cyclosporine A (see Abstract 119-95-61–2), which typically occurs within the first 2 months of transplantation. Chronic, stable renal insufficiency and persistent hypertension are the fate of some patients who experience an initial decline followed by stabilization of renal function. There is no evidence that plasmapheresis or IgG help.—F.H. Epstein, M.D.

Neurohormonal and Hemodynamic Changes in Severe Cases of the Ovarian Hyperstimulation Syndrome
Balasch J, Arroyo V, Fábregues F, Saló J, Jiménez W, Paré JC, Vanrell JA (Hosp Clínic i Provincial, Univ of Barcelona, Spain)
Ann Intern Med 121:27–33, 1994   119-95-60–4

Background.—Severe ovarian hyperstimulation syndrome (OHSS) is a potentially life-threatening complication that occurs in 2% of women undergoing induced ovulation for in vitro fertilization. It is thought to result from increased capillary permeability, particularly within the ovarian circulation, which leads to the escape of intravascular fluid into the peritoneal cavity and subsequently reduced intravascular volume. There have been few investigations assessing the importance of systemic hemodynamics in this syndrome. The systemic hemodynamics, endogenous vasoactive neurohormonal factors, and renal function in OHSS were investigated in a prospective longitudinal study.

Method.—Thirty-one women with severe OHSS participated. During the syndrome, measurements were taken of mean arterial pressure; cardiac output; peripheral vascular resistance; hematocrit concentration; renal function; plasma renin activity; plasma aldosterone; norepinephrine; antidiuretic hormone; atrial natriuretic peptide and estradiol levels; and urinary concentrations of prostaglandin E_2 and 6-keto-prostaglandin F_1. The same measurements were done 4–5 weeks after recovery.

Results.—During OHSS, patients showed increased hematocrits (mean of the paired difference, .047; 95% confidence interval (CI), .029–0.064), decreased arterial pressures (-16.6 mm Hg; CI, -19.8 to -13.6), increased cardiac output (2.6 L/min; CI, 2.13–3.17), and reduced peripheral vascular resistance, compared with 4 weeks after recovery. Significantly increased levels of plasma renin activity and plasma concentrations of aldosterone, norepinephrine, antidiuretic hormone, and atrial natriuretic peptide levels were also associated with OHSS. Hemoconcentration occurred in 16 patients but not in the remaining 15, despite the fact that both groups showed similar values for arterial pressure, cardiac output, and peripheral vascular resistance. However, women with hemoconcentration showed higher levels of renin, norepinephrine, and antidiuretic hormone.

Conclusion.—The pathogenesis of OHSS is more complex than was previously thought. In addition to hemoconcentration resulting from the escape of fluid to extravascular spaces, the syndrome is consistently associated with significant arteriolar vasodilation. Because both disorders occur simultaneously, the result is a hyperdynamic circulatory dysfunction that typically brings arterial hypotension, increased cardiac output, reduced peripheral vascular resistance, and intense stimulation of the renin-angiotensin and sympathetic nervous systems, along with antidiuretic hormone. This in turn is counterbalanced by increased renal production of vasodilator prostaglandins, maintaining renal perfusion and glomerular filtration rates within normal limits. However, these systems encourage renal sodium and water retention, which contributes to edema.

▶ This fascinating syndrome is common enough on the wards of modern ob-gyn services that specialize in in vitro fertilization, but most internists are unfamiliar with it. It is characterized by rapidly accumulating ascites and edema, sometimes with pleural effusion, often together with severe abdominal pain referable to enlarged ovaries with ruptured, bleeding follicles. The ascitic fluid is high in protein, cytokines, and perhaps other agents that increase capillary permeability, such as vascular endothelial growth factor (1). Plasma renin is very high, and salt is retained. The syndrome resembles pregnancy in that cardiac output is high and systemic vascular resistance is low, possibly as a result of the high levels of circulating ovarian hormones. Acute renal failure may complicate the picture, especially if nonsteroidal anti-inflammatory drugs (NSAIDs) are given for pain, because they inhibit the renal synthesis of prostaglandins, which act as the first intrarenal line of defense of kidney function when renal perfusion is threatened (2).—F.H. Epstein, M.D.

References

1. McClure N, Healy DL, Rogers PA, et al: Vascular permeability growth factor as capillary permeability agent in ovarian hyperstimulation syndrome. *Lancet* 344:235–236, 1994.
2. Balasch J, Carmona F, Llach J, et al: Acute prerenal failure and liver dysfunction in a patient with severe ovarian hyperstimulation syndrome. *Hum Reprod* 5:348–351, 1990.

Eosinophils in Urine Revisited
Ruffing KA, Hoppes P, Blend D, Cugino A, Jarjoura D, Whittier FC (Pitt County Mem Hosp, Greenville, NC; Northeastern Ohio Univ, Rootstown; Affiliated Hosp, Canton, Ohio)
Clin Nephrol 41:163–166, 1994   119-95-60–5

Background.—In the past, authorities have suggested that eosinophiluria may be a useful test for diagnosing acute interstitial nephritis

---

Sensitivity and Specificity of > 1/100 Eosinophils in the
Urine for Patients With and Without the Diagnosis of AIN

	+AIN	−AIN
+TEST	6	10
(greater than 1% eosinophils)		
−TEST	9	26
(less than 1% eosinophils)		

$n = 51$. The sensitivity for this group of patients is 40%, and the specificity is 72%.

(Courtesy of Ruffing KA, Hoppes P, Blend D, et al: *Clin Nephrol* 41:163–166, 1994.)

(AIN). The use of urinary eosinophil analysis as a diagnostic indicator is attractive because the only other method for diagnosing AIN is renal biopsy. The sensitivity and specificity of this analysis are still in question.

Methods and Findings.—One hundred forty-eight patients with pyuria were initially studied. The patients were consecutively hospitalized and selected because they had white blood cells in the urine. Four percent had urinary eosinophilia of more than 1 eosinophil per 100 cells. None of these patients had AIN; therefore, the false positive rate was 4% and the specificity, 96%. However, in a select group of patients in whom AIN was suspected by a nephrology consultant, eosinophils were found in the urine of 6 of 15 patients with a confirmed diagnosis of AIN and in 10 of 36 patients with a different renal diagnosis. In this group, the sensitivity of this analysis was 40% and the specificity, 72%, with a positive predictive value of only 38% (table). Both Hansel's and Wright's stain were used to detect eosinophils.

Conclusions.—The positive predictive value of eosinophiluria in a screening sample was too low and the number of false positives and negatives in a select group too high to confirm the diagnosis of AIN. It cannot accurately be used alone in making this diagnosis.

▶ This conclusion agrees with my own experience. Urinary eosinophilia may not be present in patients with interstitial nephritis and, if eosinophils are seen in the urinary sediment, they are not necessarily specific for that condition. Renal biopsy is the best way to make the diagnosis of acute interstitial nephritis.—F.H. Epstein, M.D.

61 Acute Renal Failure

Effects of Atrial Natriuretic Peptide in Clinical Acute Renal Failure
Rahman SN, Kim GE, Mathew AS, Goldberg CA, Allgren R, Schrier RW, Conger JD (Univ of Colorado Health Sciences Ctr, Denver)
Kidney Int 45:1731–1738, 1994   119-95-61–1

Introduction.—Several animal studies found that treatment with atrial natriuretic peptides (ANP) can reduce the severity and/or hasten recovery in experimental models of ischemic and nephrotoxic acute renal failure (ARF). The pharmacologic properties of ANP make the agent ideally suited to counteract reduced glomerular perfusion and tubular obstruction, two proposed pathophysiologic mechanisms of glomerular filtration rate (GFR) reduction in ARF. The potential benefits of ANP therapy were examined in 53 patients with ARF.

Methods.—Patients from 3 hospitals who had been given a diagnosis of established intrinsic ARF entered the study. Criteria for entry included an increase in serum creatinine of more than 0.7 mg/dL/day for at least 3 days, to a level of more than 2.5 mg/dL; urinary Na greater than 20

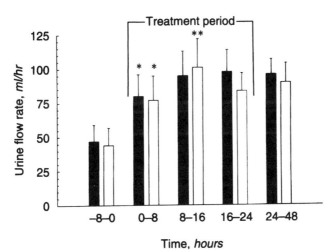

Fig 61–1.—Changes in mean urine flow rates for group I (ANP, *solid bar*) and group II (control, *open bar*) patients with treatment. Significant increases in the urine flow rates in both groups occurred in the first 8 hours of treatment (*$P < .05$). There was a further increase in urine flow rate between 8 and 16 hours of treatment only in group II (**$P < .05$). (Courtesy of Rahman SN, Kim GE, Mathew AS, et al: *Kidney Int* 45:1731-1738, 1994.)

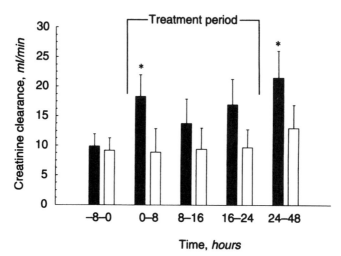

Fig 61–2.—Changes in creatinine clearances in group I (ANP, *solid bar*) and group II (control, *open bar*) patients with treatment. There was a significant increase in creatinine clearance in the first 8 hours of treatment only in group I compared with baseline and group II (*P < .05). The creatinine clearance increase was again significantly greater in group I than the preinfusion or corresponding group II value during the 24 hours after treatment. There were no significant changes in creatinine clearance in group II. (Courtesy of Rahman SN, Kim GE, Mathew AS, et al: *Kidney Int* 45:1731–1738, 1994.)

mEa/L; a urine to serum creatinine ratio less than 20: and urinary sediment typical of acute tubular necrosis. Those in group I were treated with human ANP with or without diuretics. Group II patients were treated with or without diuretics and no ANP. Administration of ANP was either intrarenally through catheters placed in both renal arteries (.08 μg/kg/min for 8 hours) or IV at an initial dose of .08 μg/kg/min, which was increased in 30-minute steps to a final dose of .16 to .24 μg/kg/min for 24 hours. Diuretic infusion (IV furosemide or mannitol given for 24 hours) was begun at the same time as ANP. Creatinine clearance was measured to detect changes in effective GFR.

Results.—The 2 groups were similar in age, sex, etiology of ARF, and entry serum creatinine and creatinine clearance. The mean urine flow rates significantly increased in both groups during the first 8 hours of treatment (Fig 61–1). Overall, there were no differences in urine flow rate between group I and II patients before, during, or after treatment. Creatinine clearance, however, increased significantly in group I patients during the first 8 hours of ANP therapy and by 24 hours after discontinuing therapy. Group II patients showed no corresponding increase in creatinine clearance (Fig 61–2). Significantly fewer patients required dialysis in group I (23%) than in group II (52%). There was a nonsignificant trend toward improved survival in group I.

Conclusion.—Short-term parenteral infusions of ANP improved creatinine clearance and significantly reduced the need for dialysis in patients with established intrinsic ARF. Mortality was lower in patients who received ANP (17% vs. 35%), but the difference was not significant.

▶ After all the work that Dr. John Conger and his conscientious crew of collaborators at 3 affiliated hospitals went through to collect 53 patients with ARF over a period of at least 3 years, I'm sorry that I am underwhelmed by the results. Atrial natriuretic peptide just didn't seem to make much of a difference in this series, in which it was given after the diagnosis of ARF was established. Moreover, you will note that the average urine flow in these patients at baseline, both treated with ANF and untreated, was more than 1,000 mL/day—not exactly oliguric renal failure. Dr. Conger tells me that in the patients with true oliguric acute renal failure—less than 400 mL/day of urinary output—no trend to benefit of any kind was noted. These negative results are in accord with the failure of ANF to improve early renal function in transplanted kidneys (1). It's too bad, because you'd think that a vasodilator with specific renal receptors that increases GFR promptly in normal kidneys would be just the thing for the presumed functional glomerular shutdown in acute renal failure. Evidently, once ARF is established, changes occur within the damaged kidney that are very difficult to reverse acutely.—F.H. Epstein, M.D.

Reference

1. Ratcliffe PJ, Richardson AJ, Kirby JE, et al: Effect of intravenous infusion of atriopeptin 3 on immediate renal allograft function. *Kidney Int* 39:164–168, 1991.

Transplant-Associated Thrombotic Microangiopathy: The Role of IgG Administration as Initial Therapy
Hochstetler LA, Flanigan MJ, Lager DJ (Univ of Iowa, Iowa City)
Am J Kidney Dis 23:444–450, 1994   119-95-61–2

Background.—Thrombotic microangiopathy may be clinically apparent as thrombotic thrombocytopenic purpura (TTP) or hemolytic uremic syndrome (HUS). Hemolytic uremic syndrome/thrombotic thrombocytopenic purpura carries mortality rates as high as 50%. Among the many treatments that have been tried, IV IgG has reportedly benefited adult patients with TTP.

Two Cases.—Two transplant recipients with cyclosporine-associated thrombotic microangiopathy were successfully treated by IV IgG as cyclosporine was continued. One patient who had juvenile-onset diabetes received a renal-pancreas graft, and the other patient received a liver allograft for cryptogenic cirrhosis. Graft function was maintained in both patients, and neither had recurrent microangiopathy.

Clinical Series.—Twenty-one of 512 cadaver kidney recipients (4.1%) had clinical symptoms of HUS/TTP and supportive histopathologic findings. Eleven of the patients had diabetes. All the patients had received prednisone, azathioprine, and cyclosporine as immunosuppression. Hemolytic uremic syndrome/thrombotic thrombocytopenic purpura was diagnosed from 2 to 56 days (mean, 28 days) after transplantation. The patients were not universally febrile or cognitively compromised, and the laboratory findings varied widely. Cyclosporine was withdrawn in 10 cases and the dose was reduced in 6 others. Nevertheless, 5 patients (24%) died and 7 transplants were removed. New IgM anti-cytomegalovirus antibody developed in 42% of the patients during the acute illness.

Conclusion.—Intravenous IgG administration may be an effective means of treating transplant recipients who have HUS/TTP while maintaining graft function.

▶ While the administration of IgG coincided with remission of the signs of TTP in the 2 patients cited here, I am not impressed with its general usefulness in producing improvement in this post-transplant syndrome associated with cyclosporine treatment. In this report, the low dose of cyclosporine was reduced further in one patient in conjunction with IgG therapy, and in both patients active cytomegalovirus infection appeared to be at least partly responsible for the microangiopathic picture. The paper is important, however, because it calls attention to a fairly common cause of renal deterioration occurring up to 2 months after transplantation in patients receiving cyclosporine A. The diagnosis should be suspected when microangiopathic hemolytic anemia, an elevated lactic dehydrogenase level, thrombocytopenia, and a falling platelet count are present. A definitive diagnosis can be made from the renal biopsy specimen, which shows platelet-fibrin thrombi in small blood vessels and glomerular capillaries. This vascular pathology is part of the spectrum of cyclosporine toxicity and has also been seen in patients treated with FK-506. Concurrent cytomegalovirus infection may predispose to the syndrome, and it should be noted that vasculitis is a recognized feature of systemic cytomegalovirus disease (1). Because the picture is not easily distinguished from acute vascular rejection, even on biopsy, many patients are treated by reducing or withdrawing cyclosporine A and giving OKT3 (Ortho Biotech Inc., Raritan, NJ) for rejection. Perhaps, as these authors suggest, IgG should also be tried.—F.H. Epstein, M.D.

Reference

1. Golden MP, Hammer SM, Wanke CA, Albrecht MA: Cytomegalovirus vasculitis: Case reports and review of the literature. *Medicine* 73:246–255, 1994.

Unilateral Nephrectomy and Cisplatin as Risk Factors of Ifosfamide-Induced Nephrotoxicity: Analysis of 120 Patients
Rossi R, Gödde A, Kleinebrand A, Riepenhausen M, Boos J, Ritter J, Jürgens

H (Univ Children's Hosp, Münster, Germany)
J Clin Oncol 12:159–165, 1994   119-95-61–3

Introduction.—Patients treated with ifosfamide for childhood malignancies are at risk for subsequent renal damage. Complete renal Fanconi's syndrome is reported to occur with a frequency of 1.4% to 5% after ifosfamide, but severe tubular dysfunction is more common. Children treated with chemotherapy including ifosfamide were studied to identify risk factors for renal damage.

Patients and Methods.—The 120 patients had a median age of 11 years at the start of treatment. All had not been receiving chemotherapy for at least 3 months (median, 13 months) and were free of malignant disease at the first renal examination. Ewing's/soft tissue sarcoma (33 cases) and osteosarcoma (24 cases) were the most common primary diagnoses. The median cumulative dose of ifosfamide was 30 g/m². In addition to this drug, 68 patients had been treated with gentamicin, 57 with methotrexate, and 51 with cisplatin. The glomerular filtration rate and serum bicarbonate levels were measured and proximal tubular function assessed in all patients during follow-up.

Results.—Results of all renal tests were normal in only one third of the patients. Proximal tubular dysfunction, as measured by percent amino acid reabsorption, was present in 66.3% of the patients; fractional reabsorption of phosphate yielded a 38.3% rate of dysfunction. Glomerular impairment and acidosis were less frequent findings. Seven patients had renal Fanconi's syndrome resulting in hypophosphatemic bone disease, and 15 had generalized tubulopathy. Both disorders were diagnosed over a wide range of time (.5 to 7.3 years) after completion of chemotherapy. Unilateral nephrectomy had been performed in 10 patients, and this procedure was the single most important risk factor for renal dysfunction. Cisplatin also increased the risk for ifosfamide-mediated nephrotoxicity.

Conclusion.—Ifosfamide is widely used in the treatment of childhood malignancy. This series of patients treated with the drug had a high incidence of renal abnormalities. Renal Fanconi's syndrome was identified in 5.7% and severe tubular dysfunction in another 12.5%. Unilateral nephrectomy and concomitant cisplatin significantly increase the risk of ifosfamide-induced nephrotoxicity.

▶ Ifosfamide is widely used in treating malignancies in children because of its supposed efficacy as compared with cyclophosphamide. The drug is accumulated by proximal tubules and, as a result, the renal toxicity that it causes is characterized by proximal tubular dysfunction, i.e., Fanconi's syndrome. Hypophosphatemia with renal phosphate wasting is the most common manifestation, and aminoaciduria is also frequently seen. Glucosuria and acidosis are less often encountered, and frank azotemia is rare. Cisplatinum is often administered simultaneously as part of the cancer chemotherapy regimen, and because platinum toxicity is specifically localized to the straight portion of the proximal tubule, this combination especially predisposes to the toxic Fanconi's syndrome. In many patients the damage is permanent, and oral phosphate supplements are indicated to bring the serum phosphorus to or toward normal levels. Because a reduction in renal mass increases the risk of ifosfamide toxicity, this drug should be given to patients with caution and in reduced dosage after unilateral nephrectomy.—F.H. Epstein, M.D.

62 Chronic Renal Failure

The Effects of Dietary Protein Restriction and Blood-Pressure Control on the Progression of Chronic Renal Disease
Klahr S, for the Modification of Diet in Renal Disease Study Group (Washington Univ, St Louis, Mo)
N Engl J Med 330:877–884, 1994   119-95-62–1

Objective.—Animal studies have found that protein restriction and and control of hypertension can delay the progression of renal disease.

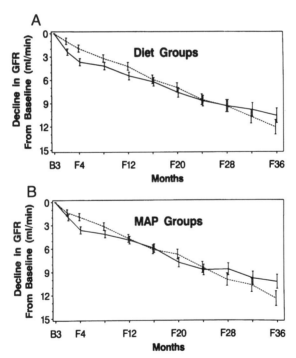

Fig 62–1.—Estimated mean (± SE) decline in the glomerular filtration rate from baseline (B) to selected follow-up times (F) in study 1. **A**, patients assigned to the usual-protein diet (*dashed line*) are compared with those assigned to the low-protein diet (*solid line*). **B**, patients assigned to the usual-blood-pressure group (*dashed line*) are compared with those assigned to the low-blood-pressure group (*solid line*). To correct for any bias introduced by stopping points, the mean declines were estimated by the maximum-likelihood method with a two-slope model for the covariance matrix of the serial measurements of the glomerular filtration rate. (Courtesy of Klahr S, for the Modification of Diet in Renal Disease Study Group: *N Engl J Med* 330:877–884, 1994.)

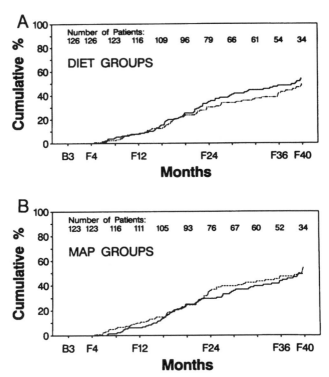

Fig 62–2.—The occurrence of end-stage renal disease (ESRD) or death in patients in study 2. **A,** patients assigned to the low-protein diet (*solid line*) are compared with those assigned to the very-low-protein diet (*dashed and dotted line*) (P = .62). **B,** patients in the usual-blood-pressure group (*dash line*) are compared with those in the low-blood-pressure group (*solid line*) (P = .33). The numbers below each panel indicate the total number of patients in the 2 groups being compared at each baseline (B) or follow-up (F) visit. The relative risk of ESRD or death was .93 (95% confidence interval, .65–1.33 for the patients assigned to the very-low-protein diet as compared with those assigned to the low-protein-diet, and it was .85 (95% confidence interval, .6–1.22) for the patients in the low-blood-pressure group, as compared with those in the usual-blood-pressure group. (Courtesy of Klahr S, for the Modification of Diet in Renal Disease Study Group: N Engl J Med 330:877–884, 1994.)

Studies of this issue in humans have been hampered by methodologic problems. The results of the Modification of Diet in Renal Disease (MDRD) Study, in which 840 patients with various renal diseases were randomized as to dietary protein intake and blood pressure control, were reported.

Methods.—The MDRD Study consisted of 2 randomized, multicenter trials. The first trial included 585 patients, all with glomerular filtration rates of 25 to 55 mL/min/1.73 m². They received either a usual-protein or a low-protein diet, consisting of 1.3 vs. .58 g/kg/day. They were also assigned to a usual - or low-blood pressure group, with mean arterial pressure values of 107 and 92 mm Hg, respectively. In the second study, glomerular filtration rates were lower: 13 to 24 mL/min/1.73 m². One group received a low-protein diet of .58 g/kg/day, whereas the other received a very low-protein diet of .28 g/kg/day. Blood pressure groups were the same as in the first study. The patients were evaluated monthly over a mean follow-up of 2.2 years, based on the intention to treat.

Results.—The first study showed no difference between diet or blood pressure groups in the mean projected 3-year decrease in glomerular filtration rate. The low-protein group and the low-blood pressure group did show a more rapid decline in glomerular filtration rate during the first 4 months of the study, after which the decline showed (Fig 62–1). The second study revealed a marginally slower decline in the very low-protein group than in the low-protein group. However, no difference was observed in time to end-stage renal disease or death (Fig 62–2). Patients in the low-blood pressure group of both studies who had more advanced proteinuria at baseline had a significantly slower rate of decline in glomerular filtration rate. All of the protein restriction and blood pressure interventions were well tolerated.

Conclusions.—A low-protein diet may slow the decline in renal function somewhat in patients with moderate renal insufficiency. In patients with more severe renal insufficiency, a very low-protein diet does not even have this small benefit. In patients with urinary protein excretion of more than 1 g/day, maintaining blood pressure at a low level may be of some benefit.

▶ The most important stimulus to the organization of this huge study of protein restriction in more than 1,500 patients with renal insufficiency was the clear demonstration that a low-protein diet slows the progression of renal disease in rats (1). It's apparent from the present paper that restriction of dietary protein has far less dramatic effects on human renal disease—the outcome after 2–3 years was essentially the same in patients whose diet was severely restricted in protein as in their controls. Consistent with the well-known short-term effect of a protein meal to increase glomerular filtration rate (GFR), an immediate consequence of protein restriction was a slight *fall* in GFR, presumably functional in nature, followed by a slightly slower decline than that observed in control patients eating more protein. Five and 10 months after completion of the original 3-year study, a cohort of 302 patients was reexamined, but again, no statistically significant difference attributable to protein restriction was evident (2).

A reasonable conclusion for the working clinician, I think, is that if there is any effect of protein restriction of this degree (0.3 to 0.5 g of protein per kg per day) on the progression of human renal failure, it is small and, at least for several years, not important. Therapeutic efforts and the patients' energy, resources, and resolve will be better spent in controlling blood pressure, especially, perhaps, with inhibitors of the action or formation of angiotensin II. Other strategies to reduce the slow but inexorable progress of glomerular and interstitial scarring deserve investigation.—F.H. Epstein, M.D.

References

1. Brenner BM: Nephron adaptation to renal injury or ablation. *Am J Physiol* 249:F324–F337, 1985.
2. Levey AS, Beck GI, Caggiula AW, et al: Trends toward a beneficial effect of a low protein diet during additional follow-up in the modification of diet in renal disease study (Abstract). *J Am Soc Nephrol* 5:336, 1994.

The Effect of Angiotensin-Converting-Enzyme Inhibition on Diabetic Nephropathy

Lewis EJ, for the Collaborative Study Group (Rush-Presbyterian-St Luke's Med Ctr, Chicago)
N Engl J Med 329:1456–1462, 1993   119-95-62–2

Background.—Patients with diabetic nephropathy have a progressive decline in renal function. Antihypertensive drugs may slow this decline. Whether captopril has kidney-protecting properties independent of its effect on blood pressure in patients with diabetic nephropathy was determined.

Methods.—Four hundred nine patients were enrolled in a randomized, controlled study. Eligibility criteria included age between 18 and 49 years; insulin-dependent diabetes mellitus for at least 7 years, with an onset before age 30 years; diabetic retinopathy; and urinary protein excretion of 500 mg/day or more. All patients meeting these criteria during a single examination were eligible, regardless of previous blood-pressure status or a previous need for antihypertensive medication. Captopril, 25 mg, was given three times daily to 207 patients, and placebo was given to 202 patients, for a median of 3 years.

Findings.—Serum creatinine levels doubled in 25 patients given captopril and in 43 patients given placebo. Associated decreases in the risk of the serum creatinine concentration doubling were 48% in all patients receiving captopril, 76% in the subgroup whose baseline serum creatinine level was 2 mg/dL, 55% in the subgroup whose concentration was 1.5 mg/dL, and 17% in the subgroup whose concentration was 1 mg/dL. The mean rate of decline in creatinine clearance was 11% per year in patients given captopril and 17% in those given placebo. In patients whose baseline serum creatinine levels were 1.5 mg/dL or higher, creatinine clearance dropped by a mean of 23% per year in the captopril group and 37% per year in the placebo group. Captopril therapy was associated with a 50% decrease in the risk of combined end points of death, dialysis, and transplantation independent of the small disparity in blood pressure between groups (Fig 62–3).

Conclusions.—Captopril protects against renal function deterioration in patients with insulin-dependent diabetic nephropathy. It is significantly more effective than blood-pressure control alone.

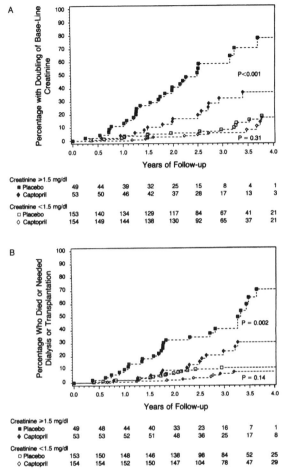

Fig 62–3.—Cumulative incidence of events in patients with diabetic nephropathy in the captopril and placebo groups, according to the baseline serum creatinine concentration. A total of 102 patients had a baseline serum creatinine concentration of ≥ 1.5 mg/dL, and 307 had a baseline serum creatinine concentration below 1.5 mg/dL. **A,** the cumulative percentage of patients in each subgroup who had a doubling of the serum creatinine concentration to at least 2 mg/dL is shown. **B,** the cumulative percentage of patients in each subgroup who died or required dialysis or renal transplantation is shown. The *numbers* at the bottom of the figure are the numbers of patients in each subgroup at risk for the event at baseline and after each 6-month period. (Courtesy of Lewis EJ, for the Collaborative Study Group: N Engl J Med 329:1456-1462, 1993.)

▶ It is well known that a decrease in glomerular capillary pressure generally diminishes proteinuria, and angiotensin-converting enzyme (ACE) inhibitors tend to be more effective than other antihypertensive agents in decreasing protein excretion, because they selectively dilate the efferent glomerular arteriole in addition to producing systemic vasodilatation. What has not been known previously, however, is whether over the long term ACE inhibitors do a better job than other means of controlling blood pressure in reducing the rate of progression of chronic renal failure. This paper strongly suggests that they do, at least in insulin-dependent diabetes with proteinuria. Note that the beneficial effect of captopril to postpone progression of renal insufficiency was most pronounced in patients who already had some diminution in renal function (serum creatinine greater than 1.5 mg/dL). In those with less marked renal impairment, the advantage of captopril was not statistically significant, though perhaps with a follow-up longer than 4 years a significant difference would emerge.

The beneficial effect of ACE inhibition is probably related at least in part to the actions of angiotensin II to promote endothelial and medial proliferation in small blood vessels and to induce expression of transforming growth factor-beta (TGF-β), which in turn stimulates scar formation and the synthesis of extracellular matrix (1). Angiotensin-converting enzyme inhibition (this time with enalapril) has also been shown to have a long-term stabilizing effect on plasma creatinine in adult-onset diabetic patients whose blood pressure is normal (2) and in nondiabetic patients with nephrotic proteinuria (3), especially those with IgA nephropathy (4). A caveat is that soon after treatment is initiated, both in normotensive and hypertensive patients, creatinine clearance often falls—a functional change that is usually reversible when the medication is discontinued but which may be dangerous for patients who are already close to the brink of renal failure.—F.H. Epstein, M.D.

References

1. Kagami S, Border WA, Miller DE, Noble NA: Angiotensin II stimulates extracellular matrix protein synthesis through induction of transforming growth factor-beta expression in rat glomerular mesangial cells. *J Clin Invest* 93:2431–2437, 1994.
2. David RM, Savin H, Jutrin I, et al: Long-term stabilizing effect of angiotensin-converting enzyme inhibition on plasma in creatinine and on proteinuria in normotensive type II diabetic patients. *Ann Intern Med* 118:577–581, 1993.
3. Praga M, Hernandez E, Montoya C, et al: Long-term beneficial effects of angiotensin-converting enzyme inhibition in patients with nephrotic proteinuria. *Am J Kidney Dis* 20:240–248, 1992.
4. Cattran DC, Greenwood C, Ritchie S: Long-term benefits of angiotensin-converting enzyme inhibitor therapy in patients with severe immunoglobulin A nephropathy: A comparison to patients receiving treatment with other antihypertensive agents and to patients receiving no therapy. *Am J Kidney Dis* 23:247–254, 1994.

Systemic Distribution of β_2-Microglobulin–Derived Amyloidosis in Patients Who Undergo Long-Term Hemodialysis: Report of Seven Cases and Review of the Literature

Gal R, Korzets A, Schwartz A, Rath-Wolfson L, Gafter U (Golda Med Ctr, Petah Tiqva, Israel)
Arch Pathol Lab Med 118:718–721, 1994　　　　　119-95-62-3

Background.—Patients undergoing long-term hemodialysis may have a form of amyloidosis, termed hemodialysis-associated amyloidosis

(HAA), in which β_2-microglobulin is the principal protein component of amyloid. The osteoarticular system is predominantly affected. Patients who are affected may have carpal tunnel syndrome, bone cysts, or destructive spondyloarthropathy.

Objective.—Visceral amyloid deposits were sought in 20 patients autopsied after having received hemodialysis for 4 years or longer. The 16 men and 4 women were aged 40–80 years. Seven of the 20 patients had been receiving dialysis for longer than 10 years. Cuprophane dialyzers were used exclusively.

Findings.—All 7 patients who underwent dialysis for longer than 10 years, but none of the 13 treated for shorter times, had visceral HAA. Amyloid was found chiefly in the blood vessel walls. The heart and gastrointestinal tract each were involved in 6 of 7 cases, and the lungs were involved in 5 cases. The deposits either encircled the vessels and replaced the muscular layer or bulged into the vessel lumen. Two patients who underwent dialysis for 20 and 21 years, respectively, had massive visceral amyloid deposits. The deposits stained positively with antiserum to β_2-microglobulin and negatively with antisera to amyloid protein A, kappa and lambda light chains, and prealbumin.

Conclusion.—Visceral HAA is found only after 10 or more years of hemodialysis and involves mainly the blood vessels of the heart, gastrointestinal tract, and lungs.

▶ The favorite site of β_2-microglobulin deposition in hemodialysis-related amyloidosis is, of course, the bones and joints, with carpal tunnel syndrome its most common clinical manifestation. This useful autopsy study reminds us that visceral amyloidosis may also complicate the long-term retention of β_2-microglobulin, especially in patients who have been dialyzed for more than 10 years. The distribution of amyloid in such patients is mainly in the walls of blood vessels, particularly in the gastrointestinal (GI) tract, lungs, and heart. The important clinical consequences most often involve the GI tract, occasionally causing intestinal perforation. It is interesting and surprising that the spleen is spared in this form of amyloidosis.—F.H. Epstein, M.D.

Impairment of Cardiac Function and Energetics in Experimental Renal Failure

Raine AEG, Seymour A-ML, Roberts AFC, Radda GK, Ledingham JGG (John Radcliffe Hosp, Oxford, England)
J Clin Invest 92:2934–2940, 1993   119-95-62-4

Background.—During chronic renal failure, cardiac energetics may be abnormal, leading to impaired cardiac performance and increased susceptibility to ischemia. Because interpretation of studies performed in vivo may be complicated by reflex neural and hormonal effects, cardiac function, energetics, and susceptibility to ischemia were examined in experimental chronic uremia in vitro, using an isolated working heart preparation and ^{31}P nuclear MR (^{31}P NMR) imaging of hearts perfused by a modified Langendorff technique.

Methods and Findings.—Renal impairment was produced via subtotal nephrectomy in male Wistar rats. Sham-operated rats served as controls. Cardiac output of isolated hearts perfused with Krebs-Henseleit buffer was significantly lower at all levels of preload and afterload in the renal failure rats at 4 weeks after nephrectomy, as compared with the pair-fed, sham-operated control animals. In control rats, increased cardiac output paralleled increases in perfusate calcium (from .73 to 5.61 mmol/L), whereas uremic hearts failed in high calcium perfusate. The ^{31}P NMR spectra from hearts of renal failure and control rats during 30-minute normoxic Langendorff perfusion showed that basal phosphocreatine was decreased by 32% to 4.7 μmol/g wet wt. In addition, the phosphocreatine to adenosine triphosphate ratio was also reduced by 32% in uremic hearts. A notable reduction in phosphocreatine was observed in the uremic hearts during low flow ischemia. An accompanying marked increase of inosine into the coronary effluent was also observed (14.9 vs. 6.1 μM).

Conclusions.—Cardiac function is impaired in experimental renal failure, in association with aberrant cardiac energetics and increased susceptibility to ischemic damage. These derangements may be influenced by disordered myocardial calcium utilization.

▶ These experiments on the isolated hearts of rats with uremia of 4 weeks' duration bear on the clinical question of "uremic cardiomyopathy." There is some skepticism about whether such an entity exists, apart from the disturbances in cardiac function to be expected from anemia, hypertension, hypocalcemia, and fluid overload. The improvement in cardiac function observed in uremic patients after dialysis, for example, can be explained almost entirely by the rise in serum calcium achieved by dialysis (1).

The conclusion of this paper is that the experimental uremic state does indeed induce marked impairment of myocardial function that cannot be explained by anemia, hypertensive hypertrophy, or changes in the concentration of calcium perfusing the heart. Moreover, the changes were not mimicked simply by increasing to uremic levels the concentration of urea or creatinine in the fluid used to perfuse hearts from normal control rats. In addition, hearts from uremic animals were far more susceptible to ischemia than control hearts. It would be of great interest to see whether, for example, dietary control of serum phosphorus or intermittent dialysis to reduce uremia would normalize these cardiac abnormalities.—F.H. Epstein, M.D.

Reference

1. Henrich WL, Judron JM, Nixon JV: Increased ionized calcium and left ventricular contractility during hemodialysis. N Engl J Med 310:19–23, 1984.

Socioeconomic Status and End-Stage Renal Disease in the United States

Young EW, Mauger EA, Jiang K-H, Port FK, Wolfe RA (Univ of Michigan, Ann Arbor; US Renal Data System Coordinating Ctr)
Kidney Int 45:907–911, 1994   119-95-62–5

Introduction.—A number of recent studies have documented considerable variations in the incidence of treated end-stage renal disease (t-ESRD) in the United States. These variations are related to demographic factors such as race, age, sex, and place of residence. Blacks are known to have a higher incidence of t-ESRD and a lower socioeconomic status than whites. It was hypothesized that socioeconomic status might explain some of the effects of race on t-ESRD incidence.

Methods.—The United States Renal Data System (USRDS) was used to obtain demographic characteristics of incident cases of t-ESRD from 1983 to 1988. Socioeconomic status was based on the average race-specific, per capita income of the county of residence. The incidence of t-ESRD for individuals younger than 60 years of age was modeled as a log-linear function of socioeconomic and demographic factors.

Results.—Blacks made up 38% of the 80,172 incident cases of t-ESRD. For both blacks and whites, the majority of patients were men in the group 40-60 years of age. Relatively few white patients lived in counties with an average income less than $10,000, whereas relatively few blacks lived in counties with an average income more than $25,000.

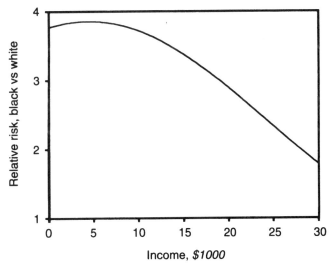

Fig 62–4.—Relative high risk of t-ESRD for blacks relative to whites at different levels of average race-specific, per capita county income. (Courtesy of Young EW, Mauger EA, Jiang K-H, et al: *Kidney Int* 45:907–911, 1994.)

After adjustment for other covariates, the adjusted incidence of t-ESRD varied significantly by geographic region for both races. Overall, there was an inverse relationship between the incidence of t-ESRD and income level. The relative risk at the lowest income level (as much as $10,000) was 1.21 for whites and 1.10 for blacks. At the highest income levels
(> $25,000), the relative risk of t-ESRD was .77 for whites and .69 for blacks. Without adjustment for per capita county income, the relative risk for blacks compared to whites was 3.78 (Fig 62–4). Adjustment for income lowered the relative risk for blacks to 3.38.

Conclusion.—Differences in socioeconomic status between blacks and whites explain some, but not most, of the racial differences in the incidence of t-ESRD. The inverse association between incidence of t-ESRD and socioeconomic status may be mediated by blood pressure, diabetes, and urban environmental characteristics. Although the majority of patients lived in urban counties, blacks were more likely than whites to live in an urban environment.

▶ End-stage renal disease hits hardest among the poor and the elderly. Men are more susceptible than women, and blacks more so than whites. That is the gist of most epidemiological studies dealing with chronic renal failure. The effect of poverty is definite, but the reasons are not clear; they may have to do with crowding, infection, or inadequate preventive and treatment measures. The incidence of renal failure rises with age, as would be expected of any chronic disease in which scarring progresses over time. The predisposing effect of the male sex must have a biological cause that we do not yet understand; it is apparent in other animals as well as in man. The special susceptibility of blacks is not entirely explained by their socioeconomic distribution, and it may be related to a racial propensity to hypertension or to small inherited differences in inflammatory or desmoplastic response.—F.H. Epstein, M.D.

63 Hypertension

Linkage of the Angiotensinogen Gene to Essential Hypertension
Caulfield M, Lavender P, Farrall M, Munroe P, Lawson M, Turner P, Clark AJL
(St Bartholomew's Hosp, London; Royal Postgraduate Med School, London)
N Engl J Med 330:1629–1633, 1994   119-95-63–1

Background.—The renin-angiotensin system has an important role in regulating vascular tone and cardiovascular remodeling, as well as salt and water homeostasis. As such, it is involved in the control of blood pressure. Angiotensinogen, or renin substrate, is a key part of the system. It is cleaved by renin to yield angiotensin I, which in turn is cleaved by angiotensin-converting enzyme to form angiotensin II. Observations that plasma angiotensinogen levels correlate with blood pressure and track through families indicate that angiotensinogen may have a role in the development of essential hypertension.

Objective and Methods.—To determine whether the angiotensinogen gene on chromosome 1q42-43 is linked with essential hypertension, samples of DNA were obtained from 63 white families of European origin in which at least 2 persons had essential hypertension. When possible, affected cousins, nephews, nieces, and half-siblings were investigated. Linkage was sought using a dinucleotide-repeat sequence flanking the angiotensinogen gene as a marker. The affected-pedigree-member approach to linkage analysis was used. Linkage also was sought for 2 molecular variants of the angiotensinogen gene, one encoding threonine rather than methionine at position 235 (M235T), and the other encoding methionine rather than threonine at position 174 (T174M).

Findings.—Significant linkage was established between essential hypertension and the angiotensinogen-gene locus (Fig 63–1). Linkage was maintained in family members having diastolic blood pressures higher than 100 mm Hg, as well as in both male-male and female-female pairs. No association was found between essential hypertension and either M235T or T174M.

Conclusion.—Regions within or near the angiotensinogen gene on chromosome 1q42-43 now have been linked with essential hypertension.

▶ Clinicians have long known that essential hypertension runs in families and is therefore probably inherited. However, the fact that there is a continuous (i.e., smooth) distribution curve of blood pressure in the population indicates that the genetic basis of essential hypertension is polygenic and thus does not follow simple mendelian patterns of inheritance. Several genes probably

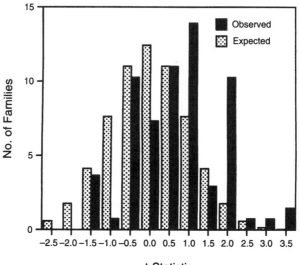

t-Statistic

Fig 63–1.—Distribution of the observed and expected frequencies of shared alleles, as indicated by the t-statistic, in 63 multiplex families with essential hypertension. The t-statistic tests whether affected relatives share alleles at the angiotensinogen locus more often than would be expected by chance. The observed scores are shifted to the right, suggesting a linkage between the angiotensinogen gene and essential hypertension. (Courtesy of Caulfield M, Lavender P, Farrall M, et al: N Engl J Med 330:1629–1633, 1994.)

interact with environmental stimuli; to produce hypertension in those predisposed. Candidate genes might well include those associated with the renin-angiotensin system, e.g., those encoding for angiotensinogen, renin, angiotensin II receptors or angiotensinogen-converting enzyme.

This study and an earlier one (1), both limited to Caucasians, suggest an association between mutations that are either in or close to the angiotensinogen gene, and essential hypertension. Its significance is enhanced by reports that the mutations of the angiotensinogen gene are detected in disproportionate numbers in human pre-eclampsia (2), by the observation that elevated blood pressure tracks with high plasma levels of angiotensinogen in families (3), and by the production of hypertension in transgenic mice with overexpression of the angiotensinogen gene (4).

These findings are placed in perspective by an accompanying editorial in the *New England Journal of Medicine:* "Whenever a linkage-based analytic algorithm is used, we must remember that the test encompasses not only the candidate gene, but also an entire chromosomal region that contains tens or even hundreds of other genes. Thus, the present data are entirely compatible with the possibility of linkage to an as yet unidentified gene in close proximity to the angiotensinogen gene on chromosome 1, thereby raising another note of caution for proper interpretation of the data: demonstration of linkage by itself, even if confirmed, can never implicate one particular gene . . . Although the consistent tenor of a series of papers instills some confidence, it does not outweigh concern aroused by methods and statistical analysis that are less than robust. We need larger-scale, prospective investigations that will provide the analytic stringency essential to the study of polygenic disease" (5).

The next abstract (Abstract 119-95-63-2) provides an encouraging bit of confirmation. The same molecular variant of the angiotensinogen gene has now been shown to be significantly more common in hypertensive patients in Japan than in normotensive Japanese controls.—F.H. Epstein, M.D.

References

1. Jeunemaitre X, Soubrier F, Kotelvtsev YV, et al: Molecular basis of human hypertension: Role of angiotensinogen. *Cell* 71:169–180, 1992.
2. Ward K, Hata A, Jeunemaitre X, et al: A molecular variant of angiotensinogen associated with pre-eclampsia. *Nat Genet* 4:59–61, 1993.
3. Watt GCM, Harrap SB, Foy CJW, et al: Abnormalities of glucocorticoid metabolism and the renin-angiotensin system: A four-corners approach to the identification of genetic determinants of blood pressure. *J Hypertens* 10:473–482, 1992.
4. Kimura S, Mullins JJ, Bunnemann B, et al: High blood pressure in transgenic mice carrying the rat angiotensinogen gene. *EMBO J* 11:821–827, 1992.
5. Lindpaintner K: Genes, hypertension, and cardiac hypertrophy. *N Engl J Med* 23:1678–1679, 1994.

Angiotensinogen as a Risk Factor for Essential Hypertension in Japan

Hata A, Namikawa C, Sasaki M, Sato K, Nakamura T, Tamura K, Lalouel J-M (Nagoya City Univ, Japan; Yamanashi Med Univ, Japan; Univ of Utah, Salt Lake City)

J Clin Invest 93:1285–1287, 1994   119-95-63-2

Background.—Elevated rates of essential hypertension and cerebrovascular accidents among the Japanese population results from the high level of sodium intake. However, genetic factors involving the renin-angiotensin system have also been implicated in essential hypertension. In Caucasians, a common molecular variant of angiotensinogen (AGT), the precursor of the potent vasoactive hormone angiotensin II, appears to be a marker for a genetic predisposition to essential hypertension. The same variant is now reported to be associated with essential hypertension in Japanese patients.

Methods.—One hundred and five patients with a mean age of 61 years and 81 normotensive controls with a mean age of 34 years were studied. All patients had established hypertension defined by a systolic blood pressure (BP) > 160 mm Hg and/or a diastolic BP > 95 mm Hg. None had secondary hypertension, renal disease, or diabetes mellitus. Hybridization of enzymatically amplified DNA with allele-specific oligonucleotides determined genotypes at residues 174 and 235 of AGT.

Results.—Allele T235 was significantly more common among hypertensive patients than in normotensive controls, with 79% of patients and 54% of controls homozygous for this allele. Normotensive Japanese showed a much higher frequency of allele T235 than normotensive Caucasians. The frequency of allele M174 did not significantly differ between patients and controls and was similar to the frequency reported for Caucasians.

Conclusion.—Allele T235 may behave as a global risk factor for essential hypertension in humans. However, it is not known whether T235 exerts this effect directly or serves as a marker for molecular variants of AGT that have yet to be identified. It may be that T235 is a marker for a salt-sensitive form of essential hypertension, given the involvement of AGT in salt homeostasis.

▶ The high incidence of the homozygous state for the suspect T235 angiotensinogen gene in *normotensive* Japanese controls (54% in normotensives vs. 79% in hypertensives) makes it virtually certain that other unmeasured environmental or genetic factors must be interacting in an important way with the T235 gene, if that gene is indeed a significant marker of susceptibility to high blood pressure.—F.H. Epstein, M.D.

The Diagnosis and Treatment of Baroreflex Failure

Robertson D, Hollister AS, Biaggioni I, Netterville JL, Mosqueda-Garcia R, Robertson RM (Vanderbilt Univ, Nashville, Tenn; Univ of Colorado Health Sciences Ctr, Denver)
N Engl J Med 329:1449–1455, 1993   119-95-63–3

Introduction.—The syndrome of baroreflex failure has often been confused with autonomic failure. The latter condition, however, is frequently associated with severe orthostatic hypotension, whereas baroreflex failure is dominated by volatile hypertension. The causes, clinical spectrum, and treatment were clarified in a prospective evaluation of 11 patients with dysfunction of the arterial baroreflexes.

Patients and Methods.—The patients identified were part of a group of approximately 500 patients evaluated for autonomic or blood pressure problems. Baroreflex failure was characterized by the inability of exogenous vasoactive substances to alter heart rate. Symptoms included severe, labile hypertension and hypotension, often with headache, flushing, and emotional instability. Those with diagnosed baroreflex failure underwent hemodynamic monitoring and biochemical, physiologic, and pharmacologic testing. Also studied were 12 normal subjects and 20 patients—8 with essential hypertension and 12 with autonomic failure resulting from the Bradbury-Eggleston syndrome.

Results.—The causes of baroreflex failure were neck irradiation in 3 cases, bilateral carotid-body tumors in 4 cases, section of a glossopharyngeal nerve in 1 case, bilateral destruction of the nucleus tractus solitarii in 1 case, and unknown in 2 cases. Maximal systolic blood pressures ranged from 164 to 280 mm Hg, and minimal systolic pressures from 58 to 96 mm Hg. The highest blood pressures were associated with the most severe symptoms. During blood pressure surges, plasma norepinephrine and epinephrine concentrations sometimes were many times normal. Excessive pressor and tachycardic responses to the mental arithmetic and cold pressor tests and marked hypersensitivity to clonidine were present in all patients. Most findings in patients with baroreflex failure differed substantially from those in normal subjects and patients with essential hypertension and autonomic failure. Clonidine therapy was effective in reducing the frequency of attacks and the blood pressure and heart rate in attacks that did occur.

Conclusion.—Baroreflexes originate in the great vessels of the neck and thorax, and serve to prevent an excessive rise or fall in arterial pressure. Patients with otherwise unexplained labile hypertension should be evaluated for the syndrome of baroreflex failure. Responsiveness to clonidine and phenylephrine can help to distinguish the syndrome from other disorders.

▶ The characteristic clinical features of this unusual syndrome, including paroxysmal labile hypertension, headaches, and sweating, closely resemble those of pheochromocytoma, and the levels of catecholamines in plasma and urine may approach those seen in that disease. The distinguishing feature of patients with baroreflex failure is the failure of heart rate either to decrease when systolic blood pressure is elevated by 25 mm Hg by stepwise bolus injections of phenylephrine or to increase when systolic pressure is lowered by the same amount by nitroprusside. Most patients have a history of neck irradiation or surgical operations on the neck in which bilateral glossopharyngeal/vagus nerve damage was incurred; in others there is a familial predisposition to paragangliomas involving the carotid body, but in a few the cause is not apparent. The best treatment is clonidine, which lowers the level of plasma norepinephrine in patients with baroreflex failure, but not in those with pheochromocytoma. The authors speculate that baroreflex failure may be the cause of labile hypertension in some patients with essential hypertension, and that seems to have been the case in one patient whom we have studied.—F.H. Epstein, M.D.

Percutaneous Transluminal Renal Angioplasty in the Management of Hypertension and Renal Failure in Patients With Renal Artery Stenosis
Tykarski A, Edwards R, Dominiczak AF, Reid JL (Western Infirmary, Glasgow, Scotland)
J Hum Hypertens 7:491–496, 1993   119-95-63-4

Introduction.—Percutaneous transluminal renal angioplasty (PTRA) has become an accepted method of treatment for patients with hypertension resulting from renal artery stenosis. There is relatively little information, however, on the role of this procedure in the treatment of renal failure. Patients with significantly impaired renal function before PTRA were assessed for the effects of the procedure on blood pressure (BP) control and renal function.

Patients and Methods.—Between February 1990 and March 1992, 30 patients with at least 70% stenosis of the renal artery underwent 43 PTRA procedures. All were admitted with uncontrolled hypertension and/or renal impairment. In 63% of patients the cause of stenosis was bilateral atherosclerosis. Patients were given 5,000 IU of heparin intra-arterially after a 5-F catheter was advanced across the stenosis. If the catheter could not be advanced because of the severity of stenosis, a bolus of isosorbide dinitrate (100 μg) was injected into the renal artery, and a 5-F balloon catheter was used. The procedure was repeated if results were suboptimal. Aspirin (300 mg daily) was taken as antiplatelet therapy for 6 months.

Results.—Twenty-four of the 30 patients had a successful procedure in at least one renal artery and were followed for at least 4 months, with a mean follow-up of 10 months. Technical success of PTRA was defined as a residual stenosis of 50% or less on the postdilation angiogram. Patients were considered cured of renovascular hypertension if diastolic BP was less than 90 mm Hg without antihypertension medication. Improvement in renal function was defined as a reduction of at least 20% in plasma creatinine concentration. The initial technical success rate of PTRA was 81%; after 10 months, the overall success rate was 79%. Initially, 88% showed an initial benefit, with 71% considered cured and 17% with improved renovascular hypertension. After 10 months, however, the rate of cure was 38% and the rate of improvement was 33%. Renal function was improved in 68% of those who had renal insufficiency before PTRA. Patients with bilateral severe atheromatous disease were less likely to experience an improvement of BP control or renal function.

Conclusion.—The benefits of PTRA were confirmed. A high proportion of patients showed satisfactory improvement of BP control, and further deterioration of renal function was prevented in many cases. Both arteries should be dilated in patients with bilateral stenoses. Complications were few (9%), but the risk/benefit profile should be considered for each patient before PTRA.

▶ These results of balloon angioplasty in renal artery stenosis that was predominantly atherosclerotic in origin are a little better than those reported by others—but not much. About a third of patients were cured of their hypertension when studied 4–24 months after the procedure. Of particular interest is their report that ostial lesions within the renal artery proper responded as well as those distal to the ostium; that has not been the experience of other centers. However, they caution that aortic atheromatous plaques close to the ostium have a less favorable prognosis. Patients with bilateral renal artery stenosis and renal insufficiency form a special category in which angioplasty might be useful in temporarily staving off dialysis by providing some improvement in renal function, even though incomplete. In 13 such patients in whom the procedure was attempted, serum creatinine fell by 20% in 7; i.e., about 50% of patients.—F.H. Epstein, M.D.

Alcohol and Blood Pressure: The INTERSALT Study
Marmot MG, Elliott P, Shipley MJ, Dyer AR, Ueshima H, Beevers DG, Stamler R, Kesteloot H, Rose G, Stamler J (Univ College, London; London School of Hygiene and Tropical Medicine; Northwestern Univ, Chicago; et al)
BMJ 308: 1263–1267, 1994   119-95-63–5

Objective.—Some studies suggest a relationship between alcohol consumption and increased blood pressure, but it is not clear whether this reflects only an acute pharmacologic effect. The association of alcohol use and blood pressure was explored in 4,844 men and 4,837 women, aged 20–59 years, who were enrolled in INTERSALT, an international 50-center epidemiologic study. Alcohol consumption was recorded on each of 7 days before standardized blood pressure measurements were acquired.

Findings.—A positive association linking heavy alcohol use with blood pressure was documented at 35 of the 48 centers where at least some participants reported consuming at least 300 mL/wk of alcohol. The overall association was significant at the highest level of alcohol intake. After adjusting for key confounding factors, men drinking 300–499 mL/wk of alcohol had blood pressures that averaged 2.7/1.6 mm Hg higher than nondrinkers. For men taking at least 500 mL/wk, the difference averaged 4.6/3 mm Hg. Men who drank heavily and episodically had more marked increases in blood pressure. Women who drank at least 300 mL/wk had blood pressures 3.9/3.1 mm Hg higher than women who did not drink.

Implication.—If reducing alcohol use can lessen even a low-order excessive risk of elevated blood pressure, the effects on morbidity and mortality might be substantial.

▶ This huge international study of more than 9,000 men and women confirms the notion that heavy alcohol consumption—defined as 3 to 4 or more drinks per day—is associated with an increase in blood pressure. The mechanism of the effect is not yet clear, but it is probably multiple. Alcohol withdrawal always stimulates sympathetic nerve activity, a phenomenon seen in exaggerated form in the sweating and tremulous patient with delirium tremens. In addition, the acute administration of a moderate dose (50 mL) of alcohol increases blood pressure, heart rate, and sympathetic activity recorded directly from the peroneal nerve (1). Because some individuals are more susceptible than others, even modest social drinking may contribute to "essential hypertension" in certain patients. Advising patients to go "on the wagon" is one of the first steps in the nonpharmacological approach to hypertension.—F.H. Epstein, M.D.

Reference

1. Grassi GM, Somors VK, Renk WS, et al: Effects of alcohol intake on blood pressure and sympathetic nerve activity in normal humans: A preliminary report. *J Hypertens Suppl* 7:320–321, 1989

Increased Expression of Vascular Angiotensin II Type 1A Receptor Gene in Glucocorticoid-Induced Hypertension
Sato A, Suzuki H, Nakazato Y, Shibata H, Inagami T, Saruta T (Keio Univ, Tokyo; Vanderbilt Univ, Nashville, Tenn)
J Hypertens 12:511–516, 1994   119-95-63–6

Background.—Glucocorticoids have a role in regulating blood pressure and may contribute to hypertension. The increase in blood pressure in steroid-treated rats is lessened by an angiotensin-converting enzyme inhibitor, and the pressor response to angiotensin II is enhanced in patients with Cushing's syndrome. In cultured vascular smooth muscle cells, glucocorticoid induces the expression of angiotensin II type 1 (AT_1) receptor messenger RNA (mRNA) and increases the number of AT_1 receptors.

Objective and Methods.—The influence of dexamethasone on the expression of vascular AT_1 receptor mRNA was studied in rats given an oral dose of .1 mg daily. Expression of AT_1 receptor by rat aortic cells was determined by the Northern blot hybridization technique. The effects of enalapril maleate, an angiotensin-converting enzyme inhibitor, also were examined.

Results.—Systolic blood pressure began to increase after 3 days of dexamethasone treatment, and the increase was significant on day 5. The level of vascular AT_{1A} receptor mRNA, which initially was difficult to detect, began to increase on day 2 and rose further on day 5. Concurrent treatment with enalapril lessened the blood pressure response but did not prevent the increase in receptor expression.

Conclusion.—Vascular hypersensitivity to angiotensin II in glucocorticoid-induced hypertension may reflect in part the increased expression of vascular AT_{1A} receptor.

▶ It's still not clear why glucocorticoids induce high blood pressure. During the first few days of administration, there usually is a small increase in cardiac output and, often, in plasma volume, but these changes do not seem sufficient to account for the significant increases in both systolic and diastolic pressure frequently seen with chronic administration of glucocorticoids, especially in patients with renal disease (1). This paper suggests one possible mechanism—an increase in the expression of the mRNA message for angiotensin II receptors in the vasculature, presumably leading to an increase in the number of such receptors in arterioles and the consequent development of hypersensitivity to circulating angiotensin II. Such hypersensitivity has been demonstrated in patients with Cushing's syndrome (2) but not in normal men treated for 5 days with adrenocorticotropic hormone (3). If true, it might be possible to treat glucocorticoid-induced hypertension with angiotensin-converting enzyme inhibitors or angiotensin-receptor antagonists.—F.H. Epstein, M.D.

References

1. Whitworth JA: Mechanisms of glucocorticoid-induced hypertension. *Kidney Int* 31:1213–1224, 1987.
2. Saruta T, Suzuki H, Honda M, et al: Multiple factors contribute to the pathogenesis of hypertension in Cushing's syndrome. *J Clin Invest* 62:275–279, 1986.
3. Whitworth JA, Connell JMC, Lever AF, Fraser R: Pressor responsiveness in steroid-induced hypertension in man. *Clin Exp Pharmacol Physiol* 13:353–358, 1986.

A 5-Year Prospective, Observational Study of the Withdrawal of Antihypertensive Treatment in Elderly People
Ekbom T, Lindholm LH, Odén, A Dahlöf B, Hansson L, Wester P-O, Scherstén B (Lund Univ, Dalby, Sweden; Univ of Göteborg, Sweden; Univ of Uppsala, Sweden; et al)
J Intern Med 235:581–588, 1994   119-95-63–7

Objective.—It often is not difficult to initiate life-long medical treatment, but the decision to withdraw medication may be much more difficult. A multicenter, observational study was done to determine the course of hypertension after the withdrawal of antihypertensive therapy in 333 patients with hypertension, aged 70–84 years, who were followed up for 5 years. Approximately two thirds of the patients were women; the mean patient age was 75 years.

Management.—If the blood pressure increased to a hypertensive level during a 3-month washout, placebo was continued for one month. Patients whose supine systolic blood pressure was 180–230 mm Hg and whose diastolic blood pressure was 90 mm Hg, or who had a diastolic blood pressure of 105–120 mm Hg regardless of the systolic blood pressure while receiving placebo, were randomized into the withdrawal study. Many patients were receiving a diuretic just before withdrawal. Beta-blockers were withdrawn incrementally over a few days to minimize the sympathetic rebound.

Results.—One fifth of the patients remained without treatment during 5 years of follow-up. While untreated, patients' total mortality risk was lower than that for the general Swedish population when matched for age and gender. The risk of cardiovascular events also was lower than during treatment. Initial treatment with a low dose of a single drug and relatively low blood pressure before withdrawal predicted a successful outcome.

Conclusion.—If frequent monitoring is feasible, elderly patients with hypertension can safely have antihypertensive therapy withdrawn.

▶ The main message from this careful Swedish study of 333 hypertensive patients over the age of 70 is that, with frequent checkups, withdrawal of antihypertensive drugs can be tried without an increased risk of cardiovascular events or increase in mortality. About 40% of elderly hypertensives whose drugs were stopped remained without any indications for resumption of treatment for one year. Half of those continued normotensive for a full 5 years. These results substantiate earlier suggestions about the relative safety of a trial of withdrawing drug therapy (1).—F.H. Epstein, M.D.

Reference

1. Alderman MH, Lamport B: Withdrawal of drug therapy: A component of the proper management of the hypertensive patient, in Laragh JH, Brenner BM (eds): *Hypertension: Pathophysiology, Diagnosis and Management*. New York, Raven Press, 1990, pp 2301–2308.

Hypertension-Related Renal Injury: A Major Contributor to End-Stage Renal Disease
Walker WG (Johns Hopkins Univ, Baltimore, Md)
Am J Kidney Dis 22:164–173, 1993   119-95-63–8

Objective.—Hypertensive and diabetic nephropathy now account for 57% of new cases of end-stage renal disease (ESRD). Their increasing incidence and the magnitude of the 2 presentations combined make it clear that any significant reduction in the overall incidence of ESRD will require reversal of the trend. Hypertension, hyperlipidemia, protein intake and, possibly, genetic factors all play important roles in the initiation and progression of renal damage, and all affect intervention and prevention strategies. Available clinical information relevant to some of these issues was reviewed.

Discussion.—The data indicate highly significant associations between blood pressure and the rate of renal function loss; the role of hypertension is presumed to be causal, although the mechanism is unknown. According to serum creatinine data from the Multiple Risk Factor Intervention Trial, 5% of hypertensive men show an annual decline in renal function of 3% or more. Older men, black men, and men with initially higher levels of hypertension have even greater rates of loss. Antihypertensive treatment to maintain diastolic blood pressure at less than 95 mm Hg has been shown to protect renal function in nonblacks but not in blacks, even at similar levels of blood pressure reduction.

A longitudinal study of diabetic patients found that hypertension, plasma antiogensin II, and aldosterone all independently predicted accelerated loss of renal function in diabetic nephropathy. The use of diuretics as part of antihypertensive treatment may aggravate the situation. As long as systolic blood pressure was maintained at less than 140 mm Hg, renal function did not deteriorate significantly. No significant association was identified between cholesterol level and progressive renal damage, although this issue requires further study.

Summary.—Hypertension appears to play a major role in the progression of ESRD. Adequate blood pressure control appears to be very important, in both essential and diabetes-related hypertension. In both hypertensive and diabetic nephropathy, effective antihypertension treatment promises to reduce the incidence of ESRD.

▶ While it is now generally accepted that hypertension accelerates the decline in renal function in patients with kidney disease and that hypertensive vascular disease is presently one of the two leading causes of end-stage renal failure, the fact is that essential hypertension, especially of the mild variety (blood pressure less than 150/95), is exceedingly common in Western societies and generally causes no renal impairment. Ninety-six percent of men with mild to moderate hypertension in the Multiple Risk Factor Intervention Trial (MRFIT) study had a negligible decline in renal function or none at all when followed for 5 years, and that encouraging percentage would have been even higher for white women. Because the outlook is less optimistic for blacks and for patients with diabetes, these are the groups that should be especially targeted for antihypertensive treatment in the hope of ultimately decreasing the incidence of chronic renal failure.—F.H. Epstein, M.D.

64 Transplantation

Long-Term Efficacy and Safety of Cyclosporine in Renal-Transplant Recipients
Burke JF, Pirsch JD, Ramos EL, Salomon DR, Stablein DM, Van Buren DH, West JC (Thomas Jefferson Univ Hosp, Philadelphia; Univ of Wisconsin, Madison; Brigham and Women's Hosp, Boston; et al)
N Engl J Med 331:358–363, 1994   119-95-64–1

Introduction.—Cyclosporine reportedly produces a progressive toxic nephropathy, but it also tends to preserve renal function by preventing rejection.

Objective.—The overall effects of cyclosporine on graft rejection and renal function were evaluated by reviewing data on 1,663 renal transplant recipients treated at 6 centers. Cyclosporine was given in an initial daily dose of 8-10 mg/kg, along with antilymphocyte antibody at some of the centers. Maintenance treatment usually included cyclosporine, azathioprine, and prednisone.

Findings.—The mean daily dose of cyclosporine decreased from 6 mg/kg after 3-6 months to 3 mg/kg more than 5 years after transplantation. The drug was withdrawn in 149 patients; in 30 of them it was withdrawn because of nephrotoxicity. The mean serum creatinine from 6 months to 4 years after transplantation was 1.90 mg/dL. The mean increase in patients followed for 3 years was .2 mg/dL, and the overall median change for all patients was less than .001 mg/dL per month. Rejection at any interval significantly compromised graft survival, and rejection also affected later graft function. Patients with relatively high serum cyclosporine levels had better renal function in the first and third years after transplantation.

Conclusion.—Cyclosporine is not a cause of progressive nephropathy in renal transplant recipients.

▶ Renal transplantation usually offers long-term—but not permanent—relief from renal failure. Hence, the causes of chronic graft failure are receiving considerable attention. The most common cause of chronic graft failure is rejection. Although counterintuitive, the application of cyclosporine to renal transplant recipients has greatly decreased the incidence of early graft failure due to rejection, but it has not improved the duration of graft function among those transplants that are functioning one year post-transplantation.

The primary course of later (chronic) graft loss is believed to be chronic rejection. The tempo of chronic graft failure correlates strikingly with donor and recipient histoincompatibility. In keeping with the concept that chronic graft loss is due to immunologic graft injury, this report demonstrates that patients with early "successfully" treated early rejection episodes are especially prone to hastened, chronic graft failure.

Might cyclosporine-induced nephrotoxicity also contribute to late graft failure? This retrospective study attempts to analyze the influence of cyclosporine cloning upon rejection and late graft function. The doses of cyclosporine utilized in patients enrolled in this study have been implicated as causing nephrotoxicity in the treatment of patients with autoimmune disease. In this analysis, however, there was no discernible correlation between cyclosporine dose and graft dysfunction or hastened graft loss. These properly and conservatively interpreted experiments have been injudiciously interpreted by others as providing evidence that cyclosporine does not cause chronic nephrotoxicity. This study does not provide such evidence since cyclosporine may produce a beneficial effect in dampening the tempo of chronic rejection that is offset by an equally powerful nephrotoxic effect.—T.B. Strom, M.D.

Incidence of Non-Hodgkin Lymphoma in Kidney and Heart Transplant Recipients

Opelz G, for the Collaborative Transplant Study (Univ of Heidelberg, Germany)

Lancet 342:1514–1516, 1993   119-95-64–2

Introduction.—Organ transplant recipients experience a high rate of non-Hodgkin's lymphoma (NHL) because of treatment with immunosuppressive drugs. Little information is available regarding the incidence and risk of NHL in such patients; therefore, assessment of the risk of NHL in kidney and heart transplant patients was indicated.

Methods.—At least 1 year of follow-up information on post-transplant immunosuppressive therapy was obtained for 45,141 kidney transplant patients and 7,634 heart transplant patients.

Results.—In the first year, 194 NHL cases were reported, and in subsequent years, 123 additional cases occurred. The incidence of NHL was higher among heart transplant patients. It was also more common in North America than in Europe for both heart and kidney transplant patients. There was a higher incidence of NHL in patients receiving antithymocyte/antilymphocyte globulin (ATG/ALG) or monoclonal anti–T-cell antibody (OKT3), as well as in those patients receiving cyclosporine and azathioprine together, with or without steroids.

Discussion.—The rates of NHL among kidney and heart transplant recipients are, respectively, 20 and 120 times higher than the rates in the general population. The incidence rate in heart transplant patients is higher most likely because more aggressive immunotherapy is pursued. The higher incidence of NHL in North America is unexplained.

Conclusion.—There is an increased risk of NHL in the first year after transplant for recipients receiving prophylactic antibody treatment.

▶ This is an important article. For every increase in the magnitude of immunosuppressive therapy there is a corresponding increase in the incidence of non-Hodgkin's lymphoma (NHL). Two maintenance drug protocols are widely employed: (1) a two-drug (cyclosporine plus corticosteroid) protocol; and (2) a three-drug protocol consisting of cyclosporine (in lower doses) plus azathioprine plus corticosteroid. The three-drug protocol, although utilizing lower cyclosporine doses than the two-drug protocol, is associated with a higher incidence of NHL. A much higher incidence of NHL is evident in patients receiving highly immunosuppressive antilymphocyte antibodies (polyclonal or monoclonal).

As post-transplant B-cell lymphomas are believed to result from Epstein-Barr (EBV) virus–driven B-cell proliferation (1), it seems likely that immunosuppression blunts antiviral immunity, thereby leading to B-cell transformation by EBV.—T.B. Strom, M.D.

Reference

1. York LJ, Qualtiere LF: Cyclosporine abrogates virus-specific T-cell control of EBV-induced B-cell lymphoproliferation. *Viral Immunol* 3:127–136, 1990.

International Standardization of Criteria for the Histologic Diagnosis of Renal Allograft Rejection: The Banff Working Classification of Kidney Transplant Pathology
Solez K, Axelsen RA, Benediktsson H, Burdick JF, Cohen AH, Colvin RB, Croker BP, Droz D, Dunnill MS, Halloran PF, Häyry P, Jennette JC, Keown PA, Marcussen N, Mihatsch MJ, Morozumi K, Myers BD, Nast CC, Olsen S, Racusen LC, Ramos EL, Rosen S, Sachs D, Salomon DR, Sanfilippo F, Verani R, von Willebrand E, Yamaguchi Y (Univ of Alberta, Canada; Walter Mackenzie Centre, Edmonton, Alberta, Canada)
Kidney Int 44:411–422, 1993   119-95-64–3

Background.—Standardizing allograft biopsy interpretation is important in guiding treatment in transplant recipients and helping to establish an objective rejection end point in clinical trials. In 1991, a group of renal pathologists, nephrologists, and transplant surgeons met in Banff, Canada, to construct a schema for nomenclature and classification of renal allograft pathology. During the next year, the schema was revised considerably; the results were presented.

Standardization of Criteria for the Histologic Diagnosis of Renal Allograft Rejection.—In the Banff group schema, intimal arteritis and tubulitis are the main lesions indicating acute rejection. Glomerular, interstitial, tubular, and vascular lesions of acute and chronic rejection are defined and scored on a scale of 0 to 3+. This scoring enables an acute and/or chronic numerical coding for each biopsy. A score is also determined for arteriolar hyalinosis, an indicator of cyclosporine toxicity. The main diagnostic categories are normal, hyperacute rejection, borderline changes, acute rejection, chronic allograft nephropathy, and "other." These categories can be used with or without the quantitative coding system.

Conclusions.—The goal of the Banff group was to construct a schema in which a given biopsy grade would indicate a prognosis for a treatment response or long-term function. The clinical implications of the new standardized schema must now be proved in further studies. This classification should facilitate international uniformity in the reporting of renal allograft pathology and the performance of multicenter studies of new treatments in renal transplantation. Ultimately, it should lead to improvement in the management and care of renal transplant recipients.

▶ Many clinicians have voiced concern that the criteria for the pathologic diagnosis of rejection vary with the skill and predisposition of the given pathologist. Data collection in multicenter trials has been troubled by the disagreements among participating centers about the criteria to make a diagnosis of rejection. While a renal biopsy should provide the gold standard, biopsies have often yielded only one element of a complex assortment of criteria needed to establish a diagnosis of rejection. A brave attempt has been made and the highly reasonable standards proposed are set forth in this report.

Because of the sometimes patchy nature of rejection (I have seen circumstances in which patients have responded beautifully to antirejection therapy and one biopsy core shows minimal cellular infiltrates while the other shows florid rejection), this schema may be plagued by a significant number of false negatives. The shortcomings of the standard histologic review of the biopsy specimen as a means to diagnose rejection has spurred several laboratories to apply molecular biological techniques to the biopsy in an effort to obtain information about the proclivities of the invading leukocytes.—T.B. Strom, M.D.

Heightened Intragraft CTL Gene Expression in Acutely Rejecting Renal Allografts

Lipman ML, Stevens AC, Strom TB (Beth Israel Hosp, Boston; Harvard Med School, Boston)
J Immunol 152:5120–5127, 1994   119-95-64–4

Background.—The immune mechanisms underlying cellular allograft rejection rely on the activities of donor-specific T lymphocytes. The possibility that CTL and delayed type hypersensitivity-like mechanisms play a role in the effector phase of the host immune response has long been suggested. The relationship between activated CTLs and rejection was further explored.

Methods and Findings.—Gene expression of 3 CTL-derived effector molecules in renal allograft biopsy specimens were analyzed. Intragraft gene transcript levels for granzyme B, perforin, and TIA-1 were determined and correlated with the immunologic status of the allograft, and categorized as acute cellular rejection, chronic rejection, elements of both, or no evidence of rejection. In snap-frozen biopsy specimens, total ribonucleic acid (RNA) was extracted and the messenger RNA converted to complementary by reverse transcription. Competitive template polymerase chain reactor methods were used to quantify these levels. Intragraft granzyme B and perforin transcripts were greatly restricted to biopsy specimens in acute cellular rejection. Although TIA-1 expression was more ubiquitous, significantly higher transcript levels occurred in the acute rejection category.

Conclusions.—The finding of these transcripts in samples of acute cellular rejection implicates CTL in its pathogenesis. Intragraft CTL-specific transcript levels may be useful as rejection markers.

▶ The clinical diagnosis of rejection requires evidence of graft dysfunction and the conspicuous presence of graft-invasive mononuclear leukocytes. The differential diagnosis of renal graft dysfunction is complicated by the presence of a mononuclear leukocyte interstitial nephritis in virtually every allograft. The presence of an extensive interstitial nephritis during an episode of graft dysfunction is a reliable indication that rejection is manifest, whereas the presence of *modest* graft infiltration during an episode of *modest* graft dysfunction presents a major diagnostic problem.

Routine histology can document the extent of leukocyte graft infiltration. This technique is not informative as to the functional attributes of the leukocytes invading the graft. It seems reasonable to assume that any rejection causing mononuclear leukocytes to invade a graft will express pro-inflammatory properties. Since these pro-inflammatory properties result from de novo gene activation, pro-inflammatory mononuclear leukocytes (including activated helper and/or cytotoxic T lymphocytes) express genes not expressed by resting mononuclear leukocytes. Hence, several laboratories have probed renal allografts for the presence of gene transcripts encoding a variety of pro-inflammatory proteins.

In this study, Lipman et al. utilize a protocol that employs reverse transcription to catalyze the production of complementary DNA from intragraft RNA in the first step. Subsequently, a quantitative competitive template polymerase chain reaction technique is executed to quantify precisely the intragraft expression of genes that are expressed exclusively by cytotoxic lymphocytes. Expression of the granzyme B and perforin genes is strongly associated with the diagnosis of rejection. This study reconfirms conclusions reached by the authors in a previous report that employed less sophisticated methods.—T.B. Strom, M.D.

Gamma-Interferon Gene Expression in Human Renal Allograft Fine-Needle Aspirates

Nast CC, Zuo X-J, Prehn J, Danovitch GM, Wilkinson A, Jordan SC (Cedars-Sinai Med Ctr, Los Angeles; Univ of Calif, Los Angeles)

Transplantation 57:498–502, 1994   119-95-64–5

Introduction.—There is poor understanding of the immunologic mechanisms involved in acute transplant rejection. Certain cytokines, including gamma-interferon (γ-IFN), have been found in the urine of patients experiencing rejection. To study cytokine expression in transplant patients, fine-needle aspirates (FNA) were examined for the presence of γ-IFN messenger RNA (mRNA), using reverse transcription polymerase chain reaction (RT-PCR).

Methods.—The FNAs were available from 15 patients who experienced allograft dysfunction from 5 days to 8.5 months after renal transplantation, and from control normal and irreversibly rejected kidneys. The number of lymphocytes was counted, and the percentage of tubular cells expressing major histocompatibility complex (MHC) class II antigen was calculated in each aspirate. RT-PCR was performed with aliquots from each aspirate in separate experiments using γ-IFN. Control RT-PCR experiments were performed using cyclophylin or insulin primers. Associations between the RT-PCR findings and clinical diagnosis were studied.

Results.—Cyclophylin transcript was detected in all aspirates, as were adequate numbers of lymphocytes. Five of the 15 patients were clinically determined to be undergoing acute rejection. Aspirates from these 5 had elevated lymphocytes, positive tubular cell MHC class II expression, and elevated γ-IFN. Two patients who were not showing signs of clinical rejection, but who had significantly and weakly amplified γ-IFN transcript in their aspirates, had rejection episodes 3 days and 1 week later. The γ-IFN transcript could not be detected in aspirates from patients with acute tubular necrosis, acute cyclosporine nephrotoxicity, or clinically treated and resolved rejection.

Discussion.—These findings suggest that PCR analysis of γ-IFN mRNA in FNAs may provide sensitive and specific early diagnosis of acute rejection. Expression of γ-IFN was amplified in 2 patients before clinical signs of rejection were manifest, suggesting that these patients could be treated before significant graft injury occurs.

▶ Nast et al. also utilized a reverse transcriptase-polymerase chain reaction technique to evaluate renal allograft specimens. In this analysis, FNAs were examined for the presence of intragraft γ-IFN gene expression. Although the study cannot be considered definitive, it suggests that intragraft expression of the γ-IFN gene, a powerfully pro-inflammatory cytokine, precedes clinical evidence of rejection. If these conclusions can be confirmed and validated, it may be possible to detect and abort rejection episodes before graft dysfunction becomes evident.—T.B. Strom, M.D.

RANTES Chemokine Expression in Cell-Mediated Transplant Rejection of the Kidney

Pattison J, Nelson PJ, Huie P, von Leuttichau I, Farshid G, Sibley RK, Krensky AM (Stanford Univ, Calif)
Lancet 343:209–211, 1994   119-95-64–6

Introduction.—The role of RANTES (regulated upon activation, normal T cell expressed and secreted), a chemotactic cytokine specific for T cells, monocytes, and eosinophils produced by T cells, fibroblasts, mesangial cells, and renal tubular epithelial cells when activated by inflammatory mediators, was examined in cell-mediated transplant rejection.

Methods.—Thirty-five renal allograft biopsy specimens were examined using the VL2 antirecombinant human RANTES monoclonal antibody and the 4-layer peroxidase/antiperoxidase immunoperoxidase method.

Results.—The RANTES messenger RNA (mRNA) and protein were identified in 17 of the 20 cellular rejection specimens. The localization of RANTES to the endothelium and complex formation along peritubular capillaries suggested the presence of an endothelial receptor.

Discussion.—Chemokines cause aggregation of inflammatory cells and attract monocytes; RANTES encourages cell migration and binds to endothelium. Interleukin-1, tumor necrosis factor, and T cells activate the expression of RANTES which, in turn, attracts T cells and monocytes to the site of inflammation. The T cells then secrete additional RANTES, worsening the inflammatory response.

Conclusion.—In sum, RANTES is an important mediator of immune response and may play an important role in allograft rejection.

▶ It appears that RANTES is a chemokine, i.e., a rather small cytokine with strong chemoattractant properties exerted upon T cells and monocytes. Hence, RANTES also can be considered pro-inflammatory. Intragraft expression of RANTES mRNA and protein was strongly correlated with acute rejection episodes. In this analysis an in situ hybridization technique was used to identify and localize the site of gene expression. Although the polymerase chain reaction technique utilized in the previous studies may be more sensitive and more amenable to precise quantitation, the technique does not identify the site of gene expression. In situ hybridization uses tagged nucleic acid sequences to bind to and thereby identify the site of specific mRNAs.—T.B. Strom, M.D.

Long-Term Acceptance of Major Histocompatibility Complex Mismatched Cardiac Allografts Induced by CTLA4Ig Plus Donor-Specific Transfusion

Lin H, Bolling SF, Linsley PS, Wei R-Q, Gordon D, Thompson CB, Turka LA
(Univ of Michigan, Ann Arbor; Bristol-Myers Pharmaceutical Research Inst, Seattle, Wash; Howard Hughes Med Inst, Univ of Chicago)

J Exp Med 178:1801–1806, 1993   119-95-64–7

Background.—Underlying the process of allograft rejection is activation of T cells by antigen, which requires both engagement of the T-cell receptor by antigen and costimulatory signals delivered through other T-cell surface molecules such as CD28. A soluble recombinant fusion protein, CTLA4Ig, blocks the engagement of CD28 by B7, its natural ligand. Administration of this immunoglobulin blocks antigen-specific immune responses both in vitro and in vivo. Its administration to rats for 1 week at the time of cardiac allograft transplantation has resulted in a median allograft survival time of 30 days, although most of the grafts eventually were rejected.

Objective.—An attempt was made to achieve consistent long-term cardiac allograft survival in rats using both CTLA4Ig and donor-specific cell transfusion (DST) at the time of transplantation.

Results.—Grafts consistently survived for longer than 2 months when donor-specific transfusion was given at the time of transplantation and was followed in 2 days by a single dose of CTLA4Ig. The recipients exhibited delayed responses to donor-type skin transplants, whereas they had normal rejection responses to third-party skin transplants. In addition, they tolerated donor-matched second cardiac allografts well; the histologic findings of rejection were minimal.

Implication.—A combination of donor-specific transfusion and CTLA4Ig, administered at about the time of cardiac transplantation, is followed by prolonged and frequently indefinite allograft survival.

▶ In the past several years, there has been a resurgence of interest in suppressor-type immune activity. The field has gained new-found respectability because basic immunologists have found insights that may apply to the suppressor-type immune activity that is so evident in animal models. Perhaps the key observation in this regard is the finding that T-cell activation is a two-step process. The first signal is provided by antigenic stimulation of the T-cell receptor for antigen, and the second signal is received through the cognate interactions that take place between transmembrane T-cell and antigen-presenting cell surface proteins. In the event that naive T cells are stimulated by antigen alone, T-cell paralysis ("anergy") is fostered. A particularly potent second signal for T-cell activation is delivered through the interaction of antigen-presenting cell B7 proteins with the T-cell CD28 protein.

The B7 proteins can also be recognized by CTLA4, a protein that is expressed primarily upon activated T cells. Although this protein has a higher affinity for B7 than CD28, the stimulatory second signal is delivered primarily through the engagement of CD28 and B7. A soluble form of CTLA4 has been used by Turka and his colleagues to coat B7 and prevent engagement of all surface CD28 and B7 proteins in rodent graft recipients. This regimen was used in concert with donor blood transfusions—a manipulation long known to foster donor-specific immune suppression—to achieve long-term engraftment of cardiac allografts that does not require long-term immuno-suppression. A similar strategy has more recently yielded striking results in a renal transplant model. This strategy has captured the fancy of many workers in the field.—T.B. Strom, M.D.

65 Dialysis

The Effects of the Dialysis Membrane on Cytokine Release
Zaoui P, Hakim RM (Université de Grenoble, France; Vanderbilt Univ Med Ctr, Nashville, Tenn)
J Am Soc Nephrol 4:1711–1718, 1994   119-95-65-1

Objective.—Because previous studies of plasma cytokine levels in patients undergoing hemodialysis have yielded mixed results, a prospective crossover study was planned to study the influence of the type of dialysis membrane used on the elaboration of cytokines by peripheral blood mononuclear cells (PBMNC).

Methods.—Eight patients receiving hemodialysis were dialyzed for sequential 2-week periods with new cuprophane membranes, a low-flux, low-complement-activating membrane, and again cuprophane membranes. The ability of PBMNC to elaborate cytokines in response to phytohemagglutinin was determined after each exposure period. The cytokines measured included interleukin (IL)-1β, tumor necrosis factor-α, IL-2, and soluble IL-2 receptors.

Results.—The ability of stimulated PBMNC to form all the measured cytokines was significantly reduced after each period of exposure to cuprophane membranes. Higher levels were found after dialysis with a biocompatible membrane and, after 2 weeks, the responses were nearly normal.

Conclusion.—Hemodialysis with cuprophane membranes is associated with attenuated mononuclear-cell responses to mitogen stimulation and the elaboration of lower levels of cytokines that were nearly normalized by dialysis with a biocompatible membrane.

▶ This paper documents that the immune response of stimulated mononuclear cells is defective in patients dialyzed with a cuprophane membrane, but is very much less so with a polymethylmethacrylate (PMMA) membrane that is more biocompatible. Another study showed that cuprophane membranes result in increased postdialysis serum levels of tumor necrosis factor (TNF-α) in a way that doesn't occur with a more biocompatible polyacrylonitrile AN69 membrane (1). More importantly, Hakim et al. (2) have recently shown that biocompatibility may translate into better patient outcome. This randomized study of patients with acute renal failure found that those dialyzed with a more biocompatible PMMA membrane developed less oliguria and recovered renal function better than those utilizing a cuprophane membrane. Patient survival was also better in those patients with initial non-oliguric renal failure who were dialyzed with the more biocompatible membrane.—R.S. Brown, M.D.

References

1. Canivet E, Lavaud S, Wong T, et al.: Cuprophane but not synthetic membrane induces increases in serum tumor necrosis factor-alpha levels during hemodialysis. *Am J Kidney Dis* 23:41–46, 1994.
2. Hakim RM, Wingard RL, Parker RA: Effect of the dialysis membrane in the treatment of patients with acute renal failure. *N Engl J Med* 331:1338–1342, 1994.

Continuous Venovenous Hemodiafiltration Compared With Conventional Dialysis in Critically Ill Patients With Acute Renal Failure
Bellomo R, Boyce N (Monash Med Centre, Clayton, Victoria, Australia; Presbyterian Univ, Pittsburgh, Pa)
ASAIO J 39:M794–M797, 1993   119-95-65-2

Introduction.—Continuous venovenous hemodiafiltration (CVVHD) may offer all the advantages of continuous arteriovenous hemofiltration but, due to safer vascular access and improved dialysis clearance, may reduce the expected morbidity of critically ill patients. A single double-lumen IV catheter is used for access, and a peristaltic pump is added to maintain blood flow through the filter.

Objective.—The results of CVVHD in 76 critically ill patients with acute renal failure were compared with those previously achieved in 84 patients in intensive care who underwent either intermittent hemodialysis or peritoneal dialysis. The groups were similar in age, gender, and the number of failing organs, but Acute Physiology and Chronic Health Evaluation (APACHE) II scores indicated more severe illness in the patients treated by CVVHD. The patients were treated at the same center and represented similar case mixes.

Results.—Azotemia and hyperphosphatemia were better controlled by CVVHD than by conventional dialysis (CD) after 24 hours. Plasma urea levels were lower when CVVHD was initiated because of the readiness with which this method is implemented in the ICU. Compared with those receiving CD, more patients in the CVVHD group received full parenteral nutrition as planned and required. Oliguria lasted an average of 2 weeks in patients managed by CVVHD and 23 days in the CD group. Although the patents treated by CVVHD were more severely ill, the survival rate was higher than that with CD. For patients with less than 4 failing organs or APACHE II scores below 29 (an intermediate degree of illness) the difference in survival was significant.

Conclusion.—Continuous venovenous hemodiafiltration is a superior approach to CD for critically ill patients who have acute renal failure.

▶ Continuous arteriovenous hemofiltration (CAVH) or hemodiafiltration (CAVHD) has been considered a preferable renal replacement modality to CD in critically ill patients in surgical or medical intensive care units. The survival rate with CAVH has been shown to be better in some critically ill patients with acute renal failure (1). However, continuous venovenous hemodiafiltration (CVVHD) doesn't require the risk of arterial access needed for CAVH (or CAVHD), and the higher blood flow rates achieved with pumping used for CVVHD allow better dialysis clearance and higher ultrafiltration rates.

The authors of this study have shown that CVVHD may improve the management of critically ill patients compared to CD, but the use of a retrospective patient group receiving CD and the lack of statistical significance of the overall survival rate leaves room for confirmation of the findings in a prospective fashion. Furthermore, it is possible that the differences shown may be explained by the more biocompatible membranes used for CVVHD than CD in the past, which may not be seen when CD is done with biocompatible dialyzers (see Abstract 119-95-65–1).—R.S. Brown, M.D.

Reference

1. Kruczynski K, Irvine-Bird K, Toffelmire EB, Morton AR: A comparison of continuous arteriovenous hemofiltration and intermittent hemodialysis in acute renal failure patients in the intensive care unit. *ASAIO J* 39:M778–M781, 1993.

Continuous Ambulatory Peritoneal Dialysis and Hemodialysis: Comparison of Patient Mortality With Adjustment for Comorbid Conditions

Held PJ, Port FK, Turenne MN, Gaylin DS, Hamburger RJ, Wolfe RA (The United States Renal Data System, Bethesda, Md; Univ of Michigan, Ann Arbor; Princeton Univ, New Jersey; et al)
Kidney Int 45:1163–1169, 1994   119-95-65–3

Objective.—Mortality rates were determined for 1,725 prospective diabetic patients and 2,411 patients without diabetes who, in 1986–1987, had end-stage renal disease and underwent either continuous ambulatory peritoneal dialysis (CAPD) or hemodialysis (HD).

Methods.—Mortality rates were adjusted for a number of patient characteristics, including age, diabetic status, and the presence of comorbid conditions at the time end-stage renal disease began. Mortality in relation to the type of dialysis was analyzed by the Cox proportional hazards method. The patients were followed from 30 days to 2–4 years after the onset of illness.

Findings.—Among nondiabetic patients there was no significant difference in the relative mortality risk between those selected for CAPD and those treated by HD. In diabetic patients, however, adjusted mortality was higher in those having CAPD; the relative risk was 1.26. With use of the Cox model to adjust for pretreatment risk factors, nondiabetic patients undergoing CAPD and HD had 1-year survival estimates of 91.8% and 90.6%, respectively, and 2-year rates of 78% for both treatment groups. Diabetic patients had similar survival rates at 1 year, but at 2 years those having CAPD had a survival rate of 54% compared with 64.6% for those undergoing HD.

Conclusion.—Individuals with diabetes who have end-stage renal disease appear to live longer when maintained with HD than when managed by CAPD.

▶ Held et al. have utilized data from the Case Mix Severity Special Study of the United States Renal Data System to document a growing suspicion that diabetic patients treated with CAPD may have a higher mortality rate over time than those on hemodialysis HD. Since the study adjusted mortality for co-morbid conditions at initiation of treatment, the explanation for the difference in treatment effect may be either that unmeasured co-morbid conditions affected selection of CAPD or HD (though co-morbidity would be thought to increase the 1-year mortality in addition to that at 2 years) or that CAPD is a less effective modality for diabetics. Since another study has reported better survival with CAPD rather than with HD in young diabetics (1) and because many patients have noted a better quality of life on CAPD, it seems wise to allow strong patient preference for CAPD to be a deciding factor in treatment modality. However, it behooves the physician to be mindful of the predictors of poor dialysis outcome, i.e., inadequate dialysis dose and low serum albumin level, which may indicate a need to switch from CAPD to HD.—R.S. Brown, M.D.

Reference

1. Nelson CB, Port FK, Wolfe RA, Guire KE: Comparison of continous ambulatory peritoneal dialysis and hemodialysis patient survival with evaluation of trends during the 1980's. *J Am Soc Nephrol* 3:1147–1155, 1992.

Survival Among Mexican-Americans, Non-Hispanic Whites, and African-Americans With End-Stage Renal Disease: The Emergence of a Minority Pattern of Increased Incidence and Prolonged Survival
Pugh JA, Tuley MR, Basu S (Univ of Texas, San Antonio; Audie L Murphy Mem Veterans Hosp, San Antonio, Tex)
Am J Kidney Dis 23:803–807, 1994   119-95-65–4

Background.—Mexican-Americans are currently the second largest minority in the United States, and their numbers are increasing 5 times faster than the rest of the population. Their incidence of end-stage renal disease (ESRD) is threefold higher than that in non-Hispanic whites, and the rate of diabetic ESRD is increased sixfold. The comparative rates are similar to those reported for African-Americans.

Objective and Methods.—Survival rates were compared for these ethnic groups using data from the Texas Kidney Health Program for the years 1975–1985. The database included 88% to 90% of all patients starting to receive renal replacement therapy in Texas. The patients were followed until death or for 3 years after successful transplantation; 12% of patients were lost to follow-up. The final study population included 5,386 non-Hispanic whites, 3,162 Mexican-Americans, and 3,422 African-Americans. Both life-table analysis and age-adjusted analysis using the Cox proportional hazards model were done.

Observations.—In most age groups, Mexican-Americans survived somewhat better than non-Hispanic whites. African-Americans aged 30 years and older had progressively better survival. After adjustment for age, these ethnic differences persisted for all causes combined, for patients with diabetes and hypertension, and for those given hemodialysis at a center. Multivariate analysis confirmed a survival advantage for Mexican-Americans after controlling for age, type of disease, treatment, and the size of the treatment center. Older African-Americans exhibited a similar survival advantage. Among patients given renal replacement therapy, both of these groups survived better than non-Hispanic whites.

Discussion.—Minority groups appear to have ESRD comparatively often but to survive better with dialysis treatment. More vigorous preventive efforts may be appropriate for minority groups. A better understanding of how minority status influences survival might help in finding ways of improving the survival of non-Hispanic white patients.

▶ It has been well recognized that African-Americans have an increased incidence of ESRD, but a better survival on dialysis, than whites. This Texas study points out that a similar pattern of increased incidence of ESRD but better 5-year survival rates on dialysis are also found for Mexican-Americans compared to non-Hispanic whites. Voluntary withdrawal from dialysis, thought to occur in an increased percentage of non-Hispanic whites, could not account for the mortality differences, as withdrawal caused a very low percentage of deaths in this study. A decreased percentage of minority patients transplanted, which would leave healthier minority patients on dialysis, cannot explain the survival differences in older dialysis patients, who are usually not considered for transplantation. Studies to elucidate the factors contributing to the higher rate of ESRD and to the lower mortality rate on dialysis in minority patients compared to non-Hispanic whites would be helpful.—R.S. Brown, M.D.

A New Treatment for Dialysis-Related Amyloidosis With β2-Microgloubulin Adsorbent Column

Nakazawa R, Azuma N, Suzuki M, Nakatani M, Nankou T, Furuyoshi S, Yasuda A, Takata S, Tani N, Kobayashi F (Tokatsu Clinic Hosp, Matsudo; Kaneka Corp, Osaka; Kobayashi Eye-Clinic, Tokyo, Japan)

Int J Artif Organs 16:823–829, 1993   119-95-65–5

Introduction.—Accumulation of β_2-microglobulin in the serum is the cause of dialysis-related amyloidosis (DRA), one of the most disabling complications of long-term hemodialysis. The use of highly permeable membranes in dialysis can remove greater amounts of β_2-microglobulin than cuprophane membranes but not as much as is synthesized. The use of a β_2-microglobulin selective adsorbent for the treatment of DRA was evaluated in a clinical trial.

Methods.—The subjects were 19 patients receiving long-term hemodialysis with DRA, all of whom had amyloid osteoarthropathy. Treatment was with a direct hemoperfusion (DHP) column containing 350 mL of the adsorbent, connected in series with a highly permeable polyacrylonitrile (PAN AN69) membrane dialyzer. This treatment was given 3 times a week for 1 week in 11 patients, for 4 weeks in 5 patients, for 6 months in 1 patient, and for 1 year in 2 patients.

Results.—Percent reduction of β2-microglobulin was greater than 65% for the 16 patients treated for 1 or 4 weeks and 72% to 76.5% for the 3 patients treated for more than 6 months. After each treatment session, β_2-microglobulin levels were always less than 10 mg/L, sometimes falling to as little as 3.4 mg/L and with significant lowering of the pretreatment levels. The total amounts of β2-microglobulin removed per session averaged from 158 to 257 mg in the 3 patients treated for over 6 months. The column amounted for about 90% of the β_2-microglobulin removed, but adsorption capacity was retained for up to 5 hours of therapy. Clinical evaluations performed in 3 patients showed a favorable effect of treatment on joint symptoms and ocular fundus in 2.

Conclusions.—A new method of treatment for DRA using a β_2-microglobulin adsorbent column may delay the progression of DRA in patients undergoing long-term hemodialysis and should be considered for wider application. The ocular fundus may be a useful early diagnostic marker for DRA and for monitoring of the therapeutic effect of β2-microglobulin removal on amyloid deposition.

▶ The inability to adequately remove β_2-microglobulin (β_2-M) with conventional hemodialysis or peritoneal dialysis appears to be the major cause of DRA in long-term dialysis patients. Marked morbidity due to carpal tunnel syndrome and dialysis-associated osteoarthropathy has been linked to the deposition of β_2-M amyloid in bone, synovial tissue, and articular cartilage in such patients. Attempts to increase the removal of β_2-M have met with only limited success as newer high flux dialyzers using polysulfone or polymethylmethacrylate membranes have increased β_2-M clearance but have failed to boost the removal up to the level of synthesis, in part due to stimulation of β_2-M generation and to membrane adsorption of β_2-M (1). Likewise, the lower β_2-M levels seen in patients on peritoneal dialysis appear to be explained by residual renal clearance rather than enhanced peritoneal clearance (2). The authors of this study have proposed a novel adsorption column that can be placed in a series before the hemodialyzer to augment β_2-M removal. Although they have documented in a small group of patients that the column is effective at decreasing the serum β_2-M levels and is well tolerated, a controlled study will be needed to confirm a beneficial effect on the clinical manifestations of DRA to justify its cost.—R.S. Brown, M.D.

References

1. Lian JD, Cheng CH, Chang YL, Hsiong CH, Lee CJ: Clinical experience and model analysis on *beta*-2 microglobulin kinetics in high-flux hemodialysis. *Artif Organs* 17:758–763, 1993.
2. Amioci G, Virga G, Da Rin G, et al: Serum *beta*-2 microglobulin level and residual renal function in peritoneal dialysis. *Nephron* 65:469–471, 1993.

High Prevalence of Hepatitis C Virus (HCV) RNA in Dialysis Patients: Failure of Commercially Available Antibody Tests to Identify a Significant Number of Patients With HCV Infection

Bukh J, Wantzin P, Krogsgaard K, Knudsen F, Purcell RH, Miller RH and the Copenhagen Dialysis HCV Study Group (Natl Inst of Allergy and Infectious Diseases, Bethesda, Md; Natl Inst of Health, Bethesda, Md; Hvidovre Hosp, Copenhagen, Denmark; et al)

J Infect Dis 168:1343–1348, 1993 119-95-65–6

Background.—After effective measures for controlling the spread of hepatitis B virus (HBV) were introduced into dialysis units, patients incurred an increased risk of liver disease from hepatitis C virus (HCV). A relatively high rate of anti-HCV antibody has been described in patients undergoing dialysis, but antibody titers do not distinguish between past and current HCV infection. A very sensitive and specific method now is available for identifying HCV RNA.

Objective.—Sera from 340 patients undergoing dialysis in eastern Denmark were tested for anti-HCV using a first-generation enzyme-linked immunosorbent assay (ELISA) and also with a second-generation assay. Hepatitis C virus RNA was identified using a complementary DNA (cDNA) polymerase chain reaction assay. Only 2 of the patients were positive for HBV surface antigen.

Results.—The second-generation ELISA demonstrated anti-HCV antibody in 8% of patients. All but 1 of those patients had HCV RNA identified in their sera. Eight other patients receiving dialysis who were ELISA-negative also had detectable HCV RNA. Sixteen of 35 HCV-infected dialysis patients had positive results with a second-generation recombinant immunoblot assay. More than 60% of patients with ongoing liver disease had evidence of HCV infection.

Conclusion.—In these patients undergoing dialysis, the finding of anti-HCV antibody in serum was closely associated with HCV viremia, but viremia also is found in a significant number of antibody-negative patients. Hepatitis C virus infection might cause more than half of all ongoing liver disease in these patients.

▶ The authors document several important findings: First, a second-generation ELISA anti-HCV antibody test usually detects dialysis patients with active HCV viremia as detected by the polymerase chain reaction (PCR) assay for HCV RNA. Second, the ELISA test is much superior to the second-generation recombinant immunoblot assay (RIBA) for anti-HCV antibodies. Furthermore, some potentially infectious dialysis patients with HCV RNA in their blood are not detected by either antibody assay. These results are similar to those of a study in the United States (1). Altogether, hepatitis C accounted for over 60% of the liver disease in these Danish patients on dialysis, similar to the proportion of hepatitis C causing non-A, non-B hepatitis in other geographic areas.—R.S. Brown, M.D.

Reference

1. Kuhns M, de Medina M, McNamara A, et al: Detection of hepatitis C virus RNA in hemodialysis patients. *J Am Soc Nephrol* 4:1491–1497, 1994.

Frequency and Outcome of Pregnancy in Women on Dialysis
Hou SH (Rush Med College, Chicago)
Am J Kidney Dis 23:60–63, 1994   119-95-65-7

Introduction.—Pregnancy has been an infrequent occurrence in women on dialysis, and its outcome is uncertain. There is a substantial risk of maternal complications and spontaneous abortion. Because the care of patients undergoing dialysis has changed in recent years, the frequency and outcome of pregnancy in women with end-stage renal disease were examined in a survey of approximately 10% of the dialysis units in the United States.

Methods.—A questionnaire sent to 206 dialysis units in 10 states was returned by 194 units. Data requested included the number of women, aged 18–44 years, treated in the unit, the number and outcome of pregnancies, duration of dialysis, and use of erythropoietin at the time of conception. More detailed questionnaires were sent to units reporting a pregnancy.

Results.—The 194 units cared for 1,281 women of childbearing age. Almost 25% of these units had cared for a pregnant patient at one time. Twenty of 60 reported pregnancies occurred during the 2-year survey period, for a rate of 41.5%. Conception was most common during the first year on dialysis. Only 37% of the pregnancies reported resulted in surviving infants, although in 24 pregnancies that occurred after 1990, 52% of infants survived. Spontaneous abortion occurred in 44% and elective abortion occurred in 8% of all pregnancies. Pregnancy success was not related to dialysis modality or the use of erythropoietin. Only 1 of the 19 infants for whom gestational age was known reached term.

Conclusion.—Pregnancy in patients on dialysis still entails risks for the mother and infant. Although more infants are surviving now than in the past, spontaneous abortion and premature birth are common. Pregnancy is dangerous for women undergoing dialysis, and there is a question of whether surviving infants will have normal growth and development. Such women should be counseled on the risks of pregnancy and the need for contraception if pregnancy is not desired. Even after many years of dialysis, pregnancy remains possible.

▶ The surprising thing to me about this survey is the frequency of pregnancy in women of childbearing age who are on dialysis—about one eighth that of normal women who do not have renal failure. It is essential, therefore, to provide contraceptive counseling to enable patients to understand the risks of pregnancy and to avoid unwanted pregnancies. From one half to two thirds of pregnancies in women on dialysis will be unsuccessful, and premature delivery is the rule. Twenty percent of infants who came to term were below the tenth percentile in growth. The maternal complication rate is substantial; in this series of 39 pregnancies continued past the first trimester, there were 2 episodes of malignant hypertension, 2 severe hemorrhagic complications, and 1 episode each of disseminated intravascular coagulation, respiratory failure, and diabetic ketoacidosis. Nevertheless, for some women on dialysis who do become pregnant, these relatively high risks may be acceptable.—F.H. Epstein, M.D.

66 Sodium, Potassium, Water, and Acid-Base

Angiotensin II Suppression is a Major Factor Permitting Excretion of an Acute Sodium Load in Humans

Singer DRJ, Markandu ND, Morton JJ, Miller MA, Sagnella GA, MacGregor GA (St George's Hosp, London)

Am J Physiol 266:F89–F93, 1994

119-95-66-1

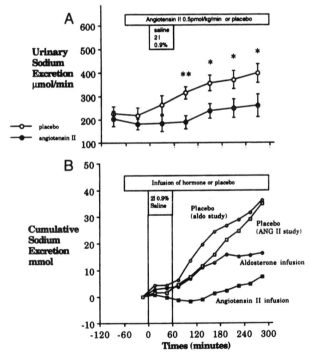

Fig 66–1.—A, effects of ANG II infusion (.5 pmol/kg/min) vs. placebo on urinary Na⁺ excretion before, during, and for 4 hours after infusion of 2 L of .9% saline ($n = 8$). ANG II vs. placebo: analysis of variance, $F = 5.5$, $P < .04$; time effect: $F = 11.4$, $P < .001$. ANG II vs. placebo: $*P < .05$; $**P < .01$. **B,** cumulative increase in urinary Na⁺ excretion vs. baseline during and for 4 hours after infusion of 2 L of .9% saline for ANG II infusion and control infusion ($n = 8$, present study) and for aldosterone infusion and control infusion ($n = 8$, previous study). (Courtesy of Singer DRJ, Markandu ND, Morton JJ, et al: *Am J Physiol* 266:F89–F93, 1994.)

Objective.—Previous studies have presented evidence that atrial natriuretic peptide and aldosterone suppression are among the mechanisms involved in response to sodium loading. A double-blind placebo-controlled study was designed to examine the role of circulating angiotensin II (ANG II) in the excretion of an acute sodium load in normal humans.

Methods.—The study participants were eight normotensive volunteers, 4 men and 4 women, ranging in age from 20 to 31 years. Dietary sodium intake was standardized at 150 mmol/day on each study day. Randomization was to a double-blind infusion of ANG II or placebo on the sixth day of each diet period. Blood was sampled under both conditions. An initial oral water load was followed by a 6-hour IV infusion of ANG II in 0.9% saline or placebo. During the second hour of this infusion, 2 liters of 0.9% saline were infused over 60 minutes. Participants were supine and fasting throughout the 8-hour studies. Urine samples were obtained with subjects standing to micturate.

Results.—Plasma ANG II decreased to 40% to 60% of basal values obtained on the control day, and a mean of 35 mmol of Na^+ (11.4% of the Na load) was excreted in the 5 hours after the start of the saline infusion. Plasma aldosterone also fell by about 50% during saline infusion. Infusion of ANG II to maintain plasma ANG II levels close to basal values (mean 6.6 pmol/L) resulted in a significant decline in Na^+ excretion to a mean of 7 mmol in the same period. Angiotensin II had no significant effect, compared with placebo infusion, on changes in urine flow during and after saline infusion. During ANG II infusion, plasma aldosterone levels closely paralleled changes in ANG II levels. Preventing the decrease in aldosterone levels by low-dose intravenous infusion of aldosterone alone affected the excretion of a sodium load much less than did the replacement of ANG II (Fig 66–1).

Conclusion.—Suppression of circulating ANG II levels is of major importance for the excretion of an acute sodium load. Maintenance of ANG II levels by low-dose infusion completely prevented the expected decrease in plasma aldosterone levels. Angiotensin II has direct actions on Na^+ excretion in addition to its effects on aldosterone.

▶ The simple question, "Why do we excrete a sodium load?" has some complicated answers. Important players that interact to produce natriuresis when salt intake is increased include a tendency for blood pressure, glomerular filtration rate, and renal blood flow to rise; an increase in renal synthesis of dopamine; heightened renal prostaglandin formation (especially PGE_2), increased renal synthesis of P-450 products of arachidonic acid metabolism; raised circulating concentrations of cardiac peptides; enhanced renal production of urodilatin; a reduction in renal sympathetic neural activity; and, of course, a decrease in the circulating levels of renin, ANG II, and aldosterone. Renal excretion of urodilatin (the "cardiac peptide" made by the kidney) was closely correlated with sodium excretion during the two days following a saline infusion in experiments like those reported here (1), implying a key role for urodilatin in the renal response to salt loading.

This paper clearly illustrates that if ANG II levels are not allowed to fall after a salt load, the expected increase in salt excretion, at least during the first four hours, is virtually abolished. Furthermore, the effect of replacing ANG II is far greater than anticipated from its action on the adrenal synthesis of aldosterone, as shown in Figure 66–1. Therefore, ANG II, even at its rather low, usual concentration in plasma, must be increasing sodium reabsorption (probably in the proximal tubule)—a chronic effect made apparent when its level is lowered by saline infusion.—F.H. Epstein, M.D.

Reference

1. Drummer C, Gerzer R, Heer M, et al: Effects of an acute saline infusion on fluid and electrolyte metabolism in humans. *Am J Physiol* 262:F744–F754, 1992 (Abstracted in the 1993 YEAR BOOK OF MEDICINE, pp 664–667).

Diuretic Therapy for Hypertension and the Risk of Primary Cardiac Arrest

Siscovick DS, Raghunathan TE, Psaty BM, Koepsell TD, Wicklund KG, Lin X, Cobb L, Rautaharju PM, Copass MK, Wagner EH (Univ of Washington, Seattle; Univ of Alberta, Edmonton; Ctr for Health Studies, Seattle)
N Engl J Med 330:1852–1857, 1994   119-95-66–2

Background.—High doses of thiazide diuretic drugs may increase the risk of sudden death from cardiac causes in patients undergoing treatment for hypertension. Low-dose thiazide treatment may reduce the risk of coronary heart disease. The association between thiazide treatment for hypertension and the occurrence of primary cardiac arrest was examined.

Methods.—The case subjects were 114 persons with hypertension who had a primary cardiac arrest between 1977 and 1990. The control subject were 535 persons with hypertension.

Findings.—The risk of primary cardiac arrest among patients treated with combined thiazide and potassium-sparing diuretics (triamterene or spironolactone) was lower than that among patients treated with a thiazide without a potassium-sparing agent (odds ratio, 0.3; 95% confidence interval, 0.1 to 0.7). Compared with low-dose thiazide treatment, moderate-dose therapy was associated with a moderate increase in risk and high-dose therapy with a greater increase in risk. Adding a potassium-sparing drug to low-dose thiazide treatment was associated with a decrease in cardiac arrest risk.

Conclusions.—Both thiazide dose and the addition of potassium-sparing agents affect the risk of primary cardiac arrest in patients undergoing hypertension treatment. These findings may explain the differences in the effect of antihypertensive treatment on mortality from coronary heart disease in previous research.

▶ These results strongly support the combined use of a potassium-sparing diuretic like triamterene when thiazides are employed to treat hypertension. It seems very likely that the protection afforded by triamterene or its equivalent (e.g., amiloride or spironolactone) is due to the avoidance of hyperkalemia, but there are two caveats. The first is that simple potassium supplementation was not shown in this study to lower the risk of cardiac arrest. The second is that absorption of a thiazide is reduced by more than half when it is combined with a potassium-sparing diuretic drug. So the action of triamterene might conceivably have been merely to lower the effective dose of thiazide. In addition to potassium depletion, one reason why high doses of diuretics may predispose to arrhythmias and sudden death is that salt depletion increases sympathetic nervous system activity.—F.H. Epstein, M.D.

Requirement of Human Renal Water Channel Aquaporin-2 for Vasopressin-Dependent Concentration of Urine
Deen PMT, Verdijk MAJ, Knoers NVAM, Wieringa B, Monnens LAH, van Os CH, van Oost BA (Univ of Nijmegen, The Netherlands; Univ Hosp Nijmegen, The Netherlands)
Science 264:92–95, 1994   1 1 9-95-66–3

Background.—The ability to clone water-selective channels has made it possible to investigate renal water transport at the molecular level. Urine concentration in mammals is regulated by the antidiuretic hormone vasopressin. When vasopressin binds to its V2 receptor, water channels are formed in the apical membranes of collecting duct cells. In nephrogenic diabetes insipidus (NDI), the kidney fails to concentrate urine in response to vasopressin. Mutations in the gene encoding the V2 receptor have been found in X-linked NDI.

A Second Water Channel.—A man with autosomal recessive NDI was discovered to be a compound heterozygote for 2 mutations in the gene encoding the water channel aquaporin-2, which is expressed only in the collecting duct. The abnormal response to vasopressin was limited to the kidney in this patient, i.e., the level of von Willebrand's factor in plasma rose normally in response to the V2 agonist dDAVP. The coding region for the V2 receptor exhibited no potentially harmful mutation. The authors therefore tested the hypothesis that in this variant patient with NDI with an intact vasopressin V2 receptor, the disease was caused by mutation of the *aquaporin-2* gene. When both wild-type *aquaporin-2* complementary DNA and the 2 mutated *aquaporin-2* complementary DNAs were cloned into *Xenopus* oocytes, each of the mutations resulted in a nonfunctional water channel protein.

Conclusion.—In man, aquaporin-2 is the vasopressin-controlled water channel.

▶ In the classic, X-linked form of inherited nephrogenic diabetes insipidus (limited to males), the V2 vasopressin receptor is abnormal, so that neither vasopressin nor its V2-specific analog, dDAVP, can act on the collecting duct to concentrate the urine or on vascular endothelium to release clotting factors. Some patients with congenital NDI, however, do not fit this pattern—they may be female or may respond to dDAVP with a normal increase in circulating von Willebrand's factor (1). In these individuals a defect distal to the V2 receptor is likely, and in the patient reported in this study, it turned out to be a compound heterozygous defect in the collecting duct's water channel, nicknamed *aquaporin-2*. I was taught in medical school that all cell membranes were freely permeable to water, but as we now know, that is so only if they contain specialized pores called aquaporins, which permit the passage of water. In contrast to *aquaporin-2*, *aquaporin-1* is in the membranes of erythrocytes and proximal tubules of the kidney. It is not controlled by vasopressin, and mutations in it would not be predicted to cause nephrogenic diabetes insipidus.—F.H. Epstein, M.D.

Reference

1. Moses AM, Miller JL, Levine MA: Two distinct pathophysiological mechanisms in congenital nephrogenic diabetes insipidus. *J Clin Endocr Metab* 66:1259–1264, 1988.

Renal Tubular Dysfunction in Chronic Alcohol Abuse: Effects of Abstinence

De Marchi S, Cecchin E, Basile A, Bertotti A, Nardini R, Bartoli E (Univ of Udine, Italy; Gen Hosp, San Vito al Tagliamento, Italy; Inst of Hygiene, Udine, Italy)

N Engl J Med 329:1927–1934, 1993   119-95-66–4

Introduction.—A variety of electrolyte and acid-base disturbances may occur in patients with alcoholism, including hypophosphatemia, hypomagnesemia, hypocalcemia, hypokalemia, metabolic acidosis, and respiratory alkalosis. The relationship between these disorders—which often play a central role in morbidity and may contribute to mortality—and renal tubular dysfunction is unclear.

Methods.—The association between renal dysfunction and electrolyte and acid-base disorders in alcoholism was examined. Sixty-one persons with chronic alcoholism who had little or no liver disease volunteered for and completed 4 weeks of withdrawal therapy. The biochemical constituents of blood and renal function were measured before and after abstinence in all patients. Forty-two normal controls were also studied.

Results.—Electrolyte disorders at admission included hypophosphatemia and hypomagnesemia in 30% of the patients with alcoholism, hypocalcemia in 21%, and hypokalemia in 13%. A range of simple and mixed acid-base disorders was seen in 36% of the patients. Of 20 patients with

Urinary Values in Patients Who Have Alcoholism With Impaired or Normal Renal Acidification on Admission and After 4 Weeks of Abstinence

URINARY MEASURE	IMPAIRED ACIDIFICATION (N = 17)		NORMAL ACIDIFICATION (N = 44)	
	ADMISSION	ABSTINENCE	ADMISSION	ABSTINENCE
Fasting pH	7.0±0.4†	5.9±0.4	6.3±0.3	6.1±0.4
Minimal pH‡	5.7±0.4†	5.0±0.4	5.1±0.2	4.6±0.4
Bicarbonate (mmol/24 hr)	11.2±4.8†	3.6±1.2	3.8±1.2	2.6±0.6
Titratable acidity (mmol/24 hr)	18±4.8†	43±20	30±9	44±7
Ammonium (mmol/24 hr)	18±5.2†	36±10	31±13	35±7
Net total acid (mmol/24 hr)§	24±7.6†	75±12	56±16	76±17
Phosphate (g/24 hr)	0.37±0.1 ‖	0.53±0.1	0.59±0.12	0.68±0.13
Creatinine (g/24 hr)	1.37±0.3	1.40±0.4	1.36±0.7	1.43±0.4
Sodium (mmol/ 24 hr)	132±29	141±25	133±37	138±33

Note: Values are means ± SD. To convert values for phosphate to millimoles per 24 hours, multiply by 32.29; to convert values for creatinine to millimoles per 24 hours, multiply by 8.8.
* $P < .001$ for the comparison with the value obtained in the same patients after 4 weeks of abstinence.
† Measured during the calcium chloride acid-loading test.
§ Calculated by subtracting the value for bicarbonate from the sum of the values for titratable acidity and ammonium.
‖ $P < .01$ for the comparison with the value obtained in the same patients after 4 weeks of abstinence.
(Courtesy of De Marchi S, Cecchin E, Basile A, et al: N Engl J Med 329:1927–1934, 1993.)

metabolic acidosis, 16 had alcoholic acidosis. Defects in renal tubular function varied widely and included decreases in threshold and maximal reabsorptive ability for glucose in 38% of the patients and in renal threshold for phosphate excretion in 36%; increased fractional excretion of β_2-microglobulin in 38%, uric acid in 12%, calcium in 23%, and magnesium in 21%; and aminoaciduria in 38%. A tubular acidification defect was seen in 28% of the patients, whereas 8% had impaired urinary concentrating ability. In patients who did not have normal urinary acidification, the mean values on admission for net acid excretion, titratable acidity, and ammonium were lower than those in the patients with normal urinary acidification (table), but improved after 4 weeks of abstinence. Forty-one percent of the patients had increased urinary excretion of N-acetyl-β-D-glucosaminidase and 34% had increased urinary excretion of alanine aminopeptidase. All of the electrolyte, acid-base, and renal tubular function abnormalities resolved after 4 weeks of abstinence. On admission, the alcoholic patients had higher levels of plasma renin, aldosterone, cortisol, and catecholamines than did normal subjects, but they had lower plasma concentrations of parathyroid hormone.

Conclusions.—Patients with chronic alcoholism have a wide range of mild, transient, renal tubular defects that may play a role in their serum electrolyte and acid-base abnormalities. The nephrotoxicity of alcohol may be unrelated to any associated liver disease. The prognostic importance of the tubular damage can not be easily assessed.

▶ The serum bicarbonate is frequently low when an alcoholic patient is admitted to the hospital, and this can sometimes be attributed to respiratory alkalosis, a common accompaniment of alcohol withdrawal. However, only 2 patients in this series of 61 had primary respiratory alkalosis, and only 4 more who were in fact acidemic had a $PaCO_2$ below that predicted by the usual respiratory response to metabolic acidosis (1). There seems little doubt, therefore, that alcohol induced a transitory, reversible impairment of renal tubular function, manifested in many patients as a reduced ability to secrete acid (i.e., renal tubular acidosis), and in a few as renal glycosuria, phosphaturia, and aminoaciduria. It is still uncertain whether the tendency of some alcoholic patients to lose magnesium in the urine to the point of developing hypomagnesemia is the cause or the result of their low circulating levels of parathyroid hormone, frequently detected in this series.—F.H. Epstein, M.D.

Reference

1. Albert MS, Dell RB, Winters RW: Quantitative displacement of acid-base equilibrium in metabolic acidosis. *Ann Intern Med* 66:312–322, 1967.

First Morning Urine pH in the Diagnosis of Renal Tubular Acidosis With Nephrolithiasis

Chafe L, Gault MH (Mem Univ, St John's, Newfoundland)
Clin Nephrol 41:159–162, 1994   119-95-66–5

Objective.—The accuracy of the fasting first morning urine pH in predicting the result of the ammonium chloride loading test was assessed in a study of recurrent renal stone-formers. A pH $\geq$ 6.10 in 2 fasting morning urines was hypothesized to predict a failure to acidify normally to pH < 5.25 after ammonium chloride; pH < 6.10 in at least 1 fasting first morning urine was hypothesized to predict normal acidification.

Methods.—These values were tested in 96 recurrent renal stone-formers and 14 non–stone-forming controls. In 46 patients, the stones were composed predominantly of calcium phosphate; 30 patients had predominantly calcium oxalate stones and 20 had stone composition between these oxalate:phosphate ratios or included different stones in both categories. No research subject was taking medications, and all had negative urine culture and normal serum chloride and potassium, peripheral blood hemoglobin, pH, and bicarbonate.

Results.—All 14 non–stone-forming controls and 86 of 96 stone-formers acidified their urine normally to a pH < 5.25 after ammonium chloride. The 10 stone-formers who failed to acidify their urine to the designated value had predominantly calcium phosphate stones. Nine of these 10 patients had a pH ≥ 6.10 for both a single and a second first morning urine, yielding a sensitivity of 90%. Nineteen of 100 individuals with a pH < 5.25 after ammonium chloride had a single fasting first morning urine pH ≥ 6.10; only 4 of 100, however, had abnormal fasting first morning pH ≥ 6.10 on 2 occasions, yielding a specificity of 96% for the 2 urines.

Conclusion.—Renal tubular acidosis is strongly suggested by the finding of 2 fasting, first morning urines both with a pH ≥ 6.10. These patients should undergo ammonium chloride loading as well, because the positive predictive value of the 2 first morning urine pH tests was only 69%. The sensitivity of fasting first morning urine pH to predict failure to acidify to pH < 5.25 after ammonium chloride was 90%. Ammonium chloride loading would be unnecessary in patients with a pH of < 6.10 for either of the 2 first fasting specimens.

▶ Distal renal tubular acidosis (RTA) predisposes to renal stones because of the tendency of calcium salts to precipitate in an alkaline urine. The condition may be inherited or caused by a variety of forms of interstitial nephritis affecting the medulla. It is characterized by failure to acidify the urine normally in the face of an acid load. Normal persons easily excrete a urine that is more acidic than a pH of 5.25 when systemic acidosis is present. In patients with the complete form of distal RTA, with low serum bicarbonate and blood pH, a spot urine with a pH greater than 5.25 is sufficient to make the diagnosis. However, persons with incomplete distal RTA often have normal values of blood pH, bicarbonate, and other electrolytes, so that one calls for an ammonium chloride loading test, in which acidosis is produced by the administration of 0.1 g of NH_4Cl per kilogram by mouth, followed by the determination of urinary pH at 2, 4, and 6 hours after the acid load. This paper shows that this elaborate acid loading test can be safety bypassed by testing the pH of two first morning urines (which should be acidic in normal subjects). If both have a pH less than 6.1, the patient does not have distal RTA; if they are greater than 6.1, the likelihood of distal RTA is strong.—F.H. Epstein, M.D.

67 Calcium and Phosphorus

Brief Report: Inhibition of Renal Phosphate Transport by a Tumor Product in a Patient With Oncogenic Osteomalacia
Cai Q, Hodgson SF, Kao PC, Lennon VA, Klee GG, Zinsmiester AR, Kumar R
(Mayo Clinic and Found, Rochester, Minn)
N Engl J Med 330:1645–1649, 1994   119-95-67–1

Introduction.—Tumor-induced osteomalacia is a rare disorder characterized by hypophosphatemia, hyperphosphaturia, and a low plasma level of 1,25-dihydroxyvitamin D. The biochemical and pathologic abnormalities resolve on removal of the tumor. The tumors responsible are thought to secrete a substance that inhibits renal tubular phosphate reabsorption, but it is not clear whether the factor interacts directly with the renal tubular cells.

Case Report.—Woman, 47, had noted aching in her arms and legs for 7 years and was found to have moderately week proximal limb muscles as well as a 2 × 1.5-cm soft tissue mass in the distal part of the anterior thigh. A low serum phosphate and a high alkaline phosphatase level were found, and an iliac bone biopsy specimen demonstrated osteomalacia. The left proximal femur fractured spontaneously the following year, when the thigh mass—which had become larger—was removed and was found to be a sclerosing hemangioma. The fracture healed postoperatively, limb weakness was less marked, and the serum phosphate level rose to normal. Lower limb pain returned along with a mass at the original site 16 years later. The maximal ability of the renal tubules to reabsorb phosphorus divided by the glomerular filtration rate (TmP/GFR) was impaired. Osteomalacia again was demonstrated, and a mass of similar pathology was removed. Again the patient improved clinically and biochemically, although the serum osteocalcin level was elevated.

Observations.—Medium from tumor-cell cultures significantly inhibited phosphate transport in cultured opossum kidney cells. The medium did not have the effect of bovine parathyroid hormone 1-34 in augmenting the accumulation of cyclic adenosine monophosphate in these cells. Nevertheless, parathyroid hormone–like immunoreactivity in tumor-cell medium was twice as high as in control medium. The factor was shown to have a low molecular weight and to be heat-labile. When tumor fragments were implanted in nude mice, the serum phosphate declined.

Conclusion.—Culture medium conditioned by the growth of sclerosing hemangioma cells from this patient with oncogenic osteomalacia inhibited phosphate transport in renal epithelial cells.

▶ The phenomenon of tumor-induced osteomalacia—an exceptionally rare syndrome described in a total of only about 70 patients worldwide—has a physiological significance far beyond its numerical frequency. Our kidneys are the main agents controlling the level of inorganic phosphate in circulating blood, and they respond promptly to changes in dietary intake of phosphorus by altering tubular reabsorption of phosphate from the glomerular filtrate. What tells them to do this? It seems likely that the message is humoral and that it is distinct from parathyroid hormone or parathyroid-related protein (PTRP), because phosphate excretion can be regulated by the kidney without changes in the level of calcium or of cyclic adenosine monophosphate (cAMP) in blood or urine.

The factor isolated by Dr. Kumar and his associates at Mayo is a prime candidate for such a hormone. Its overproduction by the tumor leads to excessive loss of phosphate in the urine and hypophosphatemia. The profound hypophosphatemia in turn shuts off 1,24-hydroxy D_3 synthesis by the kidneys, and both phenomena together produce osteomalacia and muscle weakness. An exploration of the physiology of these unusual tumors may, I believe, clarify the normal mechanisms of phosphate metabolism in the same way Jerome Conn's description of a single patient with aldosterone-producing tumor almost 40 years ago illuminated our understanding of sodium and potassium excretion. An editorial in the same issue of the *New England Journal of Medicine* (1) speculates that the phosphate-wasting described in this brief report might be relevant to the more common (but still rare) syndrome of hereditary X-linked osteomalacia, characterized by hypophosphatemic rickets, but as yet there is no proof for this hypothesis.—F.H. Epstein, M.D.

Reference

1. Econs MJ, Drezner MK: Tumor-induced osteomalacia: Unveiling a new hormone. N Engl J Med 330:1679–1681, 1994.

Effects of Oral vs. Intravenous Calcitriol on Serum Parathyroid Hormone Levels in Chronic Hemodialysis Patients
Chan R, Gleim GW, DeVita MV, Zabetakis PM, Michelis MF (Lenox Hill Hosp, New York City)
Dial Transplant 22:736–745, 1993   119-95-67–2

Rationale.—Oral and parenteral preparations of calcitriol are available for controlling the serum parathyroid hormone (PTH) in patients undergoing hemodialysis who have secondary hyperparathyroidism develop. Intravenous treatment is much more costly than oral dosing, but some believe that oral treatment is less effective.

Study Plan.—The effects of oral and intravenous calcitriol administration on the serum PTH level were studied in a prospective series of 26 patients undergoing chronic hemodialysis. Serum immunoreactive PTH (iPTH) levels were monitored over 3 months of calcitriol therapy. The dose was adjusted to maintain a serum level of calcium of 10.5 to 11.5 mg/dL.

Results.—Serum levels of iPTH decreased significantly both in patients given oral calcitriol (0.5 to 1.0 μg/day) and in those treated intravenously (0.5 to 3 μg, 3 times per week). The average decrease was 40% with oral treatment and 58% in patients treated intravenously, not a statistically significant difference. The serum calcium increased to a similar degree in the 2 groups. The serum calcium and iPTH levels at the end of the study correlated significantly in orally treated patients but not in those given calcitriol intravenously.

Conclusions.—Oral and intravenous treatment with calcitriol are both effective ways of controlling the serum iPTH in hemodialysis patients. It is appropriate to consider patient compliance and cost when deciding what form of treatment to use in a given case.

▶ Both oral and intravenous calcitriol are effective in reducing secondary hyperparathyroidism and its deleterious consequences on the skeleton. The chief mechanism is probably exerted via the action of calcitriol to raise serum calcium to the upper normal range, but it is likely that vitamin D_3 also suppresses parathyroid secretion by a direct action on parathyroid cells. There has been some disagreement as to whether the intravenous route might have special advantages as a more effective direct suppressor of PTH secretion, so in this study the two routes of administration were compared in 13 subjects each. No statistically significant difference was detected; serum calcium rose and circulating PTH fell in both groups. Some have suggested that the vitamin D be administered in "pulse" fashion so as to achieve high peak levels in the circulating blood. Presumably this helps to suppress PTH secretion via calcitriol receptors on hyperplastic parathyroid glands (1–3). In this study, however, daily oral dosing was used. While the number of patients in each group was small and the variances large, so that a small difference might not have been detected, it seems likely that if there is a difference, it is not important from a clinical standpoint. Moreover, the cost of intravenous calcitriol ($31.92 for 1 μg IV 3 times a week) vs. the cost of oral calcitriol ($10.57 for 0.5 μg daily) is substantial. I vote for routine use of the oral preparation.—F.H. Epstein, M.D.

References

1. Fukagawa M, Obazaki R, Takano K, et al: Regression of parathyroid hyperplasia by calcitriol-pulse therapy in patients on long-term dialysis. *N Engl J Med* 523:421–422, 1990.
2. Martin KJ, Ballal S, Domoto D, et al: Pulse oral calcitriol for the treatment of hyperparathyroidism in patients on CAPD (abstract). *J Am Soc Nephrol* 1:587, 1990.

3. Reichel H, Szabo A, Uhl J, et al: Intermittent vs continuous administration of 1,25-dihydroxyvitamin D$_3$ in experimental renal hyperparathyroidism. *Kidney Int* 44:1259–1265, 1993.

Bilateral Vocal Cord Paralysis Secondary to Treatment of Severe Hypophosphatemia in a Continuous Ambulatory Peritoneal Dialysis Patient

Lye WC, Leong SO (Natl Univ Hosp, Singapore)
Am J Kidney Dis 23:127–129, 1994   119-95-67–3

Case Report.—Woman, 61, had end-stage renal disease related to non–insulin-dependent diabetes and was very malnourished and had uremic symptoms when first seen. Continuous ambulatory peritoneal dialysis was instituted, but the nutritional intake remained inadequate. A flulike illness developed after 4 months of dialysis; the patient was weak and unable to walk. Blood urea was 42 mg/dL; creatinine, 3.5 mg/dL; serum potassium, 1.7 mEq/L; and serum phosphorus, .9 mg/dL. The patient was given potassium replacement and 3 g of phosphorus as sodium phosphate over 48 hours. After 2 days she was obtunded and in respiratory distress, and examination revealed tetany and carpopedal spasm. The vocal cords were adducted and immobile. The serum phosphorus at this time was 10.1 mg/dL, and the ionized calcium was 2.6 mg/dL. The serum magnesium was .5 mg/dL. Calcium chloride and magnesium sulfate were given IV and the patient improved clinically. Vocal cord motion eventually returned to normal.

Interpretation.—This patient's initial weakness and inability to walk were ascribed to hypophosphatemia and hypokalemia, but hypomagnesemia also may have been a factor. Rebound hyperphosphatemia developed when phosphate was administered and, along with hypomagnesemia, led to marked hypocalcemia and tetany.

Recommendation.—Correction of hypophosphatemia should be based on estimates of phosphate balance. This is especially important for patients with renal failure. The serum calcium also should be closely monitored, and hypomagnesemia should be ruled out before phosphate is administered.

▶ This interesting case emphasizes the susceptibility of uremic patients to hypocalcemia when the compensatory mechanisms that normally resist a fall in serum calcium are inhibited. In this patient with renal failure, the administration of phosphate to treat symptomatic hypophosphatemia led to an abnormally elevated serum phosphorus because excess phosphate could not be excreted in the urine. Serum calcium was reciprocally depressed, and its level could not be sustained because a secondary and compensatory increase in parathyroid hormone secretion was blocked by hypomagnesemia. The result was life-threatening tetany. We have recently seen another application of this principle in an elderly man, treated with etidronate for osteoporosis, who developed acute renal failure. The etidronate prevented mobilization of bony calcium as serum phosphate rose in the course of acute renal failure, and as a result, serum calcium plunged to very low levels (1).—F.H. Epstein, M.D.

Reference

1. Bacon N, Clark BA: Etidronate in acute renal failure (abstract). *J Am Soc Nephrol* 5:365, 1994.

PART EIGHT

RHEUMATOLOGY

STEPHEN E. MALAWISTA, M.D.

68 Rheumatoid Arthritis

Introduction

This year we learn that hydroxychloroquine (Abstract 119-95-68–1) and sulfasalazine (Abstract 119-95-68–2) are indeed each moderately effective in early rheumatoid arthritis; that men with Felty's syndrome (like patients with Sjögren's syndrome) have an increased risk of developing non-Hodgkin's lymphoma (Abstract 119-95-68–3); that long-term mortality in patients with rheumatoid arthritis is predictable according to simple questionnaire and joint count measures (Abstract 119-95-68–4); and that low dose prednisone induces in patients with rheumatoid arthritis a rapid axial bone loss that is largely reversible (Abstract 119-95-68–5).

Noted in passing: Clinical experimental studies seeking more effective therapy for rheumatoid arthritis, including a number of antibodies (e.g., to tumor necrosis factor-α [1, 2], intracellular adhesion molecule-1 [3], CD5 [4], CD 4 [5, 6]), an interleukin-2 fusion toxin (7), gammalinolenic acid (8, 9), omega-3 fatty acids (10), type II collagen (11), and minocycline (12); a review of HLA-DRB1 alleles as severity markers in rheumatoid arthritis (13), and a review of second-line drug therapy for rheumatoid arthritis (14).

Stephen E. Malawista, M.D.

References

1. Elliott MJ, Maini RN, Feldman M, Long-Fox A, Charles P, Katsikis P, Brennan FM, Walker J, Bijl H, Ghrayeb J, Woody JN: Treatment of rheumatoid arthritis with chimeric monoclonal antibodies to tumor necrosis factor α. *Arthritis Rheum* 36:1681–1690, 1993.
2. Dinarello CA, Rosenberg IH: Rheumatoid cachexia: Cytokine-driven hypermetabolism accompanying reduced body cell mass in chronic inflammation. *J Clin Invest* 93:2379–2386, 1994.
3. Kavanaugh AF, Davis LS, Nichols LA, Norris SH, Rothlein R, Scharschmidt LA, Lipsky PE: Treatment of refractory rheumatoid arthritis with a monoclonal antibody to intercellular adhesion molecule 1. *Arthritis Rheum* 37:992–999, 1994.
4. Fishwild DM, Strand V: Administration of an anti-CD5 immunoconjugate to patients with rheumatoid arthritis: Effect on peripheral blood mononuclear cells and *in vitro* immune function. *J Rheumatol* 21:596–604, 1994.
5. van der Lubbe PA, Reiter C, Breedveld FC, Krüger K, Schattenkirchner M, Sanders ME, Riethmüller G: Chimeric CD4 monoclonal antibody cM-T412 as a therapeutic approach to rheumatoid arthritis. *Arthritis Rheum* 36:1375–1379, 1993.
6. Moreland LW, Pratt PW, Bucy RP, Jackson BS, Feldman JW, Koopman WJ:

Treatment of refractory rheumatoid arthritis with a chimeric anti-CD4 monoclonal antibody: Long-term followup of CD4+ T cell counts. *Arthritis Rheum* 37:834–838, 1994.

7. Sewell KL, Parker KC, Woodworth TG, Reuben J, Swartz W, Trentham DE: DAB$_{486}$IL-2 fusion toxin in refractory rheumatoid arthritis. *Arthritis Rheum* 36:1223–1233, 1993.

8. Leventhal LJ, Boyce EG, Pharm D, Zurier RB: Treatment of rheumatoid arthritis with gammalinolenic acid. *Ann Intern Med* 119:867–873, 1993.

9. Phinney S: Potential risk of prolonged gamma-linolenic acid use. *Ann Intern Med* 120:692, 1994 (letter).

10. Geusens P, Wouters C, Nijs J, Jiang Y, Dequeker J: Long-term effect of Omega-3 fatty acid supplementation in active rheumatoid arthritis: A 12-month, double-blind, controlled study. *Arthritis Rheum* 37:824–829, 1994.

11. Trentham DE, Dynesius-Trentham RA, Orav EJ, Combitchi D, Lorenzo C, Sewell KL, Hafler DA, Weiner HL: Effects of oral administration of Type II collagen on rheumatoid arthritis. *Science* 261:1727–1730, 1993.

12. Kloppenburg M, Breedveld FC, Terwiel JP, Mallee C, Dijkmans BAC: Minocycline in active rheumatoid arthritis. *Arthritis Rheum* 37:629–636, 1994.

13. Weyand CM, Goronzy JJ: HLA-DRB1 alleles as severity markers in RA. *Bull Rheum Dis* 43:5–8, 1994.

14. Cash JM, Klippel JH: Second-line drug therapy for rheumatoid arthritis. *N Engl J Med* 330:1368–1375, 1994.

Hydroxychloroquine Compared With Placebo in Rheumatoid Arthritis: A Randomized Controlled Trial

Clark P, Casas E, Tugwell P, Medina C, Gheno C, Tenorio G, Orozco JA (Universidad Nacional Autonoma de Mexico, Mexico City; Univ of Ottawa, Ont, Canada)

Ann Intern Med 119:1067–1071, 1993   119-95-68-1

Background.—Antimalarial agents long have been used to treat some rheumatic disorders such as lupus. A number of double-blind, placebo-controlled trials of antimalarial therapy for rheumatoid arthritis were done in the 1950s and early 1960s, yielding some evidence of efficacy but no definitive results.

Study Plan.—In a randomized trial, hydroxychloroquine was compared with placebo in 121 patients, aged 18 and older, in whom rheumatoid disease had begun after age 16 years, and who had at least 5 actively inflamed joints. The patients had failed to respond to at least 2 salicylate or nonsteroidal anti-inflammatory agents. Hydroxychloroquine was given in a dose of 400 mg daily during the 24-week study, which used a double-blind, parallel design.

Results.—Patients complied well with taking active drug or placebo. Joint scores improved to a significant degree in hydroxychloroquine-treated patients (Fig 68–1). Both patient and physician ratings of global change indicated superior results with hydroxychloroquine compared with placebo. There were no changes in the use of aspirin analgesics or nonsteroidal anti-inflammatory drugs. Side effects were comparably fre-

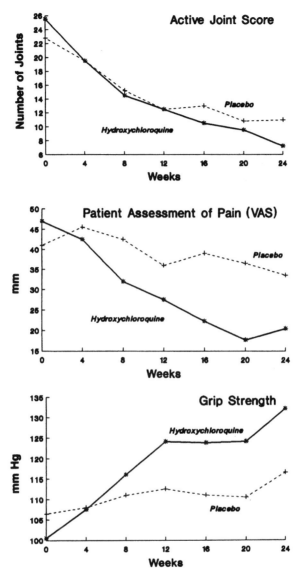

Fig 68–1.—Raw mean scores for joint scores, patient assessment of pain, and grip strength variables for each visit and each treatment group. *Abbreviation;* VAS, visual analogue scale. (Courtesy of Clark P, Casas E, Tugwell P, et al: *Ann Intern Med* 119:1067–1071, 1993.)

quent in the actively treated patients and placebo recipients. No patient had ocular toxic effects from hydroxychloroquine.

Conclusion.—Hydroxychloroquine appears to confer a modest but useful degree of benefit on patients with early rheumatoid arthritis. It may be an appropriate first choice for a second-line drug for patients who fail to respond to nonsteroidal anti-inflammatory agents.

▶ In this 6-month, double-blind, randomized trial, hydroxychloroquine proved more effective than placebo in early rheumatoid arthritis. Note that the study was designed to examine as homogenous a group as possible—one with mild disease; 80% of the patients were functional class 1 (the best category), and 93% of them had 5 or fewer radiographic erosions. It is among these patients that the often modest effects of hydroxychloroquine—the least toxic of the second-line agents—are used to best advantage (1).

Improvement in the placebo group, although significantly less than that in those who received hydroxychloroquine, reminds us how important appropriate controls are in assessing drug efficacy. The authors attribute most of this effect to the nature of the patient population, as spontaneous improvement is not uncommon in early disease. To this may be added the increased attention that people in studies receive. A watched pot may never boil, but watched patients with rheumatoid arthritis generally do better than those who are left to themselves.—S.E. Malawista, M.D.

Reference

1. Harris ED Jr: Hydroxychloroquine is safe and probably useful in rheumatoid arthritis. *Ann Intern Med* 119:1146–1147, 1993.

Sulfasalazine in Early Rheumatoid Arthritis

Hannonen P, Möttönen T, Hakola M, Oka M (Central Hosp, Jyväskylä, Finland)
Arthritis Rheum 36:1501–1509, 1993   119-95-68–2

Background.—Treatment for rheumatoid arthritis (RA) remains empirical, with an emphasis on alleviating symptoms and controlling inflammation. More aggressive treatment during the early stages of RA has been proposed, but controlled studies are lacking. The efficacy and tolerability of sulfasalazine (SSZ) for the treatment of early RA were examined.

Methods.—The study sample comprised 78 adult patients with RA, all of whom had been symptomatic for less than one year. All were receiving a stable dose of nonsteroidal anti-inflammatory drugs. Patients were randomized to receive either SSZ, beginning at a dose of 500 mg/day and gradually increasing to 2,000 mg/day, or placebo. The 2 groups were compared in terms of clinical, laboratory, and scintigraphic findings after up to 48 weeks of treatment.

Results.—At last follow-up, 9 patients in each group were in remission. Almost all clinical variables favored SSZ treatment, especially for number of swollen joints (Figs 68-2 and 68-3). This trend was apparent as early as 4 weeks after the start of treatment. There was a greater dif-

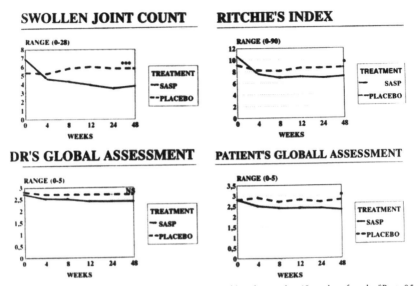

Fig 68–2.—Mean changes in primary efficacy variables during the 48 weeks of study. *P < .05; ***P < .001; *Abbreviations:* NS, not significant; SASP, sulfasalazine. (Courtesy of Hannonen P, Möttönen T, Hakola M, et al: *Arthritis Rheum* 36:1501-1509, 1993.)

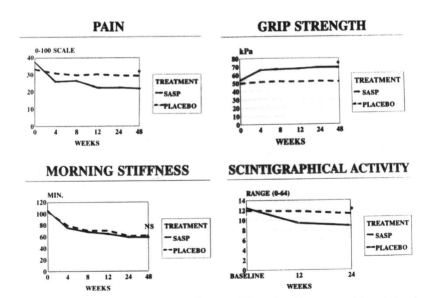

Fig 68–3.—Mean changes in secondary efficacy variables and activity score on joint scintigraphy during the 48 weeks of study. *P < .05. *Abbreviations:* NS, not significant; SASP, sulfasalazine. (Courtesy of Hannonen P, Möttönen T, Hakola M, et al: *Arthritis Rheum* 36:1501-1509, 1993.)

ference in treatment effect for seronegative patients with early RA receiving SSZ. In the first 24 weeks of treatment, scintigraphic scores decreased significantly more in patients taking SSZ. Thirty-three percent of the SSZ group vs. 22% of the placebo group showed no radiographic progression at the end of the study, but the trend was not significant.

Conclusion.—Sulfasalazine appears to be an effective treatment for patients with early RA. It has a rapid onset of action and may slow the development of joint erosion. Unfortunately, in most cases, the disease progresses despite SSZ treatment. Although there are many side effects, most patients are able to continue with treatment.

▶ Sulfasalazine has been in and out of fashion in the past half-century. Specifically designed in the 1930s to treat "rheumatic polyarthritis," which was thought to be bacterial in origin, SSZ is split by colonic bacteria into a poorly absorbed anti-inflammatory moiety, 5-aminosalicylic acid, and sulfapyridine; the latter is metabolized in the liver by acetylation. The drug lost favor in the treatment of RA in the 1940s, only to be rediscovered in the late 1970s. It is useful in the treatment of seronegative spondyloarthropathies (1), and in this study it is shown to be effective, although not dramatically so, in early (meaning ≤ 1 year's duration) RA. All test parameters improved except morning stiffness and doctor's global assessment (Figures 68–2 and 68–3). Like methotrexate, SSZ has the advantage of working relatively fast for a second-line agent; most of the changes in this study occurred within the first 4 weeks of the trial.

Side effects (2, 3) are common, occurring in perhaps 50% of patients, usually in the first 4 months of treatment; but only about half of such episodes lead to discontinuation of the drug (and many fewer in the current group). Most common are rash, nausea, abdominal pain, central nervous system disturbances, and blood dyscrasias, particularly in patients with glucose-6-phosphate dehydrogenase deficiency. The apparently greater effects of the drug on seronegative patients with early RA (vs. seropositive patients) needs confirmation.—S.E. Malawista, M.D.

References

1. 1994 YEAR BOOK OF MEDICINE, p 788.
2. Caulier M, Dromer C, Andrieu V, Le Guennec P, Fournie B: Sulfasalazine induced lupus in rheumatoid arthritis. *J Rheumatol* 21:750–751, 1994.
3. Gran JT, Myklebust G: Toxicity of sulfasalazine in rheumatoid arthritis: Possible protective effect of rheumatoid factors and corticosteroids. *Scand J Rheumatol* 22:229–232, 1993.

Incidence of Cancer Among Men With the Felty Syndrome

Gridley G, Klippel JH, Hoover RN, Fraumeni JF Jr (Natl Cancer Inst, Bethesda, Md; Natl Inst of Arthritis, Musculoskeletal and Skin Diseases, Bethesda, Md)

Ann Intern Med 120:35–39, 1994   119-95-68-3

Background.—Approximately 1% of patients with rheumatoid arthritis have Felty's syndrome, which is characterized by neutropenia, splenomegaly, and recurrent infections. Most follow-up studies of patients with rheumatoid disease indicate no increase in the incidence of cancer apart from an approximate doubling of the incidence of lymphoproliferative malignancies, but these studies have not focused on the Felty syndrome.

Objective and Methods.—In a retrospective cohort study, the frequency of cancer was estimated in patients with Felty's syndrome who were discharged from Veterans Affairs hospitals in 1969–1990. The 906 white male veterans in the study were followed for as long as 20 years and for an average of 6 years. Their average age when first hospitalized for Felty's syndrome was 61 years. Standardized incidence ratios (SIRs) were estimated for specific types of cancer.

Observations.—The overall twofold increase in cancers represented higher-than-expected numbers of all common types of cancer other than prostatic cancer. Four types of neoplastic disease were clearly increased compared with Veterans Affairs (VA) and Surveillance, Epidemiology, and End Results (SEER) Program rates: non-Hodgkin's lymphoma, leukemia, malignant melanoma, and lung cancer. Multiple myeloma and Hodgkin's disease also were more frequent than expected, but fewer than 5 cases of these cancers were seen. Cancer risk did not vary with the age at the time Felty's syndrome was diagnosed or with the number of hospitalizations for Felty's syndrome. The risk of non-Hodgkin's lymphoma was somewhat higher in patients who underwent splenectomy. The SIR for all cancers was 2.09, and that for non-Hodgkin's lymphoma was 12.8. The increased risk of leukemia held only for the first 5 years after initial hospitalization for Felty's syndrome.

Conclusion.—The increased risk of non-Hodgkin's lymphoma associated with Felty syndrome is comparable to that associated with the Sjögren syndrome. Similar immunostimulatory mechanisms may be responsible.

▶ Compared with patients with straightforward rheumatoid arthritis, those with Felty's syndrome tend to have more severe progressive destructive disease despite little objective synovitis; a higher frequency of extra-articular disease, including vasculitis; and greater mortality, especially from infection (1). To this we can now add a much higher risk for non-Hodgkin's lymphoma – twelvefold vs. twofold — one that is comparable to that seen in Sjögren's syndrome. As noted by the authors, the disadvantages of this retrospective cohort study are incomplete follow-up and ascertainment of cancers, the likely skewed representation of patients who use Veterans Affairs hospitals, the fact that hospital patients are sicker than outpatients, the lack of global confirmation of diagnoses (Felty's syndrome could not be confirmed in 16%

of the patients with lymphoma), and incomplete treatment information. With regard to the last point, the high risk for non-Hodgkin's lymphoma does not seem explainable by treatment; only one lymphoma patient was listed as having received a cytotoxic agent (azathioprine), and no one was listed as having received methotrexate, which may be associated with a reversible non-Hodgkin's lymphoma (2). The authors suggest that an increased susceptibility to various forms of cancer, and especially to non-Hodgkin's lymphoma, may relate to features of Felty's syndrome, such as the low neutrophil count, splenic dysfunction, increased susceptibility to infection, or more aggressive rheumatoid disease, that are not found in other patients with rheumatoid arthritis.—S.E. Malawista, M.D.

References

1. 1991 YEAR BOOK OF MEDICINE, p 684.
2. 1994 YEAR BOOK OF MEDICINE, p 760.

Prediction of Long-Term Mortality in Patients With Rheumatoid Arthritis According to Simple Questionnaire and Joint Count Measures
Pincus T, Brooks RH, Callahan LF (Vanderbilt Univ, Nashville Tenn)
Ann Intern Med 120:26–34, 1994   119-95-68-4

Background.—Rheumatoid arthritis affects between 0.5% and 1% of the United States population. Whether simple quantitative questionnaires to assess activities of daily living and joint counts provide reliable information in identifying increased probability of mortality over the subsequent 15 years was investigated.

Method.—Seventy-five patients with rheumatoid arthritis were studied during the fall of 1973. Evaluation included examining age, demographic variables, clinical variables, mean joint count level, stiffness, responses to questions involving activities of daily living, and physical assessment of functional status. The patients were followed up for 15 years, and the relative risk for mortality was calculated according to each baseline variable.

Results.—Although a few deaths were seen in the first few years of the study, the standard mortality ratios were 1.86 at 5 years, 1.92 at 10 years, and 1.62 at 15 years. Survival rates were lower in patients who were older and in patients with fewer than 12 years of formal education. No significant difference was seen in survival according to duration of disease. Patients with more than 30 joints involved did not survive as long as patients with fewer than 10 joints involved: less than 50% at 5 years and less than 30% at 15 years, compared with 90% at 5 years and more than 70% at 15 years, respectively (Fig 68–4). Patients who experienced more stiffness also showed a decreased survival rate. Patients who recorded the highest level of functional status on an activities-of-daily-living questionnaire had a greater rate of survival than those with the poor-

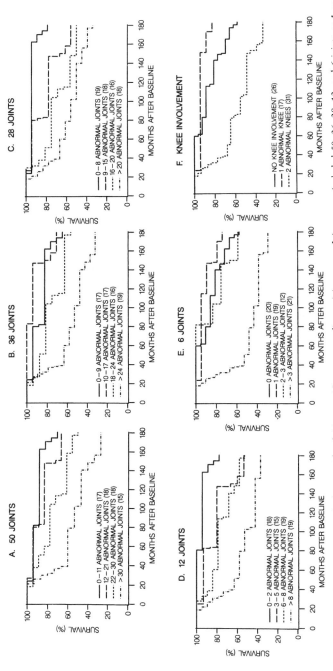

Fig 68-4.—Survival in 75 patients with rheumatoid arthritis over 15 years, according to joint counts. Joint counts included 50, 36, 28, 12, and 6 joints or 1 or 2 knees. (Courtesy of Pincus I, Brooks RH, Callahan LF: *Ann Intern Med* 120:26–34, 1994.)

A. 87 ADL QUESTIONS

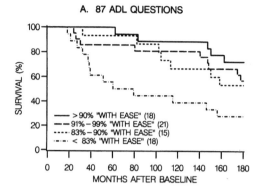

B. 20 ADL QUESTIONS (SIMULATED HAQ)

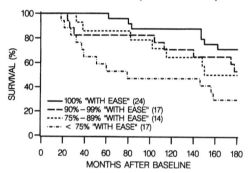

C. 8 ADL QUESTIONS (SIMULATED MHAQ)

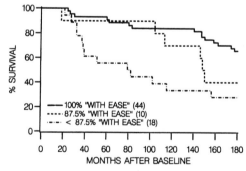

Fig 68–5.—Survival in 75 patients with rheumatoid arthritis over 15 years, according to responses to questions about ADL with 87, 20, or 8 included activities. *Abbreviations: ADL,* activities of daily living; *HAQ,* Health Assessment Questionnaire; *MHAQ,* modified HAQ. (Courtesy of Pincus T, Brooks RH, Callahan LF: *Ann Intern Med* 120:26–34, 1994.)

est functional status: 90% survived for 5 years and 70% for 15 years, compared with fewer than 50% for 5 years, and none for 15 years, respectively (Fig 68–5).

Conclusion.—Higher mortality rates can be expected of patients with rheumatoid arthritis who have more severe clinical disease, higher joint count, and poorer status in questionnaire scores and in physical measures of functional status. Quantitative functional status questionnaires and joint counts are an efficient means of identifying severe rheumatoid arthritis, and can be done in a short time (10 to 15 minutes) in any clinical setting.

▶ Significant predictors of mortality in rheumatoid arthritis included age, formal education level, joint count, activities-of-daily-living questionnaire scores, disease adjustment scores, morning stiffness, comorbid cardiovascular disease, grip strength, modified walking time, and button (manipulation) test. Five-year survival in patients with the poorest status according to these quantitative measures was 40% to 60%. To put these figures in perspective, note that they are comparable to expected survival at that time of patients with three-vessel coronary disease or with stage 4 Hodgkin's disease.

It is becoming increasingly difficult to claim that appropriate measurements are too complicated to perform in a practice setting. Simplified measures taking little time, such as a count using only 28 joints (1) and a questionnaire using only 8 activities of daily living, were similar to the more elaborate traditional measures for predicting mortality (Figures 68–4 and 68–5).

This study did not involve an inception cohort but, rather, a clinical cohort whose average duration of disease was 12 years. The authors rightly suggest prospective studies with inception cohorts to see whether these variables are useful predictors for patients early in disease. Moreover, given that rheumatoid arthritis may progress to levels at which clinical markers predict rather high mortality rates within 5 years, they support the possible value of early aggressive therapy designed to prevent progression to these levels. An appropriate subset of patients for such therapeutic trials might be those who seem immunogenetically likely to have a more difficult course (2).—S.E. Malawista, M.D.

References

1. Fuchs HA, Pincus T: Reduced joint counts in controlled clinical trials in rheumatoid arthritis. *Arthritis Rheum* 37:470–475, 1994.
2. 1994 YEAR BOOK OF MEDICINE, p 755.

Low-Dose Prednisone Induces Rapid Reversible Axial Bone Loss in Patients With Rheumatoid Arthritis

Laan RFJM, van Riel PLCM, van de Putte LBA, van Erning LJTO, van't Hof MA, Lemmens JAM (Univ Hosp Nijmegen, The Netherlands)
Ann Intern Med 119:963–968, 1993   119-95-68-5

Background.—Previous findings on the effects of low-dose glucocorticoid agents on bone in patients with rheumatoid arthritis (RA) are controversial. The positive effects of glucocorticoid drugs on the inflammatory process and on physical activity may outweigh their negative effects on bone.

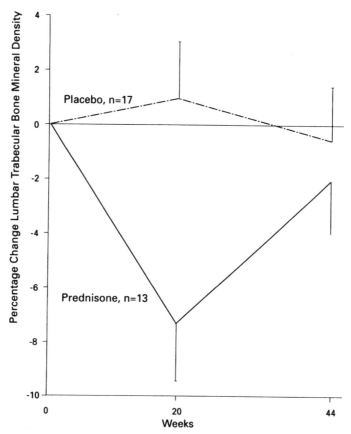

Fig 68–6.—Mean changes in lumbar, trabecular bone mineral density during and after low-dose prednisone treatment in a subset of patients who did not use prednisone between weeks 20 and 44. The change (mean ± SE) in bone mineral density was measured using dual-energy, quantitative CT. The prednisone dose was 10 mg/day from week 0 to 12 and was tapered between weeks 12 and 20. (Courtesy of Laan RFJM, van Riel PLCM, van de Plutte LBA, et al: *Ann Intern Med* 119:963–968, 1993.)

Methods.—Forty patients with active RA were enrolled in a double-blind, placebo-controlled, randomized study. All began receiving intramuscular gold salts and then were randomly assigned to prednisone or placebo. The prednisone dose, initially 10 mg/day, was tapered between weeks 12 and 20. The patients were followed-up for 24 weeks after the end of therapy.

Findings.—The effects of prednisone on disease activity and functional capacity were favorable. However, trabecular bone mineral density declined in the patients given prednisone between baseline and week 20. Placebo-treated patients evidenced little change. The prednisone group had a greater mean bone loss than the placebo group. After prednisone was discontinued, trabecular bone mineral density increased between weeks 20 and 44 (Fig 68–6). After placebo withdrawal, there was little change. The mean improvement in the prednisone group was 6.8% higher than that in the placebo group. Cortical bone mineral density did not change greatly in either period in either group.

Conclusion.—In patients with active RA, low-dose glucocorticoid drugs result in marked vertebral trabecular bone loss in the initial months of treatment. Bone loss appears to be partly reversible after treatment is discontinued.

▶ In this randomized controlled study, low-dose corticosteroid therapy given over 5 months (10 mg once daily for 3 months, tapered to zero over 2 months) produced significant lumbar trabecular (but not lumbar cortical) bone loss, which was largely reversible over the following 6 months. We do not know if much longer courses would also be reversible, but in a recent cross-sectional study of postmenopausal women with RA (1), bone mineral density (BMD) in ex-users of low-dose corticosteroids was similar to that of never-users. In that study, there was a baseline reduction in BMD at the hip (femoral head) but not the lumbar spine (they did not distinguish cortical from trabecular bone) in postmenopausal women with RA compared with postmenopausal controls; treatment with steroids resulted in further lowering of bone density at both sites.

Rheumatologists vary in their use of low-dose corticosteroids for RA (2), but few would argue that the lowest dose consistent with one's therapeutic goals is not to be sought. Long-term low-dose (≥ 5 mg per day) prednisone therapy does seem to be associated with the development of specific adverse events (e.g., fracture, gastrointestinal events, infection) in a dose-dependent fashion (3) (although, at least when the taper is down to 5 mg per day, continued suppressioon of the hypothalamic-pituitary-adrenal axis does not seem to be one of them [4]). As the authors note, the marked decrease in bone mass in the initial months of therapy suggests that prevention (see, e.g., Reference 5) be considered from the beginning and throughout corticosteroid therapy.—S.E. Malawista, M.D.

References

1. Hall GM, Spector TD, Griffin AJ, Jawad ASM, Hall ML, Doyle DV: The effect of rheumatoid arthritis and steroid therapy on bone density in postmenopausal women. *Arthritis Rheum* 36:1510–1516, 1993.
2. Criswell LA, Redfearn WJ: Variation among rheumatologists in the use of prednisone and second-line agents for the treatment of rheumatoid arthritis. *Arthritis Rheum* 37:476–480, 1994.
3. Saag KG, Koehnke R, Caldwell JR, Brasington R, Burmeister LF, Zimmerman B, Kohler JA, Furst DE: Low dose long-term corticosteroid therapy in rheumatoid arthritis: An analysis of serious adverse events. *Am J Med* 96:115–123, 1994.
4. La Rochelle GE Jr, La Rochelle AG, Ratner RE, Borenstein DG: Recovery of the hypothalamic-pituitary-adrenal (HPA) axis in patients with rheumatic diseases receiving low-dose prednisone. *Am J Med* 95:258–264, 1993.
5. 1994 YEAR BOOK OF MEDICINE, p 820.

69 Systemic Lupus Erythematosus

Introduction

This chapter deals with mothers at risk for congenital heart block and for other neonatal lupus syndromes in their children (Abstract 119-95-69–1), the reliability of histologic scoring for lupus nephritis (Abstract 119-95-69–2), and the apparent protective effect of inactive lupus at the onset of pregnancy to the development of lupus flares during pregnancy (Abstract 119-95-69–3).

Noted in passing: The use of ANAs and antibodies to DNA in clinical diagnosis (1); antibodies to defined antigens in the systemic rheumatic diseases (2); and a general review of systemic lupus erythematosus (3).

Stephen E. Malawista, M.D.

References

1. Reichlin M: ANAs and antibodies to DNA: Their use in clinical diagnosis. *Bull Rheum Dis* 42:3–5, 1993.
2. Reichlin M: Antibodies to defined antigens in the systemic rheumatic diseases. *Bull Rheum Dis* 42:4–6, 1993.
3. Systemic lupus erythematosus. *Med Prog Technol* 330:1871–1879, 1994.

Identification of Mothers at Risk for Congenital Heart Block and Other Neonatal Lupus Syndromes in Their Children: Comparison of Enzyme-Linked Immunosorbent Assay and Immunoblot for Measurement of Anti-SS-A/Ro and Anti-SS-B/La Antibodies

Buyon JP, Winchester RJ, Slade SG, Arnett F, Copel J, Friedman D, Lockshin MD (New York Univ, Hosp for Joint Diseases, Hosp for Special Surgery; Cornell Univ, Columbia Presbyterian Med Ctr, New York; Univ of Texas Health Sciences Ctr, Houston; et al)

Arthritis Rheum 36:1263–1273, 1993   119-95-69–1

Background.—Neonatal lupus is an example of passively acquired autoimmunity in which maternal IgG autoantibodies cross the placenta, which may result in congenital heart block and death or permanent injury to the fetus. Transient manifestations of neonatal lupus include photosensitive cutaneous lesions, cytopenias, and hepatic inflammation. The

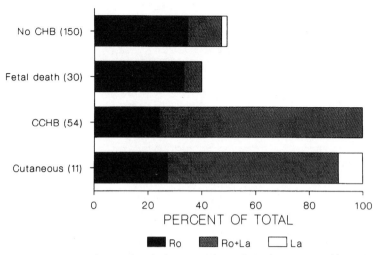

Fig 69–1.—Frequency of maternal antibodies to SS-A/Ro and SS-B/La as measured by ELISA. Sera were obtained from 4 groups of women: 150 women with autoimmune diseases who gave birth to healthy children without congenital heart block (*No CHB*), 30 with autoimmune diseases whose pregnancies ended in fetal death, 54 who gave birth to children with CHB, and 11 women who gave birth to children with transient cutaneous or other manifestations of neonatal lupus in the absence of CHB (*Cutaneous*). Four mothers had antibodies to SS-B/La in the absence of antibodies to SS-A/Ro; 2 had healthy children, 1 had a child with cutaneous neonatal lupus, and 1 had a pregnancy ending in fetal death secondary to myocarditis and another healthy infant (here included in control group of mothers with healthy children). For anti–SS-A/Ro antibodies, P < .001, CHB vs. healthy; P < .01, cutaneous vs. healthy. For anti–SS-B/La antibodies or the combination of anti–SS-A/Ro and anti–SS-B/La antibodies, P < .001, CHB vs. healthy and cutaneous vs. healthy. (Courtesy of Buyon JP, Winchester RJ, Slade SG, et al: *Arthritis Rheum* 36:1263–1273, 1993.)

identification of a maternal antibody profile that confers the highest risk for delivering a child with neonatal lupus was attempted. A previous study of mothers of children with heart block used a sodium dodecyl sulfate (SDS) immunoblot optimized to separate the 48-kd SS-B/La from the 52-kd SS-A/Ro and was able to detect antibodies to all components of the SS-A/Ro, SS-B/La system. The most frequently identified reactivity was to the 48-kd SS-B/La protein, and the presence of the combination of antibodies demonstrable to both the 48-kd SS-B/La polypeptide and the 52-kd SS-A/Ro component conferred the highest relative risk. Whether these findings are obtained when examining other manifestations of neonatal lupus was investigated. Also, how frequently this antibody profile results in the birth of a normal child was determined.

Method.—Sera were obtained from 4 groups of women: 57 whose children had congenital heart block; 12 whose children had transient dermatologic or hepatic signs of neonatal lupus but no detectable cardiac involvement; 152 with systemic lupus erythematosus and related autoimmune disease, whose children were normal; and 30 with autoimmune disease whose pregnancy resulted in miscarriage, fetal death, or early postpartum death unrelated to neonatal lupus. The antibodies to

SS-A/Ro and SS-B/La were assessed by enzyme-linked immunosorbent assay (ELISA) and by SDS-immunoblot.

Results.—Forty-seven percent of women with healthy children had antibody to SS-A/Ro, as did 43% of women whose pregnancies had resulted in fetal death. In contrast, 100% of the mothers of children with congenital heart block and 91% of the mothers of children with neonatal cutaneous lupus had antibodies that reacted with SS-A/Ro. High titers of anti-SS-A/Ro antibodies were seen more frequently in mothers of children with heart block or transient neonatal lupus than in mothers of the other 2 groups. Maternal antibodies to SS-B/La were present in 76% of the heart block group, 73% of the cutaneous neonatal lupus group, 15% of the group with healthy children, and 7% of the fetal death group (Fig 69-1). The SDS-immunoblot showed that sera from 91% of the heart block group mothers who had antibodies to SS-A/Ro, but not to SS-B/La, recognized at least 1 SS-A/Ro antigen, with significantly greater reactivity against the 52-kd component. In contrast, only 62% of the anti-SS-A/Ro positive, anti-SS-B/La negative responders in the healthy group recognized the 52-kd and/or 60-kd component. Although mothers of children with heart block or cutaneous manifestations of lupus showed no unique anti-SS-A/Ro response, only 1% of the healthy infants had mothers with antibodies directed to both the 52-kd SS-A/Ro and 48-kd SS-B/La antigens and not to the 60-kd SS-A/Ro antigen.

Conclusion.—Women with antibodies to both SS-A/Ro and SS-B/La are at increased risk of having a child with neonatal lupus, particularly if the anti-SS-A/Ro response identifies the 52-kd component on SDS-immunoblot. Women who have low titers of anti-SS-A/Ro antibodies and only recognize determinants that are altered by conditions of SDS-immunoblot are less likely to give birth to a child with neonatal lupus. No distinct pattern of antibody response was seen that differentiated mothers at risk for giving birth to infants with permanent versus transient signs of neonatal lupus, which suggests that the presence of transferred antibodies is associated with injury in a variety of different target tissues.

▶ What these authors are after is a predictor algorithm for use in counseling, based on the fine specificity patterns of maternal anti–SS-A/Ro and anti–SS-B/La antibodies that are associated with the birth of a child with transient or permanent manifestations of neonatal lupus syndromes. They have had considerable success in assessing the overall risk for neonatal disease, although the profiles of antibody responses in mothers' sera did not distinguish children who would develop transient manifestations from those who would develop heart block.

How would these workers advise us to work up an "autoimmune" mother? They would begin with an ELISA (more sensitive than immunodiffusion) to look for antibodies to SS-A/Ro and SS-B/La. With a negative ELISA the workup is done, as they would consider the likelihood of a pregnancy complicated by neonatal lupus to be small-to-nonexistent. If the ELISA is positive for antibodies to both SS-A/Ro and SS-B/La, the risk is established and, again, the workup is over, because further analysis by immunoblot, a more cumbersome and expensive technique, adds very little specificity or predictive value. The best use of the immunoblot is in the sera of mothers with antibodies to SS-A/Ro but not to SS-B/La, as this ELISA pattern is also found in many women with healthy children. Antibodies that "blot" appear to characterize mothers of children with neonatal lupus, and this specificity cannot be predicted unambiguously simply by the finding of high-titer anti-SS-A/Ro antibodies on the ELISA.

The authors point out some interesting possibilities for future work. Heart block, though rare, is potentially treatable in utero (1). Serial echocardiography, employed during the presumed period of fetal vulnerability, 18–26 weeks of gestation, might suggest myocarditis by the finding of decreased contractility in addition to associated secondary changes, such as an increase of cardiac size, pericardial effusion, and tricuspid regurgitation. With current information, they would consider such a study in mothers whose sera contain antibodies to SS-B/La on initial screen by ELISA, and/or reactivity on immunoblot to either of the SS-A/Ro antigens, particularly the 52-kd component.—S.E. Malawista, M.D.

Reference

1. Buyon JP, Swersky SH, Fox HE, Bierman FZ, Winchester RJ: Intrauterine therapy for presumptive fetal myocarditis with acquired heart block due to systemic lupus erythematosus: Experience in a mother with a predominance of SS-B(La). *Arthritis Rheum* 30:44–49, 1987.

Reliability of Histologic Scoring for Lupus Nephritis: A Community-Based Evaluation

Wernick RM, Smith DL, Houghton DC, Phillips DS, Booth JL, Runckel DN, Johnson DS, Brown KK, Gaboury CL (Providence Med Ctr, Portland Veterans Affairs Med Ctr, Oregon Health Sciences Univ, Portland; et al)
Ann Intern Med 119:805–811, 1993   115-95-69-2

Background.—Diffuse proliferative glomerulonephritis is the most severe form of lupus nephritis. However, histologic features of this disorder vary widely, making it difficult to decide on treatment or to predict renal outcome. The National Institutes of Health (NIH)–modified semiquantitative histologic scoring system has been widely used to assess the potential reversibility of lesions and to predict therapeutic response. The reliability of activity and chronicity index scoring by pathologists who routinely read renal biopsy specimens in a community setting was evaluated.

Method.—Twenty-five renal biopsy specimens were obtained from patients with a clinical diagnosis of systemic lupus erythematosus with diffuse proliferative glomerulonephritis. Five pathologists, all experienced in reading renal biopsy specimens, assessed the 25 specimens and scored

Scoring System for Histologic Features
of Renal Biopsy Specimens

Activity index
  Glomerular abnormalities
    Cellular proliferation
    Leukocyte infiltration
    Fibrinoid necrosis or karyorrhexis†
    Cellular crescents†
    Hyaline thrombi, wire loops
  Tubulointerstitial abnormalities
    Mononuclear cell infiltration
Chronicity index
  Glomerular abnormalities
    Glomerular sclerosis
    Fibrous crescents
  Tubulointerstitial abnormalities
    Interstitial fibrosis
    Tubular atrophy

Note: Each component is scored on a scale from 0 to 3.
† Weighted by a factor of 2.
(Courtesy of Wernick RM, Smith DL, Houghton DC, et al: *Ann Intern Med* 119:805-811, 1993.)

them based on the system developed by Pirani and colleagues. Each specimen was assessed for 10 components, of which 6 constitute an activity index and 4 a chronicity index (table). Each individual component is scored 0 (normal), 1, 2, or 3 (severe abnormality). Fibrinoid necrosis and cellular crescents are weighted by a factor of 2 in calculating the activity index. The maximum activity index is 24 points and the maximum chronicity index is 12 points. Each specimen was blindly and independently read by each pathologist. Of the 5 pathologists, 4 participated in a second blind assessment 8 to 9 months later. Reliability was measured by percentage agreement, intraclass correlation coefficient or kappa statistic, and individual reader effect on the group arithmetic mean.

Results.—The mean chronicity index score ranged from 2.3 to 4.8, and the mean activity index score varied from 5.8 to 11.4. Pairs of readers were within 1 point for the chronicity index and within 2 points for the activity index in 50% of cases. Risk group assignments based on chronicity index (3 strata) and activity index (2 strata) were concordant in 59% and 76% of cases, respectively. For individual components, intraclass correlation coefficients for inter-reader agreement were .58 for the chronicity index and 0.52 for the activity index. Intrareader agreement was higher than inter-reader agreement, but mean intraclass correlation coefficients exceeded 0.70 for only 1 of the 10 index components. Repeated readings showed chronicity index scores that were more than 1 point discordant in 45% of cases and activity index scores that were more than 2 points discordant in 43% of cases. Risk group assignment was seen to change on the basis of chronicity index and activity index in 36% and 21% of cases, respectively.

Conclusion.—The NIH-modified scoring system for lupus nephritis can only be moderately reproduced in a nonreferral setting. When used to predict renal outcome, it may result in misleading predictions of risk for renal failure and response to therapy.

▶ Cytotoxic drugs, which bear their own risks of morbidity, are generally used in lupus nephritis subject to activity and chronicity scores obtained from histologic sections of kidney biopsy specimens (table). In general, these indices are thought to be of high predictive value for progressive renal failure; a high chronicity index portends refractoriness to aggressive therapy, while active lesions are thought to be potentially reversible.

This study undercuts any complacency we may have had about depending on community based pathological scoring as a basis for treatment decisions. As the authors point out, small differences in chronicity index scoring may profoundly alter risk-group assignment and subsequent estimates of a patient's likelihood of developing renal failure and of responding to aggressive immunosuppressive therapy. Discordance in scoring among their pathologists was too frequent to yield reliable guidance for patient management. They believe that biopsy specimens should be scored by nephrologists working in a quality-controlled reference center, for whom scoring reliability and, ideally, validity have been shown. (For an analysis of renal biopsy vs. clinical predictors of long-term outcome in lupus nephritis, see Reference 1).—S.E. Malawista, M.D.

Reference

1. 1991 YEAR BOOK OF MEDICINE, p 698.

Lupus and Pregnancy Studies
Urowitz MB, Gladman DD, Farewell VT, Stewart J, McDonald J (Univ of Toronto, Wellesley Hosp, Toronto; Univ of Waterloo, Ont, Canada)
Arthritis Rheum 36:1392–1397, 1993   119-95-69-3

Background.—There is still controversy about whether pregnancy in patients with systemic lupus erythematosus (SLE) predisposes to flare of the underlying disease. Prepregnancy factors that are prognostic for the onset of active disease during and after pregnancy were examined.

Method.—A total of 46 patients with 79 pregnancies were compared with matched, nonpregnant patients with SLE. They were examined for clinical features that could be evaluated as potential prognostic factors, including duration of SLE, the score on the SLE Disease Activity Index (SLEDAI), and presence of major organ involvement. Active disease was defined as an SLEDAI score of equal to or greater than 2. A flare was

Systemic Lupus Erythematosus Disease Activity at Onset of Pregnancy as a Prognostic Factor for Active Lupus During Pregnancy, in 61 Pregnancies

	Active disease at onset (n = 44)	Inactive disease at onset (n = 17)
Active disease/flare during pregnancy	36*	7
Inactive disease during pregnancy	8	10

*P = .003 vs. pregnancies in which disease was inactive at onset.
(Courtesy of Urowitz MB, Gladman DD, Farewell VT, et al: *Arthritis Rheum* 36:1392–1397, 1993.)

considered to be an increase of 2 or more absolute units on the SLE-DAI.

Results.—Among the group of 79 pregnancies, age, disease duration, pregnancy number, duration of steroid therapy, and use of steroid or other disease-suppressive medications did not distinguish between those who had a flare from those who did not. Hypertension before pregnancy was associated with flare in 3 of 4 patients. However, major organ involvement was not a predictor of flare. The presence of active disease at pregnancy onset was significantly correlated with active disease during pregnancy. Of the total group of pregnancies, 61 resulted in delivery. Within this group the same results were seen: 44 of the women who delivered had active disease at onset, and in 36 of these the disease remained active or flared. Of the remaining 17 patients in whom SLE was inactive at onset, only 7 had a flare, whereas the disease remained inactive in 10 (table). When the pregnant patients with SLE were compared with the nonpregnant women with SLE, the frequency of lupus flares was similar in both groups. However, disease activity at pregnancy onset again played a major role in determining flare. The flare rate in the controls with initially active disease did not differ significantly from the flare rate in the controls with initially inactive disease; however, the flare rate in pregnant patients with initially active disease was substantially higher than that among pregnant patients with inactive disease.

Conclusion.—Disease activity at onset of pregnancy is a determining factor of flare during pregnancy. Women with SLE who are considering pregnancy should be counseled about persistently active SLE or flare in SLE, based on the status of their disease activity at onset. The physician and the patient should try to achieve inactive disease at the onset of pregnancy to provide optimum protection in later months.

▶ There is increasing evidence against the old saw that SLE tends to flare during pregnancy or in the immediate postpartum period (1). However, these authors have provided a new wrinkle: They found that inactive disease at the onset of pregnancy led to fewer flares during pregnancy than did active disease at onset (table), while in nonpregnant controls, the presence or absence of active disease at a given time did not lead to numbers of flares that were significantly different from each other. In other words, pregnancy and *inactive* lupus together *protected* against flares. No other clinical or laboratory features were predictive of flare during pregnancy, except for hypertension (at onset or occurring during pregnancy), but the numbers of affected patients were small. The basis for this putative protective effect is unclear, and the observation needs confirmation. It also is not clear that one should go to extraordinary therapeutic lengths to produce inactivity in someone planning to become pregnant.—S.E. Malawista, M.D.

Reference

1. 1990 YEAR BOOK OF MEDICINE, p 635.

70 Spondyloarthropathy and Reactive Arthritis

Introduction

In this chapter, we examine the high frequency of silent inflammatory bowel disease in spondyloarthropathy (Abstract 119-95-70–1), and the benefits of recognizing diffuse idiopathic skeletal hyperostosis (DISH) in routine chest films (Abstract 119-95-70–2).

Noted in passing: Three additional *Shigella flexneri* strains associated with enteric disease and reactive arthritis carry a so-called pHS-2 plasmid encoding an HLA-B27 mimetic peptide (1). This finding supports the molecular mimicry hypothesis for the induction of reactive arthritis, whereby a bacterial protein containing the HLA-B27 mimetic peptide would act as the arthritogenic trigger because of its similarity to a host protein (i.e., HLA-B27). This formulation presupposes that normal tolerance to the B27-derived peptide is broken, presumably during enteric infection.

Stephen E. Malawista, M.D.

Reference

1. Stieglitz H, Lipsky P: Association between reactive arthritis and antecedent infection with *Shigella flexneri* carrying a 2-Md plasmid and encoding an HLA-B27 mimetic epitope. *Arthritis Rheum Dis* 36:1387–1391, 1993.

High Frequency of Silent Inflammatory Bowel Disease in Spondyloarthropathy

Leirisalo-Repo M, Turunen U, Stenman S, Helenius P, Seppälä K (Helsinki Univ Central Hosp, Univ of Helsinki, Finland)
Arthritis Rheum 37:23–31, 1994
119-95-70–1

Background.—The spondylarthropathies are a group of seronegative arthritides, ranging from acute to chronic, that frequently are associated with the presence of HLA-B27. Some patients subsequently have frank ankylosing spondylitis, possibly because of persistent infection or a chronic locus of inflammation. Gastrointestinal infection has been implicated in worsening of chronic ankylosing spondylitis. About 4% of patients have ulcerative colitis or Crohn's disease.

Objective.—Ileocolonoscopy was performed in 118 patients with joint or back symptoms and 24 with uncomplicated acute bacterial gastroenteritis. Thirty-two of the former patients had reactive arthritis; 11 had definite or classic rheumatoid arthritis; and 18 had miscellaneous rheumatic disorders.

Findings.—Endoscopic abnormalities were found in 44% of patients with spondyloarthropathy and 6% of those with other inflammatory arthritides. One fifth of the patients with spondyloarthropathy and none of the others had changes in the ileum. Inflammatory bowel disease was diagnosed endoscopically in 19% of patients with arthritis. One fourth of patients with chronic spondyloarthropathy had possible or definite Crohn's disease. One patient with rheumatoid arthritis and one with chronic uroarthritis had changes of ulcerative colitis. The frequency of chronic inflammatory change correlated with the duration of arthritis, in contrast to the patients with acute bacterial gastroenteritis. Endoscopic findings of inflammation in the ileum and colon correlated poorly with the histologic findings. No association was found between bowel changes and either the presence of HLA-B27 or a history of nonsteroidal anti-inflammatory drug use in the past month.

Conclusion.—Early changes of Crohn's disease appear to be more prevalent in patients with spondyloarthropathy, especially when chronic, than in those with other forms of arthritis. Whether the same agent or agents are responsible for changes at both sites remains to be determined.

▶ The seronegative spondyloarthropathies, often associated with inheritance of the HLA-B27 gene, include ankylosing spondylitis, reactive arthritis, Reiter's syndrome, spondylitis and peripheral arthritis associated with psoriasis or inflammatory bowel disease, juvenile-onset spondyloarthropathy, and other conditions that are less well-defined. Investigative use of the ileocolonoscope in these disorders, as pioneered by a Belgian group followed in these pages (1–3), has indicated that subclinical bowel inflammation is common, a finding confirmed in the current Finnish study. As in earlier work, these changes are not attributable to the nonsteroidal anti-inflammatory agents (NSAIDs) that many of these patients require. There was again no association between endoscopic abnormalities and the use of NSAIDs, which in any case generally induce lesions in the mid–small intestine rather than in the terminal ileum or colon. Moreover, endoscopic lesions characteristic of Crohn's disease were seen only in patients with spondyloarthropathies, not in other patients taking NSAIDs.

Histologically (as opposed to endoscopically), the findings did not segregate as neatly as had those of the earlier workers (3), who correlated chronic lesions, for example, with (1) frequent episodes of diarrhea, serum markers of inflammation, reduced axial mobility, sacroiliitis, bamboo spine, and destructive joint lesions; (2) acute lesions, with the fecal carriage of specific organisms and with undifferentiated reactive arthritis, especially the enterogenic forms of reactive arthritis; and (3) no gut lesions, with urogenital inflammation or urogenital reactive arthritis. The current workers especially differed in their finding of what they considered to be chronic lesions in significant numbers of controls with rheumatoid arthritis. We will have to see more work to explain these discrepancies.

Of course, the implication of this line of endeavor is that chronic infectious/inflammatory gut lesions may provide an immunologic breach that allows bacterial antigens from the gut to disseminate and cause disease.—S.E. Malawista, M.D.

References

1. 1985 YEAR BOOK OF MEDICINE, p 754.
2. 1990 YEAR BOOK OF MEDICINE, p 643.
3. 1993 YEAR BOOK OF MEDICINE, p 702.

Chest Radiographs as a Screening Test for Diffuse Idiopathic Skeletal Hyperostosis
Mata S, Hill RO, Joseph L, Kaplan P, Dussault R, Watts CS, Fitzcharles M-A, Shiroky JB, Fortin PR, Esdaile JM (Montreal Gen Hosp; McGill Univ, Montreal, PQ, Canada)
J Rheumatol 20:1905–1910, 1993   119-95-70-2

Background.—Diffuse idiopathic skeletal hyperostosis (DISH) is a frequent rheumatic disorder that may often go overlooked or may be misin-

Thoracic Vertebrae	DISH Present Study (%)	DISH Resnick (%)	DISH Utsinger (%)
\multicolumn{4}{c}{Distribution of Involved Thoracic Vertebrae in the 45 Patients With DISH and From the Literature}
T1	0	24	25
T2	2	33	34
T3	16	44	37
T4	31	58	60
T5	53	70	76
T6	78	78	80
T7	93	91	94
T8	100	94	96
T9	100	96	97
T10	100	93	95
T11	84	87	94
T12	55	74	90

Abbreviation: DISH, diffuse idiopathic skeletal hyperostosis.
(Courtesy of Mata S, Hill RO, Joseph L, et al: *J Rheumatol* 20:1905–1910, 1993.)

terpreted as spondylosis. No more than 10% of those affected have abnormalities on skeletal radiography, and the clinical features are not distinctive.

Objective and Methods.—The value of chest radiography in screening for DISH was examined in 45 patients who met established diagnostic criteria for the disorder and in 106 control subjects. Forty-five controls had thoracic spondylosis, 16 had ankylosing spondylitis, and 45 had normal thoracic spine radiographs. Chest radiographs were read independently initially and again 2 months later.

Results.—The distribution of disease in the thoracic spine resembled that in published reports except for less frequent involvement from T1 through T5 (table). Chest radiograph readings were 77% sensitive and 97% specific in diagnosing DISH, and had positive and negative predictive values of 91%. Both inter-rater and intrarater reliability were high. Patients with DISH whose radiographs were read as negative had significantly less extensive disease than the others.

Conclusion.—Experienced radiologists are able to diagnose DISH quite reliably from chest radiographs.

▶ The disorder known as DISH (diffuse idiopathic skeletal hyperostosis; ankylosing hyperostosis; Forestier/Rotes-Querol disease) may be as dramatic radiographically as it is generally unimportant clinically (1). Because DISH is evident in routine 2-view chest films and occurs in up to 10% of the elderly, it is a condition that needs to be recognized by internists so that, in the asymptomatic patient, it can then be left alone.

The radiologic picture is one of flowing calcification and ossification along the anterolateral aspect of at least 4 contiguous vertebral bodies, with (cf. other spondyloses) relative preservation of disc height. The most commonly involved thoracic vertebrae are shown in the table. Unlike inflammatory spondyloarthropathies, there is no sacroiliitis or ankylosis of apophyseal (spinal diarthrodial) joints. There may be associated pelvic and peripheral osteophytes and ligamentous calcification. Appreciation of this syndrome when it shows up in the chest film of a patient who is not complaining of it will save the patient a good deal of additional radiation and expense.—S.E. Malawista, M.D.

Reference

1. Hutton C: DISH. . .a state, not a disease? *Br J Rheumatol* 28:277–278, 1989.

71 Sclerosing Syndromes

Introduction

Here we consider autoantibody reactive with RNA polymerase III in systemic sclerosis (Abstract 119-95-71–1); intravenous iloprost infusion in the treatment of Raynaud's phenomenon secondary to systemic sclerosis (Abstract 119-95-71–2); and sequelae of the eosinophilia-myalgia and toxic oil syndromes (Abstract 119-95-71–3).

Stephen E. Malawista, M.D.

Autoantibody Reactive With RNA Polymerase III in Systemic Sclerosis
Okano Y, Steen VD, Medsger TA Jr (Univ of Pittsburgh School of Medicine, Pennsylvania)
Ann Intern Med 119:1005–1013, 1993   119-95-71–1

Background.—Systemic sclerosis (SSc), an autoimmune disease, is characterized by a wide spectrum of clinical, pathologic, and serologic abnormalities. In over 90% of the patients, antinuclear antibody is produced spontaneously. In over 30%, the autoantigens to which antinuclear antibodies are directed are not known. The clinical significance of anti-RNA polymerase III antibody in patients with SSc was determined.

Methods.—Two hundred fifty-two consecutive new patients with SSc, 150 patients with other connective tissue diseases, and 20 healthy volunteers were studied for the presence of anti-RNA polymerase III antibody (Fig 71-1). Immunoprecipitation, immunoblotting, and immunodepletion studies were performed.

Findings.—Serum specimens from 23% of the patients with SSc reacted with RNA polymerase III. By contrast, none of the specimens from either control group reacted. In 40 of the 57 reacting specimens, immunoprecipitation studies also demonstrated RNA polymerase I and/or II. Anti-RNA polymerase III antibody was found in sera from 45% of the 111 patients with diffuse cutaneous involvement of SSc (dcSSc), in 6% of 114 patients with SSc and limited cutaneous involvement, and in none of the 27 patients with an SSc overlap syndrome. Among patients with dcSSc, anti-RNA polymerase III antibody was more common than antitopoisomerase I antibody. Patients with anti-RNA polymerase III antibody had a significantly greater mean maximum skin thickness score

799

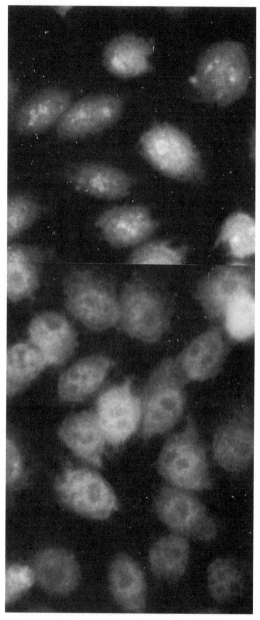

Fig 71–1.—Indirect immunofluorescence test for antinuclear antibody using HEp-2 cells as substrate. Serum specimens from patients with systemic sclerosis were diluted 1:40 with phosphate-buffered saline and used as the first antibody. (**Top**) Immunofluorescence shows nucleolar staining, suggesting that serum contains antinuclear antibody that is apparently identical to the anti-RNA polymerase I antibody shown with antinucleolar staining by Reimer and colleagues. (**Bottom**) Immunofluorescence shows nuclear speckled staining without nucleolar staining. (Courtesy of Okano Y, Steen VD, Medsger TA Jr: *Ann Intern Med* 119:1005–1013, 1993.)

and significantly lower frequencies of telangiectasias, inflammatory myopathy, restrictive lung disease, and serious cardiac abnormalities than did patients with antitopoisomerase I antibody.

Conclusion.—In many patients with SSc with diffuse or extensive cutaneous involvement, anti-RNA polymerase III antibody serves as a new marker autoantibody. This discovery fills a major gap in the identification of specific serum autoantibodies in SSc. Confirmation of these findings by additional research is needed.

▶ Systemic sclerosis (scleroderma) continues to sort itself out according to which antinucleolar or antinuclear antibodies are produced (1, 2). These markers, which are generally mutually exclusive, appear early and can be used, for example, to help identify which patients with the vasospastic disorder known as Raynaud's phenomenon will go on to develop connective tissue disease (3, 4) (most patients will not). They also define clinical subsets that tend to have different patterns of organ involvement and, therefore, different prognoses. In a recent study of Japanese patients (5), cumulative survival rates at 10 years after diagnosis of SSc (and major organ involvement linked to cause of death) were 93% in patients with anticentromere antibodies (biliary cirrhosis), 72% in those with anti-U1 RNP (isolated pulmonary arterial hypertension and cerebral hemorrhage), 66% in those with anti-DNA topoisomerase-1 (pulmonary interstitial fibrosis), and 30% in those with anti-RNA polymerases I, II, and III (cardiac and renal involvement). With these and other workers' (1, 6, 7) demonstration of RNA polymerases I, II, and III as targets for autoantibodies, the authors can now identify the antigen against which serum antinuclear antibodies are directed in more than 85% of patients in the United States with SSc.

Because there is still a considerable range in the clinical features of patients with SSc who have antibodies against a given autoantigen, workers are beginning to look for further distinguishing characteristics within antibody subsets (8). Immunoreactivity to a particular epitope on the topoisomerase-1 molecule, encompassing amino acid residues 658-700 and termed ER4, was associated with diffuse cutaneous SSc, progressive pulmonary interstitial fibrosis, and poor prognosis for 15-year survival when compared to other patients with autoantibodies to topoisomerase-1. Moreover, Japanese patients with ER4 reactivity frequently displayed the DR2/DRw52 phenotype, thus linking autoantigenic epitopes determined by molecular analysis to a clinical application.—S.E. Malawista, M.D.

References

1. 1992 Year Book of Medicine, p 649.
2. 1993 Year Book of Medicine, p 707.
3. 1990 Year Book of Medicine, p 653.
4. 1992 Year Book of Medicine, p 645.
5. Kuwana M, Kaburaki J, Okano Y, Tojo T, Homma M: Clinical and prognostic associations based on serum antinuclear antibodies in Japanese patients with systemic sclerosis. *Arthritis Rheum* 37:75–83, 1994.
6. Kuwana M, Kaburaki J, Mimori T, Tojo T, Homma M: Autoantibody reactive

with three classes of RNA polymerases in sera from patients with systemic sclerosis. *J Clin Invest* 91:1399–1404, 1993.

7. Hirakata M, Okano Y, Pati U, Suwa A, Medsger TA Jr, Hardin JA, Craft J: Identification of autoantibodies to RNA polymerase II: Occurrence in systemic sclerosis and association with autoantibodies to RNA polymerases I and II: *J Clin Invest* 91:2665–2672, 1993.

8. Kuwana M, Kaburaki J, Mimori T, Tojo T, Homma M: Autoantigenic epitopes on DNA topoisomerase I: Clinical and immunogenetic associations in systemic sclerosis. *Arthritis Rheum* 36:1406–1413, 1993.

Intravenous Iloprost Infusion in Patients With Raynaud Phenomenon Secondary to Systemic Sclerosis: A Multicenter, Placebo-Controlled, Double-Blind Study

Wigley FM, Wise RA, Seibold JR, McCloskey DA, Kujala G, Medsger TA Jr, Steen VD, Varga J, Jimenez S, Mayes M, Clements PJ, Weiner SR, Porter J, Ellman M, Wise C, Kaufman LD, Williams J, Dole W (The Johns Hopkins Univ School of Medicine, Baltimore, Md; Robert Wood Johnson Med School, New Brunswick, NJ; West Virginia Univ, Morgantown; et al)

Ann Intern Med 120:199–206, 1994   119-95-71–2

Background.—Most patients with systemic sclerosis also have Raynaud's phenomenon. Iloprost is a prostacyclin analogue with vasodilating and platelet inhibitory effects. The first double-blind, placebo-controlled, parallel group, multicenter study of the efficacy of iloprost in patients with Raynaud's phenomenon caused by systemic sclerosis was reported.

Methods.—One hundred thirty-one patients with systemic sclerosis, aged 20 to 79 years, were randomly assigned to receive 1 of 2 parallel treatments of 5 daily sequential, 6-hour IV iloprost infusions, 0.5 to 2 ng/kg per minute, or a similar amount of placebo. Frequency of Raynaud's attacks, the Raynaud's phenomenon severity score, physician's overall rating of treatment effect, and digital cutaneous lesion healing were determined.

Results.—One hundred twenty-six patients completed the 5-day infusion, and 114 completed at least 6 weeks of follow-up. With iloprost, the mean weekly number of Raynaud's attacks declined by 39.1% compared with 22.2% with placebo, for a significant difference. The mean percentage of improvement in a global Raynaud's phenomenon severity score during the 9-week follow-up was higher in the iloprost group than in the placebo group, at 34.8% and 19.7%, respectively. The overall physician rating of treatment effect indicated greater improvement with iloprost than placebo after 6 and 9 weeks. After 3 weeks, 14.6% more patients who were given iloprost had 50% or more lesions heal compared with patients given placebo. During the infusion, 92% of the patients in the iloprost group had one or more side effects compared with 57% in the placebo group.

Conclusions.—This is the largest placebo-controlled study of iloprost infusion in patients with systemic sclerosis. Findings indicate that iloprost is effective in the short-term palliation of severe Raynaud's phenomenon in this patient population.

▶ With each successive successful study, iloprost, a relatively stable analogue of prostacyclin with vasodilating and platelet-inhibitory effects, presumably comes closer to approval by the Food and Drug Administration for the treatment of Raynaud's phenomenon and its complications (1–3). In this multicenter, randomized, parallel placebo-controlled, double-blind study, there were significant improvements compared to controls, in the mean weekly number of Raynaud's phenomenon attacks, in mean global severity scores, and in physicians' overall ratings of the effect of treatment at weeks 6 and 9. In earlier work there was significantly improved healing of cutaneous lesions, including ulcers, paronychia, or fissures (3); in this study, there was only a trend in that direction.

Unlike the common and largely benign vasospastic disorder referred to as Raynaud's *disease*, Raynaud's *phenomenon* associated with systemic sclerosis is also typified by progressive fibrosis of the intima and luminal narrowing in the digital arteries and precapillary arterioles. Most available vasodilators have been incompletely effective, as one might expect when there are fibrotic structural changes. One of the more interesting properties of iloprost is the ability of a 3- or (as employed here) 5-day course to initiate changes that appear to last for many weeks, without residual active drug being present. As pointed out by these authors, these continued benefits may be due to prolonged alterations in vascular geometry or patency, or in function of endothelium or of vascular smooth muscle cells. We can look forward to longer-term studies of intermittent therapy with this promising agent.—S.E. Malawista, M.D.

References

1. 1990 YEAR BOOK OF MEDICINE, p 654.
2. 1993 YEAR BOOK OF MEDICINE, p 599.
3. 1994 YEAR BOOK OF MEDICINE, p 793.

Chronicity of the Eosinophilia-Myalgia Syndrome: A Reassessment After Three Years

Kaufman LD (The State Univ of New York, Stony Brook)
Arthritis Rheum 37:84–87, 1994
119-95-71–3

Background.—Eosinophilia-myalgia syndrome (EMS) was first identified in 1989. The early manifestations of this multisystem disorder have been described by several studies, but the long-term manifestations require definition.

Chronic Sequelae of Eosinophilia-Myalgia Syndrome in a Cohort
of 63 Patients, of Whom 57 Were Followed Up for a Mean
of 36 Months

	No. (%)	
Manifestation	At presentation	At followup
Fever	30/56 (54)	Resolved
Weight loss	33/53 (62)	Resolved
Fatigue	50/54 (93)	52/57 (91)
Myalgia	58/60 (97)	40/57 (70)
Muscle cramping	43/48 (90)	43/57 (75)
Dyspnea with or without cough	41/61 (67)	24/57 (42)
Arthralgia†	36/57 (63)	31/57 (54)
Neuropathic findings‡	32/56 (57)	32/52 (62)
Proximal muscle weakness§	33/57 (58)	21/53 (40)
Alopecia	35/62 (56)	6/57 (11)
Xerostomia	30/60 (50)	15/56 (27)
Scleroderma-like changes	26/58 (45)	25/57 (44)
Hyperpigmentation	NM	24/57 (42)
Tremor	NM	6/57 (11)
Neurocognitive symptoms	NM	49/57 (86)

Abbreviation: NM, not manifested until more than 1 year after onset of disease.
Note: The denominator for each parameter reflects the number of patients for whom data were available.
† Two patients had arthritis (see text).
‡ Paresthesias with objectively demonstrated hypesthesias, with or without abnormal nerve conduction velocity results.
§ With or without abnormal electromyography results.
(Courtesy of Kaufman LD: *Arthritis Rheum* 37:84-87, 1994.)

Methods.—A cohort of 57 patients with EMS were followed up at a single center for 21-64 months from the disease onset. All had ingested L-tryptophan and had eosinophilia. The symptoms associated with EMS were assessed every 3-6 months, and any additional complaints were identified and followed.

Results.—Only 2 patients had no symptoms at the end of the study; 50 patients had more than 3 symptoms. Persistent symptoms included (in order of prevalence) fatigue, muscle cramping, myalgia, paresthesias with hypesthesias, articular symptoms, scleroderma-like skin changes, and proximal muscle weakness (table). The patients with EMS had distinctive muscle cramping, which was resistant to therapeutic agents. Most of the patients with proximal muscle weakness showed evidence of myopathy. Pulmonary symptoms appearing in some patients appeared to be caused by muscle weakness. New disease manifestations were identified after the first year of illness, including neurologic complications—cognitive difficulties in 86% of the patients and tremor in 4 patients.

Discussion.—Eosinophilia-myalgia syndrome has serious long-term symptoms, many of them disabling. These symptoms vary in severity during the course of the disease, with periods of improvement followed by relapse. There may be a bias in the perception of severity of symptoms in patients who are referred; it is possible that some patients with EMS may have mild cases that resolve. However, most patients still being treated have chronic symptoms.

▶ The eosinophilia-myalgia syndrome, associated with the ingestion of certain batches of products containing L-tryptophan and first described in 1989, last appeared in these pages in 1991 (1), where I described its clinical features and compared it to eosinophilic fasciitis, localized forms of scleroderma, and the toxic oil syndrome (2). The epidemic has subsided and is no longer in the news, but almost all those afflicted with it continue to have significant disability (table).

Victims of the toxic oil syndrome, which appeared in Spain in 1981 and was related to the intake of rapeseed cooking oil sold in bulk, included 19,748 persons (~ 15 times as many individuals as contracted EMS), of whom 457 died. Its major features were noncardiac pulmonary edema, skin rash, myalgia, eosinophilia, joint contractures, scleroderma, sicca syndrome, polyneuropathy, and pulmonary hypertension. In an 8-year follow-up of 332 patients who lived in Colmenar Viejo (Madrid, Spain) (2), the disease was usually severe and disabling during the first 2 years, but the clinical condition of most patients improved subsequently. At the end of the follow-up period, there were 10 deaths (3%) thought to be related to the syndrome, and 47% of the patients had some kind of complaint, albeit subtle in most cases (e.g., muscle cramps, chronic musculoskeletal pain, psychological stress). Sixteen percent showed organ involvement—most importantly, widespread interstitial infiltrates, non-nectrotizing angiitis, endothelial proliferation, and tissue fibrosis. We can hope that many of the sequelae of EMS will also attenuate with time.—S.E. Malawista, M.D.

References

1. 1991 YEAR BOOK OF MEDICINE, p 705.
2. Alonso-Ruiz A, Calabozo M, Perez-Ruiz F, Mancebo L: Toxic oil syndrome: A long-term follow-up of a cohort of 332 patients. *Medicine* 72:285–295, 1993.

72 Crystal-Associated Arthritis

Introduction

Here we examine the implications of gout without elevated concentrations of serum urate (Abstract 119-95-72-1), and consider the advantages of using adrenocorticotropic hormone for the treatment of acute gouty arthritis (Abstract 119-95-72-2).

Noted in passing is a recent, brief review of gout (1).

Stephen E. Malawista, M.D.

Reference

1. Sells LL, German DC: An update on gout. *Bull Rheum Dis* 43:4–7, 1994.

Gout Without Hyperuricemia
McCarty DJ (Med College of Wisconsin, Milwaukee)
JAMA 271:302–303, 1994   119-95-72-1

Background.—In rare cases, patients seen with acute gouty arthritis have persistently normal serum urate levels.

Case Report.—Man, 88, was seen with pain and swelling in his right foot. These symptoms had persisted for about 3.5 months. A presumptive diagnosis of gout was made, despite a serum uric acid level of 6.3 mg/dL. Three weeks earlier, this level had been 5.8 mg/dL. A month after symptom onset, the patient had been hospitalized with a presumptive diagnosis of cellulitis and osteomyelitis of the right foot and given broad-spectrum antibiotics. During this treatment, the patient's uric acid levels ranged from 4.9 to 6.1 mg/dL. Subsequently, the patient underwent aspiration of the first metatarsophalangeal joint, which yielded yellow, blood-stained fluid showing negatively birefringent needle-shaped crystals both within leukocytes and free. Serum uric acid levels at this time were 6.4 and 6.7 mg/dL. Past hospital records were obtained and analyzed. Altogether, the patients had had 13 serum uric acid measurements between 1980 and 1992. All were within normal limits.

Conclusion.—There appear to be 4 situations in which normouricemia accompanies gouty arthritis. First, there are patients, like the one presented here, who never have urate levels high enough to saturate their serum at 37°C. In addition, patients with hyperuricemia from a known causal factor, such as obesity, alcoholism, or diuretic use, may become normouricemic when this factor is eliminated. Patients may also have normal urate levels of the time of an attack because of the accompanying uric acid diuresis. Finally, patients may have acute attacks with normal urate levels caused by treatment with allopurinol or a uricosuric agent. Clinicians should view gout and hyperuricemia as separate phenomena.

▶ Before getting carried away by this case, let's review a few clinical facts of gout. The majority of patients with gout do have elevated levels of serum urate, and the higher the concentration, the more likely the patients are (statistically, at least) to have attacks of acute gouty arthritis and to develop frank tophaceous involvement. However, most hyperuricemic individuals never develop gout, and the treatment of asymptomatic hyperuricemia is generally bad practice. The solubility of urate in plasma at 37°C is roughly the same as the upper limit of normal as defined by 2 SD above the mean of normal individuals (e.g., near 7 mg%). One unanswered question regards what it is in hyperuricemic individuals that usually maintains the serum urate in supersaturated solution.

The patient in this study has the converse situation: with 13 normal serum urate levels measured over 12 years and no history of diuretic or of alcohol ingestion, he seems never to have had hyperuricemia, and yet he had negatively birefringent needle-shaped crystals (characteristic of sodium urate crystals) taken from an affected joint, and an x-ray film suggesting replacement of bone by tophi. Although one might speculate that his serum is peculiarly unable to keep urate in solution, I would favor the speculation favored by Dr. McCarty, who, by the way, knows as much about gout as anyone. The solubility of urate decreases with temperature; at 30°C it is only 4.5 mg% (1). Moreover, body temperature decreases with distance from the core; peripheral joints of the lower extremity are probably closer to 30°C than to 37°C. Thus, I agree with the author: ". . .that crystals nucleated and grew to form tophi because of the physicochemical saturation of his underperfused, relatively cool, aged tissues."

The appreciation of gout without hyperuricemia is of more than academic interest. This patient suffered months of unnecessary pain and was subjected to the inherent dangers of massive mistaken antibiotic therapy. His second hospitalization cost $12,617.—S.E. Malawista, M.D.

Reference

1. Loeb JN: The influence of temperature on the solubility of monosodium urate. *Arthritis Rheum* 15:189–192, 1972.

ACTH Revisited: Effective Treatment for Acute Crystal Induced Synovitis in Patients With Multiple Medical Problems
Ritter J, Kerr LD, Valeriano-Marcet J, Spiera H (Mt Sinai School of Medicine, New York; Univ of Southwest Florida, Tampa)
J Rheumatol 21:696–699, 1994   119-95-72-2

Introduction.—Traditionally, acute crystal-induced synovitis is treated with nonsteroidal anti-inflammatory drugs (NSAIDs) and colchicine, both of which are potential causes of serious side effects. Parenteral adrenocorticotropic hormone (ACTH) therapy has proved effective in patients with medical complications, but this approach has not been widely used.

Study Plan.—Thirty-three patients with confirmed acute gout and 5 with documented acute pseudogout were treated for 43 episodes of acute crystal-induced synovitis. The indications for using ACTH included congestive heart failure, chronic renal insufficiency, gastrointestinal bleeding, and no response to NSAIDs or colchicine. Patients who had failed to respond to NSAIDs also were treated. Most episodes were treated with 40 units of ACTH every 8 hours, but doses that were twice as high were given to some patients. The ACTH was injected intravenously, intramuscularly, or subcutaneously. Colchicine, 0.6 mg PO daily, was given prophylactically in conjunction with 30 episodes.

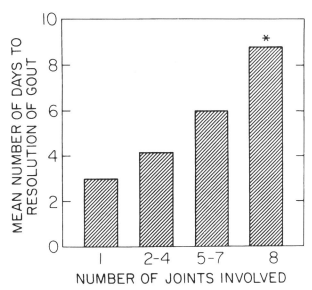

Fig 72–1.—Comparison of the number of joints involved and the days to resolution in inpatients with gout treated with ACTH. *Asterisk* indicates the slope is .8680 and $P = .0012$, showing that the length of treatment with ACTH increased as the number of joints increased. (Courtesy of Ritter J, Kerr LD, Valeriano-Marcet J, et al: *J Rheumatol* 21:696–699, 1994.)

Results.—All 5 episodes of pseudogout resolved in an average of 4 days. All but one of the 38 episodes of acute gout resolved when ACTH was given. The time to resolution increased with the number of joints involved (Fig 72–1). Four patients relapsed, although 3 of them had received colchicine. Four patients became hypokalemic during ACTH treatment, and 4 diabetic patients had worsening glycemic control and required more insulin. Four patients had mild fluid overload, but pulmonary edema did not develop in any of them.

Conclusion.—Treatment of acute crystal-induced synovitis with ACTH is effective and safe.

▶ Adrenocorticotropic hormone, first shown to be effective in the treatment of acute gouty arthritis in 1950, fell out of favor and indeed, NSAIDs, intravenous colchicine or, occasionally, corticosteroids (1) suffice for the large majority of patients. However, these authors have made a good case for ACTH in the often aged patients with multiple medical problems, including congestive heart failure, chronic renal insufficiency, or gastrointestinal bleeding. The regimen described worked in 37 of 38 patients (97%) with acute gout, as well as in all 5 (100%) with acute pseudogout. The average number of days to complete resolution, 5.5 days for gout (the time varied according to the number of joints involved; see Figure 72–1) and 4.2 for pseudogout, is competitive with other treatments. The most common tapering schedule was ACTH, 40 units (= 40 mg) q8h, q12h, qd, and off, with a taper occurring on each day that there was improvement, defined by a decrease in signs of synovitis or an increase in range of motion. The authors stress the importance of monitoring electrolytes (for hypokalemia), fluid status (for overload), and blood glucose (for hyperglycemia; in this study, only a problem in known diabetics). All adverse effects were easily controlled.—S.E. Malawista, M.D.

Reference

1. 1994 YEAR BOOK OF MEDICINE, p 797.

73 Vasculitis

Introduction

This chapter deals with the the effect of previous corticosteroid treatment on biopsy findings in giant cell (temporal) arteritis (Abstract 119-95-73-1), an apparent connection between chronic nasal carriage of *Staphylococcus aureus* and rates of relapse of Wegener's granulomatosis (Abstract 119-95-73-2), the effect of surgical cleansing of skin on the pathergy phenomenon in Behçet's syndrome (Abstract 119-95-73-3), and the clinical characteristics of a large group of patients with Takayasu's arteritis studied at the Mayo Clinic (Abstract 119-95-73-4).

Noted in passing: Another committee's attempts to name and define the most common forms of noninfectious systemic vasculitis (1), quickly taken to task (2).

Stephen E. Malawista, M.D.

References

1. Jennette JC, Falk RJ, Andrassy K, Bacon PA, Churg J, Gross WL, Hagen EC, Hoffman GS, Hunder GG, Kallenberg CGM, McCluskey RT, Sinico RA, Rees AJ, van Es LA, Waldherr R, Wiik A: Nomenclature of systemic vasculitides: Proposal of an international consensus conference. *Arthritis Rheum* 37:187–192, 1994.
2. Lie JT: Nomenclature and classification of vasculitis: Plus ça change, plus c'est la même chose. *Arthitis Rheum* 37:181–186, 1994.

How Does Previous Corticosteroid Treatment Affect the Biopsy Findings in Giant Cell (Temporal) Arteritis?

Achkar AA, Lie JT, Hunder GG, O'Fallon WM, Gabriel SE (Mayo Clinic and Foundation, Rochester, Minn; Univ of California, Davis)

Ann Intern Med 120:987–992, 1994   119-95-73–1

Purpose.—In patients with suspected giant-cell, or temporal, arteritis, the physician must often decide whether to begin preventive corticosteroid therapy right away or to await the results of temporal artery biopsy therapy. Some studies suggest that the histologic signs of arteritis may be masked after only 1 week of corticosteroid therapy, whereas others indicate that the histologic signs persist after longer courses of corticosteroids. The effects of previous corticosteroid therapy on the results of temporal artery biopsy were analyzed.

Methods.—The study included 535 patients undergoing temporal artery biopsy over a 4-year period. The clinical data included the dose and duration of corticosteroid therapy before biopsy. Biopsy slides were reviewed by a pathologist who was unaware of the clinical data and the original pathologic diagnosis. Rates of positive biopsy were compared for the 249 patients with and the 286 without previous corticosteroid therapy, with adjustment for clinical and laboratory characteristics.

Results.—Thirty-five percent of patients who did receive prebiopsy corticosteroids and 31% of those who did not had positive biopsy results. The steroid-treated patients were likely to have clinical features that were suggestive of arteritis. On adjustment for clinical and laboratory findings by logistic regression analysis, no relationship between biopsy positivity rate and corticosteroid treatment was found.

Conclusion.—No difference was found in the rates of positive temporal artery biopsy in patients who did and did not receive corticosteroids before biopsy was performed. It is still possible that corticosteroids modify the histologic characteristics of temporal artery biopsies. For patients with clinical signs of giant cell arteritis, even if they have received previous corticosteroid therapy, confirmatory temporal artery biopsy is a reasonable next step.

▶ When a patient over 50 presents with such symptoms as headache, loss of vision, and jaw claudication, perhaps in combination with polymyalgia rheumatica, one is properly inclined to begin high-dose corticosteroids sooner rather than later, to prevent irreversible complications such as blindness. However, there is a concern that corticosteroids will suppress the confirming histological evidence that many (but not all) physicians want when they are embarking on an extended course of steroid therapy. Some clinicians avoid the problem by not doing biopsies at all; they reason that false negative biopsies are common enough that, once having decided to treat, they would not be influenced by negative histology.

The Mayo experience is different, largely because of their aggressive approach to the biopsy. They remove a full 3 to 4 cm of the more clinically suspicious temporal artery (others have often taken only ≤ 1 cm); examine multiple levels in frozen sections; and if there is no evidence of vasculitis, take the other temporal artery at the same sitting for similar scrutiny both immediately and in permanent sections. In patients with negative biopsy specimens under these exacting conditions, unless there are dramatic clinical symptoms (e.g., visual loss), these authors tend to not treat with corticosteroids; in an earlier study of such patients followed for a median of 6 years (1), only 9% eventually required them.

In this retrospective, non–population-based study (91% of their patients were referred), the authors cannot and *do* not claim that corticosteroids do not alter the histology of temporal arteritis; in fact, significantly more of patients treated for more than 14 days had atypical vasculitis (e.g., no giant cells) than did those who were untreated. They do show rather nicely that if you want histologic confirmation of temporal arteritis, the fact that the patient has begun corticosteroids should not discourage you from looking for it.—S.E. Malawista, M.D.

Reference

1. Hall S, Persillin S, Lie JT, O'Brien PC, Kurland LT, Hunder GG: The therapeutic impact of temporal artery biopsy. *Lancet* 2:1217–1220, 1983.

Association of Chronic Nasal Carriage of *Staphylococcus aureus* and Higher Relapse Rates in Wegener Granulomatosis
Stegeman CA, Tervaert JWC, Sluiter WJ, Manson WL, de Jong PE, Kallenberg CGM (Univ Hosp Groningen, The Netherlands)
Ann Intern Med 120:12–17, 1994   119-95-73–2

Background.—Treatment of Wegener's granulomatosis with cyclophosphamide in combination with corticosteroids has proved to be highly successful in achieving remission. However, the subsequent course of the disease is highly variable, and most patients experience relapses. Possible risk factors for this relapse were investigated, including chronic nasal carriage of *Staphylococcus aureus* and serial antineutrophil cytoplasmic antibody (ANCA) levels in patients with Wegener's granulomatosis.

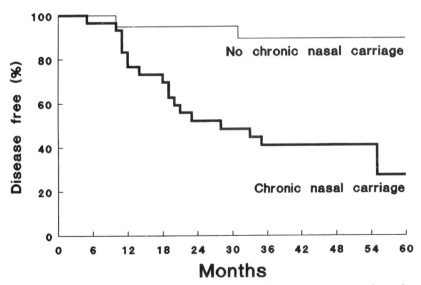

Fig 73–1.—Disease-free interval of 57 patients with Wegener's granulomatosis, grouped according to *S. aureus* carrier status. The disease-free interval was counted from the beginning of the most recent period of disease activity (either initial diagnosis or relapse; P < .001). (Courtesy of Stegeman CA, Tervaert JWC, Sluiter WJ, et al: *Ann Intern Med* 120:12–17, 1994.)

Clinical Features of 23 First Relapses in 57 Patients With Wegener's
Granulomatosis, According to *S. aureus* Nasal Carrier Status

Clinical Feature	Chronic Nasal Carriage (n = 36)	No Chronic Nasal Carriage (n = 21)
	n	
Patients with relapses	21	2
Progressive glomerulonephritis	7	
Pulmonary lesions	12	1
Nasal or upper-airway lesions	20	2
Miscellaneous		
Mononeuritis multiplex	1	
Episcleritis	4	
Tracheal stenosis	1	

(Courtesy of Stegeman CA, Tervaert JWC, Sluiter WJ, et al: *Ann Intern Med* 120:12–17, 1994.)

Method.—The study included 71 patients with biopsy-proven Wegener's granulomatosis who were followed up for 18 months. At each 4- to 6-week clinic visit, blood samples were taken for ANCA determinations, and a swab culture of the anterior nares was obtained. Occurrence of infections and relapses of Wegener's granulomatosis were identified according to strict predefined criteria.

Results.—Of the 71 patients who entered the study, analysis was completed for 51. Forty-two of these patients were found to have nasal cultures that grew *S. aureus,* and 36 were chronic nasal carriers. No significant differences in clinical characteristics were seen between the groups with and without chronic nasal carriage of *S. aureus*. However, 21 of the 36 patients with chronic nasal carriage of *S. aureus* had 1 or more relapses, whereas only 2 of 21 without chronic nasal carriage had a relapse (Fig 73–1). Nasal upper-airway lesions, progressive glomerulonephritis, and pulmonary lesions were most frequently associated with relapse (table). A total of 54 of the 57 patients had c-ANCA with specificity for proteinase-3 at some point. During the study, the median number of ANCA determinations per patient was 29. Twenty-two of 33 patients who were persistently or intermittently positive for ANCA experienced relapse compared with only 1 of 21 persistently negative patients. No significant correlation was seen between relapses of Wegener's granulomatosis and diagnosed upper airway infections.

Conclusion.—Chronic nasal carriage of *S. aureus* in a group of 57 patients with Wegener's granulomatosis followed for between 1 and 3.5 years led to the identification of a group of patients that were more prone to relapses of the disease. This study indicates a role for *S. aureus* in the pathophysiology, i.e., development of Wegener's granulomatosis relapse and a potential clue for treatment.

▶ The authors remind us that an important role for an infectious agent or agents in the induction of Wegener's granulomatosis was first suggested by Friedrich Wegener himself when he described the illness in 1936. In this study, relapses of disease were associated with chronic nasal carriage of *S. aureus* and not with clinically apparent infection. The contrarian argument would be that *S. aureus*, rather than triggering relapses, may be more likely to colonize nasal tissues that are already beset by low-grade subclinical disease activity, i.e., they are already on the road to relapse. As the authors point out, studies aimed at eliminating nasal carriage of *S. aureus* are warranted to see if relapses may be prevented. One may further ask whether the remissions reported in some patients following treatment with sulfamethoxazole-trimethoprim (1) correlate positively with nasal carrier status.—S.E. Malawista, M.D.

Reference

1. 1993 YEAR BOOK OF MEDICINE, p 718.

Effect of Surgical Cleaning of the Skin on the Pathergy Phenomenon in Behçet's Syndrome

Fresko I, Yazici H, Bayramiçli M, Yurdakul S, Mat C (Cerrahpasa Med Faculty, Istanbul, Turkey)
Ann Rheum Dis 52:619–620, 1993　　　　　　　　　119-95-73–3

Background.—The pathergy reaction, a nonspecific cutaneous hypersensitivity seen almost exclusively in patients with Behçet's syndrome, is induced by the insertion of a sterile needle into an alcohol-cleansed forearm, after which the formation of a papule or pustule is observed. It has not yet been determined whether the sterile needle introduces any agent(s) into the epidermis or dermis during penetration. Surgical cleansing of the skin was thus evaluated for its effect on the pathergy phenomenon in patients with Behçet's syndrome.

Patients and Methods.—Three groups of patients fulfilling the classification criteria for Behçet's syndrome were investigated. One forearm of each patient was cleansed with an alcohol pad only. The other arm was cleansed for 4 minutes with either 10% povidone-iodine in 93 patients, 100% chlorhexidine solution in 47 patients, or 4% aqueous chlorhexidine solution in 42 patients. The pathergy reaction was induced at 2 sites on each forearm. Sterile gloves were used when inserting the needle at the surgically cleansed sites. All puncture sites were covered with sterile pads immediately after the puncture, and these were removed at 24 hours. The pathergy reactions were read blindly at 48 hours by 2 independent observers.

Results.—The pathergy reaction was noted in 27% of the forearm cleansed with povidone-iodine before needle insertion, compared to 48% in arms cleansed with the standard alcohol pad. In forearms cleansed with 100% chlorhexidine, the prevalence of the pathergy was reduced from the 59% noted in the conventionally cleaned forearms to 36%. No significant changes were observed when the 4% aqueous chlorhexidine solution was used.

Conclusion.—In patients with Behçet's syndrome, surgical cleansing of the forearm with disinfectants of various concentrations decreases the prevalence of a positive pathergy test. This suggests that there is more involved in the production of the pathergy phenomenon than only disruption of the epidermal or dermal structural integrity.

▶ Behçet's syndrome, originally described by a Turkish dermatologist in 1937 as a triad of aphthous oral and genital ulcerations with uveitis, is now recognized as a multisystem disease that can involve skin, joints, veins, arteries, the gastrointestinal tract, meninges, and brain. Some cases of recurrent aphthous stomatitis and aphthous vulvitis in young women may be incomplete forms of the syndrome. The disease is both more frequent and more aggressive in the Middle and Far East than in North America, as is the phenomenon of pathergy, which, in this study, is reported from Istanbul. A number of recent lines of evidence favoring a pathogenetic role of bacterial antigens makes this paper worth noting (see also Abstract 119-95-73-2). In addition, Behçet's syndrome needs periodic mention here (1) for purposes of anamnesis of a disorder that is not often seen but is not to be missed.—S.E. Malawista, M.D.

Reference

1. 1991 YEAR BOOK OF MEDICINE, p 713.

Takayasu Arteritis
Kerr GS, Hallahan CW, Giordano J, Leavitt RY, Fauci AS, Rottem M, Hoffman GS (Natl Inst of Allergy and Infectious Diseases, Bethesda, Md; Natl Insts of Health, Bethesda, Md; George Washington Univ Hosp, Washington, DC)
Ann Intern Med 120:919–929, 1994.   119-95-73-4

Series.—Sixty patients seen over 20 years with a diagnosis of Takayasu's arteritis were followed prospectively for a median of 5.3 years. All but 2 patients were females. Three fourths were whites and 10% were Asians. Fifteen patients were lost to follow-up.

Clinical Findings.—The median age when symptoms developed was 25 years; one third of the group were juveniles. Symptoms often were present for several months before the diagnosis was made. The most common clinical finding, present in 80% of patients, was a bruit, which was most frequent in the carotid vessels. One third of the patients were lightheaded or dizzy, most often in relation to vertebral artery stenosis. About half the patients had musculoskeletal and joint symptoms. Visual disorders were associated with both common carotid and vertebral artery disease. Heart disease developed in nearly 40% of patients. Angiograms typically demonstrated long stenotic lesions.

Management.—Patients with active disease received oral glucocorticoid treatment for months, at which time a cytotoxic drug was added unless the patient was controlled on alternate-day steroid therapy. The drugs used included cyclophosphamide, azathioprine, and methotrexate.

Outcome.—About half the 70 courses of glucocorticoid treatment, given to 48 patients, led to remission of disease. Twenty-five patients received cytotoxic therapy in addition, and 40% of them responded at least once. Forty-five percent of 60 evaluable patients had at least one relapse. Thirty patients had a total of 79 vascular operations, most often bypass procedures. Eleven patients underwent 20 percutaneous transluminal angioplasties. Three fourths of 34 patients followed over the long term had some morbidity and 2 patients died (one was a suicide).

Conclusions.—In North America, Takayasu's arteritis is a rare disorder with varible clinical findings that responds unpredictably to treatment. A majority of patients have required repeated courses of treatment, and most have incurred a substantial degree of morbidity.

▶ This is the largest cohort of patients with Takayasu's arteritis studied so far in the United States. The diagnosis of this rare disorder of young people was based on the presence of symptoms and signs of ischemic, inflammatory large-vessel disease, as well as supportive arteriographic findings (Fig 73–3). Other causes of large-vessel abnormalities were excluded based on clinical and sometimes laboratory criteria, including: (1) inflammatory aortitis (e.g., syphilis, tuberculosis, systemic lupus erythematosus, rheumatoid arthritis, spondyloarthropathies, Buerger's, Behçet's, Cogan's, and Kawasaki's diseases or syndromes, and giant cell arteritis); (2) developmental abnormalities (e.g., Ehlers-Danlos and Marfan's syndromes); and (3) other aortic abnormalities (e.g., neurofibromatosis, ergotism, radiation fibrosis).

Vascular ischemic symptoms are the hallmark of this illness: bruit, claudication or diminished pulses. The authors emphasize that a young patient with hypertension should be further evaluated for extremity claudication, cerebral ischemia, and renal artery stenosis. Most patients with Takayasu's arteritis have multiple abnormalities of the aorta, its branches, or both. Angiography is considered the gold standard in delineating abnormal vessels in this disorder. Two recent papers deal with the treatment of Takayasu's arteritis, with methotrexate when glucocorticoids alone have not produced a sustained remission (1; from the same group) and with percutaneous transluminal angioplasty of the descending thoracic and abdominal aorta (2).—S.E. Malawista, M.D.

References

1. Hoffman GS, Leavitt RY, Kerr GS, Rottem M, Sneller MC, Fauci AS: Treatment of glucocorticoid-resistant or relapsing Takayasu arteritis with methotrexate. *Arthritis Rheum* 37:578–582, 1994.
2. Rao SA, Mandalam KR, Rao VR, Gupta AK, Joseph S, Unni MN, Subramanyan R, Neelakandhan KS: Takayasu arteritis: Initial and long-term follow-up in 16 patients after percutaneous transluminal angioplasty of the descending thoracic and abdominal aorta. *Radiology* 189:173–179, 1993.

74 Infectious Arthritis

Introduction

This chapter addresses the treatment of Lyme arthritis (Abstract 119-95-74-1) and its diagnosis by the polymerase chain reaction (PCR) (Abstract 119-95-74-2), the problem of polyarticular septic arthritis (Abstract 119-95-74-3), and the occurrence of *Pneumocystis carinii* pneumonia in the course of connective tissue disease (Abstract 119-95-74-4).

Noted in passing are the application of PCR to the diagnosis of gonococcal arthritis, another joint infection from which organisms are difficult to culture (1, 2); the risks and costs of empiric antibiotic therapy of patients with fibromyalgia and fatigue and a positive serologic test for Lyme disease (3, 4); a primarily European genotype of *Borrelia burgdorferi* associated with the development of acrodermatitis chronica atrophicans, a lesion seen principally in Europe (5, 6); and reviews of HIV infection and rheumatic disease (7) and of tuberculosis of bone and joints (8).

Stephen E. Malawista, M.D.

References

1. Liebling MR, Arkfeld DG, Michelini GA, Nishio MJ, Eng BJ, Jin T, Louie JS: Identification of *Neisseria Gonorrhoeae* in synovial fluid using the polymerase chain reaction. *Arthritis Rheum* 37:702–709, 1994.
2. Use of the polymerase chain reaction to study arthritis due to *Neisseria gonorrhoeae*. *Arthritis Rheum* 37:710–717, 1994.
3. Lightfoot RW Jr, Luft BJ, Rahn DW, Steere AC, Sigal LH, Zoschke DC, Gardner P, Britton MC, Kaufman RL: Empiric parenteral antibiotic treatment of patients with fibromyalgia and fatigue and a positive serologic result for Lyme disease: A cost-effectiveness analysis. *Ann Intern Med* 119:503–509, 1993.
4. A joint statement of the American College of Rheumatology and the Council of the Infectious Diseases Society of America: Appropriateness of parenteral antibiotic treatment for patients with presumed Lyme disease. *Ann Intern Med* 119:518, 1993.
5. Canica MM, Nato F, du Merle L, Mazie JC, Baranton G, Postic D: Monoclonal antibodies for identification of *Borrelia afzelii* sp. nov. associated with late cutaneous manifestations of Lyme borreliosis. *Scand J Infect Dis* 25:441–448, 1993.
6. van Dam AP, Kuiper H, Vos K, Widjojokusumo A, de Jongh BM, Spanjaard L, Ramselaar ACP, Kramer MD, Dankert J: Different genospecies of *Borrelia burgdorferi* are associated with distinct clinical manifestations of Lyme borreliosis. *Clin Infect Dis* 17:708–717, 1993.
7. Winchester RJ: HIV infection and rheumatic disease. *Bull Rheum Dis* 43:5–8, 1994.
8. Grosskopf I, David AB, Charach G, Hochman I, Pitlik S: Bone and joint tuberculosis: A 10-year review. *Isr J Med Sci* 30:278–283, 1994.

Treatment of Lyme Arthritis

Steere AC, Levin RE, Molloy PJ, Kalish RA, Abraham JH III, Liu NY, Schmid CH (New England Med Ctr, Boston; Tufts Univ, Boston; Little Rock Diagnostic Clinic, Ark; et al)

Arthritis Rheum 37:878–888, 1994   119-95-74-1

Objective.—An attempt was made, in patients aged 13 years and older with a diagnosis of Lyme arthritis, to determine whether the disorder is controlled by oral treatment with doxycycline or amoxicillin plus probenecid. In addition, the efficacy of intravenous ceftriaxone was examined in patients whose arthritis persisted despite antibiotic treatment.

Management.—Forty patients with at least one actively inflamed joint were randomized to receive either doxycycline in a dose of 100 mg given twice daily for 30 days, or 500 mg of both amoxicillin and probenecid 4 times daily. Nonsteroidal anti-inflammatory drugs were allowed to be taken by patients with marked joint inflammation, but intra-articular steroids were not. Two patients who failed to respond to oral treatment and 14 other patients who had not improved when given recommended antibiotic regimens received ceftriaxone intravenously in a dose of 2 g daily for 2 weeks.

Results.—Arthritis resolved within 1 to 3 months in 18 of 20 patients randomized to receive doxycycline and in 16 of 18 who received amoxicillin. Five patients, 4 of whom had received amoxicillin, later had neurologic involvement. None of the 16 patients given intravenous ceftriaxone therapy responded within 3 months. Patients who had had more and longer episodes of arthritis were less likely than others to respond. The HLA-DR4 specificity and IgG reactivity with the OspA protein of *Borrelia burgdorferi* also were adverse prognostic factors.

Recommendations.—Patients with Lyme arthritis who lack neurologic involvement should receive oral antibiotic treatment. Anti-inflammatory drugs and 1 or 2 intra-articular steroid injections may be tried if arthritis persists. If painful joint swelling continues or function is restricted, arthroscopic synovectomy may be helpful.

▶ This is the most informative paper yet on the treatment of Lyme arthritis. We learn that 18 of the 20 patients treated with doxycycline (90%) and 16 of the 18 who completed the amoxicillin regimen (89%) had resolution of their arthritis within 1–3 months after entry in the study. Waiting out the 3 months is important; the awareness that resolution takes time will avoid additional unnecessary antibiotics. Ceftriaxone has been viewed by some workers as superior to penicillin for arthritis, so it is interesting to note that (a largely different set of 16) patients with persistent arthritis, despite previous oral antibiotics or parenteral penicillin, did not respond to intravenous ceftriaxone either. Both HLA-DR4 specificity and outer-surface protein A (OspA) immunoreactivity correlated with a general lack of response to antibiotic therapy.

A major concern about oral therapy is the later development of neurologic disease. Indeed, in this study, such disease developed in 5 of the patients when arthritis was no longer present. Three patients developed subtle sensory symptoms weeks to months after study entry, and electromyograms showed diffuse polyneuropathy. The other two developed subtle memory impairment 2 and 3 years after entry; cerebrospinal fluid showed elevated total protein and production of intrathecal antibody to the spirochete. However, we are currently more aware of such subtle impairments than when this study began. Indeed, in retrospect, all 5 patients recalled minor dysesthesias or memory impairment *at the time of study entry*. Today, such patients would have had electromyography or lumbar puncture on initial presentation, and positive results would have led directly to parenteral therapy (all 5 patients, by the way, were treated successfully with a month of ceftriaxone).

So an initial trial of oral antibiotics for Lyme arthritis without symptommatic neurologic involvement seems clinically reasonable. Not the last to thank you for this approach will be your HMO. A 1-month course of doxycycline or amoxicillin costs about $60; intravenous ceftriaxone for the same period will cost 50 to 100 times as much, or more.—S.E. Malawista, M.D.

Detection of *Borrelia burgdorferi* DNA by Polymerase Chain Reaction in Synovial Fluid from Patients With Lyme Arthritis

Nocton JJ, Dressler F, Rutledge BJ, Rys PN, Persing DH, Steere AC (Tufts Univ, Boston; Mayo Found, Rochester, Minn; New England Med Ctr, Boston, Mass)

N Engl J Med 330:229–234, 1994   119-95-74-2

Objective.—*Borrelia burgdorferi* is difficult to culture from synovial fluid. In this study, the use of polymerase chain reaction (PCR) to detect *B. burgdorferi* DNA in joint-fluid samples was evaluated.

Methods.—Over a 17-year period, samples of synovial fluid were collected from 88 patients with Lyme arthritis and 64 control patients with other forms of arthritis. The samples were tested, in a blinded fashion, in 2 separate laboratories by using 4 sets of primers and probes, including 3 that targeted plasmid DNA encoding outer-surface protein A (OspA) and 1 that targeted a portion of the chromosomal DNA encoding 16S ribosomal RNA.

Results.—*Borrelia burgdorferi* DNA was detected in 85% of patients with Lyme arthritis but in none of the control patients (Table 1). The three OspA sets each detected *B. burgdorferi* DNA in 75% to 89% of the positive PCR results, and the results were moderately concordant in the 2 laboratories. Of the 73 patients with Lyme arthritis who were untreated or treated with only short courses of oral antibiotics, 70 (96%) had positive PCR results (Table 2). In contrast, only 7 (37%) of 19 patients who received either parenteral antibiotics or long courses of oral antibiotics had positive PCR results; none of these patients had received more than 2 months of oral antibiotics or 3 weeks of IV antibiotics. In

TABLE 1.—Polymerase Chain Reaction (PCR) in Synovial Fluid From Case and Control Patients

	PRIMER–PROBE SETS				
	SET 1	SET 2	SET 3	SET 4	ANY SET†
	no. of patients				
Lyme arthritis (n = 88)					
Positive PCR results	57	56	67	42	75
Negative PCR results	31	32	21	46	13
Other arthritis (n = 64)					
Positive PCR results	0	0	0	0	0
Negative PCR results	12	12	57	57	64

Note: Test results from the initial sample from each patient are shown. Samples that contained inhibitors of PCR amplification were excluded. Laboratory 1 tested all initial and serial samples from patients with Lyme arteritis and all identically stored control samples with primer-probe sets 1 and 2. Laboratory 2 tested the initial sample from each patient with Lyme arthritis, 5 of the identically stored control samples, and an additional 52 control samples from their institution with primer-probe sets 3 and 4.

(Courtesy of Nocton JJ, Dressler F, Rutledge BJ, et al: N Engl J Med 330:229-234, 1995.)

10 patients with chronic arthritis despite multiple courses of antibiotic therapy, 7 had consistently negative PCR results in all post-treatment samples.

Conclusion.—This study demonstrates that PCR testing can detect *B. burgdorferi* DNA in synovial fluid from patients with Lyme arthritis, and

TABLE 2.—Polymerase Chain Reaction (PCR) Results, According to Antibiotic Treatment

ANTIBIOTIC TREATMENT	PATIENTS		SAMPLES	
	TOTAL NO.*	NO. (%) PCR-POSITIVE	TOTAL NO.	NO. (%) PCR-POSITIVE
No antibiotics	45	43 (96)	59	54 (92)
Tested before antibiotics	16	15 (94)	26	25 (96)
Tested after short course of oral antibiotics (<1 mo)	12	12 (100)	15	15 (100)
Total, short course or none	73	70 (96)	100	94 (94)
Tested after parenteral or long courses of oral antibiotics (≥1 mo)	19	7 (37)†	26	7 (27)†

* Three patients from whom samples were obtained before antibiotic treatment and one patient from whom the sample was obtained after a short course of antibiotics also had samples obtained after parenteral antibiotic treatment. Thus, for this analysis, the total number of patients was 92 rather than 88.

P < .001 for the comparison of parenteral or long courses with short courses or no therapy.

(Courtesy of Nocton JJ, Dressler F, Rutledge BJ, et al: N Engl J Med 330:229-234, 1994.)

the sensitivity of each of the 3 OspA primer-probe sets is high. This test may prove useful in making therapeutic decisions for patients with persistent Lyme arthritis despite multiple courses of antibiotic therapy.

▶ Recovery of *B. burgdorferi* by culture of synovial fluid from patients with Lyme arthritis is extremely rare. Although such patients generally have high titers of specific antibody, they may have (or recall) no other stigmata of Lyme disease. This meticulous study indicates that PCR will be useful in diagnosis and perhaps also in evaluating the efficacy of antibiotic therapy in Lyme disease (see also References 1–3). The latter depends upon spirochetal DNA not persisting (as protein perhaps does) long after the bacteria are killed. I can offer evidence from infected mice, in which tissues are both culture- and PCR-positive, that DNA does not persist (4). When the mice were treated with sterilizing doses of antibiotics, their tissues (skin and bladder) became PCR-negative directly after treatment. If humans behave similarly— and this needs to be shown for particular compartments such as joint and subarachnoid spaces—then a positive PCR after treatment would suggest that the spirochete has not been eradicated. (A negative result means that spirochetal DNA has, at the very least, been knocked down below levels detectable by PCR.)

A major caveat here is to know who is doing the PCR; false positives are very common unless extreme precautions, such as those developed in the Persing laboratory and used here (multiple DNA targets, 2 different laboratories, isopsoralen sterilization of amplified material), are employed. The only methodological quibble in this paper is with accession of samples. The Yale specimens, at least, which date from 1975, were aliquoted in an open laboratory, without special precautions (we currently access specimens for PCR in a different building). However, *B. burgdorferi* was not cultured there until the early 1980s, controls were uniformly negative, and it is doubtful that contamination was a major problem here.

Why are PCR-positive joint fluids almost always culture-negative? I think there is a clue in a recent finding of ours (5), in which plasmid DNA (coding for OspA and outer-surface protein B [OspB]) was amplified much more frequently from Lyme arthritis joint fluid than was genomic DNA (coding for 16S RNA and flagellin), even though the latter is at least as detectable as the former from cultured spirochetes. Of possible explanations for this "target imbalance," I favor the following: Garon and colleagues have studied membrane defects (blebs) that appear on the surface of spirochetes during growth in culture, and especially after the addition of specific antiserum. These membranous vesicles are shed into culture medium and, when purified, are found to contain, along with various membrane-related proteins, plasmid DNA but not genomic DNA. Thus, it is possible that in Lyme arthritis patients, the organism itself is sequestered in synovial tissue, releasing plasmid-rich blebs into the synovial fluid. The release of antigens into the synovial space might also amplify the inflammatory response in the virtual absence of organisms, explaining the difficulty in culturing them from synovial fluid.

Time will tell, but this explanation is attractive because it addresses successfully the clinical facts of Lyme arthritis.—S.E. Malawista, M.D.

References

1. Bradley JF, Johnson RC, Goodman JL: The persistence of spirochetal nucleic
   acids in active Lyme arthritis. *Ann Intern Med* 120:487–489, 1994.
2. Rahn DW: Lyme disease: Where's the bug? *N Engl J Med* 330:282–283, 1994.
3. Sigal LH: The polymerase chain reaction assay for *Borrelia burgdorferi* in the
   diagnosis of Lyme disease. *Ann Intern Med* 120:520–521, 1994.
4. Malawista SE, Barthold SW, Persing DH: Fate of *Borrelia burgdorferi* DNA in
   tissues of infected mice after antibiotic treatment. *J Infect Dis* 170:1312–1316,
   1994.
5. Persing DH, Rutledge BJ, Rys PN, Podzorski DS, Reed KR, Mitchell PN, Liu B,
   Fikrig E, Malawista SE: Target imbalance: Disparity of *Borrelia burgdorferi* genetic material in synovial fluid from Lyme arthritis patients. *J Infect Dis*
   169:664–668, 1994.

Polyarticular Septic Arthritis
Dubost J-J, Fis I, Denis P, Lopitaux R, Soubrier M, Ristori J-M, Bussiere J-L,
Sirot J, Sauvezie B (Hôpital Gabriel-Montipied Clermont-Ferrand, France;
Hôpital Nord, Cebazat, France; Hôtel-Dieu, Clermont-Ferrand, France)
Medicine 72:296–310, 1993   119-95-74-3

Objective.—Polyarticular septic arthritis (PASA) is a rare condition.
Between 1979 and 1991, 25 patients with PASA were seen, accounting
for 16.6% of all cases of nongonococcal septic arthritis. These cases
were compared with those of PASA and monoarticular septic arthritis
(MASA) reported in the literature.

Findings.—In patients with PASA, average age of the patients was 62
years, and none was younger than 50. An average of 4 joints was involved, most frequently the knee, elbow, and shoulder. *Staphylococcus
aureus* was the most frequent causative agent. Joint aspirations were positive in 92% of patients with PASA and 95% of those with MASA, but the
frequency of positive blood cultures was significantly greater in PASA
(76% vs 33%) (Table 1). Fever and severe leukocytosis were not common. Concurrent rheumatic diseases occurred frequently in PASA but
rarely in MASA. The most frequent underlying disease in PASA was rheumatoid arthritis that was typically advanced and erosive and treated with
steroids. Mortality was 32% in PASA compared with 4% in MASA. Analysis of 184 cases of PASA reported in the literature showed that 1 in 2
cases of PASA was associated with rheumatoid arthritis, and blood cultures were positive in most cases. More recently, PASA was associated
with systemic lupus erythematosus, and disease involved streptococci or
gram-negative bacilli more than staphylococci. However, prognosis remained poor over the past 40 years, with 30% mortality (Table 2). Overall, age greater than 50 years, rheumatoid arthritis as an underlying disease, and disease of staphylococcal origin were associated with poor

TABLE 1.—Comparison of 25 Patients With PASA and 95
With MASA

Characteristics	PASA No. (%)		MASA No. (%)	P
No.	25		95	
Age (mean)	62.4		59.1	
>60 yr	14 (56)		54 (57)	
No. males	13 (52)		64 (67.4)	
Site				
Hip	20*	6.9**	18.9†	
Knee	72*	27.5**	40†	
Ankle	24*	9.8**	6.3†	
Tarsus	4*	1**	8.4†	
MTP	8*	2.9**	1†	
Shoulder	36*	9.8**	14.7†	
Elbow	40*	11.8**	3.2†	
Wrist	32*	11.8**	5.3†	
MCP, PIP	32*	16.7**	2.1†	
SC + AC	8*	2**	0†	
Hip or knee pros- thesis	16*	4.9**	14.7†	
Temp. <37.5°C	5 (20)		17/91 (18.7)	
Organism cultured				
S. aureus	20 (80)		59 (62.1)	0.05
S. coagulase neg.	1 (4)		6 (6.3)	
Streptococci	1 (4)		18 (18.9)	0.05
Pneumocci	1 (4)		2 (2.1)	
Gram-negative bacilli	1 (4)		8 (8.4)	
Positive blood cul- tures	19 (76)		31 (32.6)	0.001
Underlying disease				
RA	13 (52)		6 (6.3)	0.001
SLE	1 (4)		1 (1)	
Steroid therapy	12 (48)		4 (4.2)	0.001
Diabetes mellitus	3 (12)		15 (15.8)	
Surgical treatment	11 (44)		21 (22.1)	0.02
Fatal cases	8 (32)		4 (4.2)	0.001

* Percentage of patients with disease in this location.
** Frequency of this location as a percentage of all 102 locations.
In MASA, the percentage of patients and frequency of location (* and ** in PASA) are identical, as there is only one location in each case of MASA.
Abbreviations: PASA, polyarticular septic arthritis; MASA, monoarticular septic arthritis; MTP, metatarsophalangeal joint; MCP, metacarpophalangeal joint; PIP, proximal interphalangeal joint; SC, sternoclavicular; AC, acromioclavicular.
(Courtesy of Dubost J-J, Fis I, Denis P, et al: Medicine 72:296-310, 1993.)

TABLE 2.—Characteristics of PASA in the Literature, by Decade of Publication

Characteristic	Before 1960 No. (%)	1961–70 No. (%)	1971–80 No. (%)	1981–90 No. (%)
No.	20	42	58	64
Age (yr)	47.9	58.6	53.9	50.5
No. males	14 (70)	21 (50)	28 (48.3)	35 (54.7)
No. joints involved	4.25	3.33	3.02	3.97
Organism*				
S. aureus	14 (70)	20 (47.6)	21 (36.2)	14 (21.9)
Streptococci	1 (5)	5 (11.9)	5 (8.6)	20 (31.3)
Pneumococci	0	3 (7.1)	9 (15.5)	6 (9.4)
Gram negative bacilli	2 (10)	8 (19)	19 (32.8)	21 (32.8)
Positive blood cultures	9/14 (64.3)	19/27 (70.4)	28/36 (77)	43/52 (82.7)
Underlying disease				
Rheumatoid arthritis	14 (70)	21 (50)	27 (46.6)	18 (28.1)
Systemic lupus erythematosus	0	2 (4.8)	6 (10.3)	8 (12.5)
Steroid therapy (%)†	4 (28.6)	13 (56.5)	17 (51.5)	14 (53.8)
Diabetes mellitus	0	5 (12)	5 (8.6)	7 (10.9)
Surgical treatment	8/20 (40)	16/35 (45.7)	23/47 (48.9)	27/51 (52.9)
Fatal cases	7/20 (35)	14/42 (33.3)	15/54 (27.8)	18/63 (28.6)

* Other (rare) microorganisms were not tabulated.
† Percentage of patients with rheumatoid arthritis and systemic lupus erythematosus taking steroids.
(Courtesy of Dubost J-J, Fis I, Denis P, et al: *Medicine* 72:296–310, 1993.)

prognosis in PASA. In a subgroup of PASA with rheumatoid arthritis, male patients were more frequently affected, and most lesions resulted from staphylococci whose source was skin lesions.

Summary.—Polyarticular septic arthritis is commonly associated with rheumatoid arthritis and staphylococcal infection. Blood cultures are often positive, supporting the concept of hematogenous seeding. Prognosis remains poor. It appears that PASA may be a consequence of longer delays in diagnosis and treatment.

▶ This study of 25 patients with nongonococcal PASA, studied over 13 years (Table 1), comes from a primary and secondary reference center of a predominantly rural French province, where drug abuse and AIDS are still rare. The results are similar to those of 184 additional patients culled from the literature and presented by decade (Table 2). The patients in question often had an underlying rheumatoid arthritis (13 of 25), which was often advanced, erosive, and being treated with corticosteroid therapy. Ten patients had one or more extraarticular septic lesions. Large joints were often involved, 4 of them on average (range, 2–14); knee, hip, and shoulder joints accounted for 73% of all locations. Although cultures of joint fluid were positive in over 90% of both poly- and monoarticular septic arthritis, blood cultures were much more often positive in the former (76% vs. 33%). However, sometimes lacking were fever (5 of 25) and leukocytosis (10 of 25); 3 patients were leukopenic. Mortality in polyarticular septic arthritis was an ap-

palling 32% (vs. 4% with monoarticular involvement, Table 1), and that figure has been essentially constant over 4 decades (Table 2).

One would like more precise data on the delay in diagnosis when someone
who already has a noninfectious chronic polyarthritis complains of increased
multiple joint pains. Without a high index of suspicion in such patients, infections are often missed, even when only a single joint is involved. The best
approach is, of course, a careful history and physical examination, and a low
threshold for joint aspiration, smear, and culture.—S.E. Malawista, M.D.

Pneumocystis Carinii **Pneumonia in the Course of Connective Tissue Disease: Report of 34 Cases**

Godeau B, Coutant-Perronne V, Huong DLT, Guillevin L, Magadur G, de
Bandt M, Dellion S, Rossert J, Rostoker G, Piette J-C, Schaeffer A (Hôpital
Henri Mondor, Créteil, France; Hôpital La Pitié, Paris; Hôpital Avicenne,
Bobigny, France; et al)
J Rheumatol 21:246–251, 1994   119-95-74–4

Introduction.—*Pneumocystis carinii* (PCP) pneumonia has recently
received attention because of its association with AIDS, but it is also observed in other immunosuppressed patients. An attempt was made to
determine the circumstances, clinical features, and outcome of PCP in
patients with connective tissue diseases (CTD) but no HIV infection.

Patients and Methods.—Researchers retrospectively analyzed the records of all patients with PCP and CTD who were hospitalized during a
10-year period in adult medical units of 5 university hospitals. An en-

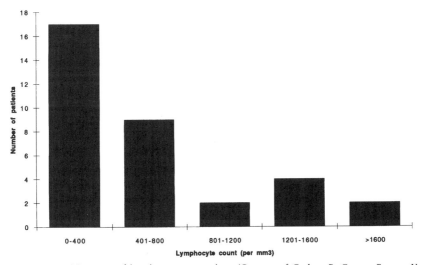

Fig 74–1.—Histogram of lymphocyte count values. (Courtesy of Godeau B, Coutant-Perrone V,
Huong DLT, et al: *J Rheumatol* 21:246–251, 1994.)

Short-Term Outcome and Underlying Connective
Tissue Disease

Connective Tissue Disease	Survivors/Number of Patients
Wegener's granulomatosis	7/12
Poly/dermatomyositis	2/5
Systemic lupus erythematosus	4/6
Polyarteritis nodosa	4/4
Rheumatoid arthritis	2/2
Adult onset Still's disease	1/1
Pemphigus	1/2
Pemphigoid	1/1
Sarcoidosis	1/1

(Courtesy of Godeau B, Coutant-Perrone V, Huong DLT, et al: *J Rheumatol* 21:246–251, 1994.)

zyme-linked immunosorbent microtest was used to exclude HIV-infected patients. Of almost 3,000 cases of CTD recorded during the study, 34 patients with PCP were evaluated. The 18 women and 16 men had a mean age of 52 years at PCP onset. The clinical and biological features of each patient were assessed, and short- and long-term outcomes were recorded. Special attention was given to the doses of corticosteroids and cytotoxic drugs received during the 60 days before the onset of PCP.

Results.—The most common diagnoses in the group were Wegener's granulomatosis (12), systemic lupus erythematosus (6), and poly/dermatomyositis (5). Most (74%) patients were seen with PCP within 8 months after the diagnosis of CTD. Thirty-two of 34 were receiving corticosteroids at the time of diagnosis of PCP; 19 had received cyclophosphamide and 5 were treated with methotrexate. The presentation of PCP was acute. Most patients were lymphocytopenic at onset (Fig 74–1), and half required intensive care for respiratory failure. A diagnosis of PCP was established in all patients by microscopic analysis of bronchoalveolar lavage. Coinfection was present in 7 cases. With the exception of one patient who initially was treated with intravenous pentamidine, therapy consisted of trimethoprim-sulfamethoxazole (TMP-SMX). Five patients had severe reactions to TMP-SMX. Eleven of 34 patients died; only one death was not due to infectious complications. Survival by underlying CTD is detailed in the table. Ten of the 23 survivors received secondary prophylaxis for PCP. Neither these patients, nor those who did not receive secondary prophylaxis, had had a relapse of PCP after mean follow-up of 22 months.

Conclusion.—This type of pneumonia is rare in patients with CTD. It should be suspected, however, if such patients are lymphocytopenic and are receiving cytotoxic agents and corticosteroids. The authors recommend that patients with CTD who present with fever, pulmonary infiltrates, hypoxemia, and lymphopenia undergo immediate bronchoalveolar lavage.

▶ Last year (1), we reviewed 6 patients with systemic lupus erythematosus (SLE) and PCP, whose risk factors for infection were a marked lymphocytopenia and high-dose corticosteroid and cytotoxic drug therapy. We concluded that prophylactic antibiotic therapy might be considered for total lymphocyte counts < 350/mm³. Now we have a 10-year retrospective study of almost 3,000 patients with a variety of connective tissue diseases from 10 adult medical units (5 internal medicine, 3 rheumatology, 2 nephrology, 1 dermatology) in 5 French university hospitals. Their risk factors were the same as those in the earlier study of SLE; 31 of 34 (91%) were lymphocytopenic (< 1,500/mm³, Figure 74–2). The estimated numbers of patients followed in these units during that period include 750 for SLE, 1,500 for rheumatoid arthritis, 250 for poly/dermatomyositis, and 100 for Wegener's granulomatosis. We are not told the lymphocyte counts of these denominators. The incidence of PCP in these various illnesses was low (less than 2%), except for Wegener's granulomatosis (12%)—perhaps because those with the latter illness were more likely to have received initial high-dose corticosteroids and long-term cyclophosphamide therapy.

The presentation of PCP in these individuals was acute and not specific, with a mean duration of symptoms of 6 days; high-grade fever was not masked by corticosteroid treatment. Acute respiratory failure was frequent, and half the patients required admission to ICUs. This clinical picture mimics that of immunocompromised patients with hematologic malignancies or cancer who acquire PCP, as opposed to patients with AIDS, whose PCP tends to develop more insidiously. Eleven patients died (table), largely from other infections after admission to intensive care units; only 3 died of PCP alone (adult respiratory distress syndrome, 2; pneumothorax, 1). Considering a mortality of one third in this study, empiric therapy for PCP, at least in the most severely lymphocytopenic patients with these illnesses, is defensible and perhaps desirable; it might be more so if the authors logged in the lymphocyte counts of the huge majority of their patients who avoided PCP.—S.E. Malawista, M.D.

Reference

1. 1994 YEAR BOOK OF MEDICINE, p 776.

75 Other Topics

Introduction

Our potpourri of other topics includes the risk of connective-tissue diseases and other disorders after breast implantation (Abstract 119-95-75-1); a controlled trial of high-dose intravenous immunoglobulin infusions as treatment for dermatomyositis (Abstract 119-95-75-2); calcific tendinitis in the proximal thigh (Abstract 119-95-75-3); fat necrosis as an unusual cause of polyarthritis (Abstract 119-95-75-4); and the benefits and disadvantages of joint hypermobility among musicians (Abstract 119-95-75-5). In addition, I have commented on an abstract dealing with the prediction of bone density from vitamin D receptor alleles that appears elsewhere in the YEAR BOOK, and I have included it as a special reference.

Noted in passing are 2 articles on fever, one of which is an attempt to place it in an evolutionary setting (1) and the other of which is a discussion of its dependence on humoral cues from the body, its orchestration largely by the hypothalamus, and the coordination of a wide range of autonomic, endocrine, and behavioral responses (2). Also included are reviews both of fever occurring with polyarthritis (3) and acute monoarthritis (4), an examination of the basic and clinical correlates of glucocorticoid therapy for immune-mediated diseases (5), and a review of antibodies to defined antigens in the systemic rheumatic diseases (6).

Stephen E. Malawista, M.D.

References

1. Mackowiak PA: Fever: Blessing or cure? A unifying hypothesis. *Ann Intern Med* 120:1037–1040, 1994.
2. Saper CB, Breder CD: The neurologic basis of fever. *N Engl J Med* 330:1880–1886, 1994.
3. Pinals RS: Polyarthritis and fever. *N Engl J Med* 330:769–774, 1994.
4. Baker DG, Schumacher HR Jr: Acute monoarthritis. *N Engl J Med* 329:1013–1020, 1993.
5. Boumpas DT, Chrousos GP, Wilder RL, Cupps TR, Balow JE: Glucocorticoid therapy for immune-mediated diseases: Basic and clinical correlates. *Ann Intern Med* 119:1109–1208, 1993.
6. Reichlin M: Antibodies to defined antigens in the systemic rheumatic diseases. *Bull Rheum Dis* 42:4–6, 1993.

Risk of Connective-Tissue Diseases and Other Disorders After Breast Implantation

Gabriel SE, O'Fallon WM, Kurland LT, Beard CM, Woods JE, Melton LJ III
(Mayo Clinic and Found, Rochester, Minn)
N Engl J Med 330:1697–702, 1994   119-95-75-1

Background.—Possibly 2 million American women have had breast reconstruction or augmentation since the advent of the silicone gel-filled breast prosthesis. Reports of connective tissue disease and autoimmune disease after breast augmentation led the Food and Drug Administration to recommend a moratorium in 1992, but case reports are not strong evidence of a causal relationship.

Objective.—A retrospective population-based study was performed to determine the risk of specified disorders after breast implantation in women living in Olmstead County, Minnesota, in 1964 to 1991.

Study Population.—Each of 749 women given a breast implant during the period under review was matched with 2 community control women evaluated medically within 2 years of the date of implantation and who were within 3 years of the study patient's age. The case women were followed for a mean of 7.8 years, and the 1,498 control women for 8.3 years. The case subjects had received a total of 1,840 implants, 78% of which were silicone devices.

Findings.—Connective tissue disease was diagnosed in 5 case subjects and 10 control women, for a relative risk of 1.06. The relative risk that a case subject would have signs or symptoms of arthritis was 1.35, but only morning stiffness was significantly more frequent in women with a breast implant (relative risk, 1.81).

Conclusion.—These findings fail to affirm an association between breast implants and connective tissue disease.

▶ The settlement for women claiming disability from certain rheumatic and other diseases due to silicone breast implants, described as being in process in the 1994 YEAR BOOK OF MEDICINE (1), has now been approved, to the tune of about $4.25 billion. It applies to implantees who have one of these disorders or who should develop one of them over the next 30 years. Studies (2), reviews (3, 4), and editorials (5, 6) on the subject continue to appear; of the studies, the one abstracted here, which does not find in implantees an increase in the diseases studied, is the best so far.

The Mayo Clinic maintains records of virtually everyone who resides in Olmstead County, Minnesota; these records are accessible by indexes to clinical and pathological diagnoses and surgical procedures. For each case there were 2 age-matched controls; for each woman receiving an implant after a mastectomy for breast cancer, there were 2 additional local controls who had undergone mastectomy for breast cancer but did not have a breast implant. Furthermore, because these workers screened and reviewed the symptoms and laboratory results directly, they could include events that met their definitions, even if the attending physician had failed to make (or record) the diagnosis. For example, contrary to previous reports (1), the incidence of abnormal test results for antinuclear antibodies in implantees did not differ significantly from that of women without implants in whom the test was performed (the same was true for rheumatoid factor and for antimicrosomal antibodies).

As pointed out by the authors and in an accompanying editorial, a definitive answer to the questions proposed would require a much larger (multicenter), preferably prospective cohort study of these relatively rare disorders, with as long a follow-up as is feasible. For example, assuming the incidence of systemic sclerosis at 1.6 cases per 100,000 women, the authors calculated that to detect a doubling of the relative risk among women with implants, they would have to follow 62,000 women with implants and 124,000 women without them for an average of 10 years each. In the meantime, the makers of these prostheses, as noted, have decided to settle out of court. To find out why, first read the accompanying editorial (5), which reminds us, among other things, that one of the major ironies in the court system is that the testimony of nonexpert witnesses is held to a more factual standard than that of the experts hired by one side or the other. Then consider that occasionally there *is* evidence of a causal relationship, as when longtime symptoms and signs rapidly resolve when an implant is removed (7).—S.E. Malawista, M.D.

References

1. 1994 YEAR BOOK OF MEDICINE, p 818.
2. Giltay EJ, Moens HJB, Riley AH, Tan RG: Silicone breast prostheses and rheumatic symptoms: A retrospective follow up study. *Ann Rheum Dis* 53:194–196, 1994.
3. Cook RR, Harrison MC, LeVier RR: The breast implant controversy. *Arthritis Rheum* 37:153–157, 1994.
4. Sánchez-Guerrero J, Schur PH, Sergent JS, Liang MH: Silicone breast implants and rheumatic disease: Clinical, immunologic, and epidemiologic studies. *Arthritis Rheum* 37:158–168, 1994.
5. Angell M: Do breast implants cause systemic disease? Science in the courtroom. *N Engl J Med* 330:1748–1749, 1994.
6. Hochberg MC: Silicone breast implants and rheumatic disease. *Br J Rheumatol* 33:601–604, 1994.
7. Ryan EH, Moore WJ: Silicone breast implants and atypical autoimmune disease. *Ann Int Med* 119:1053–1054, 1993.

A Controlled Trial of High-Dose Intravenous Immune Gloubulin Infusions as Treatment for Dermatomyositis
Dalakas MC, Illa I, Dambrosia JM, Soueidan SA, Stein DP, Otero C, Dinsmore ST, McCrosky S (Natl Inst of Health, Bethesda, Md)
N Engl J Med 329:1993–2000, 1993   119-95-75-2

Introduction.—Dermatomyositis is clinically distinct from other inflammatory myopathies because of the rash it causes. The condition can

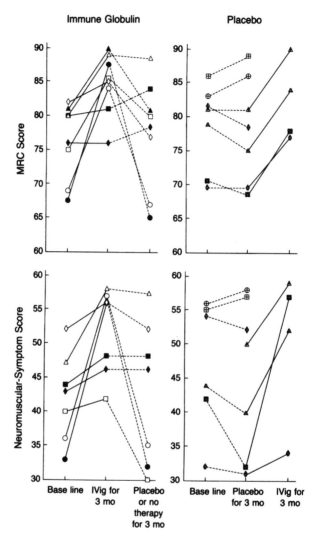

Fig 75-1.—Effect of intravenous immuno globulin (IVig) in a placebo-controlled crossover study of 15 patients with dermatomyositis. *Solid lines,* treatment with IVig; *dashed lines,* no treatment, or administration of placebo. The neuromuscular symptom scores were not available for one patient in each group. (Courtesy of Dalakas MC, Illa I, Dambrosia JM, et al: N Engl J Med 329:1993-2000, 1993.)

become resistant to therapy and lead to serious physical disabilities. In seeking a more effective and safe immunotherapy, researchers conducted a controlled study of high-dose intravenous immunoglobulin. This agent has been beneficial in the treatment of other neuromuscular diseases and in 3 small pilot studies in patients with dermatomyositis.

Patients and Methods.—Fifteen patients with a mean age of 36 years took part in the study. All had active disease that was unresponsive or

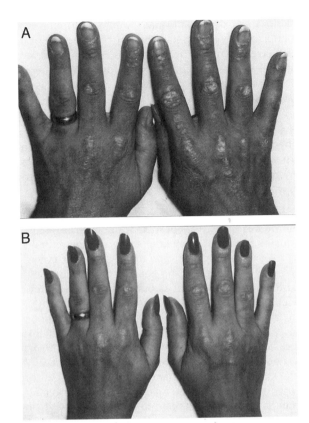

Fig 75–2.—Hands of a patient with dermatomyositis before (**A**) and after (**B**) treatment with intravenous immunoglobulin. The shiny, scaly, chronic rash, characteristically affecting the knuckles but not the phalanges, is markedly improved after therapy, for the first time in 10 years. (Courtesy of Dalakas MC, Illa I, Dambrosia JM, et al: *N Engl J Med* 329:1993–2000, 1993.)

poorly responsive to high-dose prednisone or another immunosuppressant. The patients experienced progressive muscle weakness and were impaired in their performance of the activities of daily living. In the double-blind study, 8 patients were randomly assigned to receive immunoglobulin and 7 to placebo. Muscle biopsies were performed before and after the treatment protocol. Responses were measured by using various muscle strength scales and through photographs of the rash.

Results.—The treatment and placebo groups were similar in duration of disease, neuromuscular symptoms, immunosuppressive therapy, and serum creatine kinase level. The group that received immunoglobulin had a significant improvement in muscle strength and neuromuscular symptoms after 3 months of therapy (Fig 75–1). Patients with severe muscle weakness who had required wheelchairs were able to run and climb stairs. In contrast, placebo patients showed no change overall, and the condition of 3 worsened. A crossover study confirmed these results.

Patients deteriorated after replacing immune globulin with placebo, whereas patients initially taking placebo experienced major improvement with the active treatment. Repeated biopsies in 5 responding patients showed a number of positive changes, including an increase in muscle-fiber diameter and an increase in the number and a decrease in the diameter of capillaries.

Conclusion.—A 3-month course of immune globulin therapy brought about marked improvement in patients with refractory dermatomyositis. Muscle strength increased, the rash cleared (Fig 75–2), and histologic and immunopathologic findings of repeated muscle biopsies resolved or showed marked improvement. Repeated treatments, approximately every 6 weeks, were needed for long-term benefit.

▶ The results of this small, well-designed, double-blind placebo-controlled trial of high-dose intravenous immunoglobulin infusion as treatment for dermatomyositis are exciting: it works, and the treatment is, in the short run, benign, unlike any other steroid-sparing agent at our disposal. *How* it works is not clear, but the current theories, as outlined by the authors, are (1) blockade of Fc receptors on the vascular wall, competing successfully for the site of attachment of immune complexes; (2) inhibition by immunoglobulin of the effector functions of activated T cells and the released cytokines and lymphokines, or its competition with MHC molecules; and/or (3) neutralization of complement neoantigens and the inhibition of formation of the membranolytic attack complex from the activated C4b and C3b fragments. How long it will work is also to be determined, although following the initial 3-month treatments, some patients seem to be doing well with additional treatments every 6 weeks. We will look forward to longer follow-up, as well as to similar studies of polymyositis and inclusion myositis. (For a recent review of therapeutic modalities in inflammatory myopathy, see Reference 1)—S.E. Malawista, M.D.

Reference

1. Oddis CV: Therapy for myositis. *Curr Opin Rheumatol* 5:742–748, 1993.

Special Reference

Morrison NA, Qui JC, Tokita A, et al: Prediction of bone density from vitamin D receptor alleles. *Nature* 367:284–287, 1994.
   ▶ See Abstract 119-95-56-1 and Dr. Utiger's discussion of this interesting paper.
   It is of special interest that if a large genetic component of bone density is predictable (estimated at 75%), then the smaller but significant nongenetic component can be addressed early, when intervention is likely to do the most good. Measures such as appropriate calcium intake, increased exercise with weights, avoidance of cigarettes and alcohol, increased vitamin D intake, and estrogen replacement after menopause become especially important for high-

risk individuals, who may thereby maximize the bone density achieved during growth, and minimize bone loss later.—S.E. Malawista, M.D.

Calcific Tendinitis in the Proximal Thigh
Hodge JC, Schneider R, Freiberger RH, Magid SK (Cornell Univ, NY)
Arthritis Rheum 36:1476–1482, 1993   119-95-75–3

Background.—Calcific tendinitis, occurring commonly in the shoulder, is uncommon in other sites. It has been reported in the tendons of the deltoid, pectoralis major, piriformis, rectus femoris muscles and, in the thigh area, in the gluteus maximus and vastus lateralis muscles. Dramatic clinical improvement can result from percutaneous steroid injection. Computed tomography guidance is recommended for precise localization of calcifications to avoid the sciatic nerve.

Methods and Findings.—Five patients, aged 31 to 57 years, with calcific tendinitis of the proximal thigh were assessed. Calcification was detected on anteroposterior radiographs in 3 patients and on "frog" lateral radiographs in all 5. The patient who underwent whole-body bone scanning had increased radiotracer activity in the thigh. Only the delayed phase showed an abnormal radiotracer activity focus in the 2 patients who underwent 3-phase bone scintigraphy. In both cases, soft tissue calcifications in the posterolateral thigh were seen on CT scans. The findings of the 2 MR assessments were positive: in 1, there was an area of signal void; in the other, there was an area of soft tissue edema in the posterolateral thigh. In 2 patients, percutaneous CT-guided steroid injection completely alleviated pain in 1–2 weeks.

Case Report.—Man, 57, sought medical attention for progressive posterolateral hip pain. He reported having intermittent pain in the right greater trochanter for 1 year. At physical assessment, he had a full range of active and passive motion with no focal tenderness. He was hospitalized and was found to have a mildly increased WBC count and a normal erythrocyte sedimentation rate. A "frog" lateral radiographic view showed calcifications in the posterolateral area and smooth erosion of the adjacent femoral cortex. Soft tissue calcifications and saucer-shaped erosion of the femoral cortex were confirmed with CT.

Conclusion.—Calcific tendinitis of the proximal thigh, a benign entity that can cause significant pain, must be distinguished from chronic or malignant diseases such as arthritis, infection, and soft tissue or cortical neoplasms. It may be self-limited, but medical intervention may help in some cases. Percutaneous steroid injection with CT guidance is recommended for these patients.

▶ This modest account of 5 patients with calcific tendinitis of the proximal thigh, a sometimes self-limited but, in any case, treatable problem, is worth emphasizing because of the unknown numbers of individuals with ill-defined thigh pain due to it, in whom the anteroposterior film, if done, was negative (as in 2 of 5 patients in this study), and who assume they "just have to live with it." In patients presenting with thigh pain, additional rheumatologic considerations include lumbar spine disease with radiculopathy; arthritis of the hip with distal radiation of pain or of the knee with proximal radiation; soft tissue lesions of skin, muscle, and supporting structures (e.g., trochanteric bursitis); and bony lesions of the femur. The fastest route to the current diagnosis is plain radiographs that include a "frog" lateral view (patient supine, hip and knee flexed, thigh abducted 40 degrees, and a central x-ray beam perpendicular to the table), as the calcium is often behind the femur. If negative, employ radionuclide imaging; one of these two modalities is very likely to provide the diagnosis. If plain films are negative but radionuclide imaging shows increased activity, define the lesion with a CT scan. Computed tomography guidance for corticosteroid injection allows precise targeting—one of the current patients required 3 "blind" injections before relief followed—and will help avoid the sciatic nerve.—S.E. Malawista, M.D.

Fat Necrosis: An Unusual Cause of Polyarthritis

Watts RA, Kelly S, Hacking JC, Lomas D, Hazleman BL (Addenbrooke's Hosp, Cambridge, UK)
J Rheumatol 20:1432–1435, 1993   119-95-75-4

Introduction.—Metastatic fat necrosis, a type of panniculitis, is found in up to 3% of patients with pancreatic disease and may be associated with synovitis and intramedullary bone necrosis. Panniculitis and synovitis sometimes occur before an attack of acute pancreatitis, making the diagnosis difficult.

Case Report.—Woman, 47, had noted painful, swollen ankles as well as reddened lumps over both shins for a week, and her right little finger also had become swollen. She had lost 10 kg in the past 2 months but generally felt well. Celiac disease had been diagnosed 20 years before, and there had been sporadic episodes of abdominal pain in the interim. Mild pancreatitis had been diagnosed 3 months before admission. The patient acknowledged taking 4 units of alcohol a day. She appeared ill and had a temperature of 38.4° C. Violaceous lumps were over the shins, right hip, and right shoulder, and there was an extensive rash resembling livedo reticularis. The sedimentation rate was 80 mm/hour, and the serum amylase level was 3,605 U/L. A skin biopsy revealed foamy macrophages and fat necrosis. The skin and joint changes resolved in a few days but subsequently, the joints became more painful and new skin lesions developed, along with abdominal pain and tenderness. The skin and joint lesions settled in the next 3 weeks. Radiography then showed multiple lucencies in both distal tibias (Fig 75–3), and MRI indicated fat necrosis at this site, as well as soft tissue abnormalities (Figs 75–4). Intra-abdominal pancreas-related collections twice were drained percutaneously. Bone texture was improved 5 months after admission,

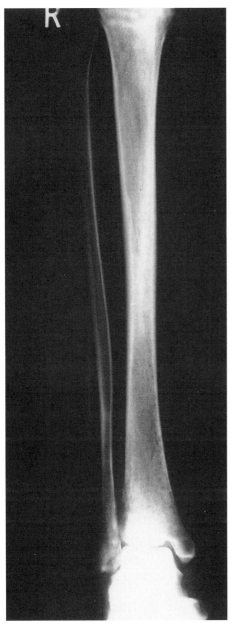

Fig 75–3.—Radiographic view of the right ankle one month after admission. Multiple medullary lucent areas with destruction of the medial tibial cortex are evident. (Courtesy of Watts RA, Kelly S, Hacking JC, et al: *J Rheumatol* 20:1432–1435, 1993.)

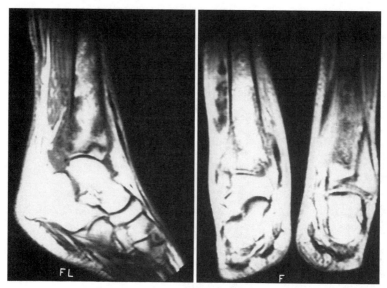

Fig 75–4.—Sagittal T1-weighted (**left**) and coronal proton-density-weighted (**right**) MR images of the ankle show multiple low-signal-intensity areas within the dital tibia and expanding the posterior cortex. Further abnormal areas lateral to the tibia are evident, indicating regions of fat necrosis in adjacent soft tissues. (Courtesy of Watts RA, Kelly S, Hacking JC, et al: *J Rheumatol* 20:1432–1435, 1993.)

and a year later, the patient was asymptomatic and had normal serum amylase level.

Discussion.—These patients typically have tender erythematous nodules that resolve without scarring in days or weeks. The polyarthritis may or may not be symmetrical. This patient had skin and joint lesions before any clinical indication of pancreatic disease. The pancreatitis resolved several weeks after the skin and joint abnormalities.

▶ When an alcoholic man presents with panniculitis, think of pancreatitis and obtain a serum amylase and biliary/pancreatic ultrasound whether or not he has abdominal pain (he frequently will not). This association is said to occur in 2% to 3% of patients with pancreatic disease. Polyarthritis is an add-on, with the triad of panniculitis with fat necrosis, polyarthritis, and pancreatic disease occurring in less than 1% of patients with acute pancreatitis or pancreatic carcinoma. (Even more rare is polyarthritis without fat necrosis elsewhere [1]).

The subcutaneous lesions tend to be more widely distributed than those of erythema nodosum, and other lesions in the differential diagnosis include lupus profundus, polyarteritis nodosa, Weber-Christian disease, and cytophagic panniculitis. Aspiration may yield liquified fat. X-rays characteristically show multiple small lucencies in the cortical regions of long bones (Fig 75–3). Magnetic resonance images are not usually necessary; I present one here only for its interest (Figs 75–4).—S.E. Malawista, M.D.

Reference

1. Ferrari R, Wendelboe M, Ford PM, Corbett WEN, Anastassiades TP: Pancreatitis arthritis with periarticular fat necrosis. *J Rheumatol* 20:1436–1437, 1993.

Benefits and Disadvantages of Joint Hypermobility Among Musicians

Larsson L-G, Baum J, Mudholkar GS, Kollia GD (Univ of Rochester, NY; Hospital for Rheumatic Diseases, Östersund, Sweden)
N Engl J Med 329:1079–1082, 1993   119-95-75-5

Introduction.—Hypermobile joints are considered helpful to ballet dancers but harmful to young athletes. Musicians may have to make fine repetitive motions involving little force, as when playing the flute or violin, or may use large muscles and considerable force, as when playing percussion instruments.

Study Design.—A 53-item questionnaire was used to gain information on work-related symptoms from 300 female and 360 male musicians. The subjects also were examined for joint hypermobility, as evidenced by passive hyperextension of the wrists to where they paralleled the forearm; passive opposition of the thumbs to where they touched the forearm (Fig 75–5); elbow and knee hyperextension of 10 degrees or more;

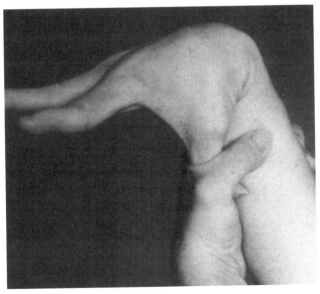

Fig 75–5.—Joint hypermobility indicated by flexion of the wrist with hyperextension of the thumb. (Courtesy of Larsson L-G, Baum J, Mudholkar GS, et al: *N Engl J Med* 329:1079–1082, 1993.)

and flexion of the trunk in the standing position so that the palms rested on the floor.

Findings.—Three fourths of the musicians had symptoms such as pain, weakness, and fatigue in their extremities on a daily basis in connection with practicing (Table 1). Those with hypermobility of specific joints were most likely to have definite symptoms. Only 5% of those with hypermobile wrists and fingers reported musculoskeletal symptoms, however, compared with 18% of those lacking hypermobile fingers. A lack of hypermobility also correlated with symptoms at the elbow, knee, and back. Hypermobility of the wrist and thumb was most prevalent in flutists, followed by violinists, cellists, and those playing wind instruments. It was least frequent in those playing the trumpet or mallet instruments. Only 2 of 19 symptomatic flutists had a hypermobile wrist and

TABLE 1.—Work-Related Joint Symptoms and
Hypermobility Among 660 Musicians, According to Joint

Joint	Hypermobility	No Hypermobility	P Value*
	no. (%) of subjects		
Wrist and fingers			
Symptoms	5 (5)	100 (18)	0.001
No symptoms	91 (95)	464 (82)	
Total	96	564	
Thumb			
Symptoms	13 (6)	38 (9)	0.28
No symptoms	207 (94)	402 (91)	
Total	220	440	
Elbow			
Elbow only			
Symptoms	1 (<1)	7 (2)	0.45
No symptoms	207 (99)	445 (98)	
Total	208	452	
Forearm			
Symptoms	16 (8)	19 (4)	0.09
No symptoms	192 (92)	433 (96)	
Total	208	452	
Knees			
Symptoms	6 (5)	1 (<1)	<0.001
No symptoms	129 (95)	527 (99)	
Total	132	528	
Spine			
Symptoms	46 (23)	50 (11)	<0.001
No symptoms	152 (77)	412 (89)	
Total	198	462	

* By Fisher's exact test for comparisons between the frequency of symptoms in subjects with hypermobility and the frequency in subjects with no hypermobility.
(Courtesy of Larsson L-G, Baum J, Mudholkar GS, et al: *N Engl J Med* 329:1079–1082, 1993.)

TABLE 2.—Activity-Related Symptoms and Hypermobility of
the Wrist and Thumb Among Flutists and Players of
Mallet Instruments

INSTRUMENT	HYPER- MOBILITY	NO HYPER- MOBILITY	TOTAL	P VALUE*
	no. (%) of subjects			
Flute				
Symptoms	2 (18)	17 (81)	19	0.002
No symptoms	9 (82)	4 (19)	13	
Total	11	21	32	
Mallet instruments				
Symptoms	7 (100)	5 (29)	12	0.005
No symptoms	0	12 (71)	12	
Total	7	17	24	

* By Fisher's exact test for comparisons between the frequency of symptoms in
subjects with hypermobility and the frequency in subjects with no hypermobility.
(Courtesy of Larsson L-G, Baum J, Mudholkar GS, et al: N Engl J Med
329:1079–1082, 1993.)

thumb (Table 2), compared to 9 of 13 who lacked symptoms. All mallet instrument players with hypermobility of these joints were symptomatic.

Interpretation.—Joint hypermobility may be an asset for musicians whose playing involves repetitive motion. The musculoskeletal symptoms associated with practice and performance may reflect either a lack of hypermobility of joints contributing to such motion or hypermobility of joints such as the knees and spine, which are associated with support function.

▶ This was fertile ground for such a project; the 660 subjects, constituting 85% of the students and 69% of the staff members of the Eastman School of Music, usually practiced their instruments 4 to 5 hours daily; 77% of them had daily symptoms such as pain, weakness, and fatigue in their extremities. The authors (see also an accompanying editorial [1]) point out that most previous studies of the medical problems of musicians have focused on the location of various symptoms, according to the instruments played, but have ignored the possible role of joint hypermobility (Fig 75–5). The current results suggest that the musculoskeletal symptoms associated with practice and performance may be due to a *lack* of hypermobility of some joints involved in intensive repetitive motion (e.g., the wrist and fingers), or to the *presence* of hypermobility of joints not involved in repetitive motion but associated with support function (e.g., the spine). Viewed in this light, joint hypermobility (or laxity), defined as a range of motion in excess of normal, is clearly an asset in the hands of a flutist, violinist, or pianist, both for facility of performance and for fewer related symptoms, but it may be a liability in his or her back. However, note the inverse relationship of hypermobility of the wrist and thumb, vs. symptoms in flutists compared to players of mallet instruments. These studies have obvious implications for the workplace in general.—S.E. Malawista, M.D.

Reference

1. Grahame R: Joint hypermobility and the performing musician. N *Engl J Med* 329:1120–1121, 1993.

Drug Index

A

Acarbose
  in diabetes, type 2, 94: 640
Acetylcholine
  in angina with normal coronary
    angiograms, coronary artery
    response to, 94: 356
N-Acetylcysteine
  in angina, and development of tolerance
    to isosorbide, 93: 334
ACTH
  therapy in acute crystal-induced
    synovitis, 95: 809
Acyclovir
  in chickenpox
    adult, 94: 878
    in children, 95: 33
  in herpes zoster, acute, 95: 33
  in HIV-infected patient, interaction with
    zidovudine, effect on progression
    to AIDS and survival, 95: 52
  in pharyngitis, herpetic, 94: 836
Adenosine
  echocardiography, stress, vs.
    dipyridamole and dobutamine,
    93: 397
  thallium imaging vs. exercise imaging,
    93: 395
    in left bundle branch block, 94: 423
  triphosphate in cystic fibrosis, 93: 111
Adrenocorticosteroids (see
    Corticosteroids)
Adrenocorticotropin
  hormone therapy in acute
    crystal-induced synovitis, 95: 809
Adriamycin (see Doxorubicin)
Albuterol
  in asthma, 93: 89
  in COPD, 95: 106
Alcohol
  injection in autonomous thyroid
    adenomas, 94: 590
Alkylating agents
  in macroglobulinemia, 94: 262
Allopurinol
  sensitivity in chronic tophaceous gout,
    93: 714
Alpha-1 antitrypsin
  aerosol, in cystic fibrosis, 93: 112
Alteplase
  (See also Plasminogen, activator, tissue)
  in pulmonary embolism, 94: 125
Altretamine
  in ovarian cancer, advanced epithelial,
    94: 294
Aluminum

hydroxide, and levothyroxine
    absorption, 93: 544
Amikacin
  in Mycobacterium avium-intracellulare
    bacteremia in AIDS, 93: 9
  in Mycobacterium haemophilum
    infection, 95: 28
  once-vs. -twice daily, 94: 876
Amiloride
  in hypertension, in elderly, 93: 627
Aminoglycosides
  in bacteremia, Enterobacter, 93: 34
  in cystic fibrosis, 94: 54
  in endophthalmitis due to
    coagulase-negative staphylococci,
    94: 896
  once-daily, 94: 877
  in pneumonia, nosocomial, in ventilated
    patients, 94: 203
5-Aminosalicylic acid
  in Crohn's disease as maintenance
    therapy, 93: 433
Amiodarone
  in heart failure, severe congestive,
    95: 438
  in tachycardia, ventricular, 94: 432
Amitriptyline
  in neuropathy, painful diabetic, 93: 581
Amoxicillin
  in Helicobacter pylori eradication
    metronidazole/ranitidine combined
      with, 94: 455
    metronidazole/tripotassium dicitrate
      bismuthate combined with, 95: 492
    omeprazole combined with, 95: 491
    omeprazole/metronidazole combined
      with, 95: 491
  in Lyme disease
    for arthritis, 95: 820; 94: xxii, xxx
    for Bell's palsy, 94: xxviii
    for carditis, 94: xxii, xxvii
    early, 94: xxii, xxiv, xxv
    during pregnancy, 94: xxii
    probenecid combined with, 93: 726
    prophylactic, 94: 807
  in pharyngitis, streptococcal, 94: 873
  prophylactic, after tick bites, 94: xxxii
Amphotericin B
  bladder irrigation for fungal urinary tract
    infection, 95: 12
  in digestive decontamination, selective,
    in mechanically ventilated patients,
    95: 153
  percutaneous instillation for hemoptysis
    in cavitary aspergilloma, 95: 150
  prophylaxis
    for fungal infection in patients at risk
      of neutropenia, 94: 890

Antiviral agents
    effect on hepatitis C virus antigen,
        94: 513
APSAC (*see* Anistreplase)
Ara-C
    in leukemia, acute lymphoblastic
        adult, 93: 237
        childhood, 95: 295
Asacol
    in Crohn's disease, as maintenance
        therapy, 93: 433
Ascorbic acid
    supplementation in
        hypercholesterolemia, 95: 362-363
Asparaginase
    in leukemia, acute lymphoblastic
        adult, 93: 236
        childhood, 95: 295
Aspirin
    in angina, unstable, 95: 379; 93: 324
    colon cancer risk and, fatal, 95: 523
    colorectal adenoma risk and, 95: 522
    colorectal cancer risk and, 95: 522
    after coronary artery disease instability
        episode, 93: 325
    in gastrointestinal bleeding, ulcer and
        nonulcer, 93: 415
    /hirudin combined with thrombolysis
        (in dog), 94: 327
    in Lyme carditis, 94: xxvi
    in myocardial infarction
        non-Q-wave, 95: 379
        suspected, 93: 310
    for thromboembolism prevention in
        atrial fibrillation, 95: 454
Atenolol
    in hypertension, in elderly, 93: 627
    in nephropathy, diabetic, 95: 676
Atrial
    natriuretic peptide treatment of acute
        renal failure, 95: 709
Auranofin
    in rheumatoid arthritis, 93: 686
Azapropazone
    peptic ulcer bleeding and, 95: 500
Azathioprine
    in Crohn's disease, 94: 475
    in heart transplantation, non-Hodgkin's
        lymphoma after, 95: 738
    in kidney transplantation
        in blacks, 93: 660
        lymphoma after, non-Hodgkin's,
            95: 738
    in rheumatoid arthritis
        combined with methotrexate, 93: 685
        vs. methotrexate, 93: 685
    in Takayasu's arteritis, 95: 817

Azidothymidine (*see* Zidovudine)
Azithromycin
    in cervicitis, chlamydial, 94: 869
    in Lyme disease, early, 94: xxii, xxiv,
        xxv; 93: 726
    in pneumonia, community-acquired,
        95: 147, 149
    in urethritis, chlamydial, 94: 869
AZT (*see* Zidovudine)
Aztreonam
    in diarrhea
        bacterial, 93: 439
        travelers', 93: 59

B

Bacillus Calmette-Guérin vaccine (*see*
        Vaccine, BCG)
BCG (*see* Vaccine, BCG)
BCNU
    in myelomatosis, 93: 256
Beclomethasone
    in asthma
        in children, effect on short term
            growth, 95: 86
        cough variant, 94: 21
        effect on bone mineral content, in
            children, 95: 84
    bronchitis, chronic, 93: 107
Beta-agonist
    in asthma, risk of death and near death
        and, 93: 87
    inhaled, response, in distinguishing
        between asthma and COPD,
        95: 103
Beta-blockers
    in angina, chronic stable, 93: 333
    in cardiomyopathy, dilated, 95: 436
    effect on aortic dilatation progression,
        95: 467
    effect on triglycerides and cholesterol,
        94: 315
    in heart failure, 95: 437
    for heart rate variability, low, 94: 431
    in hypertension
        in elderly, 93: 627
        pulmonary, primary, 94: 134
        withdrawal of, in elderly, 95: 733
    levothyroxine and quality of life,
        95: 613
    in myocardial infarction, 94: 350
Beta-carotene
    supplementation in
        hypercholesterolemia, 95: 362-363
Beta-lactams
    dosing regimens, 94: 877
    in *Enterobacter* bacteremia, 93: 34

in *Helicobacter pylori* eradication,
94: 457; 93: 40
amoxicillin combined with, effect on
duodenal ulcer recurrence, 94: 455
amoxicillin/omeprazole combined
with, 95: 491
amoxicillin/tripotassium dicitrate
combined with, 95: 492
bismuth/tetracycline combined with,
95: 491, 492
regression of gastric lymphoma after,
primary low-grade B-cell, 94: 461
Mexiletine
in arrhythmias, 94: 437
Midazolam
for sedation of critically ill, 94: 192
Minocycline
in rheumatoid arthritis, experimental,
95: 773
Misoprostol
gynecomastia and, 95: 639
in ulcer prevention, NSAID-induced
gastric and duodenal, 94: 465
Mitomycin
in esophageal cancer, 93: 411
in lung cancer, non-small cell, 95: 128
Mitoxantrone
in leukemia, acute myelogenous,
94: 251
MK-886
effect on allergen-induced airway
responses, 94: 14
Monoclonal antibody(ies)
anti-tumor necrosis factor, effect on
cytokine levels in sepsis, 94: 159
anti-Vβ, in skin and cardiac
transplantation (in mice), 94: 726
IgM, in therapy for septic shock, 93: 50
marrow purging with, and autologous
marrow transplant in acute
lymphocytic leukemia, 94: 280
therapy
in rheumatoid arthritis, 94: 751
in septic shock, 93: 50
Mono-Embolex NM
in heparin-induced thrombocytopenia
syndrome, 95: 284
Morcizine
after myocardial infarction, 93: 388
Morphine
patient-controlled, for sickle cell-related
pain, 94: 243
Mupirocin
ointment, intranasal
for elimination of *Staphylococcus
aureus* nasal carriage in health care
workers, 95: 35

-resistant *Staphylococcus aureus*
outbreak on dermatology ward
associated with environmental
reservoir, 95: 45
in staphylococcal infection, familial,
94: 877
Mustine
in Hodgkin's disease, side effects of,
94: 249

N

Nadolol
effect on morning increase in
ambulatory ischemia, 95: 398
Nalbuphine
patient-controlled, for sickle cell-related
pain, 94: 243
Naproxen
peptic ulcer bleeding and, 95: 500
Narcotics
intravenous, in sickle cell vaso-occlusive
pain crisis in adults, 94: 242
Naseptin
in staphylococcal infection, familial,
94: 877
Neomycin
in staphylococcal infection, familial,
94: 877
Nevirapine
-resistant HIV, in vitro development of,
95: 55
Niacin
immediate-release, effect on
high-density lipoprotein cholesterol
levels, 95: 362
Nicardipine
in coronary artery disease prevention
after heart transplantation, 94: 413
Nicorette, 93: 99
Nicotine
inhaler for smoking cessation, 94: 29,
30
nasal spray for smoking cessation,
94: 31
patch, 93: 99
predicting who will quit with, 95: 95
Nifedipine
in aortic regurgitation, 94: 387
in coronary artery disease prevention
after heart transplantation, 94: 413
GITS, effect on circadian patterns of
myocardial ischemia in chronic
stable angina patients, 93: 333
in hypertension
effect on cardiac hypertrophy,
95: 469

in digestive decontamination, selective,
in mechanically ventilated patients,
95: 153
topical, for digestive tract
decontamination in ICU, 93: 26
Toxin
interleukin-2 fusion, in experimental
rheumatoid arthritis, 95: 773
Tretinoin (*see* Retinoic acid, all-*trans*)
Triamcinolone
in gouty arthritis, acute, 94: 797
Triamterene
in hypertension and risk of primary
cardiac arrest, 95: 759
Tridione
anemia and, aplastic, 95: 273
Trimethoprim
acidosis due to, renal tubular, 94: 735
-induced hyperkalemia in AIDS, 94: 734
-sulfamethoxazole
in diarrhea, travelers', 93: 60
in pneumococcal disease during HIV
infection, 93: 9
in *Pneumocystis carinii* pneumonia in
connective tissue disease, 95: 827
prophylaxis for *Pneumocystis carinii*
pneumonia in AIDS, effect on
toxoplasmic encephalitis in AIDS,
95: 59
prophylaxis for *Pneumocystis carinii*
pneumonia in AIDS, primary,
94: 859
prophylaxis for *Pneumocystis carinii*
pneumonia in AIDS, secondary,
94: 861
-resistant pneumococcal infections, in
U.S., 95: 43
-resistant *Streptococcus pneumoniae*
in day care center, 94: 847
in *Salmonella* enteritis, 95: 39
in Wegener's granulomatosis, 93: 718
Tripotassium
dicitratobismuthate in *Helicobacter
pylori* eradication, 94: 457
amoxicillin/metronidazole combined
with, 95: 492
regression of primary low-grade B-cell
gastric lymphoma after, 94: 461
Trisodium phosphonoformate
in cytomegalovirus retinitis in AIDS,
93: 6
Tumor
necrosis factor, monoclonal antibody to,
effect on cytokine levels in sepsis,
94: 159

U

Urecholine
effect on delayed gastric emptying,
94: 467
Uridine
triphosphate in cystic fibrosis, 93: 111
Urokinase
in angina, unstable, 93: 323
in myocardial infarction,
thrombocytopenia after, 95: 388
Ursodeoxycholic acid
in cholangitis, primary sclerosing,
93: 493
Ursodiol
in cirrhosis, primary biliary, 95: 556

V

Vaccine
BCG
BCG infection after, in HIV-infected
children, 95: 22
with immunotherapy in colorectal
cancer, 94: 295
in normal healthy adults, 95: 20
tuberculin testing after, in children,
95: 21
hepatitis A, formalin-inactivated, in
children, 93: 451
hepatitis B, response of persons positive
for antibody to hepatitis B core
antigen, 93: 454
influenza
serologic tests for HIV, HTLV-1 and
hepatitis C after, false-positive,
93: 148
target-based model for increasing
usage in private practice, 93: 56
pneumococcal
in HIV infection, 93: 9
protective efficacy of, 93: 53
varicella, routine program for U.S.
children, cost-effectiveness of,
95: 32
Vancomycin
in *Clostridium difficile* carriers,
asymptomatic, 93: 349
in endophthalmitis due to
coagulase-negative staphylococci,
94: 896
in *Enterococcus faecalis*,
gentamicin-resistant, 93: 29
in meningitis, resistant pneumococcal,
94: 848
in pneumococcal infections, 95: 45

asymptomatic, duration of benefits,
95: 50
didanosine combined with,
alternating or simultaneous, 95: 53
effect on small intestinal mucosa,
93: 443
interaction with acyclovir, effect on
progression to AIDS and survival,
95: 52

vs. didanosine, 94: 855
prophylaxis after occupational HIV
exposure and subsequent HIV
seroconversion, 94: 857
-resistant HIV, in vitro development of,
95: 55
-resistant HIV-1 infection, 94: 856

Subject Index*

This cumulative index gives the volume (year) and page locations of subjects included in the five most recent annual editions of the YEAR BOOK. It will accumulate with each subsequent edition by deletion of the earliest year's references. The volumes (years) appear in *italic* type, preceding the page numbers and separated from them by a colon.

A

Abdomen
  pain (*see* Pain, abdominal)
  radiotherapy causing chronic
    pancreatitis, *94:* 543
  surgery, major, heparin prophylaxis for
    venous thromboembolism in,
    94: 123
  trauma combined with thoracic trauma
    as risk factor for early onset
    pneumonia, *95:* 198
  ultrasound, conventional, *vs.*
    hydrocolonic, for colon tumor
    diagnosis and staging, *93:* 447
Abortion
  spontaneous, in dialysis patients,
    95: 574
Abscess
  draining, and nosocomial transmission
    of tuberculosis, *91:* 17
  endocarditis-associated, transesophageal
    echocardiography in diagnosis,
    92: 66
  epidural, of cervical spine, MRI of,
    93: 70
Abuse
  alcohol (*see* Alcohol, abuse)
  drug (*see* Drug, abuse)
  substance (*see* Substance, abuse)
ABVD
  in Hodgkin's disease, advanced, *94:* 247
Acanthocyturia
  as marker for glomerular bleeding,
    92: 547
Acarbose
  in diabetes, type 2, *94:* 640
Acetaminophen
  in osteoarthritis of knee, *92:* 665
Acetylcholine
  in angina with normal coronary
    angiograms, coronary artery
    response to, *94:* 356
  coronary vasomotor response to, related
    to risk factors for coronary artery
    disease, *91:* 336
N-Acetylcysteine
  in angina, and development of tolerance
    to isosorbide, *93:* 334
Acid
  -base, *95:* 757-764; *94:* 731-740
    disorders in alcoholism, *95:* 761

equilibrium, renal regulation of, effect
  of sustained hyperventilation on,
  92: 601
-fast smears, sputum, in diagnosis of
  tuberculosis in AIDS patients,
  93: xxvii-xxviii
reflux in reflux esophagitis, effects of
  ranitidine/cisapride on, *94:* 451
secretion
  Helicobacter pylori and, *95:* xix-xx
  sensitivity to gastrin in duodenal ulcer
    after eradication of *Helicobacter
    pylori* and, *94:* 457
Acidosis
  alcoholic, *95:* 762
  lactic
    dichloroacetate in, *94:* 735
    osmolal gap increase in, *92:* 605
  metabolic
    effect on 1,25 $(OH)_2D$ in
      phosphorus-restricted patients,
      94: 737
    effect on growth hormone secretion
      (in rat), *94:* 739
  renal tubular
    hepatitis with, chronic active,
      presenting as hypokalemic periodic
      paralysis with respiratory failure,
      94: 739
    nephrolithiasis with, first morning
      urine pH in diagnosis of, *95:* 763
    trimethoprim causing, *94:* 735
Acinetobacter
  pneumonia in ventilated patients, and
    mortality and hospital stay, *94:* 205
Acne
  conglobata and spondyloarthropathy,
    94: 781
Acquired immunodeficiency syndrome (*see*
  AIDS)
Acrodermatitis chronic atrophicans
  Borrelia burgdorferi and, *95:* 819
Acromegaly
  bromocriptine in, long-term, *93:* 506
  in empty sella syndrome, *94:* 554
  octreotide in (*see* Octreotide, in
    acromegaly)
ACTH
  (*See also* Corticotropin)
  (4-9) analogue for prevention of
    cisplatin neurotoxicity in ovarian
    cancer, *91:* 295

Anaplastic
  large cell lymphoma, Ki-1, clinical
    features, *92:* 226
Ancylostoma caninum
  infection, occult enteric, *95:* 508
Androgenic
  alopecia and polycystic ovaries, *95:* 629
  steroids, use by body builders, *91:* 552
Androstenedione
  serum, in women with polycystic
    ovaries, *95:* 629
Anemia
  anagrelide causing, *93:* 222
  aplastic
    colony-stimulating factor in,
      granulocyte-macrophage, *92:* 199
    gamma-interferon gene expression in
      bone marrow in, *95:* 273
    graft-*vs.*-host disease and,
      transfusion-associated, *94:* 236
    hepatitis and, viral, *93:* 224
    interleukin-3 in, *92:* 200
    pesticides and, *95:* 271
    treatment, malignant tumors after,
      95: 269
  of cancer, decreased erythropoietin
    response in, *91:* 228
  in erlichiosis, *95:* 69, 72
  in hemodialysis patients, EPO in
    effect on brain and cognitive function,
      92: 593
    long-term, effect on cardiac output
      and left ventricular size, *92:* 598
  hemolytic, warm-type autoimmune, red
    cell transfusion in, *94:* 234
  of multiple myeloma, erythropoietin for,
    91: 227
  in nephropathy, late-onset bone marrow
    transplantation, *95:* 704
  refractory, prognostic factors and
    proposals for improved scoring
    system, *93:* 238
  of renal disease, end-stage,
    erythropoietin therapy in, cost
    implications to Medicare, *95:* 274
  of renal failure, chronic, erythropoietin
    in, *93:* 637; *92:* 197
  in rheumatoid arthritis, erythropoietin
    for, *92:* 168, 625
  sideroblastic, pure, prognostic factors
    and proposals for improved scoring
    system, *93:* 238
Anergic
  HIV-infected patients, risk of
    tuberculosis development among,
    95: 19
Aneurysm

  of hemodialysis arteriovenous fistula,
    color Doppler ultrasound of,
    93: 648
  intracranial, in polycystic kidney disease,
    93: 605
Angina
  N-acetylcysteine in, and development of
    tolerance to isosorbide, *93:* 334
  coronary bypass for, survival 15 to 20
    years after, *94:* 364
  isosorbide-5-mononitrate in, twice-daily,
    lack of pharmacologic tolerance
    and rebound angina with, *95:* 401
  microvascular, *94:* 355
  patients with normal coronary
    angiograms, impaired
    endothelium-dependent coronary
    vasodilatation in, *94:* 355
  serotonin in, *94:* 357
  sleep apnea and, *93:* 125
  stable
    bypass surgery for, 18-year follow-up,
      93: 348
    chronic, aspirin in, *92:* 302
    chronic, effect of nifedipine on
      circadian patterns of myocardial
      ischemia in, *93:* 333
    mortality in, silent ischemia during
      daily life as predictor of, *91:* 340
  unstable
    antithrombotic therapy in,
      combination, in nonprior aspirin
      users, *95:* 379
    aspirin in, *93:* 325
    calcium channel blockers in, *91:* 322
    reactivation after discontinuation of
      heparin, *93:* 324
    thrombolysis in, *93:* 322
    thrombus in, coronary artery,
      angioscopy of, *93:* 320
    tissue plasminogen activator in,
      95: 380
  variant, role of coronary spasm in
    development of fixed coronary
    obstructions in, *93:* 327
Angioedema
  after leucovorin/methotrexate in
    rheumatoid arthritis, *94:* 763
Angiofollicular
  lymph node hyperplasia and
    membranoproliferative
    glomerulonephritis, *94:* 671
Angiography
  central nervous system, in vasculitis,
    93: 717
  coronary

glycoprotein inhibitor of cholesterol
crystallization, isolation of, 94: 539
pain, acalculous, cholecystectomy in,
92: 437
pancreatitis, acute, endoscopic
papillotomy in, 94: 541
response, intestinal phase of, effect of
cholecystokinin receptor antagonist
on, 91: 491
sludge
pancreatitis due to, acute, 93: 495
in pregnancy, 94: 533
tract, 95: 563-564; 94: 533-539;
93: 489-494
Bilirubin
serum levels in sepsis and septic shock,
effect of high-dose
methylprednisolone on, 94: 179
Biochemical
effects of testosterone supplementation
in aging male, 94: 622
responses to interferon-α in chronic
hepatitis C, 95: 545
tests distinguishing ectopic from
pituitary ACTH dependent
Cushing's syndrome, 92: 464
variables associated with bone density in
primary hyperparathyroidism,
94: 609
Biolab Malakit
for *Helicobacter pylori*, 94: 460
Biologic
features of gut inflammation in
spondyloarthropathies, 93: 702
phenomenon of Lyme disease, 94: 807
Bioprosthetic
heart valve (*see* Valve, bioprosthetic)
Biopsy
of adrenal mass in operable lung cancer
patients, 95: 123
in arteritis, temporal, effect of previous
corticosteroids on findings, 95: 811
aspiration
fine-needle, in renal transplant
rejection, gamma-interferon gene
expression in, 95: 742
percutaneous needle, of adrenal
masses in operable lung cancer
patients, 95: 123
transtracheal, in community-acquired
pneumonia, 95: 144
bronchial
(*See also* transbronchial *below*)
in asthma during remission,
inflammatory markers in, 92: 81
mast cell histochemical characteristics
and degranulation in, in asthma,
94: 19

duodenal, in celiac disease, 95: 513
endomyocardial
for myocardial changes due to
transplant-associated coronary
arteriosclerosis, 93: 378
vs. signal-averaged ECG in detection
of heart transplant rejection,
93: 376
kidney, in lupus nephritis, 91: 698
lung, video thoracoscopic *vs.* open, in
diagnosis of interstitial lung disease,
94: 143
muscle, deltoid, in cardiomyopathy
related to alcoholic myopathy,
95: 433
synovial, bacterial antigens in, in
Yersinia-triggered reactive arthritis,
92: 642
transbronchial
(*See also* bronchial *above*)
in lung cancer diagnosis, 94: 63
after lung transplantation, 94: 149
Bio-Rad GAP Test IgG
for *Helicobacter pylori*, 94: 460
Birth
control pills (*see* Contraceptives, oral)
stillbirth after maternal Lyme disease,
94: xxxiii
Bismuth
/antibiotics, effect on duodenal ulcer
healing, 92: 382
subsalicylate in *Helicobacter pylori*
infection, 93: 40
/tetracycline/metronidazole in
Helicobacter pylori eradication,
95: 491, 492
Bisoprolol
levothyroxine therapy and quality of life,
95: 613
Bites
animal, amoxicillin/clavulanate
prophylaxis after, 91: 64
Russell's viper, effects on hormone
levels, 91: 512
tick (*see* Tick, bites)
Bjork-Shiley mechanical heart valve
vs. porcine bioprosthesis, 92: 322
Blacks
(*See also* Race)
coronary disease in, mortality rates and
risk factors, 94: 318
glomerulopathy in, collapsing, 95: 695
gonorrhea trends in 1980s in, 93: 76
Helicobacter pylori infection prevalence
in, 95: xviii
hip fracture risk in, in women, 95: 655
hypertension in, and renal function
change, 94: 705

Bruit
in Takayasu's arteritis, 95: 816

Brush
protected specimen, in diagnosis of
nosocomial pneumonia in
ventilated patients, 94: 205;
92: 129

Bucindolol
in heart failure, 95: 437

Budd-Chiari syndrome
experience and literature review,
95: 558

Budesonide
in asthma
effect on growth and pituitary-adrenal
function, in children, 95: 600
moderate and severe, 91: 81
newly detected, 92: 85
effects on serum osteocalcin, 92: 90

Bullectomy
in emphysema, idiopathic giant bullous,
95: 102

Bullous
emphysema, idiopathic giant, imaging
findings in, 95: 101

BUN
in sepsis and septic shock, effect of
high-dose methylprednisolone on,
94: 179

Bundle branch block
left, adenosine vs. exercise thallium
imaging in, 94: 423

Burkitt's lymphoma (see Lymphoma,
Burkitt's)

Burning
indoor, of charcoal briquets, causing
carbon monoxide poisoning,
95: 182

Burns
nystatin prophylaxis for Candida
infection after, 93: 52

Bursa
foreign body injury to, penetrating,
92: 672

Busulfan
in leukemia
myelogenous, chronic, 93: 243
myeloid, chronic, vs. interferon
alfa-2a, 95: 304

Bypass
cardiopulmonary
for coronary angioplasty support,
91: 346
pancreatic cellular injury after, risk
factors for, 92: 449
coronary artery
for angina, stable, 18-year follow-up,
93: 348

for angina, survival 15 to 20 years
after, 94: 364
costs of, 94: 383
effects on employment, 95: 403
effects on outcome after resuscitation
from out of hospital cardiac arrest,
93: 347
gender bias in patient selection for,
93: 338
graft patency determined by cine
MRI, 91: 383
mortality, in women, 91: 356
after myocardial infarction, one-year
results, 93: 314
myocardial viability after, thallium
imaging detecting, 94: 421
sternal wound infections after,
Rhodococcus bronchialis, 92: 27
vs. angioplasty, 94: 377
vs. angioplasty in symptomatic
multivessel coronary disease,
95: 407
gastric, for weight loss in prevention of
type II diabetes, 95: 665
procedures in Takayasu's arteritis,
95: 817

C

Ca 19.9 antigen
levels in hemochromatosis, 95: 555

Cachectin (see Tumor, necrosis factor)

Cachexia
pathogenesis, tumor necrosis factor in
(in mice), 92: 253

Caffeine
hypertension and, 93: 623

CAGE questionnaire
in alcoholism screening, 91: 475

Calciferol
exogenous, and vitamin D endocrine
status in elderly nursing home
residents, 94: 597

Calcific
tendinitis in proximal thigh, 95: 837

Calcification
adrenal, in pulmonary tuberculosis,
95: 595

Calcinosis
in CREST syndrome, effect of diltiazem
on, 92: 648

Calciotropic
hormone levels, abnormal, in
preeclampsia, 93: 561

Calcitonin
effect on osteoporotic vertebral
fracture, 93: 671

in leukemia, chronic myeloid, 94: 275
transfusion with seronegative blood
products and, 94: 270
retinitis in AIDS, foscarnet in, 93: 6
diabetes insipidus after, nephrogenic,
91: 662
Cytometry
flow, DNA, prognostic value in locally
recurrent, conservatively treated
breast cancer, 94: 288
Cytoplasmic
antibodies, antineutrophil (*see*
Antibodies, antineutrophil
cytoplasmic)
autoantibodies, antineutrophil (*see*
Autoantibodies, antineutrophil
cytoplasmic)
Cytoreductive
therapy in marrow transplantation
causing veno-occlusive disease of
liver, 94: 268, 526
Cytosine arabinoside
in Hodgkin's disease, 92: 219
in leukemia, acute, 91: 261
lymphoblastic, 93: 267
in myelodysplastic syndromes,
advanced, 91: 272
Cytotoxic
T cell-specific serine protease gene
transcripts and renal allograft
rejection, 93: 657
therapy
in breast cancer, early, 93: 279
in Hodgkin's disease, relapsed,
91: 250
in lupus erythematosus, systemic,
94: 776
in pneumonitis, cryptogenic
organizing, 93: 160
in Takayasu's arteritis, 95: 817
Cytoxan (*see* Cyclophosphamide)

D

Dacarbazine
in Hodgkin's disease, 93: 276
advanced, 94: 247
in melanoma, metastatic, 93: 287
Dactinomycin
in sarcoma, osteogenic, 93: 290
Danazol
in thrombocytopenia, autoimmune,
91: 239
Dapsone
-pyrimethamine prophylaxis against
Pneumocystis carinii pneumonia

and toxoplasmosis in HIV
infection, 94: 92
Daunorubicin
in leukemia, acute
lymphoblastic, adult, 93: 236
myelogenous, 94: 251; 92: 214
Day care center
spread of multiply resistant
Streptococcus pneumoniae at,
94: 846
DDAVP
in diabetes insipidus during pregnancy,
94: 560
DDC
alterations in pancreas cancer, 95: 574
ddC
/zidovudine in advanced HIV infection,
94: 856; 93: 7
ddI (*see* Dideoxyinosine)
D-dimer
in blood, to rule out venous
thromboembolism, 95: 131
Deafness
in infant after streptomycin for
tuberculosis during pregnancy,
94: 82
Death
(*See also* Mortality)
in arteritis, giant cell, rates and causes
of, 91: 714
asthma, and beta-agonists, 93: 87
breast cancer causing, node-positive,
effect of tamoxifen on, 94: 289
carbon monoxide poisoning, due to
indoor burning of charcoal
briquets, 95: 183
certificate accuracy in asthma, 94: 8
isoniazid-associated, 91: 197
smoking causing, 94: 29
sudden (*see* Sudden death)
Decompression
surgery
cyst, for autosomal dominant
polycystic kidney disease, 93: 607
for pituitary apoplexy, 91: 510
Decontamination
selective
antibiotics for, nonabsorbable, 93: 26
digestive, in mechanically ventilated
patients, 95: 153
for prevention of bacterial infection in
ICU, 92: 28
Defibrillator
automatic implantable cardioverter
effect on survival in coronary artery
disease patients with severely
depressed ventricular dysfunction,
92: 334

tobramycin in, aerosolized, 94: 50, 52
transmembrane conductance
regulator in pancreas, localization
of, 92: 450
marrow, effect on response to
erythropoietin in uremia, 94: 239
pulmonary
active, up to 17 years after childhood
chemotherapy with carmustine,
91: 150
idiopathic, clubbing of fingers and
smooth muscle proliferation in,
95: 173
idiopathic, determinants of
progression in, 95: 167
idiopathic, interleukin-8 gene
expression in, 93: 155
pathogenesis of, 94: 97
Filgrastim
(*See also* Colony-stimulating factor,
granulocyte)
in agranulocytosis, clozapine-induced,
95: 278
for relapse of leukemia and
myelodysplasia after marrow
transplantation, 95: 318
Filter
vena cava (*see* Vena cava, filter)
Finasteride
in prostatic hyperplasia, benign, 94: 623
Finger(s)
clubbing and smooth muscle
proliferation in idiopathic
pulmonary fibrosis, 95: 170
innervated by median nerve, sensory loss
in, in carpal tunnel syndrome,
93: 740
nodulosis on, accelerated, during
methotrexate therapy for
rheumatoid arthritis, 93: 681
-stick device, spring-loaded,
transmission of hepatitis B virus by,
93: 452
Fingerprinting
DNA, in tuberculosis, 95: 15, 16
Fish
catfish-related injury and infection,
93: 77
oil
in IgA nephropathy, 95: 699
supplementation in
cyclosporine-treated kidney
transplant recipients, 94: 727;
91: 643
Fistula
arteriovenous hemodialysis, color
Doppler ultrasound assessment of,
93: 647

Fitness
cardiorespiratory, and risk of myocardial
infarction, 95: 363
FK 506
in kidney transplantation, 91: 639
Flaviviruses
marrow failure and, 91: 232
Flecainide
in arrhythmias, 91: 378
in tachycardia, atrioventricular
re-entrant, 92: 339
Floxuridine
in colorectal cancer metastatic to liver,
91: 283
Flu
deaths due to, 94: 73
Fluconazole
in candidiasis
hepatosplenic, 93: 64
oropharyngeal, in AIDS, resistance to,
95: 61
vulvovaginal, 94: 889
in esophagitis,*Candida*, in AIDS,
94: 888
in meningitis, cryptococcal, in AIDS,
92: 16
prophylaxis
for *Candida* infections after burn
injury, 93: 53
for fungal infection in patients at risk
of neutropenia, 94: 890
for meningitis, relapsing cryptococcal,
93: 10
review of, 91: 60
in thrush, oral, in AIDS, 94: 889
in urinary tract infection, fungal, 95: 12
Fludarabine
in leukemia, chronic lymphocytic,
92: 224
loading dose/continuous infusion
schedule, 93: 244
prednisone combined with, 95: 307
in lymphoma
low-grade, 93: 258
macroglobulinemic, 91: 259
-refractory chronic lymphocytic
leukemia, 2-chlorodeoxyadenosine
in, 95: 309
-resistant chronic lymphocytic leukemia,
2-chlorodeoxyadenosine in,
93: 245
Fludrocortisone
in Addison's disease, and plasma renin
activity, 93: 523
Fluid(s)
balance, relationship between
hemodynamics, pulmonary
infiltration, and ARDS and, in

beta-blockers in, 95: 437

bucindolol in, 95: 437

chronic, angiotensin-converting enzyme inhibitors in (see Angiotensin, -converting enzyme inhibitors, in heart failure, chronic)

chronic, mild-to-moderate, ibopamine in, 94: 408

chronic, tumor necrosis factor in, circulating, 91: 373

congestive (see below)

development after enalapril in patients with reduced left ventricular ejection fractions, 93: 372

end-stage, and sudden cardiac death in familial hypertrophic cardiomyopathy, 94: 394

pleural effusions in AIDS due to, 94: 95

in renal failure patients, chronic, effect of erythropoietin in, 93: 637

sudden death and, timing of, 95: 442

failure, congestive

cardiovascular examination in, 94: 404

CPAP in, cardiac output response to, 93: 204

enalapril vs. hydralazine-isosorbide in, 92: 325

frank, due to anagrelide, 93: 222

magnesium chloride in, effect on frequency of ventricular arrhythmia, 95: 440

metoprolol in, 95: 437

neutrophil-activating peptide-2 in, 94: 211

ouabain levels in, endogenous, 93: 370

outcome in dialysis patients, 91: 651

pulmonary hypertension in, and plasma endothelin, 93: 369

severe, amiodarone in, 95: 438

sleep apnea in, CPAP for, 91: 118

survival after onset of, 94: 403

vesnarinone in, 94: 407

function

impairment in renal failure (in rat), 95: 721

normalization after regression of cardiac hypertrophy, 95: 468

in hypereosinophilic syndromes, 95: 282

hypertrophy, regression of, normalization of cardiac structure and function after, 95: 468

imaging, antimyosin antibody, in myocarditis, 92: 360

left, sympathetic denervation, for long QT syndrome, 92: 338

morbidity after noncardiac surgery, relation to perioperative myocardial ischemia, 92: 298

mortality after noncardiac surgery, relation to perioperative myocardial ischemia, 92: 298

output

erythropoietin in hemodialysis patients and, 92: 598

in ovarian hyperstimulation syndrome, 95: 705

response to CPAP in congestive heart failure, 93: 204

pacing (see Pacing)

pain during coronary angioplasty, 94: 375

palpitations and natural menopause, 93: 569

parasympathetic activity, decreased in hypertrophic cardiomyopathy, 94: 393

rate variability

in cardiomyopathy, hypertrophic, 94: 394

circadian, effect of environment on, 92: 353

risk for sudden death and, 94: 430

rhythm disturbance in Lyme disease, 94: xxvi

risk

before abdominal aortic surgery, dipyridamole-thallium imaging and gated radionuclide angiography in assessment of, 95: 444

before nonvascular surgery, assessment by echocardiography and thallium imaging, 95: 446

structure, normalization after regression of cardiac hypertrophy, 95: 468

surgery, open, HTLV-I/II infection in, transfusion-transmitted, 91: 230

tamponade, percutaneous balloon pericardiotomy for, 94: 445

testing, noninvasive, 94: 417-427

transplant (see Transplantation, heart)

valve (see Valve)

Heated

vapor, inhalation of (see Steam, inhalation)

Helicobacter pylori, 95: xvii-xxviii

acid secretion and, 95: xix-xx

-associated exaggerated gastrin release in duodenal ulcer, 92: 380

current status in diagnosis, therapy, pathology, and thinking, 95: xvii-xxviii

pure, in HIV infection,
immunoglobulin therapy in,
93: 226
transient, and parvovirus, 95: 273
magnesium, concentration in cor
pulmonale, 94: 129
transfusion in warm-type autoimmune
hemolytic anemia, 94: 234
Reflex(es)
autonomic, in syncope associated with
paroxysmal atrial fibrillation,
94: 443
baroreflex failure, diagnosis and
treatment of, 95: 728
vasoconstriction withdrawal,
paradoxical, causing
hemodialysis-induced hypotension,
94: 716
Reflux
acid, in reflux esophagitis, effects of
ranitidine/cisapride on, 94: 451
esophagitis (see Esophagitis, reflux)
gastroesophageal (see Gastroesophageal,
reflux)
vesicoureteric, medical *vs.* surgical
treatment, in children, 93: 618
Regurgitation
aortic (see Aortic, regurgitation)
mitral (see Mitral, regurgitation)
tricuspid, as marker for adverse
outcome in patients undergoing
balloon mitral valvuloplasty,
95: 422
valvular, Doppler-detected, and
regurgitant murmur, 91: 359
Rehabilitation
program, multidisciplinary pulmonary,
benefits of, 92: 111
for substance abuse, 91: 402
Reinfarction
effect of streptokinase *vs.* immediate
angioplasty on, 95: 385
Reinnervation
sensory, causing chest pain in cardiac
transplant recipients, 92: 330
sympathetic, after heart transplantation,
94: 414
Reiter's syndrome
Chlamydia in synovium in, molecular
evidence for, 93: 701
postvenereal, antibiotics in, 93: 699
Relaxation
vs. propranolol in mild hypertension,
93: 624
Renal
(*See also* Kidney)
artery stenosis, percutaneous angioplasty
in, 95: 729

cell carcinoma (see Carcinoma, renal
cell)
colic, plain abdominal x-ray in, 93: 619
complications of insulin-dependent
diabetes mellitus, and oral
contraceptives, 95: 673
crisis in systemic sclerosis, outcome of,
91: 707
hepatorenal syndrome (see Hepatorenal,
syndrome)
Renin
activity
measurement in Addison's disease,
93: 522
plasma, in ovarian hyperstimulation
syndrome, 95: 705
-angiotensin-aldosterone system
disorders, diagnosis under random
conditions, 93: 525
polycystic kidney disease and, 92: 580
in diabetes mellitus, 93: 611
plasma aldosterone-plasma renin activity
ratio in diagnosis of
renin-angiotensin-aldosterone axis
disorders, 93: 525
-sodium profile and risk of myocardial
infarction in hypertensives, 92: 578
Renovascular
hypertension, diagnostic strategies in,
91: 630
Reperfusion
after myocardial infarction (see
Myocardial infarction, reperfusion
after)
Reproductive
age, women of, and bioprosthetic *vs.*
mechanical cardiac valve
replacement, 94: 391
axis suppression in acute illness, relation
to disease severity, 94: 625
outcome of infertile patients, effect of
endometriosis on, 93: 567
system, 95: 629-641; 94: 613-626;
93: 561-572
Residual
volume
in distinguishing between COPD and
asthma, 95: 105
Respiratory
alkalosis, chronic, 92: 601
bronchiolitis-associated interstitial lung
disease, relation to desquamative
interstitial pneumonia, 91: 140
care practitioners, knowledge of
metered-dose inhaler use, 94: 9
diagnosis, 94: 137-145; 93: 187-188
distress syndrome, acute, 95: 231-259
definition, 95: 238

vs. balloon angioplasty in coronary
artery disease, 95: 415
Sterile
technique, improved, positive line
cultures in cardiovascular patients
after, 93: 19
Sternal
wound infections, *Rhodococcus
bronchialis,* after coronary bypass,
92: 27
Steroid(s)
(*See also* Corticosteroids)
anabolic
coagulation abnormalities after,
94: 233
use by body builders, 91: 552
androgenic, use by body builders,
91: 552
-dependent asthma (*see* Asthma,
corticosteroid-dependent)
-induced osteoporosis (*see*
Osteoporosis, steroid-induced)
injection, percutaneous CT guided, for
calcific tendinitis in proximal thigh,
95: 837
intravenous pulsed, in rheumatoid
arthritis, 91: 679
in lupus erythematosus, systemic, and
risk for *Pneumocystis carinii*
pneumonia, 94: 776
in nephropathy, C1q, in pulse doses, in
children, 93: 602
-resistant nephrotic syndrome,
cyclosporine in, 91: 596
tablets in chronic asthma, 94: 26, 28
tapering in acute asthma, 94: 22
therapy, burst,
hypothalamic-pituitary-adrenal
function one week after, 94: 569
in Wegener's granulomatosis, 93: 718
Stiff-man syndrome
discussion of, 92: 256
Stillbirth
after maternal Lyme disease, 94: xxxiii
Still's disease
adult-onset and juvenile-onset,
long-term evolution of, 91: 683
Stomach, 95: 485-502; 94: 455-467;
93: 413-421
(*See also* Gastric; Gastrointestinal)
Stones, 94: 741-747
bile duct, after previous
cholecystectomy, duodenoscopic
sphincterotomy for, 91: 488
biliary, ceftriaxone-associated, in Lyme
disease, 94: xxix
gallstones (*see* Gallstones)
renal (*see* Nephrolithiasis)

urinary, and ulcerative colitis, 94: 493
Stool
ras oncogene mutations in, in patients
with curable colorectal tumors,
93: 293
Streptococcal
pharyngitis (*see* Pharyngitis,
streptococcal)
pharyngotonsillitis, presumed,
Arcanobacterium haemolyticum in
children with, 94: 839
Streptococci
β-hemolytic, group C, and endemic
pharyngitis, 92: 24
Streptococcus
anginosus in pharyngitis, 94: 837
equisimilis in pharyngitis, 94: 837
milleri in pharyngitis, 94: 837
pneumoniae
antimicrobial resistance in, 94: 845
drug-resistant, multiple, spread at day
care center, 94: 846
drug-resistant, treatment and
diagnosis of infections caused by,
94: 849
meningitis, dexamethasone in, in
children, 95: 38
meningitis, in adults, 94: 881
meningitis, penicillin- and
cephalosporin-resistant, failure of
cephalosporin in, 94: 847
pleural effusions in AIDS due to,
94: 94
pneumonia due to,
community-acquired, 95: 145
pneumonia due to, in HIV-infected
patients, 95: 158
respiratory tract infection due to,
lower, 94: 76
pyogenes infection after penicillin G
prophylaxis, 92: 25
Streptokinase
intrapleural, in loculated, nonpurulent
parapneumonic effusions, 93: 165
in myocardial infarction
captopril and, 95: 390
direct thrombin inhibitor as adjunct
to, 95: 386
heparin and, 94: 328
intracranial hemorrhage after, 95: 387
suspected, *vs.* anistreplase and tissue
plasminogen activator, 93: 310
vs. alteplase, 91: 326
vs. angioplasty, immediate, 95: 384;
94: 326
Streptomycin
in tuberculosis
in AIDS, 93: xxx

long-term, and bone mineral density,
93: 545
need during pregnancy in hypothyroid
women, 91: 532
replacement therapy
blood sampling time during, effect on
thyroid hormone levels, 94: 585
lipid concentrations and, circulating,
94: 583
therapy
hyperthyroidism due to, prolonged
subclinical, and bone mass changes,
95: 610
thyrotropin measurement during,
serum, second vs. third generation
methods for, 95: 605
in thyroid carcinoma, 92: 485
Tick
bites
Lyme disease due to (see Lyme
disease)
Lyme disease prevention after,
94: xxxi-xxxii; 93: 722
exposure, erlichiosis after, 95: 70
Ixodes uriae, Lyme borreliosis cycle in,
94: 832
Tidal
irrigation in osteoarthritis of knee,
93: 735
volume, ratio of respiratory frequency
to, as predictor of ventilator
weaning outcome, 94: 199
Tinel's sign
in carpal tunnel syndrome, 93: 740
Tissue
connective tissue disease (see
Connective tissue disease)
plasminogen activator (see Plasminogen,
activator, tissue)
T lymphocytes (see T cells)
T-lymphotropic virus (see HTLV)
Tobacco
smokeless, and cardiovascular disease
mortality, 95: 368
smoking (see Smoking)
Tobramycin
aerosolized, in cystic fibrosis, 94: 50, 52
in digestive decontamination, selective,
in mechanically ventilated patients,
95: 153
topical, for digestive tract
decontamination in ICU, 93: 26
Toluene
diisocyanate-induced asthma, 92: 151
airway mucosal inflammation due to,
93: 161
Tomography
computed

in cold, common, 95: 5
in Cushing's syndrome, in children
and adolescents, 95: 599
in empty sella, 94: 555
in HIV patients with emphysema-like
pulmonary disease, 93: 146
of lung inflation, regional, in adult
respiratory distress syndrome,
95: 232
in lymphangiomyomatosis,
pulmonary, 91: 152
in pancreatitis, acute, 94: 542
in pancreatitis, chronic, 95: 565
of pituitary microadenoma, 93: 503
quantitative, of postmenopausal
vertebral bone density, 93: 552
of renal cystic disease, acquired, in
dialysis patients, 93: 608
in rhombencephalitis, Listeria
monocytogenes, 94: 883
single-photon emission (see SPECT)
in sinusitis, chronic, relation to
allergy, asthma, and eosinophilia,
95: 80
of tendinitis in proximal thigh,
calcific, 95: 837
of toxoplasmosis, CNS, in AIDS,
94: 862
of tuberculosis in HIV infection,
93: xxv
in vanishing lung syndrome, 95: 101
positron emission, fluorodeoxyglucose,
for viable myocardium, 95: 449,
450
Tonometry
gastric, vs. routine blood gas analysis for
intramural pH, 94: 138
Tophaceous
gout (see Gout, tophaceous)
Tophi
as initial manifestation of gout, 93: 715
recurrence after withdrawal of
antihyperuricemic therapy in
tophaceous gout, 93: 796
Tourniquet
deflation during total knee arthroplasty
and thromboembolism, 94: 122
Toxic
colitis in ulcerative colitis, 94: 493
dilatation in ulcerative colitis, 94: 493
effects of ipratropium bromide vs.
theophylline in COPD, 94: 42
oil syndrome, chronicity of, 95: 805
Toxicity
of antibiotic prophylaxis of tick bites,
94: xxxi
auditory, of desferrioxamine in
hemodialysis patients, 92: 597

single, results of, 95: 261
single, ventricular function after,
  transthoracic echocardiography of,
  95: 452
lung, in COPD
single, 91: 219
single *vs.* double, 92: 114
marrow, 95: 317-328; 94: 267-282;
  93: 261-278
allogeneic, increasing use of, 93: 261
in anemia, aplastic, solid cancers after,
  95: 269
autologous, after high-dose ifosfamide
  and escalating doses of carboplatin,
  92: 233
in breast cancer, 94: 287
cytomegalovirus infection after (*see*
  Cytomegalovirus, infection in
  transplant recipients, marrow)
donor, unrelated, 91: 269
donor, unrelated, closely
  HLA-matched, 91: 278
donor program for, U.S. national,
  95: 317
graft-*vs.*-host disease after (*see* Graft,
  -*vs.*-host disease, in marrow
  transplant recipients)
in Hodgkin's disease, and high-dose
  cytotoxic therapy, 91: 250
in Hodgkin's disease,
  granulocyte-macrophage
  colony-stimulating factor as adjunct
  to, 93: 223
in Hodgkin's disease, relapsed,
  93: 274; 91: 250
in leukemia, acute, as therapy for
  primary induction failure, 93: 266
in leukemia, allogeneic marrow,
  filgrastim for relapse after, 95: 318
in leukemia, lymphoblastic, acute,
  high-risk, 91: 270
in leukemia, lymphoblastic, acute, in
  first remission, 93: 267
in leukemia, lymphocytic, acute,
  CALLA-positive, autologous
  marrow and ex vivo marrow
  leukemia cell purging used in,
  94: 280
in leukemia, myeloblastic, acute,
  93: 273
in leukemia, myelocytic, 91: 268
in leukemia, myelogenous, acute,
  allogeneic marrow, 94: 252
in leukemia, myelogenous, chronic, in
  chronic phase, 93: 264
in leukemia, myelogenous, chronic,
  with unrelated donor, 94: 273;
  91: 276

in leukemia, myeloid, acute, 91: 265
in leukemia, myeloid, acute, after
  anticancer treatment in childhood,
  95: 298
in leukemia, myeloid, acute,
  autologous cryopreserved marrow,
  94: 278
in leukemia, myeloid, chronic,
  complications of, 94: 275
in lymphoid malignancy, high-grade,
  autologous marrow, 92: 235
in lymphoma, malignant, 91: 253
in lymphoma, non-Hodgkin's,
  91: 251
in lymphoma, non-Hodgkin's,
  autologous *vs.* allogeneic, 95: 321;
  94: 281
in lymphoma, non-Hodgkin's, B-cell,
  91: 254
in lymphoma, toxicity and survival
  after, 91: 248
in myelodysplastic syndromes,
  primary, 93: 239
in myeloma, multiple, autologous,
  94: 258
in myeloma, multiple, combined with
  interferon-α and melphalan,
  93: 257
nephropathy after, late-onset, clinical
  course of, 95: 704
outcome in patients requiring ICU
  support, 93: 269
in sickle cell disease, 95: 324
for thalassemia, 95: 325
veno-occlusive disease of liver and
  multiorgan failure after, 94: 268,
  525
organ, hepatitis C virus transmission by,
  92: 418
pancreas, in diabetes, ten-year
  experience with, 91: 573
race and, 92: 589
skin, survival, major histocompatibility
  complex-specific prolongation of
  (in mice), 94: 726
stem cell
autologous, in lymphoma,
  non-Hodgkin's, 95: 320
fetal human, in utero transplant (in
  sheep), 93: 228
Transsphenoidal
surgery for Cushing's disease, predicting
  relapse after, 94: 571
Transtracheal
aspiration in community-acquired
  pneumonia, 95: 144
oxygen delivery in COPD, 93: 105
Transtubular

Author Index